OXFORD MEDICAL PUBLICATIONS

DRUGS, DISEASES, AND
THE PERIODONTIUM

DRUGS, DISEASES, AND THE PERIODONTIUM

ROBIN A. SEYMOUR

AND

PETER A. HEASMAN

WITH

IAN D. M. MACGREGOR

Department of Operative Dentistry, The Dental School
University of Newcastle upon Tyne

Oxford   New York   Tokyo

OXFORD UNIVERSITY PRESS

1992

Oxford University Press, Walton Street, Oxford OX2 6DP

Oxford New York Toronto
Delhi Bombay Calcutta Madras Karachi
Petaling Jaya Singapore Hong Kong Tokyo
Nairobi Dar es Salaam Cape Town
Melbourne Auckland
and associated companies in
Berlin Ibadan

Oxford is a trade mark of Oxford University Press

Published in the United States
by Oxford University Press, New York

A catalogue record for this book is available from the British Library

Library of Congress Cataloging in Publication Data
Seymour, R. A.
Drugs, diseases, and the periodontium / Robin A. Seymour and Peter
A. Heasman.
(Oxford medical publications)
Includes index.
1. Periodontal disease.   2. Periodontium—Effect of drugs on.
3. Oral manifestations of general diseases.   I. Heasman, Peter A.
II. Title.   III. Series.
[DNLM: 1. Age Factors.   2. Dental Deposits—etiology.
3. Nutrition Disorders—complications.   4. Periodontal Diseases–
–drug therapy.   5. Periodontal Diseases—etiology.   6. Smoking–
–adverse effects.   WU 240 S521d]
RK361.S49   1992   617.6'32—dc20   91–27158
ISBN 0–19–261992–6 (hardback)

Set by Latimer Trend & Co Ltd.

Printed and bound in Hong Kong

FOREWORD

The periodontium comprises tissues which resemble those elsewhere in the body, but are adapted for specialized functions— to support the teeth in the jaws and to maintain and defend the integrity of the barrier between the internal and external environment. It is continually threatened by the accumulation of microbial plaque, but in health the host–parasite relationship is in equilibrium, resulting in the development or progression of chronic periodontal disease. In particular, a great variety of drugs and diseases may act topically or systemically to disturb the balance; the periodontium provides a situation, unique in the body, to observe the complex interplay between the internal and external environment. In addition, a wide range of systemic diseases can affect the periodontium directly and their diverse manifestations here may differ from those elsewhere in the mouth.

The growth in our knowledge of the importance of the interrelationship between internal medicine and oral disease is evidenced by advances in the field of oral medicine, reflecting those in general medicine. The latter have led to increased life expectancy and general ageing of the population, and there is little doubt that these factors will result in changing patterns of oral disease which will challenge all branches of the dental profession. To meet these challenges the dentist will require sources of up-to-date information which combine review and critical comment and provide a comprehensive reference for diagnosis, treatment, and learning. This book successfully fulfils these requirements and the authors are to be congratulated on producing a first-class text which provides a unique source of information linking periodontology, oral medicine, and contemporary biological science. Although the text is aimed primarily at the specialist in periodontology, any practitioner or student who dips into its pages will not only find answers to immediate questions but is likely to be stimulated to further enquiry and learning.

Professor J. V. Soames
Department of Oral Pathology
University of Newcastle upon Tyne

PREFACE

The periodontium is a unique structure that maintains the support of the dentition. Periodontal disease results in the breakdown of this support and thus compromises the dentition. There is overwhelming evidence that periodontal disease is caused by bacterial plaque, or more specifically by an interaction between the bacterial products and the host's immune and inflammatory responses. It is also well recognized that a variety of systemic factors can influence the response of the periodontal tissues to plaque. These include specific disease states, drug therapy, ageing, smoking, diet, and the sex hormones. In addition, certain drugs can have a beneficial effect on periodontium and its response to plaque. Obvious examples include antimicrobial agents and anti-inflammatory drugs. All of these subjects form the basis of this book, and hence its title, *Drugs, Diseases, and the Periodontium*.

The first two chapters are concerned with the pathogenesis of periodontal disease, and the role of plaque and calculus in this process. We have made no attempt to complete an exhaustive treatise on this subject. The aim is to provide the reader with a background on these topics that will facilitate understanding as to how systemic disease and drugs can affect the periodontium.

Chapters 3 and 4 cover the effects of systemic diseases and drug therapy on the periodontium. Both chapters appraise the prevalence of these problems and investigate the underlying mechanisms that predispose such patients to periodontal changes.

Age related factors and periodontal diseases are discussed in Chapter 5. These include prepubertal and juvenile periodontitis, as well as periodontal problems in the elderly.

Chapter 6 investigates the effects of cigarette smoking on the periodontal tissues, whilst Chapters 7 and 8 cover sex hormones and diet, respectively.

The final three chapters deal with the beneficial effects of drugs in the control of periodontal disease, notably anti-plaque and anti-calculus agents, antimicrobials, and anti-inflammatory drugs.

Primarily this book is aimed at the periodontologist or the dental practitioner with a special interest in periodontology. We would also hope that the postgraduate students preparing for higher degrees will find the contents useful.

Newcastle upon Tyne　　　　　　　　　　　　　　　　　　　　　　　　　　　　　　R. A. S.
December 1991　　　　　　　　　　　　　　　　　　　　　　　　　　　　　　　　　P. A. H.

CONTENTS

ACKNOWLEDGEMENTS

The authors wish to acknowledge the help and support of their colleagues from the Dental School and Hospital, Newcastle upon Tyne, and would like to record their thanks to the following: Professor J. V. Soames, Department of Oral Pathology, University of Newcastle upon Tyne, for writing the foreword to this book and his helpful comments on Chapters 1 and 3. Professor A. Rugg-Gunn, Department of Child Dental Health, for his criticisms and comments on Chapter 5. Mr J. G. Walton, for the exacting and time-consuming task of proof-reading the manuscript. The staff of the Northern Regional Drug Information Service for providing computer searches. Finally, we are indepted to Claire Grainger for her excellent typing of the manuscript.

Professor J. V. Soames and Dr I. MacLeod, Department of Oral Pathology, University of Newcastle upon Tyne, provided the illustrations for Figs 3.9, 3.10, 3.11, 3.12, 3.14, 3.15, 3.21 and 3.22. Professor J. J. Murray, Department of Child Dental Health, University of Newcastle upon Tyne, provided the illustrations for Figs 3.4 and 3.5. Dr M. Snow, Consultant Physician, Department of Medicine, Newcastle General Hospital, provided the illustrations for Figs 3.18 and 3.19. Dr M. Saxby, Senior lecturer in Periodontology, Birmingham Dental School, provided the illustration for Fig. 3.9. Mr I. Chapple, Lecturer in Periodontology, Birmingham Dental Hospital, provided the illustration for Fig. 3.20.

The following illustrations and tables have been reproduced from various journals by kind permission of the Editors and Publishers. Figs 3.6 and 3.7 reproduced from Welbury, R. Ehlers–Danlos Syndrome; historical review, report of 2 cases in one family and treatment needs. *The American Journal of Dentistry for Children* (1989), May/June 220–4. Fig. 3.13 reproduced from Parsons, E. *et al.* Wegener's granulomatosis, a distinct gingival lesion. *Journal of Clinical Periodontology* (1991), 18 (in press). Figs 3.16 and 3.17 reproduced from Glenwright, D. and Shaw, L. Histiocytosis X: an oral diagnostic problem. *Journal of Clinical Periodontology* (1988), 15, 312–15. Figs 4.3 and 4.4 reproduced from Seymour, R. A. Calcium-channel blockers and gingival hyperplasia. *British Dental Journal* (1991), 170 (in press). Fig. 4.5 reproduced from MacLeod, I. and Ellis, J. Plasma cell gingivitis related to the use of a herbal toothpaste. *British Dental Journal* (1989), 166, 375–6. Fig. 5.2 reproduced from Smith, D. G. and Seymour, R. A. Periodontal disease and treatment in the elderly: Part 1. *Dental Update* (1989), 16, 18–24. Fig. 9.3 reproduced from Bonesvoll, P. Oral pharmacology of chlorhexidine. *Journal of Clinical Periodontology* (1977), 4, 49–65. Fig. 9.4 reproduced from Bonesvoll, P. *et al.* Influence of concentration, time, temperature and pH on the retention of chlorhexidine in the human oral cavity after mouthrinsing. *Archives of Oral Biology* (1974), 19, 1025–9. Fig. 9.5 reproduced from Loe, H. *et al.* Inhibition of experimental caries by plaque prevention. *Scandinavian Journal of Dental Research* (1972), 80, 1–9. Fig. 9.6 reproduced from Cumming, B. R. and Loe, H. Optimal dosage and method of delivering chlorhexidine solution for the inhibition of dental plaque. *Journal of Periodontal Research* (1973), 8, 57–62. Figs 9.7 a,b reproduced from Siegrist, B. E. *et al.* Efficacy of supervised rinsing with chlorhexidine digluconate in comparison to phenolic and plant alkaloid compounds. *Journal of Periodontal Research* (1986), 21 (Suppl. 16), 60–73. Figs 9.8 a,b reproduced from Briner, W. W. *et al.* Assessment of susceptibility of plaque bacteria to chlorhexidine after 6 months oral use. *Journal of Periodontal Research* (1986), 21 (Suppl. 16), 53–9. Table 3.6 reproduced from Israelson, H. *et al.* The hyperplastic gingivitis of Wegener's granulomatosis. *Journal of Periodontology* (1981), 52, 81–7. Table 3.7 reproduced from Artzi Z. *et al.* Periodontal manifestations of adult onset histiocytosis X. *Journal of Periodontology* (1989), 60, 57–6. Table 4.1 reproduced from Seymour, R. A. and Jacobs, D. J. Cyclosporin and the gingival tissues. *Journal of Clinical Periodontology* (1992), 19 (in press).

Text in Chapters 4, 5, 6 and 11, has appeared in various articles written by the authors. We wish to acknowledge the editors and publishers of the following journals for allowing us to use this material. Seymour, R. A. and Heasman, P. A. Drugs and the periodontium. *Journal of Clinical Periodontology* (1988), 15, 1–16. Seymour, R. A. and Jacobs, D. J. Cyclosporin and the gingival tissues. *Journal of Clinical Periodontology* (1992), 19 (in press). Smith, D. G. and Seymour, R. A. Periodontal problems in the elderly. Part 1 and 2. *Dental Update* (1989), 16, 18–24 and 50–55. Macgregor, I. D. M. Smoking, saliva and salivation. *Journal of Dentistry* (1988), 18, 14–17. Macgregor, I. D. M. Clinical effects of smoking on oral ecology. *Clinical Preventive Dentistry* (1989), 11, 3–7. Heasman, P. A. The role of non-steroidal anti-inflammatory drugs in the management of periodontal disease. *Journal of Dentistry* (1988), 16, 247–57.

1.   The pathogenesis of periodontal disease

1.1 INTRODUCTION

Periodontal disease is a disease of the supporting structures of the teeth, notably the periodontal ligament, cementum, alveolar bone, and the various tissue components of the gingiva. There is overwhelming evidence that periodontal disease is caused by the microbial component of plaque. More precisely, the disease is a consequence of an interaction of bacterial plaque and its products with the host's inflammatory and immune responses. Thus, inflammation and various immunological changes are the features of periodontal disease. Where these changes are confined to the gingival tissues, the condition is referred to as gingivitis. Periodontitis occurs when the inflammatory changes result in disruption of the connective tissue attachment and apical migration of the junctional epithelium.

Periodontitis can be further categorized as prepubertal, juvenile (see Chapter 5), rapidly progressive, chronic adult, and refractory. This chapter provides a brief review of the clinical features, pathogenesis, histopathology, inflammatory, and immunological changes that occur in gingivitis and periodontitis.

1.2 GINGIVITIS

1.2.1 INTRODUCTION

The American Academy of Periodontology defined gingivitis as an inflammatory lesion confined to the tissues of the marginal gingiva (Aiguier *et al.* 1937). This definition still holds true today. The cause of the gingival inflammation is the accumulation of bacterial plaque at or near the gingival margin (Loe *et al.* 1965; Payne *et al.* 1975; Moore *et al.* 1982). The microbiology of plaque associated with gingivitis and the changes with respect to time are discussed later. The bacterial component of plaque produces and releases a variety of enzymes and toxins (e.g. lipopolysaccharides and lipoteichoic acid) which diffuse through the junctional epithelium and initiate inflammatory changes in the gingival connective tissue. These changes are mediated by a variety of endogenous inflammatory mediators and include histamine, the kinins, the eicosanoids from cell-membrane phospholipids, complement factors, and lysosomal enzymes released from polymorphonuclear leukocytes (PMNs).

1.2.2 DEFENCE MECHANISMS IN THE GINGIVAL SULCUS

The gingival sulcus is under a constant challenge from the oral microflora, the bacterial colonization on the tooth surface, and perhaps certain constituents of food and drink. The junctional epithelium is a unique structure, but in the presence of plaque, affords little protection to the underlying connective tissue. The oral environment together with the host's defence mechanism provide a degree of protection to the dentogingival area. These defence mechanisms include saliva, crevicular (gingival) fluid, polymorphonuclear leukocytes, and perhaps certain micro-organisms.

Saliva

Saliva production and secretion play a vital role in maintaining oral health. The constant contact between saliva and the oral mucosa serves as a flushing action, which helps to remove bacteria. Thus, only those bacteria that have the capacity to adhere to the tooth surface (pellicle) will play a role in plaque development (see Chapter 2). Saliva also contains the secretory immunoglobulin IgA, agglutinins, lysozyme, viable PMNs and lactoferrin, which interferes with bacterial adhesion and growth. Salivary IgA may inhibit or impede the colonization of bacteria on to the tooth surface. However, various streptococci produce an IgA protease that breaks down salivary IgA and facilitates tooth-surface colonization (Kilian and Reinholdt 1986). Salivary agglutinins will cause bacterial clumping and impede their adherence to tooth surfaces. Finally, saliva contains viable PMNs that are capable of phagocytosing bacteria.

Crevicular fluid

This fluid forms in the gingival connective tissues as a result of exudation from the microcirculation. The fluid percolates through the tissues and junctional epithelium into the gingival crevice (Cimasoni 1983). This unidirectional flow provides a continuous flushing action, which may serve to reduce bacterial colonization of the crevice. Production and flow of crevicular fluid increases in relation to the level of inflammation in the gingival tissues (Loe and Holm-Pedersen 1965). Indeed, the flow of crevicular fluid (as assessed by the Periotron®) has been used as an objective measure of gingival inflammation.

The composition of crevicular fluid is very similar to serum, but the constituents are at much lower concentrations. Protective components of crevicular fluid include the complement proteins, antibodies, and non-specific opsonins.

Many of the bacteria harboured in the gingival crevice will activate the host's immune response. The complement cascade forms an integral part of this response and this reaction can be activated by either the classic or alternate pathway. Activation via the classic pathway is caused by the interaction between bacteria or their products with IgG or IgM; the alternate pathway involves direct activation of C3 by various factors, including bacterial endotoxins from Gram-negative organisms.

When the complement cascade is activated, a series of biologically active fragments (peptides) are formed by cleavage. Some of the fragments, for example C3a and C5a, potentiate the inflammatory response and cause an increase in vascular permeability. C5a is a potent chemotactic factor for PMNs and monocytes, whilst C3b facilitates phagocytosis by opsonization and immune adherence. Other complement fragments have been shown to increase lymphokine production (Sandberg *et al.* 1975), stimulate prostaglandin release (Rutherford and Schenkein 1983) and induce bone resorption (Raisz *et al.* 1974). The various complement fragments also have a role in healing and connective tissue regeneration (Bordin *et al.* 1984). Activation of the entire complement cascade can lead to the lysis of Gram-negative bacteria in the presence of lysozyme.

More recent evidence has confirmed the role of complement activation in the initiation of gingival inflammation (Patters *et al.* 1989). In a study of experimental gingivitis, the percentage of C3 cleavage increased significantly with plaque accumulation and the development of gingival inflammation. This suggests that complement cleavage may be important in the initiation of gingival inflammation.

Antibodies and complement are often sufficient to destroy micro-organisms. However, PMNs can act in concert with antibody and complement. The latter opsonizes the organisms, which facilitates phagocytosis. This mechanism is most important in maintaining the health of the gingival tissues.

Polymorphonuclear neutrophils

PMNs are now considered to be the primary or first line of defence in the protection of the gingival tissues from bacterial plaque (for a review, see Miller *et al.* 1984). There is also evidence to suggest that these cells have an important role in preventing the development of gingivitis, the formation of pockets, and the progression of periodontal disease (Page 1986). There are many systemic diseases that have either an acquired or inherited defect in PMN function (e.g. diabetes mellitus, Down's syndrome, Papillon–Lefèvre syndrome, cyclic neutropenia, Chediak–Higashi syndrome, lazy leukocyte syndrome). A common feature of these disorders is an increased susceptibility to periodontal disease and often rapid periodontal destruction. This feature is linked to the defect in PMN numbers or function (see Chapter 3).

In neutropenic dogs, the extension of subgingival plaque proceeded at a faster rate than in normal dogs (Attstrom and Schroeder 1979). Although this study lasted for only a few days, it provides additional evidence for the protective role of the PMNs in preventing the progression of subgingival plaque along the root surface. Defects in PMN function have also been reported in prepubertal and juvenile periodontitis (see Chapter 5). However, the same degree of PMN dysfunction (impaired chemotaxis) has not been observed in patients with chronic inflammatory periodontal disease (Van Dyke *et al.* 1980; Gale *et al.* 1983). Functional disorders of PMN activity in chronic adult periodontitis may be caused by a local interaction between the cell and bacterial products (for a review see Seymour *et al.* 1986a).

PMNs are present throughout the junctional epithelium and gingival connective tissue in health (Attstrom 1971; Schroeder 1973) and in germ-free rats (Yamasaki *et al.* 1979). The migration of PMNs increases with the build up of plaque and the development of gingival inflammation. Many bacterial products, together with the leukotrienes and complement cleavage products, are potent chemotactic agents to PMNs.

When plaque is allowed to accumulate in the gingival sulcus, the PMNs seem to provide a barrier between the bacteria and epithelial cells. This prevents direct contact between epithelium and bacteria (Schroeder 1970). PMNs in the gingival sulcus phagocytose bacteria, protecting the tissues from bacterial attack. Phagocytosis can result in the release (spillage) of lysosomal enzymes from the PMNs, which can cause tissue damage and potentiate the inflammatory response (Attstrom 1975).

The precise role of the PMNs in the pathogenesis and progression of periodontal disease is unclear. Viable and fully functional PMNs are mandatory for maintaining the health of the periodontium. Phagocytosis is essentially a protective mechanism but results in the spillage of lysosomal enzymes, which in turn will cause further tissue damage. The interaction between certain bacteria and their products with PMNs may be an important feature in the progression of a periodontal lesion.

1.2.3 THE DEVELOPMENT OF GINGIVITIS

Studies of experimental gingivitis (Loe *et al.* 1965; Schroeder *et al.* 1975; Lindhe and Rylander 1975) have firmly established the microbial aetiology of gingivitis. The development of the clinical features of gingivitis is related to plaque accumulation, and the inflammation resolves when plaque is removed. Animal and volunteer studies have investigated the histological and cellular changes that occur in the gingival tissues during the development of gingivitis. These various sequential changes can be identified as distinct lesions, which have been designated the initial, early, and established lesions (Page and Schroeder 1976). When the lesion progresses to periodontitis, it is referred to as an advanced lesion.

The initial lesion

This lesion of experimentally induced gingivitis is basically an acute inflammatory response to the accumulation of plaque and changes can be observed 1–2 days after cessation of plaque control. The predominant changes are vascular, and include dilatation of the microvascular plexus beneath the most coronal portion of the junctional epithelium, i.e. at the base of the histological sulcus. As a consequence, there is an increase in vascular permeability and further production of crevicular fluid with enhanced neutrophil transmigration. Slight changes occur in the perivascular connective tissue matrix, with degradation of collagen by collagenases or other enzymes released from migrating PMNs. There is an exudation of plasma proteins from the circulation, which include fibrinogen, complement, and immunoglobulins. Fibrin is deposited within the peri-vascular connective tissue matrix. The cellular infiltrate (PMNs and macrophages) comprises 5–10 per cent of the marginal gingival connective tissue. All the features of the initial lesion in humans are seen at four days after the beginning of plaque accumulation.

The early lesion

The early lesion evolves from the site of the initial lesion and is seen after about one week of plaque accumulation. Its main feature is an infiltrate of small, medium, and large lymphocytes, macrophages, and a small number of plasma cells. Some 75% of the cells in this infiltrate are lympho-cytes, and they occupy between 5–15 per cent of the marginal connective tissue. There is marked collagen loss in this area. Below the marginal junctional epithelium there is an increase in vascularization. The gingival fibroblasts start to show distinct changes, which include swelling of the mitochondria, vacuolarization of the endoplasmic reticu-lum, electrolucent nuclei, and rupture of the cell mem-branes.

Changes start to occur in the junctional epithelium, with deepening of the histological sulcus and downgrowth of subgingival plaque. There is proliferation of the basal cell layer and rete peg formation. The intercellular spaces between epithelial cells are densely packed with PMNs and crevicular fluid flow reaches its maximum between 6–12 days (Lindhe *et al.* 1973). It is at this stage in the develop-ment of gingivitis that obvious clinical signs are seen.

The duration of the early lesion has not been definitely determined. In experimental gingivitis (Seymour *et al.* 1983), the early lesion was reported to occur throughout the 21-day course of the experiment. The cellular infiltrate consisted mainly of lymphocytes of which 70 per cent were T cells. This study would suggest that the duration of the early lesion is longer than previously thought (Page and Schroeder 1976).

The established lesion

In the sequential series of events, the established lesion follows the early lesion, but the timing of this is uncertain. The predominant cell types in this lesion are plasma cells and B lymphocytes. These cells appear to be located in the periphery of the lesion (Seymour and Greenspan 1979; Okada *et al.* 1983) and synthesize mainly immunoglobulins of the IgG_1 and IgG_3 subclasses. The proportion of lympho-cytes to plasma cells varies with the level of inflammation present in the tissues. In severe cases of gingivitis, there are proportionately more lymphocytes than plasma cells; con-versely, the numbers of plasma cells increase when estab-lished lesions stop bleeding on probing (Lindhe *et al.* 1980; Cooper *et al.* 1983).

The established lesion can progress to the advanced lesion (that is, periodontitis) or remain stable (Suomi *et al.* 1981). There is controversy surrounding the factors that can affect the progression of an established lesion. As the gingival lesions develop, the proportion of T cells decreases, and B

cells and plasma cells increase. This change in the lympho-cyte population may be related to change in disease activity (Seymour *et al.* 1979). Animal studies suggest that the change from an established lesion to an advanced lesion is caused by changes in the microbial flora and the develop-ment of acute inflammatory changes in the gingival tissues (Kennedy and Polson 1973; Page *et al.* 1975).

1.2.4 MICROBIOLOGY OF GINGIVITIS

In gingival health, a thin layer of plaque (< 60 μm) is found at the gingival margins. This layer consists mainly of *streptococci* (*sanguis* types) and the *Actinomyces* species—*viscosus*, *naeslundii*, and *israelii* (Slots 1977a; Loesche and Syed 1978). The subgingival flora in healthy tissues has a similar composition to plaque found above the gingival margin.

Gingivitis is associated with a greater abundance of plaque and there is a shift in composition from a microflora dominated by *streptococci* to one dominated by *Actinomyces* (Loesche and Syed 1978). The onset of gingival bleeding appears to be associated with an increase in *A. viscosus* and *Bacteroides gingivalis* (White and Mayrand 1981). In spite of these findings, there is uncertainty whether the clinical manifestations of gingivitis are related to quantitative or qualitative changes in bacterial plaque.

Studies of experimental gingivitis have shown that the composition of plaque shows little interindividual variation during the first four days (Moore *et al.* 1982). As the lesion progresses, so variation becomes more apparent. This implies that the progression of gingivitis is related to a sequential colonization in the plaque microflora rather than a quantitative increase in plaque mass.

Other investigations have suggested that the change in the cell-mediated immune response is important in the development of gingivitis (for a review see Van Palenstein Helderman 1981). This sort of change in the immune response may be mediated by the number of bacteria present in the subgingival plaque. Therefore, changes in bacterial number could exert a greater pathogenic effect on the gingival tissues as opposed to small shifts in microbial composition. These findings would support the view that the development of gingivitis is related more to quantitative changes in plaque rather than qualitative changes and therefore support the non-specific plaque hypothesis in the aetiology of gingivitis.

1.3 PERIODONTITIS

1.3.1 INTRODUCTION

The progression of an established gingivitis to the advanced lesion heralds the onset of periodontitis—an inflammatory disease of the periodontal tissues. The features of periodont-itis include loss of connective tissue attachment to the root surface and exposure of cementum; apical migration of the junctional epithelium, which can result in gingival reces-sion or pocket formation; and alveolar bone loss and an increase in tooth mobility. The progression of periodontitis is now considered episodic with bursts of disease activity followed by periods of quiescence.

The formation of a periodontal pocket allows plaque to colonize the root surface and the layer of necrotic cementum. The pocket environment facilitates the growth of anaerobic micro-organisms, and certain bacterial types have been designated 'periodontopathogens'. These bacteria have been implicated as causal in the destructive phases of periodontitis.

In this section, we will be considering the change from the established to an advanced lesion, the episodic nature of periodontal destruction, the host immune response, and cellular, biochemical, and microbial interactions that can lead to tissue resorption.

1.3.2 CONVERSION OF AN ESTABLISHED TO AN ADVANCED LESION

Longitudinal studies in both humans and animals have shown that in some cases the established gingival lesion can remain stable for months or even years, whilst others progress to destructive forms of periodontitis (Lovdal *et al.* 1958; Page *et al.* 1975; Schroeder and Lindhe 1975; Suomi *et al.* 1981). The precise nature and aetiology of this change is poorly understood, but possibly involves an interplay between several factors. Possible causes for this conversion include an alteration in the host's response, a change in the plaque microflora, and an acute inflammatory change in the gingival tissues with pocket formation.

As gingivitis progresses, there is a reduction in T cells and an increase in B cells and plasma cells. It has been suggested that this shift in lymphocyte populations is the harbinger of impending tissue destruction and is responsible for the conversion of a gingivitis to a periodontitis (Seymour *et al.* 1979). Whether the shift is related to a failure of the T cell response or enhancement of B cells has not been established. Further studies (for a review see Seymour 1987) have shown that the immunoregulatory control of T cells is important in the progression of periodontal disease.

Changes in plaque composition are apparent in the development of gingivitis (see p. 3). An increase in plaque mass will facilitate the growth of anaerobic bacteria at the tooth surface and in the gingival crevice. A change in plaque microflora could increase the antigenic challenge on the host response and cause a failure of the T cell response.

Pocket formation is related to the apical extension of bacterial plaque (Schroeder and Attstrom 1980). The root surface is covered with plaque that is difficult to remove by conventional mechanical methods. There is increased permeability of the junctional epithelium and the underlying connective tissue is readily exposed to bacterial products. Animal studies (in which periodontal lesions are produced by ligatures placed round the teeth) have shown that the conversion of a stable, established lesion to a progressive lesion is accompanied by an acute inflammatory change in the gingival connective tissue (Kennedy and Polson 1973; Schroeder and Lindhe 1975). As the progressive lesion stabilizes, the cellular infiltrate changes from a lesion dominated by PMNs to one dominated by lymphoid cells. However, findings from ligature-induced periodontitis in various

animals need to be interpreted with caution. It is not clear how applicable the changes in such lesions are to those in adult periodontitis.

Once a pocket has formed (i.e. the disease has progressed from established to advanced), the condition is no longer reversible and a new equilibrium needs to be established in the host–parasite relationship.

1.3.3 THE NATURE OF DESTRUCTION IN PERIODONTITIS

Evidence from epidemiological studies would suggest that periodontal destruction in adults with periodontitis follows a slow, progressive, linear course with disease severity showing an increase with age (Axelsson and Lindhe 1978; Loe *et al.* 1978). However, these studies provide little information on attachment loss at individual sites. In animal studies, periodontal destruction occurred at only 10 per cent of interdental sites in infected rats (Garant 1976*a*; Garant and Cho 1979). The destruction followed a 'burst' of acute inflammation, which was characterized by ulceration of the junctional epithelium and a massive infiltration of PMNs. Osteoclastic activity also showed a similar 'burst of activity', with bone destruction followed by quiescence (Garant 1976*b*).

Regular measurement of attachment levels at individual sites in an untreated human population has shown that some sites lose up to 5 mm of attachment, whilst others lose none (Goodson *et al.* 1982; Haffajee *et al.* 1983). These figures are not consistent with a continuous disease process.

Two further models have been proposed to account for the episodic or cyclical nature of periodontal destruction— 'the random burst model' and 'the asynchronous burst model' (Socransky *et al.* 1984). In the random burst model (i.e. random with respect to time), some sites are free and remain free of destruction throughout the patient's life, whilst other sites undergo a brief 'burst of activity' followed by a period of quiescence. Further bursts may in time occur at these sites. This model supports the concept that disease activity at a site is related to a local failure of the host response to control a pathogen(s) resident in the pocket. It seems likely that the failure may be related to a change in the microbial composition of subgingival plaque.

The feature of the asynchronous burst model is that certain sites remain free of disease whilst others show bursts of destruction that are asynchronous and short. Thus, in this model, multiple sites show breakdown within short periods of time, but further periods of activity could occur throughout the life of the patient's dentition.

An additional feature of periodontal destruction is that certain teeth are more likely to be affected than others. Furthermore, the pattern of tissue destruction tends to follow a bilateral distribution (Hirschfeld and Wasserman 1978; Loe *et al.* 1978). Knowing whether a site is active or not will provide for more optimal treatment (Listgarten 1986).

1.3.4 MARKERS OF DISEASE ACTIVITY

There has been much interest in obtaining a valid and reproducible marker of periodontal disease activity. Such a marker or markers would identify the patient or site at risk from periodontal destruction. Potential disease markers have been considered in a series of review articles, and topics covered include systemic predisposition (Wilton *et al.* 1988), periodontal indices (Griffiths *et al.* 1988), laboratory markers from crevicular fluid (Curtis *et al.* 1989), laboratory markers from analysis of saliva (Wilton *et al.* 1989), and the microbial analysis of subgingival plaque (Maiden *et al.* 1990).

The effects of systemic disease, drug therapy, age changes, smoking, diet, and sex hormones on the rate of periodontal destruction are discussed throughout this book. Clinical measurements and the various periodontal indices are only capable of detecting disease retrospectively. Biochemical markers of tissue breakdown and the presence of certain inflammatory mediators in crevicular fluid provide promising indicators of disease activity, in particular glycosaminoglycans and prostaglandins of the E series. Salivary analysis of various immunoglobulins and proteins is a poor prognostic indicator.

The isolation of particular periodontopathogens in relation to destructive periodontal lesions has led to the development of techniques for sampling and the rapid identification of these micro-organisms. *Bact. gingivalis* is one such pathogen, and the presence of this bacterium in subgingival plaque may be a useful indicator of disease activity.

1.4 THE IMMUNE RESPONSE IN PERIODONTAL DISEASE

The immune system is the body's major defence mechanism against infection. In basic terms, this system involves the recognition of foreign material (or antigen) by the various immunocompetent cells (macrophages and lymphocytes). Recognition is followed by the production of specific neutralizing proteins (immunoglobulins or antibodies), which provide the basis of the humoral response, or of specific cells (sensitized T lymphocytes), which are involved in cell-mediated immunity. Both systems result in the elimination of antigen.

The precise role of the various components of the immune system in the pathogenesis of periodontal disease remains an area of controversy. Several studies have suggested that the interaction between plaque antigens and the host's immune response contributes to the disease process by a variety of immunopathological mechanisms (Horton *et al.* 1972; Genco *et al.* 1974; Asaro *et al.* 1982; Taubman *et al.* 1983). Although the immune response is a protective mechanism, when inappropriately activated it could contribute towards tissue destruction. This section will consider the role of the various cellular components of the immune system in the pathogenesis of periodontal disease.

1.4.1 MACROPHAGES

These large mononuclear scavenger cells are derived from blood monocytes and play an essential role in the immune

Table 1.1 Properties of interleukin 1 that may be important in the pathogenesis of periodontal disease

Property	Reference
Induces T-cell proliferation	
Induces T-helper cells to produce and release interleukin 2	Shaw *et al.* 1980
Induces interleukin 2-receptor expression	
Enhances B-cell differentiation and antibody production	Koopman *et al.* 1978; Wood 1979
Induces fibroblast proliferation	Schmidt *et al.* 1982
Increases osteoclasts and stimulates bone resorption	Heath *et al.* 1985
Stimulates chondrocytes and fibroblasts to release collagenases and prostaglandins	Postlethwaite *et al.* 1983; Gowen *et al.* 1984; Meats *et al.* 1984

response. Macrophages are attracted to sites of inflammation by chemotactic factors that include lymphokines. In the immune response, macrophages are primarily concerned with the presentation of antigens to lymphocytes. Thus, these two cells are often in close contact.

Macrophages have a variety of functions in protecting the host's tissues, but can also participate in tissue destruction. They regulate lymphocyte function and phagocytose bacterial and other cell debris. Activated macrophages produce a variety of substances that can break down the supporting tissues. These include proteases, lysosomal enzymes, and oxidizing agents. They are also the major source of prostaglandins, which are potent stimulators of osteoclasts (Loning *et al.* 1980).

The macrophage is a major source of interleukin 1—a cytokine that regulates the activity of other cells. Production can be enhanced by bacterial lipopolysaccharide (Gery and Waksman 1972). This cytokine is also produced by B lymphocytes and squamous epithelial cells. Interleukin 1, which was formerly known as lymphocyte activation factor, acts primarily on T lymphocytes. The further properties of this cytokine that are relevant to the pathogenesis of periodontal disease are listed in Table 1.1. These findings would suggest that interleukin 1 may be an important mediator in chronic destructive periodontal disease.

1.4.2 T LYMPHOCYTES

These cells, together with macrophages, are involved in the cell-mediated immune response and delayed hypersensitivity reactions. Whether these reactions are important in tissue destruction associated with periodontal disease is a subject of debate. Animal studies suggest that T cells regulate bone loss (Heijl *et al.* 1980; Yoshie *et al.* 1983), whereas in patients with periodontal disease, the change from a stable to a progressive lesion is accompanied by a shift from a T-cell lesion to one dominated by B cells (Seymour *et al.* 1979).

Activation of T lymphocytes requires the presence of a macrophage and the release of interleukin 1. This activation results in the production of committed T cells, helper (CD4) cells, suppressor (CD8) cells, natural killer (NK) cells, and memory cells.

The interaction between T-helper and -suppressor cells may have an important regulatory control of T-cell function (Seymour 1987). A study of experimental gingivitis has shown that the proportions of CD4:CD8 cells in the perivascular infiltrate from gingival connective tissue decreased as the disease progressed (Seymour *et al.* 1986*b*). Similarly, in children with gingivitis, the CD4:CD8 ratio was reported to be 2:1 (Johannessen *et al.* 1986), whereas in adult periodontitis, this ratio was approximately 1:1 (Taubman *et al.* 1984; Cole *et al.* 1986). It has not been established whether the altered CD4:CD8 ratio is a cause or a manifestation of the disease process. However, the findings would suggest that the immunoregulatory control of T-cell activity may be important in the progression of periodontal disease.

NK cells act like cytotoxic lymphocytes that destroy target cells. They are important in viral infections and in the identification of tumour cells. The activity of these cells is augmented in chronic inflammatory periodontal disease. NK-cell activity has been shown to correlate with the severity of periodontal disease (Tsoumis and Dolby 1985). The increased activity of these cells may be related to interferon, which is produced by T-helper cells.

Activated lymphocytes are induced to release lymphokines by contact with antigen or mitogen. Lymphokines are glycoproteins with a variety of biological properties. Over a hundred different lymphokines have been identified, based upon differing properties. However, they may not be individual compounds but an identical or closely related group of molecules. Lymphokine properties and factors that are important in periodontal disease include:

- chemotactic for macrophages and PMNs,
- macrophage activation factor (MAF),
- macrophage inhibition factor (MIF),
- osteoclast activation factor (OAF),
- cytotoxicity to gingival fibroblasts (α-lymphotoxin),
- proliferation of T lymphocytes (interleukin 2).

OAF is of interest in periodontal disease because it may be part of a possible mechanism for bone resorption and collagen loss (Raisz *et al.* 1975). The production and activity of OAF appears to be prostaglandin-dependent (Yoneda and Mundy 1979). There is evidence that OAF and interleukin 1 are the same or very similar compounds (Meikle *et al.* 1986).

1.4.3 B LYMPHOCYTES

These lymphocytes are responsible for producing the humoral or antibody response of the immune system. Activation of B lymphocytes requires the participation of macrophages and the helper T cell. Once activated, the B cell undergoes clonal expansion and gives rise to an antibody-producing plasma cell and memory B cell. The result is the production of specific antibody (immunoglobulins IgG and IgM), which binds to the antigen to form an immune complex. Antibodies to a variety of periodontopathic organisms have been found in both serum and crevicular fluids of

patients with periodontal disease (for review, see Genco and Slots 1984). However, the functional capabilities of these antibodies in bacterial inhibition are poorly understood.

Antigen–antibody complexes (Ag–Ab) can be phagocytosed by PMNs or macrophages. The formation of these complexes will also activate the complement system. Phagocytosis, Ag–Ab complexes, and the complement fragments can cause the release of further biochemical mediators of inflammation, in particular prostaglandins of the E series (PGE$_2$). This is a potent stimulator of osteoclast activity and can cause significant bone resorption (Rifkin *et al.* 1980; El Attar and Lin 1981).

1.5 POSSIBLE MECHANISMS OF TISSUE DESTRUCTION IN PERIODONTAL DISEASE

The pathogenesis of periodontal disease is based upon an interaction between bacterial plaque and the host's immune and inflammatory responses. This interaction causes the activation of a variety of cellular mechanisms and the release of several biochemical mediators that have the potential to cause breakdown of the connective tissue matrix. Possible mechanisms include prostaglandin-induced osteoclast activation, interleukin 1-stimulated osteoclast and fibroblast activity, immune dysfunction, and the direct action of bacterial enzymes and toxins.

1.5.1 PROSTAGLANDINS

Macrophages and PMNs are a major source of prostaglandins in the periodontal tissues. As previously discussed, these cells can release prostaglandins of the E series (e.g. PGE$_2$) when stimulated by complement products or antigen–antibody complexes. Once released they are potent stimulators of osteoclast activity. Drugs that inhibit prostaglandin synthesis (i.e. non-steroidal anti-inflammatory agents) can markedly reduce the resorption of alveolar bone in animals and humans (Williams *et al.* 1985, 1989; Jeffcoat *et al.* 1988). These longitudinal studies support the concept that prostaglandins are important mediators of bone loss in periodontal disease, and that preventing their release inhibits the rate of bone loss. This subject is discussed in further detail in Chapter 11.

1.5.2 INTERLEUKIN 1

Connective tissue is degraded by a group of enzymes known as the metalloproteinases. In the gingival tissues, these metalloproteinases, which include collagenases, are produced by gingival fibroblasts and other cells including macrophages and PMNs. Thus, any process that results in connective tissue degradation will involve these cells and their enzymes.

Various cytokines are released after activation of the host's immune response. Interleukin 1 released by macrophages can activate both osteoblasts and fibroblasts to produce collagenases and prostaglandins (Meikle *et al.*

1986). This evidence would suggest that interleukin 1 is an important chemical messenger that can modulate tissue destruction.

1.5.3 IMMUNE DYSFUNCTION

The immune response can be regarded as having either a protective or destructive role in the pathogenesis of periodontal disease. A further model has been proposed (Shenker 1987) that suggests immune dysfunction (immunosuppression) is important in the aetiology of periodontal disease. In this model, the initial exposure of the host's tissues to a potential pathogen results in either a satisfactory immune response with elimination of the pathogen and no disease, or a poor response that allows bacterial colonization. The poor response may be attributable to failure of the host's cells to recognize the pathogen, and/or a factor produced by the pathogen that impedes the immune system. Colonization is followed by immune recovery, which could result in an immune-mediated tissue injury, or elimination of the pathogen and resolution of the disease. This model may also account for the episodic nature of periodontal disease and the anomalous finding of persistent periodontal destruction in patients with high antibody titres to various periodontopathogens.

Local immune dysfunction caused by bacterial products may be important in the pathogenesis of periodontal disease. However, patients who have systemic immunosuppression (e.g. renal transplant patients) appear to have less periodontal destruction and gingival inflammation than age- and sex-matched controls (see Chapter 3). This would suggest that certain types of systemic immunosuppression afford the patient a degree of protection against destructive periodontal disease.

1.5.4 BACTERIAL SPECIFICITY

A specific microflora has been implicated in adult patients with periodontitis (see Chapter 2). Species commonly identified in such cases include *Bact. gingivalis, intermedius,* and *forsythus, Actinobacillus actinomycetemcomitans, Selonomonas sputigen, Eikenella corrodens,* and spirochaetes (Slots 1977*b*, 1979, 1986; Speigel *et al.* 1979).

In vitro studies have shown that many of these bacteria can produce a variety of enzymes and toxins which can interfere with many cellular functions. For example, *Bacteroides* species and *A. actinomycetemcomitans* produce collagenase and other proteolytic enzymes that may contribute to local tissue destruction (Soderling and Paunio 1981; Robertson *et al.* 1982). These bacteria can also produce factors that inhibit the normal defence mechanisms in the pocket, inactivate antibodies, and prevent phagocytosis (Baehni *et al.* 1981; Shenker *et al.* 1982; Sundquist *et al.* 1982). *A. actinomycetemcomitans* secretes a leukotoxin (McArthur *et al.* 1981) and *Bact. gingivalis* can produce a lipopolysaccharide that induces destruction by a direct action on bone cells (Nair *et al.* 1983).

Although several studies show that the 'periodontopathogens' can produce a variety of 'destructive' mediators, it is not clear what contribution they make to the destructive features of periodontal disease.

1.6 SUMMARY

In this chapter, we have attempted to review the various cellular, biochemical, and immunological changes that occur in the periodontium in response to bacterial plaque. Also, we have tried to identify those changes that are important in the pathogenesis of periodontal disease. There appear to be three key areas in the pathogenesis of periodontal disease that have attracted considerable research activity over the past two decades. These include the progression of an established gingivitis to an advanced lesion, aetiological factors in the 'burst' hypothesis, and the initiation and progression of connective tissue degradation and bone loss.

The conversion of an established gingival lesion to an advanced lesion is accompanied by a change in plaque microflora, a shift in lymphocyte populations from T to B cells, and a loss of epithelial attachment with pocket formation. In some patients with indifferent plaque control, the established lesion can persist for many months, whilst in others, the progression is rapid. Such clinical findings beg the question, why are these patients responding differently? Are such differences related to the pathogenicity of their respective plaques or to the variability of their host responses? At present, it is difficult to provide conclusive answers to these questions.

Longitudinal studies in adults have shown that periodontal destruction is episodic and is characterized by bursts of activity followed by periods of quiescence. These bursts may be asynchronous or random. There is uncertainty over the site-specificity of such bursts and the factors that can initiate them. Certain bacterial species (the so-called periodontopathogens), are associated with active disease. *In vitro* studies confirm the pathogenicity of these bacteria and the ability of the enzymes and toxins to destroy the periodontal tissues. However, it remains to be confirmed whether these bacteria are the cause (initiators) or the consequence of the burst of activity. It could also be argued that bursts are related to a localized failure of the host's response. An obvious cause for such a failure is a change in antigenic challenge from the subgingival microflora.

There is overwhelming evidence that bacterial plaque activates the host's immune response. As a result, a variety of cellular and biochemical mediators are released, some of which have the potential to cause degradation of the connective tissue and alveolar bone resorption. The exact mechanisms of plaque-induced periodontal destruction is uncertain. Interleukin 1, prostaglandins of the E series, lysosomal enzymes released from macrophages, and PMNs all have the potential to modulate tissue destruction. The contribution that each of these mediators makes to periodontal breakdown has not been substantiated. In reality, all mediators may be involved.

The pathogenesis of periodontal disease remains an area of intensive research. Perhaps the only fact we can state with confidence is that the disease is caused by the accumulation of plaque. The subsequent interaction of bacteria and their products with the host's immune and inflammatory responses probably leads to tissue breakdown and the progression of the disease. A thorough understanding of the disease process is important because this will lead to more appropriate methods of control. Furthermore, this understanding will help to explain how a variety of systemic factors can influence the response of the periodontal tissues to bacterial plaque.

REFERENCES

Aiguier, J. E., McCall, J. O. and Merritt, A. H. (1937). Report of the committee on nomenclature of the American Academy of Periodontology. *Journal of Periodontology*, 8, 88–95.

Asaro, J. P., Nisengard, R., Beutner, E. H. and Neiders, M. (1982). Experimental periodontal disease—immediate hypersensitivity. *Journal of Periodontology*, 54, 23–8.

Attstrom, R. (1971). Studies on neutrophil polymorphonuclear leukocytes at the dento-gingival junction in gingival health and disease. *Journal of Periodontal Research* (suppl. 8), 7–15.

Attstrom, R. (1975). The roles of gingival epithelium and phagocytosing leukocytes in gingival defence. *Journal of Clinical Periodontology*, 2, 25–32.

Attstrom, R. and Schroeder, H. E. (1979). Effect of experimental neutropenia on initial gingivitis in dogs. *Scandinavian Journal of Dental Research*, 87, 7–23.

Axelsson, P. and Lindhe, J. (1978). Effect of controlled oral hygiene procedures on caries and periodontal disease in adults. *Journal of Clinical Periodontology*, 5, 133–51.

Baehni, P. C., Tsai, C. C., McArthur, W. P., Hammong, B. F., Shenker, B. J., and Taichman, N. S. (1981). Leukotoxic activity in different strains of the bacterium *Actinobacillus actinomycetemcomitans* isolated from juvenile periodontitis in man. *Archives of Oral Biology*, 26, 671–6.

Bordin, S., Page, R. C. and Narayanan, A. S. (1984). Heterogeneity of normal human diploid fibroblasts: isolation and characterisation of a unique phenotype. *Science*, 223, 171–3.

Cimasoni, G. (1983). *Crevicular fluid updated*. Karger, Basel.

Cole, K. L., Seymour, G. J., and Powell, R. N. (1986). The autologous mixed lymphocyte reactions (AMLR) using periodontal lymphocytes. *Journal of Dental Research*, 65, 473.

Cooper, P. G., Caton, J. G., and Polson, A.M. (1983). Cell populations associated with gingival bleeding. *Journal of Periodontology*, 54, 497–502.

Curtis, M. A. *et al.* (1989). Detection of high-risk groups and individuals for periodontal disease. Laboratory markers from analysis of crevicular fluid. *Journal of Clinical Periodontology*, 16, 1–11.

El Attar, T. M. A and Lin, H. S. (1981). Prostaglandins in gingiva of patients with periodontal disease. *Journal of Periodontology*, 56, 16–19.

Gale, K. M., Powell, R. N., and Seymour, G. J. (1983). The polymorphonuclear leukocyte chemotactic response to *Bacteroides melaninogenicus*. II. Effect of age and periodontal disease status. *Journal of Periodontal Research*, 18, 126–31.

Garant, P. R. (1976a). An electron microscopic study of periodontal tissues of germfree rats and rats monoinfected with *Actinomyces naeslundii*. *Journal of Periodontal Research*, 11 (Suppl.15), 9–79.

Garant, P. R. (1976b). Light and electron microscopic observations of osteoclastic alveolar bone resorption in rats monoinfected with *Actinomyces naeslundii*. *Journal of Periodontology*, 47, 717–23.

Garant, P. R. and Cho, M. I. (1979). Histopathogenesis of spontaneous periodontal disease in conventional rats. I. Histometric and histologic study. *Journal of Periodontal Research*, 14, 297–309.

Genco, R. J. and Slots, J. (1984). Host responses in periodontal diseases. *Journal of Dental Research*, 63, 441–51.

Genco, R. J., Mashimo, P. A., Kryger, G., and Ellison, S. A. (1974). Antibody mediated effects on the periodontium. *Journal of Periodontology*, 45, 330–7.

Gery, I. and Waksman, B. H. (1972). Potentiation of the T-lymphocyte response to mitogens. II. The cellular source of persisting mediator(s). *Journal of Experimental Medicine*, 136, 143–55.

Goodson, J. M., Tanner, A. C. R., Haffajee, A. D., Sornberger, G. C., and Socransky, S. S. (1982). Patterns of progression and regression of advanced periodontal disease. *Journal of Clinical Periodontology*, 9, 472–81.

Gowen, M., Wood, D. D., Ihrie, E. J., Meats, J. E., and Russell, R. G. G. (1984). Stimulation by human interleukin I of cartilage breakdown and production of collagenase and proteoglycanase by human chondrocytes but not human osteoblasts *in vitro*. *Acta Biochimica et Biophysica*, 797, 186–92.

Griffiths, G. S. *et al.* (1988). Detection of high-risk groups and individuals for periodontal diseases. Clinical assessment of the periodontium. *Journal of Clinical Periodontology*, 15, 403–10.

Haffajee, A. D., Socransky, S. S., and Goodson, J. M. (1983). Clinical parameters and predictors of destructive periodontal disease activity. *Journal of Clinical Periodontology*, 10, 257–65.

Heath, J. K., Saklatvala, J., Meikle, M. C., Atkinson, S. J., and Reynolds, J. J. (1985). Pig interleukin I (catabolin) is a potent stimulator of bone resorption *in vitro*. *Calcified Tissue International*, 37, 95–103.

Heijl, L., Wennstrom, J., and Socransky, S. S. (1980). Periodontal disease in gnotobiotic rats. *Journal of Periodontal Research*, 15, 405–19.

Hirschfeld, L. and Wasserman, B. (1978). A long-term survey of tooth loss in 600 treated periodontal patients. *Journal of Periodontology*, 49, 225–37.

Horton, J., Leikin, S., and Oppenheim, J. (1972). Human lymphoproliferative reaction to saliva and dental plaque deposits: an *in vitro* correlation with periodontal disease. *Journal of Periodontology*, 43, 522–7.

Jeffcoat, M. K., Williams, R. C., Reddy, M. S., English, R. L., and Goldhaber, P. (1988). Flurbiprofen treatment of human periodontitis: effect on alveolar bone height and metabolism. *Journal of Periodontal Research*, 23, 381–5.

Johannessen, A. C., Nilsen, R., Knudsen, G. E., and Kristofersen, T. (1986). *In situ* characterisation of mononuclear cells in human chronic marginal periodontitis using monoclonal antibodies. *Journal of Periodontal Research*, 21, 113–27.

Kennedy, J. E. and Polson, A. M. (1973). Experimental marginal periodontitis in squirrel monkeys. *Journal of Periodontology*, 44, 140–4.

Kilian, M. and Reinholdt, J. (1986). Interference with IgA defense mechanisms by extracellular bacterial enzymes. *Medical Microbiology*, 5, 173–208.

Koopman, W. J., Farrar, I. J., and Fuller-Bonar, J. (1978). Evidence for the identification of lymphocyte activating factor as the adherent cell-derived mediator responsible for enhanced antibody synthesis by nude mouse spleen cells. *Cellular Immunology*, 35, 92–8.

Lindhe, J. and Rylander, H. (1975). Experimental gingivitis in young dogs. A morphometric study. *Scandinavian Journal of Dental Research*, 83, 314–26.

Lindhe, J., Hamp, S. E., and Loe, H. (1973). Experimental periodontitis in the beagle dog. *Journal of Periodontal Research*, 8, 1–10.

Lindhe, J., Liljenberg, B., and Listgarten, M. (1980). Some microbiological and histopathological features of periodontal disease in man. *Journal of Periodontology*, 51, 264–9.

Listgarten, M. A. (1986). A perspective on periodontal diagnosis. *Journal of Clinical Periodontology*, 13, 175–81.

Loe, H. and Holm-Pedersen, P. (1965). Absence and presence of fluid from normal and inflamed gingiva. *Periodontics*, 3, 171–7.

Loe, H., Theilade, E., and Jensen, S. B. (1965). Experimental gingivitis in man. *Journal of Periodontology*, **36**, 177–87.

Loe, H., Anerud, A., Boysen, H., and Smith, M. (1978). The natural history of periodontal disease in man. The rate of periodontal destruction before 40 years of age. *Journal of Periodontology*, **49**, 607–20.

Loesche, W. J. and Syed, S. A. (1978). Bacteriology of human experimental gingivitis: effect of plaque and gingivitis score. *Infection and Immunity*, **21**, 830–9.

Loning, T. H., Albert, H. S., Lisboa, B. P., Burkhardt, A., and Caselitz, J. (1980). Prostaglandin E and the local immune response in chronic periodontal disease. Immunohistochemical and radioimmunological observations. *Journal of Periodontal Research*, **15**, 525–35.

Lovdal, A., Arno, A., and Waerhaug, J. (1958). Incidence of manifestations of periodontal disease in light of oral hygiene and calculus formation. *Journal of the American Dental Association*, **56**, 21–33.

McArthur, W. P., Tsai, C. C., Baehni, P. C., Genco, R. J., and Taichman, N. S. (1981). Leukotoxic effect of *Actinobacillus actinomycetemcomitans*: modulation by components. *Journal of Periodontal Research*, **16**, 159–70.

Maiden, M. F. J. *et al.* (1990). Detection of high-risk groups and individuals for periodontal diseases: laboratory markers based on the microbial analysis of subgingival plaque. *Journal of Clinical Periodontology*, **17**, 1–13.

Meats, J. E., McGuire, M. K. B., Ebsworth, N. M., Englis, D. J., and Russell, R. G. G. (1984). Enhanced production of prostaglandins and plasminogen activator during activation of human articular chondrocytes by products of mononuclear cells. *Rheumatology International*, **4**, 143–57.

Meikle, M. C., Heath, J. K., and Reynolds, J. J. (1986). Advances in understanding cell interactions in tissue resorption. Relevance to the pathogenesis of periodontal diseases and a new hypothesis. *Journal of Oral Pathology*, **15**, 239–50.

Miller, D. R., Lamster, I. B., and Chasens, A. I. (1984). Role of the polymorphonuclear leukocyte in periodontal health and disease. *Journal of Clinical Periodontology*, **11**, 1–15.

Moore, W. E. C. *et al.* (1982). Bacteriology of experimental gingivitis in young adult humans. *Infection and Immunity*, **38**, 651–67.

Nair, B. C., Mayberry, W. R., Dziak, R., Chen, P. B., Levine, M. J., and Hausmann, E. (1983). Biological effects of a purified lipopolysaccharide from *Bacteroides gingivalis*. *Journal of Periodontal Research*, **18**, 40–9.

Okada, H., Kida, T., and Yamagami, H. (1983). Identification and distribution of immunocompetent cells in inflamed gingiva of human chronic periodontitis. *Infection and Immunity*, **41**, 365–74.

Page, R. C. (1986). Gingivitis. *Journal of Clinical Periodontology*, **13**, 345–55.

Page, R. C. and Schroeder, H. E. (1976). Pathogenesis of inflammatory periodontal disease. *Laboratory Investigation*, **33**, 235–49.

Page, R. C., Simpson, D. M., and Ammons, W. F. (1975). Host tissue response in chronic inflammatory periodontal disease. IV. The periodontal and dental status of a group of aged great apes. *Journal of Periodontology*, **46**, 144–55.

Patters, M. R., Niekrash, C. E., and Lang, N. P. (1989). Assessment of complement cleavage of gingival fluid during experimental gingivitis in man. *Journal of Clinical Periodontology*, **16**, 33–7.

Payne, W. A., Page, R. C., Ogilvie, A. L., and Hall, W. B. (1975). Histopathologic features of the initial and early stages of experimental gingivitis in man. *Journal of Periodontal Research*, **10**, 51–64.

Postlethwaite, A. E., Lackman, L. B., Mainardi, C. L., and Kang, A. H. (1983). Interleukin I stimulation of collagenase production by cultured fibroblasts. *Journal of Experimental Medicine*, **157**, 801–6.

Raisz, L.G., Sandberg, A. L., Goodson, J. M., Simmons, H. A., and Mergenhagen, S. E. (1974). Complement-dependent stimulation of prostaglandin synthesis and bone resorption. *Science*, **185**, 789–91.

Raisz, L. G., Luben, R. A., Mundy, G. R., Dietrich, J. W., Horton, J. E., and Trummel, C. L. (1975). Effect of osteoclast activating factor from human leukocytes on bone metabolism. *Journal of Clinical Investigation*, **56**, 408–13.

Rifkin, B. R., Baker, R. L., and Coleman, S. J. (1980). Effect of prostaglandin E$_2$ on macrophages and osteoclasts in cultured foetal long bones. *Cell and Tissue Research*, **207**, 341–6.

Robertson, P. B., Lantz, M., Marucha, P. T., Kornman, K. S., Trummel, C. L., and Holt, S. C. (1982). Collagenolytic activity associated with *Bacteroides* species and *Actinobacillus actinomycetemcomitans*. *Journal of Periodontal Research*, **17**, 275–83.

Rutherford, R. B. and Schenkein, H. A. (1983). C3 cleavage products stimulate release of prostaglandins by human mononuclear phagocytes *in vitro*. *Journal of Immunology*, **130**, 874–7.

Sandberg, A. L., Wahl, S. M., and Mergenhagen, S. E. (1975). Interaction of soluble C3 fragments with guinea pig lymphocytes. Comparison of effects of C3a, C3b, C3c and C3d on lymphokine production by C3b-stimulated B cells. *Journal of Immunology*, **115**, 139–44.

Schmidt, J. A., Mizel, S. B., Cohen, D., and Green, I. (1982). Interleukin I, a potential regulator of fibroblast proliferation. *Journal of Immunology*, **128**, 2177–82.

Schroeder, H. E. (1970). The structure and relationship of plaque to the hard and soft tissues: electron microscopic interpretation. *International Dental Journal*, **20**, 353–81.

Schroeder, H. E. (1973). Transmigration and infiltration of leukocytes in human junctional epithelium. *Helvetica Odontologica Acta*, **17**, 6–18.

Schroeder, H. E. and Attstrom, R. (1980). Pocket formation: an hypothesis. In *The borderland between caries and periodontal disease*, (ed. T. Lehner and G. Cimasoni). Academic Press, London.

Schroeder, H. E. and Lindhe, J. (1975). Conversion of established gingivitis in the dog with destructive periodontitis. *Archives of Oral Biology*, **20**, 775–82.

Schroeder, H. E., Graf, D-B. M., and Attstrom, R. (1975). Initial gingivitis in dogs. *Journal of Periodontal Research*, **10**, 128–42.

Seymour, G. J. (1987). Possible mechanisms involved in the immunoregulation of chronic inflammatory periodontal disease. *Journal of Dental Research*, **66**, 2–9.

Seymour, G. J. and Greenspan, J. S. (1979). The phenotypic characterisation of lymphocyte subpopulations in established human periodontitis. *Journal of Periodontal Research*, **14**, 39–40.

Seymour, G. J., Powell, R. N., and Davies, W. I. R. (1979). Conversion of a stable T-cell lesion to a progressive B-cell lesion in the pathogenesis of chronic inflammatory periodontal disease: an hypothesis. *Journal of Clinical Periodontology*, **6**, 267–77.

Seymour, G. J., Powell, R. N., and Aitken, J. F. (1983). Experimental gingivitis in humans. A clinical and histologic investigation. *Journal of Periodontology*, **54**, 522–8.

Seymour, G. J., Whyte, G. J., and Powell, R. N. (1986a). Chemiluminescence in the assessment of polymorphonuclear leukocyte function in chronic inflammatory periodontal disease. *Journal of Oral Pathology*, **15**, 125–31.

Seymour, G. J., Walsh, L. J., and Gemmell, E. (1986b). Class II MHC expression and T-cell subsets in experimental chronic inflammation. *Journal of Dental Research*, **65**, 835.

Shaw, J., Caplan, B., Paetkau, V., Pilarski, L. M., Delovitch, T. L., and McKenzie, I. F. C. (1980). Cellular origins of co-stimulator (IL2) and its activity in cytotoxic T-lymphocyte response. *Journal of Immunology*, **124**, 2231–40.

Shenker, B. J. (1987). Immunological dysfunction in the pathogenesis of periodontal diseases. *Journal of Clinical Periodontology*, **14**, 481–98.

Shenker, B. J., Tsai, C. C., and Taichman, N. S. (1982). Suppression of lymphocyte responses by *Actinobacillus actinomycetemcomitans*. *Journal of Periodontal Research*, **17**, 462–5.

Slots, J. (1977a). Microflora in the healthy gingival sulcus in man. *Scandinavian Journal of Dental Research*, **85**, 247–54.

Slots, J. (1977b). The predominant cultivatable microflora of advanced periodontitis. *Scandinavian Journal of Dental Research*, **85**, 114–21.

Slots, J. (1979). Subgingival microflora and periodontal disease. *Journal of Clinical Periodontology*, **6**, 351–82.

Slots, J. (1986). Bacterial specificity in adult periodontitis: a summary of recent work. *Journal of Clinical Periodontology*, **13**, 912–17.

Socransky, S. S., Haffajee, A. D., Goodson, J. M., and Lindhe, J. (1984). New concepts of destructive periodontal disease. *Journal of Clinical Periodontology*, **11**, 21–32.

Soderling, E. and Paunio, K. U. (1981). Conditions of production and properties of the collagenolytic enzymes by two *Bacillus* strains from dental plaque. *Journal of Periodontal Research*, **16**, 513–23.

Spiegel, C. A., Hayduk, S. E., Minah, G. E., and Krywolap, G. N. (1979). Black-pigmented *Bacteroides* from clinically characterized periodontal sites. *Journal of Periodontal Research*, **14**, 376–82.

Sundquist, G., Bloom, G. D., Enberg, K., and Johansson, E. (1982). Phagocytosis of *Bacteroides melaninogenicus* and *Bacteroides gingivalis* in vitro by human neutrophils. *Journal of Periodontal Research*, **17**, 113–21.

Suomi, J. D., Smith, L. W., and McClendon, B. J. (1981). Marginal gingivitis during a sixteen week period. *Journal of Periodontology*, **42**, 268–70.

Taubman, M. A., Yoshie, H., Wetherell, J. R., Ebersole, J. L., and Smith, D. J. (1983). Immune response and periodontal bone loss on germfree rats immunized and infected with *Actinobacillus actinomycetemcomitans*. *Journal of Periodontal Research*, **18**, 393–401.

Taubman, M. A., Stoufi, E. D., Ebersole, J. L., and Smith, D. J. (1984). Phenotypic studies of cells from periodontal disease tissues. *Journal of Periodontal Research*, **19**, 587–90.

Tsoumis, C. S. G. and Dolby, A. E. (1985). Human antibody-dependent cellular cytotoxicity and natural killer cytoxicity in periodontal disease. A preliminary report. *Journal of Periodontal Research*, **20**, 122–30.

Van Dyke, T. E., Horoszewicz, A. V., Cianciola, L. J., and Gengo, R. J. (1980). Neutrophil chemotaxis dysfunction in human periodontitis. *Infection and Immunity*, **27**, 124–32.

Van Palenstein Helderman, W. H. (1981). Microbial etiology of periodontal disease. *Journal of Clinical Periodontology*, **8**, 261–80.

White, D. and Mayrand, D. (1981). Association of oral *Bacteroides* with gingivitis and adult periodontitis. *Journal of Periodontal Research*, **16**, 259–65.

Williams, R. C., Jeffcoat, M. K., Kaplan, M. L., Goldhaber, P., Johnson, M. G., and Wechter, W. J. (1985). Flurbiprofen: a potent inhibitor of alveolar bone resorption in beagles. *Science*, **227**, 640–2.

Williams, R. C., Jeffcoat, M. K., and Howell, T. H. (1989). Altering the course of human alveolar bone loss with the non-steroidal anti-inflammatory drug flurbiprofen. *Journal of Periodontology*, **60**, 485–90.

Wilton, J. M. A. *et al.* (1988). Detection of high-risk groups and individuals for periodontal diseases. Systemic predisposition and markers of general health. *Journal of Clinical Periodontology*, **15**, 339–46.

Wilton, J. M. A. *et al.* (1989). Detection of high-risk groups and individuals for periodontal disease: laboratory markers from analysis of saliva. *Journal of Clinical Periodontology*, **16**, 475–83.

Wood, D. D. (1979). Purification and properties of human B cell activating factor. *Journal of Immunology*, **123**, 2395–99.

Yamasaki, A., Nikai, H., Niitani, K., and Ijukin, N. (1979). Ultrastructure of the junctional epithelium of germ-free rat gingiva. *Journal of Periodontology*, **50**, 641–8.

Yoneda, T. and Mundy, G. R. (1979). Monocytes regulate osteoclast activating factor production by releasing prostaglandins. *Journal of Experimental Medicine*, **150**, 338–50.

Yoshie, H., Taubman, M. A., Olson, C. L., Ebersole, J. L., and Smith, D. J. (1983). Periodontal bone loss and immune characteristics of congenitally athymic and thymus cell reconstituted athymic rats. *Journal of Dental Research*, **62**, 273.

2. Dental plaque and calculus

2.1 PLAQUE

2.1.1 INTRODUCTION

Dental plaque occupies a central role as the major aetiological factor in the pathogenesis of dental caries and periodontal disease (Loe *et al.* 1965; Theilade *et al.* 1966; Von Der Fehr *et al.* 1970). Consequently, these two diseases may be prevented or successfully controlled by the complete, regular removal of plaque from tooth surfaces. Marginal gingivitis is a completely reversible condition and the introduction of plaque control procedures will resolve the inflammation and produce a state of gingival health (Egelberg 1965; Loe *et al.* 1965; Axelsson and Lindhe 1974). If the inflammatory lesion spreads to cause destruction of the periodontal fibres and resorption of alveolar bone, then the condition is no longer reversible by plaque control alone, although control will adequately prevent any further progression of the disease process (Suomi *et al.* 1971; Axelsson and Lindhe 1981).

Dental plaque has been defined as a bacterial aggregation on the teeth or other solid structures in the mouth (Dawes *et al.* 1963). It is an uncalcified, soft material which is so tenaciously adherent to the tooth surface that it resists removal by salivary flow or a gentle spray of water across its surface. The dense bacterial masses are enveloped within a matrix that originates either from the host (salivary glycoproteins), or from the bacteria themselves (extracellular polysaccharidès).

Clinically, plaque may be difficult to identify with the naked eye. Only when the deposit has reached a certain thickness can it be seen as a yellowish substance in the vicinity of the free gingival margin. Depending upon its location with respect to the gingival margin, plaque may be characterized as supragingival or subgingival and the plaque of each location has a quite distinct bacteriological composition.

2.1.2 THE COMPOSITION OF PLAQUE

Approximately 70 per cent of the volume of plaque is composed of bacterial cells. The remaining volume is made up of extracellular polysaccharides, which act as a matrix for the cellular component. The carbohydrates include dextran, which is a predominantly $\alpha 1,6$ linked variety of glucan (polymer of glucose), and mutan, which is predominantly $\alpha 1,3$ linked (Guggenheim 1970). The glucans are produced primarily by *Streptococcus mutans* and *Actinomycetes* spp. during initial plaque formation (Wood and Critchley 1966; Guggenheim and Schroeder 1967) and if the carbohydrates are enzymatically hydrolysed, then plaque formation can be significantly reduced or inhibited (Fitzgerald *et al.* 1968; Bowen 1971).

The absolute solubility of glucans in water is dependent upon the ratio of $\alpha 1,6$ and $\alpha 1,3$ groups that are present. The $\alpha 1,6$ varieties have freedom of rotation, which is due to an extra bond in the residue. This produces flexible coils of glucan molecules, which are soluble in water.

The structural relationship of the $\alpha 1,3$ linked residues is such as to produce rigid and closely packed sugar groups. They have, therefore, a tendency to form fibrous aggregates, which are insoluble in water (Rolla *et al.* 1985).

The glucans are metabolically synthesized by *Strep. mutans*, which use active glucosyltransferase (GTF) enzyme on dietary sucrose as the substrate. The GTF molecule may also play an important role in the binding of bacteria to tooth surfaces (see p. 12). Fructan (a levan) is also present in plaque matrix, although in much smaller quantities than dextrans. Fructans are 2,6 linked molecules, and are also relatively soluble in water. They serve as the nutrient reserve for plaque bacteria when levels of dietary sucrose are low.

In addition to the bacteria and matrix, plaque contains small numbers of epithelial cells and white blood cells, which probably are derived from the crevicular fluid. Other organisms may also be encountered in plaque, such as yeasts, fungi, and protozoa, although their role, if any, in the aetiology of periodontal disease is unknown.

2.1.3 THE DEVELOPMENT OF PLAQUE

If a tooth surface is thoroughly and vigorously cleaned of all soft deposits, then a structural entity that is distinct from dental plaque will begin to form within only a few minutes. This so-called acquired pellicle is an amorphous layer between 0.1 µm and 1.0 µm thick. It is composed of salivary glycoproteins that have become selectively adsorbed onto the tooth surface (Armstrong 1967; Leach 1979). The adsorbed molecules of glycoprotein may penetrate the enamel surface and this can lead to difficulty in completely removing the pellicle (and subsequently plaque) from the tooth by normal toothbrushing (Meckel 1965; Leach and Saxton 1966). The molecules of glycoprotein eventually undergo a biochemical transformation to produce a highly insoluble surface coating (Sonju and Rolla 1973). This is the base upon which supragingival plaque formation occurs.

Bacterial colonization of acquired pellicle has been reported as occurring within 24 h after tooth cleaning (Theilade and Theilade 1970), although Gram-positive cocci, epithelial cells, and leukocytes may be seen after only 4 h of pellicle formation (Brecx *et al.* 1981). The initial microbial colonization is around and within defects, irregularities, and cracks on the tooth surface (Mierau and Singer 1978; Lie 1979). Plaque then accumulates at the gingival margins in the interdental spaces and continues in a coronal direction.

A degree of specificity is involved in the adsorption of bacteria to the pellicle and two of the predominant colonizers are *Strep. sanguis* and *Strep. mitis*. These Gram-positive cocci are adsorbed to a greater extent than either *Strep. salivarius* or the Gram-negative *Veillonella* spp., even though the latter are present in higher proportions in saliva (Van Houte *et al.* 1971). A small percentage of Gram-positive rods are also present in early formed plaque. *A. viscosus* and *A. naeslundii* are amongst the most prevalent.

As the growth of plaque continues the number of bacteria increases rapidly by further adsorption from saliva and by multiplication of the bacteria that have already colonized the tooth surface. When the volume of plaque increases, there are concurrent qualitative changes in its bacterial composition (Loe *et al.* 1965; Theilade *et al.* 1966). The proportions of Gram-negative cocci and Gram-positive and -negative rods increases gradually and the percentage of Gram-positive cocci is reduced.

Filamentous and fusiform bacteria are seen in 2- to 4-day-old plaque as they eventually grow in to replace the coccal forms (Listgarten *et al.* 1975). Vibrios, spirils, and spirochaetes are in evidence a few days later (Loe *et al.* 1965). When gingivitis has developed as a clinical entity, the composition of supragingival plaque is very similar to that in chronic adult periodontal disease.

Maturation of the plaque matrix increases the proportion of Gram-negative organisms relative to the proportion of Gram-positive organisms and the respiratory characteristics of the bacteria become predominantly anaerobic. Such micro-organisms are found in the deeper layers of plaque, where growth conditions are more favourable to their metabolism (Ritz 1969).

When inflammation develops in the marginal gingival tissues they become oedematous and swollen. The primary source of nutrients of the microbial flora changes as the increased flow of crevicular fluid continuously bathes the subgingival deposits. The most apical portion of the previously supragingival plaque becomes protected within the clinically deepened gingival sulcus and may now be regarded as a subgingival deposit. The growth of subgingival plaque is enhanced by the downgrowth of bacteria into pockets from the supragingival location. This occurs by movement of discrete colonies of pioneer bacteria, by chemotaxis of motile forms, and predominantly by the migration of a continuous layer of plaque (Theilade and Attstrom 1979; Ten Napel *et al.* 1985). The environment changes to further enhance the colonization and growth of Gram-negative, anaerobic bacteria. The subgingival plaque is protected from the natural cleansing mechanisms of the mouth. A more loosely adherent bacterial layer can exist on the surface of the plaque mass.

Mature subgingival plaque contains many motile organisms. Large numbers of spirochaetes are in close contact with the anatomical wall of the gingival crevice (pocket). Bacteria that have different morphological forms are able to aggregate and so produce the characteristic 'corn cob' and 'test-tube brush' appearances (Listgarten 1976). The microbial (plaque) flora thus becomes extremely complex and almost totally anaerobic in nature. Gram-negative rods such as the black-pigmented *Bacteroides* and *Fusobacterium nucleatum* are present in significant numbers and are potentially pathogenic to the host's tissues (Slots 1977).

The periodontal destruction that can ensue may be dependent either upon the host's response to an accumulating volume of subgingival plaque, or perhaps to the presence of only a small number of strains of pathogenic organisms that have colonized the developing gingival/periodontal pocket (see p. 14).

2.1.4 MECHANISMS OF BACTERIAL ADHERENCE TO THE TOOTH SURFACES

The bacteria that initially colonize the pellicle or tooth surface must possess a specific mechanism by which they adhere either to glycoprotein or to the hydroxyapatite. Many oral bacteria have ultrastructural appendages or fimbria radiating from their surfaces, and it is likely that these are important mediators of early bacterial attachment. The fimbria have distinct lectin-like properties, which may be able to recognize specific sites within the pellicle or hydroxyapatite. One example is the ability of *Strep. mutans* to recognize β-galactoside residues of salivary glycoproteins in the pellicle (Gibbons and Qureshi 1979). Similarly, bacterial coaggregation can occur, involving surface lectins on one micro-organism and carbohydrate-containing receptors on another cell. Such mechanisms would be responsible for the observation that several different types of bacteria can be found on a tooth surface after only a few days of abstinence from tooth cleaning. Another mechanism of bacterial adherence involves the GTF molecule, which converts dietary sucrose to glucan polymers (see p. 11). GTF binds strongly to saliva-coated hydroxyapatite and may be able to bind bacteria directly to the surface. Alternatively, indirect mechanisms may involve GTF interactions with $\alpha 1,3$ glucose chains, which are produced by the adsorbed enzyme on cell surfaces (Rolla *et al.* 1983, 1985). This would explain why bacterial adherence to tooth surfaces is not improved by pre-made or commercially available glucans, as the active GTF enzyme is only available during bacterial production of glucan molecules (Van Houte and Upeslacis 1976).

It is, of course, possible that other phenomena such as electrostatic or electrodynamic forces can influence cell–tooth and cell–cell adherence, but current evidence suggests that it is the lectin–carbohydrate interaction which is of primary importance for bacterial adhesion (Van Houte 1979).

2.1.5 THE FORMATION OF PLAQUE ON ROOT SURFACES

The exposure of root surfaces in the mouth is common, either as a consequence of periodontal treatment or as a result of gingival recession. The formation of acquired pellicle and plaque on clean cementum surfaces resembles closely their development on enamel. A thin and homogeneous pellicle will cover cementum within 2 h of discontinuation of tooth cleaning. The surface of the pellicle is quickly colonized by Gram-positive cocci (Carrassi *et al.* 1989). On cementum this colonization is rather haphazard, whereas on enamel it occurs preferentially in pits and cracks on the surface (Nyvad and Fejerskov 1987 *a*, *b*). After about 24 h, rods and filaments are seen perpendicular to the surface and, as the plaque matures, the microbial population shifts from one primarily of cocci to one containing increased numbers of filamentous organisms (Carrassi *et al.* 1989).

2.1.6 FACTORS THAT AFFECT THE DEVELOPMENT AND COMPOSITION OF PLAQUE

The development of dental plaque upon a surface is directly related to the rate at which bacteria adhere to that surface and their subsequent rate of multiplication. Evidence suggests that plaque growth during the initial 24-h period is quite slow relative to the later exponential growth of organisms, which occurs over three days (Quirynen and van Steenberghe 1989). Such findings are not universal, however, as other studies have demonstrated a linear growth of dental plaque with time (Mierau and Singer 1978; Bergstrom 1981).

Clinical experience reveals that plaque will tend to accumulate beneath overhanging restorations and adjacent to tilted or crowded teeth. Such areas are protected from both natural cleansing mechanisms and toothbrushing. However, there are other factors that predispose to a marked variation in both the actual rate of development and the composition of plaque; they are pertinent to the discussion in this chapter and are described next.

Age of the subject

Brecx *et al.* (1985) made observations on the quantitative and qualitative aspects of plaque in young and elderly individuals. During the first 24 h of plaque development there was little difference in the types of bacteria seen in each group. Gram-positive coccal forms predominated but rods and filaments were also seen in small numbers. Quantitatively, fewer bacteria were found in older subjects at 4 and 8 h of plaque build-up, although this difference was no longer observed after 24 h. Results of other studies indicate that from day 1 onwards, plaque collects at a faster rate in elderly than in young subjects (Holm-Pedersen *et al.* 1975; 1980).

This suggests that there is a difference in growth rate between the two age groups, which may be due to differences in available nutrients. Alternatively, changes in the oral environment, such as a reduction in salivary flow rate with age, may be responsible (Brecx *et al.* 1985).

Diurnal variation

The growth of plaque is not constant over a 24-h day/night period. Growth rate is reduced by up to half during a 12-h night rest period. One possible explanation for this is that the bacterial colonies are starved of nutrients when salivary output is reduced during the night (Quirynen and van Steenberghe 1989).

Nature of the pellicle

The composition and structure of the acquired pellicle may influence the interaction between itself and the colonizing bacteria (Sonju and Glantz 1975). The proportion of glutamic acid residues within the glycoprotein pellicle will increase the hydrophobic nature of the integument (Leach 1979) and it has been shown that 'heavy' plaque formers have significantly larger quantities of glutamic acid in pellicle than 'light' plaque formers (Simonsson *et al.* 1987). Hydrophobic interactions between the pellicle and the bacteria are considered to be important in promoting bacterial adherence to the tooth. Streptococcal serotypes with reduced hydrophobicity have an impaired ability to adhere to hydroxyapatite *in vitro* (Westergren and Olsson 1983).

Roughness of the tooth surface

Irregularities and areas of roughness on the surfaces of teeth will encourage the early colonization of bacteria on enamel (Swartz and Phillips 1957). Irregularities include simple cracks in enamel, a pronounced enamel–cementum junction, and areas of enamel hypoplasia. After the initial colonization of the defect, plaque will continue to develop at a faster rate than upon adjacent areas of smooth enamel (Quirynen and van Steenberghe 1989).

The location of the plaque in the mouth

The existence of any microbial community depends strictly upon the interrelationship between the organisms and their immediate environment. Ecological factors, such as nutritional requirements, local oxygen levels, removal of bacteria by saliva, and antimicrobial host factors, are of primary importance in determining the composition of a microbial community at a specific site in the mouth. The marked contrast between bacterial types that are present in supra- and subgingival plaque provides one example of how ecological factors effect bacterial composition of plaque.

Further, occlusal fissure plaque has a different bacterial composition when compared with dentogingival plaque on the smooth surfaces of teeth. Total viable counts of organisms in fissure plaque remain relatively constant after about one week (Theilade *et al.* 1982), although certain qualitative changes occur with time. There is a relative increase in *Strep. mutans* and Gram-positive rods, and a reduction in *Strep. sanguis* and *salivarius*. In old fissure plaque, Gram-positive, facultative, anaerobic rods predominate (Theilade *et al.* 1982).

The bacterial composition of the plaque that forms on the surfaces of dentures is similar to that of fissure plaque and species of *streptococci* and *Actinomyces* predominate. Yeasts usually account for less than 1 per cent of the plaque organisms in patients with and and without a denture-induced stomatitis, although significantly larger numbers of yeasts are found in stomatitis patients (Budtz-Jorgensen *et al.* 1983).

Diet

The bacteria in plaque are able to metabolize dietary sugars to produce carbohydrate polymers, which provide the major constituent of plaque matrix (see p. 11). Consequently, if diets are supplemented with additional intakes of various carbohydrates, then the quantity of plaque and the rate of its formation would be expected to increase. Carlsson and Egelberg (1965) found that the addition of glucose or fructose to a carbohydrate-free diet did not increase the quantity of plaque, although sucrose supplements produced a greater plaque mass. Similar findings have been observed in other experiments (Sheinin and Makinen 1971; Rateitschak-Pluss and Guggenheim 1982). However, Folke *et al.* (1972) found that high-sucrose diets did not alter the quantity of plaque formed, although a general increase in microbial density was observed. *Strep. mutans* was also more prevalent in the plaque of subjects on high dietary-sucrose intake, but this increase was not significant. Further experiments have confirmed that *Strep. mutans* does proliferate as a result of sucrose supplementation, whereas the relative proportion of the bacteria is reduced when sucrose intake is restricted (Gehring *et al.* 1974).

Dental restorative materials

Patients who are regular dental attenders are likely to have a number of dental restorations that include different materials. The plaque-retaining capacity of materials varies and this factor must partly be related to surface roughness rather than to the actual structure or composition of the material itself (Swartz and Phillips 1957). Dental porcelain has repeatedly been shown to have a lower plaque retention than other materials (Kaqueler and Weiss 1970; Wise and Dykema 1975; Chan and Weber 1986) but the differences are reduced when all the materials are highly polished (Clayton and Greene 1970). Restorations of porcelain fused to metal are more likely to retain plaque on the exposed gold than on the porcelain (Kaqueler and Weiss 1970; Chan and Weber 1986).

Extensive polishing of amalgam does not reduce markedly its plaque-retaining ability (Laurell *et al.* 1983). However, *in vitro* studies suggest that plaque formation on different brands of amalgam does vary. Dispersion-phase alloys inhibit plaque growth, a finding which may be related to their initial-phase composition and zinc content (Dummer and Wills-Wood 1984). Increasing the copper content of amalgam, however, does not necessarily inhibit bacterial growth (Smales 1981; Dummer and Wills-Wood 1984).

Fluoride ions have been incorporated into glass-ionomer cements but their clinical effectiveness in inhibiting plaque is reduced by the relative surface roughness of the set material (Smales 1981). The effect of regular topical fluoride applications to enamel, however, is to reduce plaque formation (Dijkman *et al.* 1985).

2.1.7 PATHOGENICITY OF PLAQUE

There is an unquestionable relationship between plaque and periodontal disease. Bacteria in plaque are able to initiate an inflammatory response in the periodontal tissues by one of two mechanisms. First, by inactivating the host's response to the insult. This is achieved by the production of factors that reduce phagocytosis and intracellular killing of bacteria, degrade immunoglobulins and complement, and enhance the killing and degradation of defence cells. Secondly, bacteria produce factors that have a direct destructive effect on the host's tissues (see Chapter 1). Such factors include proteolytic enzymes, toxic metabolic products, and fatty cell-wall components (lipotechoic acids), which accumulate in plaque and produce a reservoir of potentially damaging antigenic substances. However, although the mechanisms of tissue destruction are becoming clearer, the precise role of either individual or groups of bacteria in the pathogenesis of periodontal disease has yet to be elucidated. Ongoing controversy has produced two quite extreme theories in an attempt to explain the microbial aetiology of periodontal disease.

The specific theory

According to the classical specific theory, a direct relationship exists between a single species of bacteria and the onset and progression of periodontitis. The theory has recently been broadened to suggest that between 6 and 12 microbial species are responsible for the majority of periodontal disease, and additional forms of organisms can contribute to the disease in a small percentage of the population (Socransky 1977). As an example, there is strong evidence to implicate *Actinobacillus actinomycetemcomitans* as a major pathogen in juvenile periodontitis (Tanner *et al.* 1979; Mandell 1984). Furthermore, this organism together with *Bacteroides gingivalis* and *intermedius* are suspected pathogens in active, destructive lesions of chronic adult periodontal disease (Slots 1986). However, the actinobacillus has also been isolated from groups of subjects who do not suffer from juvenile periodontitis (or any other type of disease) (Zambon *et al.* 1983), and this indicates that the organism may be harmless and indigenous in some subjects whilst being potentially pathogenic in others. Approximately 200 bacteria have now been detected in affected sites of patients with juvenile periodontitis (Moore *et al.* 1982), and these findings tend to complicate further the specific plaque theory.

From the aspect of treatment, the specific theory raises some interesting possibilities. Theoretically, by removing specific bacterial pathogens the progression of disease could be controlled, although the eradication of indigenous organisms may be difficult if not impossible to achieve (Theilade 1986). The use of antibiotics may eliminate foreign pathogens but indigenous bacteria quickly recolonize sites when the antibiotics are withdrawn. According to this theory, a non-pathogenic plaque containing only harmless, indigenous bacteria is the ideal goal and so, theoretically, the need for absolute plaque control in the management of periodontal disease would become obsolete.

The non-specific theory

Proponents of the classical version of this theory suggest that all oral bacteria are capable of producing virulence factors and that all plaque is pathogenic. Clinical signs of disease only become apparent when the amount of plaque exceeds a certain threshold beyond which the host's immune response is unable to protect the tissues. The theory does not consider it important that some organisms are more prevalent in certain disease states, or that sites of tissue destruction can be populated by a different subgingival flora when compared to apparently inactive or immune sites in the same mouth (Slots 1986).

It is possible that the precise role of plaque bacteria in the aetiology of periodontal disease is explained by a combination of both theories. When plaque is allowed to accumulate on a clean tooth in a healthy environment, gingivitis will inevitably follow within a few days. Gingivitis represents an inflammatory and immune response to a complex, non-specific, and dynamic microflora. The gingivitis may remain contained in the superficial tissues indefinitely, or it may progress to involve deeper structures and cause periodontal destruction. This progression could be the result of a variation in the host response mechanism (non-specific theory) and/or the colonization of the gingival crevice by pathogenic bacteria (specific theory). Subsequently, the continued loss of periodontal attachment tends to occur with sporadic bursts of activity at random sites in the mouth (Socransky *et al.* 1983), and such activity may be associated with the presence of one, or more likely a small group of, specifically pathogenic bacteria (Slots 1986).

2.1.8 BACTERIAL INVASION OF THE GINGIVAL TISSUES

The discovery of certain forms of bacteria and mycoplasms within the periodontal connective tissues suggests that organisms from the surface of subgingival plaque can penetrate the junctional or pocket epithelium and cause further periodontal destruction (Saglie *et al.* 1982*a*,*b*; Manor *et al.* 1984). Conversely, passive infection may have occurred during the handling of the tissues at biopsy (Saravanamuttu 1987).

If active invasion does occur, then elimination of the invading organisms may not be complete after time-honoured methods of disease management such as scaling and root planing. The organisms will survive and multiply in the tissues and antibiotic therapy may be necessary to supplement more traditional methods.

2.2 CALCULUS

2.2.1 INTRODUCTION

Dental calculus is a hard, calcified deposit that is found on teeth and other solid structures in the mouth. It is classified according to its location relative to the marginal gingiva. Hard deposits on the clinical crowns of teeth are known as supragingival calculus. This is crumbly in texture and yellowish-white in colour, although staining is not uncommon, particularly in smokers. Supragingival calculus is often formed in abundance in areas adjacent to the openings of salivary ducts, an observation that has linked its formation to physiological changes in the freshly secreted saliva.

Subgingival calculus is often visible to the naked eye as a narrow, dark-green, or black band located just apical to the free gingival margin. Such deposits are very hard and particularly resistant to removal by scaling instruments. Occasionally, subgingival calculus will become 'supragingival' in location as a result of gingival recession and periodontal disease. Subgingival calculus formation has no predilection for a particular site in the mouth, which suggests that its formation is more probably associated with the crevicular fluid rather than saliva.

2.2.2 COMPOSITION OF CALCULUS

Calculus is composed of about 80 per cent inorganic material and 20 per cent organic matter. Calcium and phosphorus constitute the major proportion of the inorganic salts but other ions such as magnesium, sodium, zinc, carbonate, and fluoride are present in variable quantities (Theilade and Schroeder 1966). The organic matrix contains approximately 36–40 per cent of nitrogenous components (protein) and 12–28 per cent carbohydrate (Little *et al.* 1961). Lipids are present in only very small amounts and are probably derived from the cell walls of bacteria that are enveloped within the calculus during its mineralization. Ultrastructural analysis of mature calculus reveals that the inorganic phase has a crystalline form; four types of crystal structure have been observed. A carbonate-containing apatite having fine, needle-shaped crystals, and magnesium- and zinc-containing, bulk-shaped fragments of Whitlockite are two of the main constituents (Driessens 1982; Kani *et al.* 1983). A third important component is the platelet-shaped crystals of octacalcium phosphate. Further, if salivary pH is low enough, rod-shaped crystals of dicalcium phosphate dihydrate (brushite) are also present (Driessens *et al.* 1985). Brushite is not present in detectable quantities in subgingival calculus (Jensen and Dano 1954; Gron *et al.* 1967), and in supragingival deposits it is more abundant in younger calculus than in older samples (Rowles 1964). This observation suggests that brushite is converted into one of the other crystalline forms as part of the maturation of calculus.

Structurally, calculus is a very porous substance that contains numerous spaces within the calcified matrix. Such spaces may represent uncalcified bacteria or conversely can be seen around individual calcified organisms themselves (Shirato *et al.* 1981).

2.2.3 ATTACHMENT OF CALCULUS TO TOOTH SURFACES

Subgingival calculus is particularly resistant to removal from the tooth surface, suggesting a strong mode of attachment between the tooth and the deposit. Calculus can be locked quite firmly into small irregularities or areas of resorption on the surface of cementum (Zander 1953). Furthermore, bacteria can penetrate enamel, dentine, or cementum as part of the caries demineralization process. If surface remineralization then follows, the invading bacteria become mineralized and indistinct from those that are embedded in the calculus which can later form on the remineralized surface (Zander 1953; Selvig 1969).

2.2.4 MINERALIZATION OF CALCULUS

The exact mechanism of calculus formation is unknown. The presence of plaque on a tooth surface is a prerequisite and it is within the soft deposit that mineralization occurs. A seed or nucleus upon which mineralization starts and crystal growth can continue has not been isolated. Bacteria have been suggested as possible candidates, although components of the intermicrobial matrix such as proteolipids may also be implicated (Lie and Selvig 1974; Sidaway 1979; Ennever *et al.* 1979). Whatever the nature of the seed, it is generally believed that some change must occur in the saliva and/or crevicular fluid before mineralization occurs. Both of these fluids continuously flow over the surface of the plaque and so small ions are able to penetrate its structure (McNee *et al.* 1982; Tatevossian and Newbrun 1983).

Saliva and most other body fluids are supersaturated with hydroxyapatite. Some of the calcium ions form complexes with carbon dioxide and other small molecules. It has been suggested that, when saliva enters the mouth CO_2 is lost and salts of calcium precipitate. This theory helps to explain why abundant quantities of calculus are found adjacent to salivary duct openings (Jenkins 1978).

The calcification of plaque may also be related to changes in the pH of saliva or of plaque itself. Resting (non-acid forming) plaque has a higher pH than the surrounding saliva (Kleinberg and Jenkins 1964). This increase in alkalinity could be caused by the production of ammonia, urea, and amines by proteolytic activity in plaque (Critchley *et al.* 1968). The increased pH would favour precipitation of calcium phosphates. Evidence for this mode of calculus formation comes from studies which have shown that subjects with high salivary urea concentrations tend to be more heavy calculus formers (Mandel and Thompson 1967; Epstein *et al.* 1980). 'Heavy' calculus formers have higher 3-day plaque levels (about $4\times$) of insoluble calcium and inorganic phosphate than do 'light' calculus formers (Mandel 1974). This demonstrates the rapidity with which seeding of crystals can occur in plaque that has only recently formed on a clean tooth surface.

2.2.5 PATHOGENICITY OF CALCULUS

The precise relationship between calculus and periodontal disease has received a considerable amount of attention in recent years. *In vivo*, calculus always has a layer of plaque on its surface and consequently it is difficult to separate the effects of these two deposits upon the periodontal tissues.

The results of long-term longitudinal studies have shown that plaque control measures alone are not as effective as when they are combined with subgingival scaling and root planing in the management of periodontal disease (Chawla *et al.* 1975; Tagge *et al.* 1975; Hellden *et al.* 1979; Cercek *et al.* 1983).

Supragingival calculus acts as a mechanical obstruction to personal oral-hygiene procedures and so prevents adequate plaque removal. Subgingival calculus, however, is at least initially the result rather than the cause of disease. Its development relies upon the apical downgrowth of supragingival plaque, which then calcifies and serves as a nidus for further plaque growth. This subgingival calculus develops in a protected, anaerobic environment that is subsequently colonized by periodontopathic organisms.

In addition to its plaque-retaining capacity, subgingival calculus, by virtue of its porosity, can absorb and act as a reservoir for antigenic material, toxins, and bone-resorbing factors of bacterial origin (Patters *et al.* 1982). Subgingival calculus may therefore have an active role in stimulating periodontal attachment loss and its removal is mandatory if successful maintenance of periodontal health is to be achieved.

REFERENCES

Armstrong, W. G. (1967). The composition of organic films formed on human teeth. *Caries Research*, **1**, 89–103.

Axelsson, P. and Lindhe, J. (1974). The effect of a preventive programme on dental plaque, gingivitis and caries in schoolchildren. Results after one and two years. *Journal of Clinical Periodontology*, **1**, 126–38.

Axelsson, P. and Lindhe, J. (1981). Effect of controlled oral hygiene procedures on caries and periodontal disease in adults. *Journal of Clinical Periodontology*, **8**, 239–48.

Bergstrom, J. (1981). Photogrammetric registration of dental plaque accumulation *in vivo*. *Acta Odontologica Scandinavica*, **89**, 275–84.

Bowen, W. H. (1971). The effects of calcium, magnesium, and manganese on dextran production by a cariogenic *Streptococcus*. *Archives of Oral Biology*, **16**, 115–19.

Brecx, M., Holm-Pedersen, P., and Theilade, J. (1985). Early plaque formation in young and elderly individuals. *Gerodontics*, **1**, 8–13.

Brecx, M., Ronstrom, A., Theilade, J., and Attstrom, R. (1981). Early formation of dental plaque on plastic films. *Journal of Periodontal Research*, **16**, 213–27.

Budtz-Jorgensen, E., Theilade, E., and Theilade, J. (1983). Quantitative relationship between yeasts and bacteria in denture-induced stomatitis. *Scandinavian Journal of Dental Research*, **91**, 134–42.

Carlsson, J. and Egelberg, J. (1965). Effect of diet on early plaque formation in man. *Odontologisk Revy*, **16**, 112–25.

Carrassi, A., Santarelli, G., and Abati, S. (1989). Early plaque colonisation on human cementum. *Journal of Clinical Periodontology*, **16**, 265–7.

Cercek, J. F., Kiger, R. D., Garrett, S., and Egelberg, J. (1983). Relative effects of plaque control and instrumentation on the clinical parameters of human periodontal disease. *Journal of Clinical Periodontology*, **10**, 46–56.

Chan, C. and Weber, H. (1986). Plaque retention on teeth with full ceramic crowns: a comparative study. *Journal of Prosthetic Dentistry*, **56**, 666–71.

Chawla, T. N., Nanda, R. S., and Kapoor, K. K. (1975). Dental prophylaxis procedures in control of periodontal disease in Lucknow (rural) India. *Journal of Periodontology*, **46**, 498–503.

Clayton, J. A. and Greene, E. (1970). Roughness of pontic materials and dental plaque. *Journal of Prosthetic Dentistry*, **23**, 407–11.

Critchley, P., Saxton, C. A., and Kolendo, A. B. (1968). The histology and histochemistry of dental plaque. *Caries Research*, **2**, 115–29.

Dawes, C., Jenkins, G. N., and Tonge, C. H. (1963). The nomenclature of the integuments of the enamel surface of teeth. *British Dental Journal*, **115**, 65–8.

Dijkman, A. G., Nelson, D. G. S., Jongelbloed, W. L., Weerkamp, A. H. and Arends, J. (1985). *In vitro* plaque formation on enamel surfaces treated with topical fluoride agents. *Caries Research*, **19**, 547–57.

Driessens, F. C. M. (1982). *Mineral aspects of dentistry*. Karger, Basel.

Driessens, F. C. M., Borggreven, J. M. P. M., Verbeeck, R. M. H., Van Dijk, J. W. E., and Feagin, F. F. (1985). On the physicochemistry of plaque calcification and the phase composition of dental calculus. *Journal of Periodontal Research*, **20**, 329–36

Dummer, P. M. H. and Wills-Wood, M. (1984). *In vitro* plaque formation on dental amalgam. *Journal of Oral Rehabilitation*, **11**, 539–45.

Egelberg, J. (1965). Local effect of diet on plaque formation and development of gingivitis in dogs. I. Effects of hard and soft diets. *Odontologisk Revy*, **16**, 31–41.

Ennever, J., Vogel, J. J., Boyan-Salyers, B., and Riggan, L. J., (1979). Characterisation of calculus matrix calcification nucleator. *Journal of Dental Research*, **58**, 619–23.

Epstein, S. R., Mandel, I., and Scopp, I. W. (1980). Salivary composition and calculus formation in patients undergoing hemodialysis. *Journal of Periodontology*, **51**, 336–8.

Fitzgerald, R. J, Spinell, D. M., and Stoudt, T. H. (1968). Enzymatic removal of artificial plaques. *Archives of Oral Biology*, **13**, 125–8.

Folke, L. E. A, Gawronski, T. H., Staat, R. H., and Harris, R. S. (1972). Effect of dietary sucrose on quantity and quality of plaque. *Scandinavian Journal of Dental Research*, **80**, 529–33.

Gehring, F., Makinen, K. K., Larmas, M., and Scheinin, A. (1974). Turku sugar studies. IV. An immediate report on the differentiation of polysaccharide-forming streptococci (*S.mutans*). *Acta Odontologica Scandinavica*, **32**, 435–44.

Gibbons, R. J. and Qureshi, J. V. (1979). Inhibition of adsorption of *Streptococcus mutans* strains to saliva-treated hydroxyapatite by galactose and certain amines. *Infection and Immunity*, **26**, 1214–17.

Gron, P., Van Campen, G. J., and Linstrom, I. (1967). Human dental calculus. Inorganic chemical and crystallographic composition. *Archives of Oral Biology*, **12**, 829–37.

Guggenheim, B. (1970). Enzymatic hydrolysis and structure of water-insoluble glucan produced by glucosyltransferases from a strain of *Streptococcus mutans*. *Helvetica Odontologica Acta*, **14** (Suppl. 5), 89.

Guggenheim, B. and Schroeder, H. E. (1967). Biochemical and morphological aspects of extracellular polysaccharides produced by cariogenic streptococci. *Helvetica Odontologica Acta*, **11**, 131–52.

Hellden, L. B., Listgarten, M. A. and Lindhe, J. (1979). The effect of tetracycline and/or scaling on human periodontal disease. *Journal of Clinical Periodontology*, **6**, 222–30.

Holm-Pedersen, P., Agerbaek, N., and Theilade, E. (1975). Experimental gingivitis in young and elderly individuals. *Journal of Clinical Periodontology*, **2**, 14–24.

Holm-Pedersen, P., Folke, L. E. A., and Gawronski, T. H. (1980). Composition and metabolic activity of dental plaque from healthy young and elderly individuals. *Journal of Dental Research*, **59**, 771–6.

Jenkins, G. N. (1978). Pellicle, plaque and calculus. In *The physiology and biochemistry of the mouth*. (4th edn), p. 403. Blackwell Scientific, London.

Jensen, A. T. and Dano, M. (1954). Crystallography of dental calculus and the precipitation of certain calcium phosphates. *Journal of Dental Research*, **33**, 741–50.

Kani, T., Kani, M., Moriwaki, Y., and Doi, Y. (1983). Microbeam X-ray diffraction analysis of dental calculus. *Journal of Dental Research*, **62**, 92–5.

Kaqueler, J. and Weiss, M. (1970). Plaque accumulation on dental restorative materials. *Journal of Dental Research*, **49** (abstr. 202).

Kleinberg, I. and Jenkins, G. N. (1964). The pH of dental plaque in the different areas of the mouth before and after meals and their relationship to the pH and rate of flow of resting saliva. *Archives of Oral Biology*, **9**, 493–516.

Laurell, L., Rylander, H. and Pettersson, B. (1983). The effect of different levels of polishing of amalgam restorations on the plaque retention and gingival inflammation. *Swedish Dental Journal*, **7**, 45–53.

Leach, S. A. and Saxton, C. A. (1966). An electron microscopic study of the acquired pellicle and plaque formed on the enamel of human incisors. *Archives of Oral Biology*, **11**, 1081–94.

Leach, S. A. (1979). A biophysical approach to interactions associated with the formation of the matrix of dental plaque. In *Dental plaque and surface interactions in the oral cavity* (ed. S. A. Leach), pp. 159–83. Information Retrieval, London.

Lie, T. (1979). Morphologic studies on dental plaque formation. *Acta Odontologica Scandinavica*, **37**, 73–85.

Lie, T. and Selvig, K. (1974). Calcification of oral bacteria—an ultrastructural study of two strains of *Bacterionema matruchotii*. *Scandinavian Journal of Dental Research*, **82**, 145–52.

Listgarten, M. A., Mayo, H. E., and Tremblay, R. (1975). Development of dental plaque on epoxy resin crowns in man. A light and electron microscopic study. *Journal of Periodontology*, **46**, 10–26.

Little, M. F., Casciani, C. and Lensky, S. (1961). The organic matrix of dental calculus. *Journal of Dental Research*, **40**, 753 (abstr. 311).

Loe, H., Theilade, E., and Jensen, S. B. (1965). Experimental gingivitis in man. *Journal of Periodontology*, **36**, 177–87.

McNee, S. G., Geddes, D. A. M., and Weetman, D. A. (1982). Diffusion of sugars and acids in human dental plaque *in vitro*. *Archives of Oral Biology*, **27**, 975–9.

Mandel, I. D. (1974). Biochemical aspects of calculus formation. II. Comparative studies of saliva in heavy and light calculus formers. *Journal of Periodontal Research*, **9**, 211–21.

Mandel, I. D. and Thompson, R. H. (1967). The chemistry of parotid and submaxillary saliva in heavy calculus formers and non-formers. *Journal of Periodontology*, **38**, 310–15.

Mandell, R. L. (1984). A longitudinal microbiological investigation of *Actinobacillus actinomycetemcomitans* and *Eikenella corrodens* in juvenile periodontitis. *Infection and Immunity*, **45**, 778–80.

Manor, A., Lebendiger, M., Shiffer, A., and Tovel, H. (1984). Bacterial invasion of periodontal tissues in advanced periodontitis in humans. *Journal of Clinical Periodontology*, **55**, 567–73.

Meckel, A. M. (1965). The formation and properties of organic films on teeth. *Archives of Oral Biology*, **10**, 585–97.

Mierau, H-D. and Singer, D. (1978). Reproduzierbarkeit der plaquebildung in dentogingivalen Bereich. *Deutsche Zahnaertzliche Zeitschrift*, **33**, 566–73.

Moore, W. E. C., Holdeman, L. V., Sonibert, R. M., Hash, D. E., Burmeister, J. A., and Ranney, R. R. (1982). Bacteriology of severe periodontitis in young adult humans. *Infection and Immunity*, **38**, 1137–48.

Nyvad, B. and Fejerskov, O. (1987a). Scanning electron microscopy of early microbial colonisation of human enamel and root surfaces *in vivo*. *Scandinavian Journal of Dental Research*, **95**, 287–96.

Nyvad, B. and Fejerskov, O. (1987b). Transmission electron microscopy of early microbial colonisation of human enamel and root surfaces *in vivo*. *Scandinavian Journal of Dental Research*, **95**, 297–307.

Patters, M. R., Landesberg, M. R. L., Johansson, L. A., Trummel, C. L. and Robertson, P. N. (1982). Bacteroides gingivalis antigens and bone resorbing activity in root surface fractions of periodontally involved teeth. *Journal of Periodontal Research*, **17**, 122–30.

Quirynen, M. and van Steenberghe, D. (1989). Is early plaque growth constant with time? *Journal of Clinical Periodontology*, **16**, 278–83.

Rateitschak-Pluss, E. M. and Guggenheim, M. (1982). Effects of a carbohydrate-free diet and sugar substitutes on dental plaque accumulation. *Journal of Clinical Periodontology*, **9**, 239–51.

Ritz, H. L. (1969). Fluorescent antibody staining of *Neisseria*, *Streptococcus* and *Veillonella* in frozen sections of dental plaque. *Archives of Oral Biology*, **14**, 1073–84.

Rolla, G., Ciardi, J. E., and Schultz, S. A. (1983). Adsorption of glucosyl transferase to saliva coated hydroxyapatite. Possible mechanism for sucrose dependent bacterial colonisation of teeth. *Scandinavian Journal of Dental Research*, **91**, 112–17.

Rolla, G., Scheie, A. A., and Ciardi, J. E. (1985). Role of sucrose in plaque formation. *Scandinavian Journal of Dental Research*, **93**, 105–11.

Rowles, S. L. (1964). The inorganic composition of dental calculus In *Bone and tooth*, Proceedings, 1st European Symposium, Oxford, 1963, (ed. H. J. J. Blackwood), pp. 175–83. Pergamon, Oxford.

Saglie, F. R., Carranza, F. A., Newman, M. G., Cheng, L., and Lewin, K. J. (1982*a*). Identification of tissue-invading bacteria in human periodontal diseases. *Journal of Periodontal Research*, **17**, 452–5.

Saglie, F. R, Newman, M. G., Carranza, F. A., and Pattinson, G. L. (1982*b*). Bacterial invasion of gingiva in advanced periodontitis in humans. *Journal of Periodontology*, **53**, 217–22.

Saravanamuttu, R (1987). Bacterial invasion of the periodontium in chronic periodontitis: the role of surgical contamination. *British Dental Journal*, **162**, 68–72.

Selvig, K. A. (1969). Biological changes at the tooth–saliva interface in periodontal disease. *Journal of Dental Research*, **48**, 846–55.

Sheinin, A. and Makinen, K. K. (1971). The effect of various sugars on the formation and chemical composition of dental plaque. *International Dental Journal*, **21**, 302–21.

Shirato, M. *et al.* (1981). Observations of the surface of dental calculus using scanning electron microscopy. *Journal of Nihon University School of Dentistry*, **23**, 179–87.

Sidaway, D. A. (1979). A microbiological study of dental calculus. III. A comparison of the *in vitro* calcification of viable and non-viable microorganisms. *Journal of Periodontal Research*, **14**, 167–72.

Simonsson, T., Ronstrom, A., Rundegren, J., and Birkhed, D. (1987). Rate of plaque formation—some clinical and biochemical chacteristics of 'heavy' and 'light' plaque formers. *Scandinavian Journal of Dental Research*, **95**, 97–103.

Slots, J. (1977). The predominant cultivable microflora of advanced periodontitis. *Scandinavian Journal of Dental Research*, **85**, 114–21.

Slots, J. (1986). Bacterial specificity in adult periodontitis. A summary of recent work. *Journal of Clinical Periodontology*, **13**, 912–17.

Smales, R. J. (1981). Plaque growth on dental restorative materials. *Journal of Dentistry*, **9**, 133–40.

Socransky, S. S. (1977). Microbiology of periodontal disease—present status and future considerations. *Journal of Periodontology*, **48**, 497–504.

Socransky, S. S., Haffajee, A. D., Goodson, J. A. M., and Lindhe, J. (1983). New concepts of destructive periodontal disease. *Journal of Clinical Periodontology*, **10**, 21–32.

Sonju, T. and Glantz, P-O. (1975). Chemical composition of salivary integuments formed *in vivo* on solids with some established surface characteristics. *Archives of Oral Biology*, **20**, 687–91.

Sonju, T. and Rolla, G. (1973). Chemical analysis of the acquired pellicle formed in two hours on cleaned human teeth. *Caries Research*, **1**, 30–8.

Suomi, J. D., Greene, J. C., Vermillion, J. R., Doyle, J., Chang, J. J., and Leatherwood, E. C. (1971). The effect of controlled oral hygiene procedures on the progression of periodontal disease in adults: results after third and final years. *Journal of Periodontology*, **42**, 152–60.

Swartz, M. and Phillips, R. (1957). Comparison of bacterial accumulations on rough and smooth enamel surfaces. *Journal of Periodontology*, **28**, 304–7.

Tagge, D. L., O'Leary, T. J., and El-Kafrawy, A. H. (1975). The clinical and histological response of periodontal pockets to root planing and oral hygiene. *Journal of Periodontology*, **46**, 527–33.

Tanner, A. C. R., Haffer, C., Brathall, G. T., Viscont, R. A., and Socransky, S. S. (1979). A study of the bacteria associated with advancing periodontitis in man. *Journal of Clinical Periodontology*, **6**, 278–307.

Tatevossian, A. and Newbrun, E. (1983). Diffusion of small ionic species in human saliva plaque fluid and plaque residue *in vitro*. *Archives of Oral Biology*, **28**, 109–15.

Ten Napel, J., Theilade, J., Matsson, L., and Attstrom, R. (1985). Ultrastructure of developing subgingival plaque in beagle dogs. *Journal of Clinical Periodontology*, **12**, 507–24.

Theilade, E. (1986). The non-specific theory in microbial aetiology of inflammatory periodontal diseases. *Journal of Clinical Periodontology*, **13**, 905–11.

Theilade, E. and Theilade, J. (1970). Bacteriological and ultrastructural studies of developing dental plaque. In *Dental plaque* (ed. W. D. McHugh), pp. 27–40, Churchill Livingstone, Edinburgh.

Theilade, E. and Theilade, J. (1985). Formation and ecology of plaque at different locations in the mouth. *Scandinavian Journal of Dental Research*, **93**, 90–5.

Theilade, E., Wright, W. H., Jensen, S. B., and Loe, H. (1966). Experimental gingivitis in man. II. A longitudinal clinical and bacteriological investigation. *Journal of Periodontal Research*, **1**, 1–13.

Theilade, E., Fejerskov, O., Karring, T., and Theilade, J. (1982). Predominant culturable microflora of human dental fissure plaque. *Infection and Immunity*, **36**, 977–82.

Theilade, J. and Attstrom, R. (1979). The distribution and ultrastructure of subgingival plaque in beagle dogs with gingival inflammation. *Journal of Periodontal Research*, **14**, 254–5.

Theilade, J. and Schroeder, H. E. (1966). Recent results in dental calculus research. *International Dental Journal*, **16**, 205–21.

Van Houte, J. (1979). Bacterial adhesion in the mouth. In *Dental plaque and surface interactions in the oral cavity* (ed. S. A. Leach), pp. 69–100. IRL Press Ltd, London and Washington DC.

Van Houte, J. and Upeslacis, V. N. (1976). Studies of the mechanism of sucrose-associated colonisation of *Streptococcus mutans* on teeth of conventional rats. *Journal of Dental Research*, **55**, 216–22.

Van Houte, J., Gibbons, R. J., and Pulkkinen, A. J. (1971). Adherence as an ecological determinant for streptococci in the human mouth. *Archives of Oral Biology*, **16**, 1131–41.

Von Der Fehr, F. R., Loe, H., and Theilade, E. (1970). Experimental caries in man. *Caries Research*, **4**, 131–48.

Westergren, G. and Olsson, J. (1983). Hydrophobicity and adherence of oral streptococci after repeated subculture *in vitro*. *Infection and Immunity*, **40**, 432–5.

Wise, M. D. and Dykema, R. W. (1975). The plaque retaining capacity of four dental materials. *Journal of Prosthetic Dentistry*, **33**, 178–90.

Wood, J. M. and Critchley, P. (1966). The extracellular polysaccharide produced from sucrose by a cariogenic streptococcus. *Archives of Oral Biology*, **11**, 1039–42.

Zambon, J. J., Christersson, L. A., and Slots, J. (1983). *Actinobacillus actinomycetemcomitans* in human periodontal disease. Prevalence in patient groups and distribution of biotypes and serotypes within families. *Journal of Periodontology*, **54**, 707–11.

Zander, H. A. (1953). The attachment of calculus to root surfaces. *Journal of Periodontology*, **24**, 16–19.

3. Systemic diseases and the periodontium

3.1 INTRODUCTION

It is now well established that the aetiological agent in periodontal disease is bacterial plaque, and a simplistic view of a model for periodontal destruction is shown in Fig. 3.1. As discussed in Chapter 1, the toxins and enzymes produced by bacterial plaque elicit inflammatory and immunological changes in the periodontal tissues at both a cellular and molecular level. These responses can be affected by a variety of systemic factors that can alter the response of the tissue to plaque. Furthermore, certain systemic disorders can have a direct effect on the periodontal tissues, and these represent the periodontal manifestations of a systemic disease. Examples of the latter would include widening of the periodontal ligament in scleroderma, or sarcoid gingivitis in sarcoidosis.

The aim of this chapter is to discuss the effect of systemic disease on the periodontal tissues and their response to bacterial plaque. The systemic factors can be considered under the following headings: endocrine, genetic, haematological, chronic granulomatous conditions, connective tissue disorders, disorders of the immune system, disorders of the reticulo-endothelial system, infections, and skin disorders. Other systemic factors that can affect the periodontal tissues include age, puberty, pregnancy, menopause, nutrition, smoking, and drug therapy. These are discussed in Chapters 4–8.

[The references in this chapter are divided into sections by disease.]

3.2 ENDOCRINE DISORDERS

3.2.1 INTRODUCTION

The endocrine glands produce hormones that control metabolism and maintain homeostasis. Hormones are substances secreted by specific tissues and transported to distant tissues where they exert their effects. The endocrine system is mostly regulated by the pituitary gland, which has a glandular component (adenohypophysis) and a neural component (neurohypophysis). Trophic hormones are produced by the adenohypophysis, which in turn regulates the activity of other endocrine glands. The secretion of trophic hormones is controlled by specific releasing factors from the hypothalamus. Production of these factors and of trophic hormones is controlled by a feedback mechanism from circulating hormones. The neurohypophysis stores and releases hormones that are produced in the hypothalamus.

3.2.2 ENDOCRINE DISORDERS AND THE PERIODONTIUM

Diabetes mellitus is the main endocrine disorder that affects the periodontium and this is considered in the next section. Likewise, the sex hormones can alter the response of the periodontal tissues to plaque and this topic is discussed in Chapter 7. Disorders of the pituitary, thyroid, and adrenal glands have little direct effect on the periodontal structures or in altering the host's response to bacterial plaque. Acromegaly, an overproduction of growth hormone, can lead to spacing of the teeth. However, the spacing is due to an increase in bone growth.

Disorders of calcium homeostasis have a minimal effect on the periodontium. Hyperparathyroid disease is associated with complete or partial loss of the lamina dura, and giant-cell lesions. The latter can appear as radiolucencies associated with the periodontal ligament. Once the parathyroid adenoma is treated, the bony lesions resolve. Other disturbances of calcium homeostasis (i.e. hypoparathyroidism, osteoporosis, and vitamin D deficiency) do not appear to have a significant effect on the periodontium.

3.3 DIABETES MELLITUS

Diabetes mellitus is a term used to describe those metabolic disorders that are characterized by glucose intolerance. The disease is usually a primary disorder, but can be related to certain endocrine abnormalities or diseases of the pancreas. Primary diabetes mellitus can be classified into two major categories – type 1, or insulin dependent (IDDM); and the more common, type 2, or non-insulin dependent.

The main feature of type 1 diabetes is a decrease in circulating insulin. It is usually of sudden onset and occurs predominantly before the age of 25 years. Symptoms include thirst, polyuria, hunger, and weight loss. The condition is controlled by daily injections of insulin. Type 2

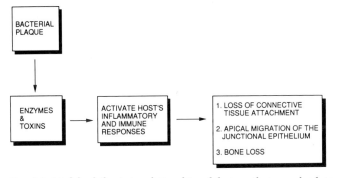

Fig. 3.1 Model of the interrelationship of factors that can lead to periodontal destruction.

diabetes is of gradual onset and mainly affects obese, middle-aged people. This type of diabetes is frequently associated with insulin resistance and is controlled by diet alone or a combination of diet and oral hypoglycaemic drugs (e.g. sulphonylureas or biguanides).

The diabetic state is often associated with vascular changes, which are referred to as early arteriosclerotic ageing. The most characteristic of these changes are found in arterioles, capillaries, and venules in a wide variety of organs and tissues. Renal, retinal, and neural changes are frequently reported.

It is now suggested that many of these vascular changes are related to disorders in the binding of serum proteins to cell membranes (Miller and Michael 1976; Chavers et al. 1981). Furthermore, a model of aberrant diabetic basement membrane has been proposed (Rohrbach and Martin 1982), which is characterized by the lack of a specific proteoglycan, heparan sulphate. The lack of heparan sulphate leaves newly formed basement membrane functionally defective and in constant need of synthesis. This would account for the observed increase in thickness of some diabetic basement membranes. Heparan sulphate also serves as a negatively charged shield preventing serum anions from permeating the membrane. Thus, diabetic membranes are not only more permeable but also more cationic. This would enable serum proteins to bind to the basement membrane rather than pass through it.

The aetiology of diabetes mellitus remains uncertain. In type 1 diabetes, there may be an abnormality of the immune system (assessed by human lymphocyte antigen (HLA) status), and/or an association with viral infections such as mumps (Handwerger et al. 1980; Asplund 1981). This finding would suggest an interrelationship between the two factors. One possibility is that future diabetics could have inherited particular complex genes. As a consequence, they could fail to eliminate an infecting virus, which in turn might destroy the pancreatic β cells, or trigger off a destructive autoimmune reaction to the insulin-producing cells (Nerup et al. 1971).

The control of the diabetic state is usually gauged by fasting blood glucose levels or a urine glucose test. The various levels used as an assessment of the degree of control (well controlled, moderate and poor) are shown in Table 3.1. These measures give an instantaneous picture of the degree of metabolic control. A further method of assessing diabetic control is the measurement of the glycosylated haemoglobin fraction, HbA_1c. This measure is an index of the long-term blood glucose levels in diabetics and is the result of the chemical condensation of HbA_1 with glucose (Bunn et al. 1976). The percentage fraction of HbA_1c thus increases during the life-span of the individual erythrocyte and is proportional to the prevailing integrated blood glucose concentration during this period. The measurement of HbA_1c therefore gives a more true picture of diabetic control during the preceding weeks and months (Gabbay et al. 1977).

Approximately 2 per cent of the population has diabetes, but in only half of these subjects is the disease recognized (Scully and Cawson 1987). Statistics show a 6 per cent annual increase in the incidence of this disease.

Table 3.1 Criteria for the various categories of control of diabetes

Control of diabetes	Fasting blood glucose level (mmol/1)	Urine glucose levels (g/24 h).	HbA_1c
Well controlled	<7.2	0–20	<10
Moderately controlled	7.3–11	20.1–39.9	10.1–11.2
Poorly controlled	>11	>40	>12

3.3.1 DIABETES MELLITUS AND PERIODONTAL DISEASE

The relationship between diabetes mellitus and periodontal disease has been extensively studied, although the findings are somewhat contradictory. Early studies suggested that the diabetic patient was more susceptible to periodontal breakdown, which was characterized by extensive bone loss, increased tooth mobility, widening of the periodontal ligament (Fig. 3.2), suppuration, and abscess formation (Swenson 1954; Burkjett and Sindoni 1959). Furthermore, animal studies have shown that experimentally induced diabetes results in a marked increase in the amount of alveolar bone loss in these animals when compared with controls (Rutledge 1940; Glickman 1946).

A synopsis of most of the investigations carried out over the past 30 years is shown in Table 3.2 (Appendix to this chapter). The studies can be divided into two main categories, those that investigated a mixed group of patients whose diabetes was controlled by a variety of methods, and those who were controlled by insulin alone (IDDM). The studies can be further categorized into those which showed that diabetics were slightly susceptible to an increased periodontal breakdown (indicated by * in the table), and those which showed a marked susceptibility to periodontal breakdown (indicated by **).

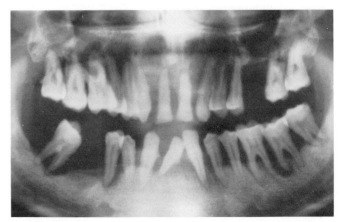

Fig. 3.2 Radiograph showing extensive periodontal bone loss in an insulin-dependent diabetic patient.

In part, some of the contradictory findings may be related to the different periodontal measurements used in the various populations of diabetics and the different methods used to assess the severity of the diabetes and its metabolic control. When all these factors are taken into account, it would appear that the well-controlled diabetic is at no greater risk from periodontal destruction than the population at large. However, several studies suggest that the poorly controlled diabetic, who shows other systemic complications (e.g. retinopathy, nephropathy) does appear to be more at risk from periodontal disease than otherwise healthy controls. Possible mechanisms for this increased susceptibility are considered below.

3.3.2 PATHOGENESIS OF DIABETES MELLITUS AND PERIODONTAL DISEASE

There are several underlying factors that accompany diabetes mellitus which may account for the apparent increased prevalence of periodontal disease in this condition. These factors can be considered under the following headings: (a) vascular changes (b) alteration in polymorphonuclear leukocyte (PMN) function; (c) changes in the biochemistry of crevicular fluid; (d) changes in the microflora of dental plaque. In many instances, the contribution of these factors in the pathogenesis of periodontal disease needs to be determined. It would seem logical to support the concept of an interplay of one or more factors contributing to the increased periodontal breakdown observed in some diabetics.

Vascular changes

The vascular changes that accompany diabetes are well recognized and account for the increased incidence of retinopathy and nephropathy. The underlying mechanism of these changes relates to the lack of heparan sulphate in basement membranes (see p. 20). Various studies have reported on vascular changes occurring in the gingival tissues of diabetics (Ray 1948; Russell 1966; Keene 1969; Hove and Stallard 1970; Lin *et al.* 1975). Changes include thickening and hyalinization of vascular walls, PAS-positive, diastase-resistant thickenings of capillary basement membranes, swelling and occasional proliferation of endothelial cells, and splitting of capillary basement membranes. These light-microscopic changes in the gingival capillaries have been supported by ultrastructural investigations, which show that the thickening of the basement membrane is characterized by an increase in an amorphous, granular and fibrillary material, with an occasional scattering of collagenous fibrils (Frantzis *et al.* 1971; Listgarten *et al.* 1974).

Diabetic-induced changes in the capillary basement membrane may have an inhibitory effect on the transport of oxygen, white blood cells, immune factors, and waste products, all of which could affect tissue repair and regeneration. The significance of the vascular changes in increasing the susceptibility of the diabetic to periodontal disease has not been fully elucidated. Some studies have failed to correlate the microangiopathic changes in the gingival vasculature with the degree and severity of periodontal destruction (Ketcham *et al.* 1975). Other investigations have suggested that there is no relationship between the vascular changes and periodontal status (McMullen *et al.* 1967; Listgarten *et al.* 1974).

PMN function

The role of PMNs in the pathogenesis of periodontal disease has been discussed in Chapter 1. Impairment of PMN function is a feature of diabetes mellitus. Disorders include reduced phagocytosis, intracellular killing, and impaired adherence (Saadoun 1980). Diabetics and their relatives also have an impaired PMN chemotactic response (Clark 1978). This suggests that the disorder is at a cellular level, although serum glucose and insulin levels can affect PMN function *in vivo*. The precise mechanism of the impaired chemotaxis has not been elucidated. Suggested causes include inhibition of the glycolytic pathway within the PMN, abnormal cyclic nucleotide metabolism, which disrupts the organization of microtubules and microfilaments, or a reduction in leukocyte membrane receptors.

Impairment of PMN chemotaxis in the gingival crevice has also been demonstrated in diabetics with severe periodontitis (Manouchehr-Pour *et al.* 1981) and also in families with a history of diabetes (McMullen *et al.* 1981). The importance of PMN dysfunction in the relationship between diabetes and periodontal disease remains to be determined.

Biochemistry of crevicular fluid

Alterations in the constituents and flow rate of crevicular fluid have been shown to be associated with diabetes. The glucose content of crevicular fluid is raised in diabetics and correlates with serum levels (Ficara *et al.* 1975). Levels of cyclic AMP are reported to be reduced in diabetics when compared with controls (Grower *et al.* 1975). These reduced levels may be a reflection of a systemic defect of cyclic AMP production.

It has also been reported that the flow rate of crevicular fluid is increased in children with diabetes (Ringelberg *et al.* 1977). Furthermore, this increase correlates with the level of gingival inflammation. The significance of the changes in crevicular fluid in diabetics in relation to the increased incidence of periodontal destruction remains to be determined. It may well be that the changes are the consequence of the disease and are not causative.

Changes in plaque microflora

Several studies have compared the microbiology and enzymic activity of dental plaque obtained from diabetics and non-diabetics. The findings from these studies are varied. Proteolytic activity of plaque has been reported to be similar in samples from both diabetics and non-diabetics (Nord *et al.* 1969), whereas hyaluronidase activity is lower in plaque from diabetics (Kjellman *et al.* 1970).

In work with alloxan-induced diabetic rats, plaque obtained from the gingival crevice produced an overgrowth of *Leptotrichia buccalis*. Endotoxins from this bacterium can stimulate gingival macrophages to produce collagenases (McNamara *et al.* 1982). However, collagenase production is also increased in germ-free diabetic rats, which suggests that the production of this enzyme is endogenously mediated (Rammamurthy and Golub 1983). An increase in collagenase production may be yet another factor that contributes to the increased incidence of periodontal breakdown observed in some diabetics.

The subgingival microflora of periodontal lesions has been investigated (Mashimo *et al.* 1983). The predominant cultivatable micro-organisms from such patients were *Capnocytophaga* spp. and 'anaerobic vibrios'. *Actinobacillus actinomycetemcomitans* was also cultivated from one-third of the patients. Mashimo *et al.* suggest that the micro-organisms found in periodontal lesions from patients with juvenile diabetes differ quantitatively from those of adult periodontitis and localized juvenile periodontitis. The flora may represent another major constellation of bacteria associated with periodontal bone loss.

In type 2 diabetes, the microbiological and immunological data suggest that *Bacteroides intermedius*, *Wolinella recta* and *Bact. gingivalis* are important in the aetiology of periodontitis associated with the diabetic state (Zambon *et al.* 1988).

The relationship between specific bacteria and periodontal destruction is a contentious issue. If specific bacteria are responsible for the increased periodontal breakdown seen in some diabetics, then such a finding should be confirmed by longitudinal studies.

3.3.3 Periodontal treatment in patients with diabetes mellitus

Nearly all diabetics respond to conventional periodontal treatment, although in certain instances, special considerations need to be applied. Diabetics are susceptible to infections (see p.20), and these can disturb the degree of metabolic control. It is therefore important that periodontal infections such as acute necrotizing ulcerative gingivitis (ANUG) or periodontal abscess be treated promptly and effectively. Similarly, if a diabetic patient requires periodontal surgery, it may be advisable to do this under antibiotic cover. Amoxycillin, 3 g, one hour before the operation would be satisfactory cover; if the patient is allergic to penicillin, then erythromycin, 1.5 g, one hour before the procedure, followed by erythromycin, 500 mg, six hours later, is a satisfactory alternative regimen.

If the patient requires a general anaesthetic, then this must be given by an experienced anaesthetist in a hospital. Also, the patient's insulin or hypoglycaemic treatment will need to be adjusted by a physician. Again, it would be advisable to carry out the surgery under antibiotic cover.

There are few reports of the response of diabetic patients to periodontal therapy. Bay *et al.* (1974) reported that the gingival response in 57 insulin-dependent diabetics to a plaque control programme was the same as in healthy controls.

The use of antimicrobial drugs in the management of periodontal disease has not been evaluated in control conditions. Animal studies in diabetic rats showed that minocycline inhibits collagenase activity in both PMNs and gingival tissues (Golub *et al.* 1983). In this study, an adolescent diabetic twin was treated with minocycline, which produced a significant reduction in gingival inflammation, crevicular fluid flow, and collagenase activity. Further appraisal of this drug in the management of periodontal disease in diabetics is therefore indicated.

3.4 GENETIC DISORDERS

3.4.1 Introduction

There is a wide range of genetic disorders that can affect the periodontium. Those considered in this section include Down's syndrome, hypophosphatasia, Papillon–Lefèvre syndrome, Ehlers–Danlos syndrome, hereditary gingival fibromatosis, the mucopolysaccharidoses, and hyperoxaluria. Some of the haematological and primary immune disorders are also inherited and these are discussed in the relevant section.

Patterns of inheritance for single-gene disorders can be autosomal dominant, autosomal recessive, or X-linked. Many of the conditions described in this section are rare, but produce significant periodontal changes.

3.4.2 Down's syndrome (mongolism)

Introduction

This syndrome, named after Langdon-Down, was first reported in 1866, and is the most common autosomal chromosome abnormality. It results from a trisomy of the twenty-first chromosome (Rappoport and Kaplan 1961). The most likely cause of this trisomy is non-dysjunction during oogenesis. Although trisomy 21 is a positive sign of Down's syndrome, it is not observed in all cases. There are mongoloids who have the normal chromosome complement of 46, but these persons probably have a reciprocal translocation of chromosome groups 13–15 and groups 21–22 (Penrose *et al.* 1960). In such cases, the defect may be transmitted by either parent, who may be a normal phenotype, but with a chromosomal complement of only 45 (Hall 1962). The risks to such mothers of having a Down's syndrome baby is in the range of 1:3 to 1:6.

The overall incidence of Down's syndrome in the population is approximately 1:700, but this increases to 1:100 if the mother is over the age of 45 (Scully and Cawson 1987).

People with the syndrome have a variety of functional disturbances: they are more prone to infections and the incidence of leukaemia is 20 times greater than in the rest of the population. Facial characteristics and dental disorders, especially periodontal problems and an increased susceptibility to ANUG, are important features.

Periodontal problems

It is now well established that those with Down's syndrome are more prone to periodontal disease and breakdown of the dental supporting structures (Plate 1, following p. 48). A common clinical finding is marked alveolar bone loss, especially around the lower incisors, which have small, conical roots (Brown 1971). Table 3.3 (Appendix to this chapter) is a synopsis of epidemiological studies of the prevalence and severity of periodontal disease in Down's syndrome. Overall, the incidence of periodontal disease is in excess of 90 per cent, and for their age, people with the syndrome are very susceptible to periodontal destruction.

Findings from the studies in Table 3.3 suggest that institutionalized persons with Down's syndrome have more periodontal disease than those cared for at home (Swallow 1964; Cutress 1971). The prevalence of periodontal disease in those cared for at home is between 50 and 60 per cent (Silimbani 1962; Gullikson 1973). This finding may be a reflection of differences in oral care in the respective places, or a combination of both environmental and systemic factors that can influence disease susceptibility (Cutress 1971). Further evidence to support this view comes from comparative studies of the incidence and severity of periodontal disease in Down's syndrome and in those who are mentally retarded (Johnson and Young 1963; Swallow 1964; Cohen and Winer 1965; Kroll *et al.* 1970; Gullikson 1973; Saxen *et al.* 1977).

Longitudinal studies of the periodontal status in Down's syndrome suggest that the rate of periodontal destruction increases with age (Brown 1978; Saxen and Aula 1982). One study reported that the rate of breakdown was 0.9 Periodontal Index units per year (Miller and Ship 1977). If these results are extrapolated, it would indicate that the whole dentition would be lost in nine years.

Early studies suggested that the distribution of periodontal destruction in Down's syndrome was uneven throughout the mouth, with the lower incisors most frequently involved (Dow 1951). Susceptibility of the teeth to bone loss is in the following order: lower incisors, upper incisors, first permanent molars, deciduous molars, premolars, and canines.

Aetiology

In an excellent review on periodontal disease in Down's syndrome, Reuland-Bosma and van Dijk (1986) state that the aetiology of the increased periodontal destruction remains obscure. However, several factors can be considered that predispose to this increased breakdown. These come under the categories of local and systemic.

Local factors

The most important local factor in the pathogenesis of periodontal destruction in Down's syndrome is bacterial plaque. Other local factors that may contribute to increased susceptibility include occlusal problems, oral habits, and changes in the composition of saliva.

Bacterial plaque.

As with other types of periodontal diseases, the presence of plaque and calculus is paramount in the aetiology of the disease. However, the amount of destruction that occurs in Down's syndrome is excessive for the age of the patient and the levels of plaque.

Quantitative investigations of the microbiology of plaque from people with Down's syndrome have had mixed findings. Black-pigmented *Bacteriodes* have been isolated from the gingival sulcus of 71 per cent of children with the syndrome, and 10 per cent of mentally retarded children (Meskin *et al*, 1968). A further study showed that counts of black-pigmented *Bacteroides* were increased in both Down's syndrome and the mentally retarded (Cutress *et al.* 1970). Further investigations are perhaps indicated to identify the role of black-pigmented *Bacteriodes* in the aetiology of periodontal destruction in Down's syndrome.

Others have made investigated streptococcal counts (Cutress 1971), the viable number of salivary anaerobic bacteria (Eastcott and Loutit 1968), and the proportions of Gram-positive and Gram-negative bacteria in plaque samples (Keyes *et al.* 1971). Their results are somewhat inconclusive. Streptococcal counts were higher in plaque samples obtained from Down's syndrome and mentally retarded subjects (30–60 per cent) than in those from healthy controls (13–22 per cent). However, counts of salivary anaerobic bacteria were lower in children with Down's syndrome when compared to their siblings. Plaque samples taken from 106 children with the syndrome showed that the composition was Gram-positive cocci 5 per cent, Gram-negative cocci 18 per cent, and diplococci 21 per cent. Very few spirochaetes were found in the samples.

Borrelia vincenti and *Bacillus fusiformis* are frequently cultivated from smears obtained from children with Down's syndrome (Brown and Cunningham 1961). This may explain the high incidence of ANUG associated with this syndrome (Brown 1973).

Occlusal problems.

The classic occlusal pattern of a child with Down's syndrome is a class III malocclusion, an anterior open bite with a lack of lip seal, a posterior cross-bite, and crowding of the lower anterior teeth. The incidence of these occlusal problems varies from study to study, but appears to be in excess of 30 per cent (Brown and Cunningham 1961; Swallow 1964; Cohen and Winer 1965; Gullikson 1973).

The high incidence of malocclusion in Down's syndrome and its relationship to the severity of periodontal destruction has not been fully investigated. Crowding will impede thorough plaque removal, but it is a contentious issue whether a relationship exists between trauma from the occlusion and an increase in the rate of periodontal breakdown (Polson 1986).

The lack of a lip seal and mouth-breathing will have a drying effect on the buccal gingiva, especially in the upper anterior region. This will make the gingival tissues more susceptible to inflammatory changes.

High frenal attachments are reported to occur more frequently in Down's syndrome. These are associated with areas of severe periodontal breakdown (Brown 1978).

Habits.

An enlarged protruding tongue is often a feature associated with Down's syndrome. True macroglossia is reported to have an incidence of 11 per cent (Cohen and Winer 1965).

The forward position of the mandible and the underdeveloped nasal and maxillary bones do not provide enough room for the tongue, hence people with Down's syndrome are more comfortable with their mouths open and the tongue protruding. Tongue thrusting is a common oral habit found in the syndrome, and has an incidence of between 52 and 83 per cent (Brown and Cunningham 1961; Swallow 1964). There does not appear to be an association between this habit and the severity of periodontal destruction (Swallow 1964).

Bruxism and thumb sucking are further oral habits that have a higher incidence in Down's syndrome than in other mentally retarded children (Gullikson 1973). Again, the relationship between these habits and the periodontal destruction has not been determined.

Saliva.
Certain changes have been reported to occur in the flow rate and composition of parotid saliva in Down's syndrome. When compared to that of mentally retarded children, saliva from children with the syndrome has a higher pH buffering capacity, and higher levels of sodium, calcium, and bicarbonate (Winer *et al.* 1965; Winer and Feller 1972). The salivary flow rate in children with Down's syndrome is reported to be half that of normal children. Submandibular salivary flow rate and composition do not appear to be affected.

The significance of the changes in parotid saliva to periodontal disease has not been evaluated. An increase in salivary pH may facilitate calculus formation, although supragingival calculus is not always a prominent feature in Down's syndrome (Brown and Cunningham 1961). The changes in saliva may be more important in the development of dental caries than in the development of periodontal disease.

Systemic factors
There are many systemic disorders that are a feature of Down's syndrome which can affect the response of the periodontal tissues to bacterial plaque. These factors can be categorized as follows: changes in the immune system, vascular changes, and nutritional factors.

The immune system.
The role of this system in the pathogenesis of periodontal disease has been discussed in Chapter 1. In Down's syndrome, defects have been reported in all the cellular components involved in the host response, i.e. PMNs, monocytes, B and T lymphocytes.

PMN function.   Many abnormalities have been reported in the PMNs obtained from people with Down's syndrome. The number of PMNs in the peripheral blood of these subjects is normal, but the cells are younger (immature). This may be related to the increased rate of cell turnover (Mellman *et al.* 1967).

There have been several reports on disorders of PMN function in Down's syndrome. These include impaired chemotaxis (Kahn *et al.* 1975), especially in institutionalized

patients (Barkin *et al.* 1980*a*), and reduced phagocytosis of *Candida albicans* (Rosner *et al.* 1973).

Other studies have reported defects in the bactericidal activity and intracellular killing of PMNs against *Staphylococcus aureus*, *Escherichia coli*, and *C. albicans* (Kretschmer *et al.* 1974; Costello and Weber 1976; Seger *et al.* 1976). Surprisingly, bactericidal activity against *Strep. pyogenes* is normal in Down's syndrome (Kretschmer *et al.* 1974). The defect in bactericidal activity may be due to a disturbance of intercellular oxidative metabolism in PMNs, especially in young children with the syndrome (Kretschmer *et al.* 1974; Eschenbach and Budenbender 1976).

Monocyte function.   The function of these cells appears to be only partly affected in Down's syndrome. Chemotaxis is impaired, but less so than PMNs (Barkin *et al.* 1980*b*). The phagocytic properties of these cells is normal in Down's syndrome, but they have a defect in opsonization. The sensitivity of monocytes to leukocyte interferon is three times greater in Down's syndrome than in normal controls. *In vitro*, this increased sensitivity prevents the maturation of monocytes to macrophages (Epstein *et al.* 1980).

B-lymphocyte function.   The number of circulating B lymphocytes in Down's syndrome appears to be normal, but the cells do show an alteration (capping) in their surface receptors to immunoglobulins and concanavalin (Naeim and Walford 1980). These changes in surface receptors are similar to those that occur in the aged (85 years and over). This suggests that in Down's syndrome there is premature ageing of the B-cell population.

Serum levels of immunoglobulins in Down's syndrome vary with age. IgM and IgD appear to be high in early childhood, whereas the levels of IgA and IgG rise with increasing age.

T-lymphocyte function.   These cells appear to be markedly affected in Down's syndrome. Counts tend to be low, especially when under the control of thymic hormonal factors. Similarly, there is impaired maturation of T lymphocytes, again due to a defect in thymic hormonal factors (Levin *et al.* 1979). The impaired maturation could be due to stress and a subsequent overloading of the immature immune system. This would lead to a depletion of the primary and secondary lymphoid organs, an increase in the circulating levels of immature T and B lymphocytes, poor mitotic effector function of T cells, and a possible defect in the suppressor T-cell system (Whittingham *et al.* 1977). Changes in T-cell maturation may be more marked in the institutionalized person with Down's syndrome, where antigenic challenge is greater. This may be one factor that accounts for the increased prevalence of periodontal destruction found in these people.

An age-related decrease in T-lymphocyte stimulation to the mitogens phytohaemagglutinin, pokeweed, and concanavalin has been reported in Down's syndrome (Seger *et al.* 1977; Nishida *et al.* 1981). This reduction in T-cell response does not appear to be related to serum factors (Rigas *et al.* 1970).

The changes in T-cell function coincide with abnormalities in the thymus gland. These include large, calcified Hassal bodies and a depletion of lymphocytes in the gland's cortex (Levin *et al.* 1979).

Relationship between changes in the immune system, Down's syndrome, and periodontal disease.

Any disorder of the immune system is likely to have an effect on the response of the periodontal tissues to bacterial plaque. Some recent investigations have tried to relate periodontal changes in Down's syndrome to defects in the immune system.

The host immune response has been investigated in a child with the syndrome and her sibling during experimental gingivitis (Reuland-Bosma *et al.* 1988a,b). An earlier and more extensive gingival inflammation occurred in the Down's child. PMNs were harvested from gingival crevicular wash-outs and peripheral blood in both subjects. They were compared for the secretion of hydrogen peroxide on stimulation, and the phagocytosis and intercellular killing of *C. albicans*. The results were similar for both children; however, an impaired chemotactic response was recorded in the child with Down's syndrome. Similarly, lymphocytes from that child showed a reduced blastogenic response to phytohaemagglutinin and pokeweed, and a lack of immune regulation leading to a prolonged helper/inducer cell activation. The investigators concluded that the various differences observed in the specific and non-specific host response mechanisms may account for the differences in gingival changes between the child with the syndrome and her sibling.

A more extensive controlled study confirmed that experimental gingivitis occurs earlier and is more extensive in Down's syndrome than normal children (Reuland-Bosma *et al.* 1986, 1988c). Cellular and morphological investigations indicate that, in Down's syndrome, there is a 40 per cent loss of gingival connective tissue, an earlier PMN response, and a delayed lymphocyte infiltration into the connective tissue subjacent to the junctional epithelium. These findings may be related to the impaired lymphocyte and PMN function that occurs in the syndrome.

Vascular changes.

Patients with Down's syndrome suffer from severe circulatory problems characterized by thin and narrow peripheral arterioles and capillaries. Their capillary fragility is high (81.1 per cent) when compared with the 19 per cent found in mentally retarded children (Dallapiccola *et al.* 1971). These vascular changes may be related to a connective tissue disorder and/or diminished platelet activity.

The impaired peripheral circulation in Down's syndrome could lead to local tissue anoxia. It has been suggested that the midline of the mandible is particularly susceptible to these vascular changes, and this may account for the increased periodontal breakdown often found around the lower incisors (Cohen 1958).

Nutritional factors.

High serum levels of vitamin C appear to be associated with rapid periodontal destruction and Down's syndrome (Tsunemitsu *et al.* 1963; Shapiro *et al.* 1969). This finding may be related to the increase in collagen synthesis reported to occur in the gingival tissues of Down's children (Claycomb *et al.* 1970). Collagen formed in the gingival tissues of these children tends to be immature, owing to a metabolic block in maturation. This may be a further factor in the aetiology of the severe periodontal disease associated with this syndrome.

Vitamin A levels have been investigated in Down's syndrome (Cutress *et al.* 1976). Their findings were that tolerance levels and absorption were normal.

Treatment

The patient with Down's syndrome presents many problems for the dental surgeon in the treatment of periodontal problems. They are more susceptible to ANUG, which should be treated with the appropriate antimicrobial therapy (metronidazole). The issues that are of paramount importance when considering their periodontal treatment are patient cooperation and acceptance of treatment, and support from family and carers. There is little information on the response of patients with Down's syndrome to periodontal therapy. Good plaque control is a prerequisite for successful treatment in any patient with a periodontal problem. However, in many instances, the person with Down's syndrome lacks the dexterity, application, or ability to carry out thorough plaque control. They are often dependent upon relatives to carry out oral hygiene measures, or on carers if they are institutionalized. Hence, the motivation and persistence of relatives are important factors if oral hygiene is to be correctly and regularly carried out. Unfortunately, it is very often the case that the parents of children with Down's syndrome are elderly and are unable to cope with an awkward and perhaps obstreperous child. This lack of cooperation makes tooth brushing a low priority.

In institutions, routine mouth care and oral hygiene may be further neglected by a shortage of staff and poor motivation. It is therefore not surprising that attempts at long-term plaque control in Down's syndrome often fail.

Chemical plaque control is an obvious alternative where mechanical plaque control is not succeeding. Again, routine use of the various antiplaque agents in children with Down's syndrome depends upon cooperation between the child and parents and/or carers. The agent must be acceptable to the patient and easy to use. Some of the antiplaque agents have an unpleasant taste, which would reduce their acceptance and further hinder cooperation. Long-term antimicrobial therapy in the control of periodontal disease in this syndrome has not been evaluated.

Conclusions

Severe periodontal destruction is a common feature of Down's syndrome. This is due to a variety of local and systemic factors that facilitate plaque accumulation and alter the response of periodontal tissues to the pathogenicity of plaque. It is difficult to put particular emphasis on any one factor. Plaque and calculus are the features that the dental surgeon can try and control, hence the emphasis of treatment must relate to the removal of these factors.

3.4.3 HYPOPHOSPHATASIA

Introduction

This is a rare familial condition, which was first described in 1948 (Rathbun 1948), and results from an inborn error of metabolism. The metabolic disorder is essentially a deficiency in the enzyme alkaline phosphatase. Other characteristics of hypophosphatasia include an abnormal mineralization of bone and dental tissues, and an increased urinary excretion of phosphoethanolamine. The disease is believed to demonstrate a typical autosomal-recessive mode of inheritance. The affected individual is homozygous for the condition, whilst both parents are heterozygous for the disease (Harris and Robson 1959). Clinically, three forms of hypophosphatasia can be recognized, based upon the age of the individual. These are:

- *Infantile.* Lesions are present at birth or within the first six months. They include softening of the bones, fever, anaemia, vomiting, and hypocalcaemia. The mortality of this form of hypophosphatasia is high, with more than half of cases dying in infancy.
- *Juvenile.* Lesions gradually become apparent after the age of 6 months and before 24 months. Bone lesions are usually mild, with bowing of the legs. There is premature loss of the deciduous teeth. This type of hypophosphatasia is usually self-limiting.
- *Adult.* Characterized by the late onset of osteoporosis, fragility of the long bones, bone pain, and sometimes a history of vitamin D-resistant rickets (Fraser 1957).

A condition known as pseudohypophosphatasia has been described, which has all the characteristic features of hypophosphatasia but the serum alkaline phosphatase levels are normal (Scriver and Cameron 1969).

Biochemical findings

Alkaline phosphatase is important for bone mineralization. The enzyme is found in osteoblasts and levels increase during phases of bone deposition. In hypophosphatasia, serum and tissue levels of the enzyme are low or absent, but osteoblasts are otherwise normal. There appears to be no consistent relationship between the severity of the disease and serum levels of alkaline phosphatase (Fraser 1957). In hypophosphatasia, phosphate activity in bone is markedly reduced in the metaphysis, periosteum, and costochondral junction (Harris and Robson 1959).

Phosphoethanolamine is found in the urine of persons with hypophosphatasia, and also in those with coeliac disease, hypothyroidism, and scurvy. Parents or relatives of siblings with hypophosphatasia also excrete some phosphoethanolamine in their urine (Harris and Robson 1959). The metabolic significance of this finding is obscure. It has been suggested that phosphoethanolamine is a breakdown product of cephalin and a substrate for alkaline phosphatase. Urinary phosphoethanolamine levels are better discriminators than measurements of serum alkaline phosphatase for detecting asymptomatic relatives who are heterozygous.

Periodontal manifestations

Several case reports have appeared since 1948 describing the periodontal and other dental manifestations of hypophosphatasia (Bruckner *et al.* 1962; Baer *et al.* 1964; Baysal 1965; Pimstone *et al.* 1966; McCormick and Ripa 1968; Casson 1969; Houpt *et al.* 1970; Beumer *et al.* 1973; Brittain *et al.* 1976; Jedrychowski and Duperon 1979; Fung 1983).

The dental features are so specific that they can be considered diagnostic (Baer *et al.* 1964). These include (a) premature exfoliation of one or more of the anterior deciduous teeth, either spontaneously or as a result of very slight trauma; (b) absence of severe clinical gingival inflammation associated with the exfoliating teeth; (c) presence of 'shell' teeth; (d) loss of alveolar bone, which is usually limited to the anterior primary teeth. Only the deciduous incisors and sometimes the canines are affected in hypophosphatasia; the permanent dentition is thought to be normal (Beumer *et al.* 1973).

Microscopically, exfoliated teeth invariably show a complete absence of cementum or only isolated areas of abnormally formed cementum (Bruckner *et al.* 1962). Fibres of the periodontal ligament are occasionally seen adhering to areas of the root surface. In these areas, there is a slight basophilic deposit on the root surface. At the ultra structural level, any remaining islands of cementum show well-defined collagen fibrils embedded in a dense organic matrix (Listgarten and Houp 1969). The cementum surface appears rough and irregular, and contains a conglomeration of spherical granules with a diameter of 0.05–1 μm. Where cementum is absent, the collagen fibres of the periodontal ligament come close to, but did not appear to connect with, the collagen fibrils of the underlying dentine.

A more extensive investigation has been made on a family manifesting hypophosphatasia (Baab *et al.* 1985, 1986). The three children (all boys) had premature loss of the deciduous incisors and canines from the age of 1½ years onwards. The involved teeth had normal formed roots, and exfoliation had occurred in the absence of clinical signs of gingival inflammation. Microbial examination in these children showed the presence of *Bact. intermedius*, *Cap. ochracea* and *Eubacterium saburreum* as the predominant forms in the subgingival plaque. Elevated levels of serum antibodies reacting to *Bact. gingivalis*, *Cap. gingivalis* and *Cap. sputigena* were found in two of the children. Investigations of neutrophil function showed that all three children had an abnormality in leukocyte chemotaxis.

These findings suggest that the lack of connective tissue attachment to the root surface may render it more susceptible to bacterial contamination by species associated with soft tissue destruction. Thus, periodontal destruction in children with hypophosphatasia may result from the same basic processes as occur in simple periodontitis (Page and Baab 1985).

Treatment

Various measures have been used in the treatment of hypophosphatasia with very little success. These include vitamins D and C, thyroid gland extract, growth hormone, thiamine chloride, cortisone, and a high-phosphate diet. Some improvement in skeletal calcification has been reported with cortisone and a high-phosphate diet (Brittain *et al.* 1976). Since the juvenile form of the disease is self-limiting, many of the skeletal lesions improve over a period of time.

Dental treatment is palliative. The prognosis for the deciduous teeth, especially the incisors and canines, is poor. For cosmetic reasons, or for space maintenance, children may require a partial denture.

3.4.4 PAPILLON–LEFÈVRE SYNDROME

This syndrome is an autosomal-recessive trait, characterized by a diffuse palmar–plantar keratosis and premature loss of both the deciduous and permanent dentitions. It was first described in 1924 (Papillon and Lefèvre 1924), and approximately 140 cases have been reported. An excellent review article has discussed 111 cases (Haneke 1979); of these, 45 cases were familial from 22 families. Consanguity of the parents was found in approximately a third of the cases. Males and females are almost equally affected and most of the reports deal with Caucasians. Papillon–Lefèvre syndrome is very rare and has an incidence of 1–4/million, although 2–4 perşons/1000 are heterozygous (Gorlin *et al.* 1964).

Parents who already have a child with this syndrome ought to be advised that there is a 25 per cent probability of any further children suffering from it. However, it is highly improbable that someone with this syndrome will have a child similarly affected.

Clinical features

The syndrome commonly affects the primary dentition (Plate 2) during the second to third years of life. Structurally, the teeth are normal and root formation is unaffected. Progressive periodontal destruction (Fig. 3.3) usually results in premature loss of the primary dentition by the age of 6 years. Teeth are lost in the order of eruption (Baer and Benjamin 1974). In many cases, the presence of lymphadenopathy at the time of examination is reported. The gingival tissues heal after loss of the deciduous teeth, but the permanent dentition erupts early. This is probably secondary to the atrophy of the alveolar bone (Haneke *et al.* 1975). A similar destructive process starts to affect the periodontal

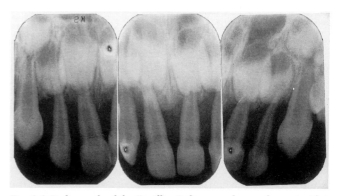

Fig. 3.3 Radiograph of the Papillon-Lefèvre syndrome shown in Plate 2; extensive bone loss affects the upper deciduous incisors.

tissues of the permanent teeth, resulting in progressive bone loss and their exfoliation.

Histopathologically, the gingival tissues manifest a picture similar to that seen in advanced lesions of adult periodontitis. Hyperplastic pocket epithelium is grossly infiltrated with PMNs and a smaller number of lymphocytes and macrophages. In the underlying connective tissue, there are large, perivascular accumulations of inflammatory cells. Plasma cells are the predominant cell type in the deeper parts of the underlying connective tissue. Ultrastructurally, these cells appear to show degenerative changes (Sloan *et al.* 1984), characterized by crystalline or spherical droplets (Russell bodies) of electron-dense material within dilated cisternae of rough endoplasmic reticulum. These observations support the view that gingival plasma cells follow a 'suicidal' pathway of differentiation (Garant and Mulvihill 1972).

The prognosis for the teeth in Papillon–Lefèvre syndrome is poor and most subjects are edentulous by the age of 16 years. More recent evidence suggests that vigorous treatment can improve the prognosis and examples are considered later.

Skin lesions

The characteristic skin lesions are diffuse, erythematous, keratotic areas on the palms and soles. Quite often, the plantar–palmar keratoses are transgredient, affecting the dorsa of the fingers and toes. Hyperhydrosis of the palms and soles, and 'non-typical' nail changes also occur with varying frequency. Histologically, the skin shows hyperkeratosis, sometimes with parakeratotic patches, acanthosis, and slight inflammatory perivascular infiltrates.

Other features

Ectopic calcifications of the falx cerebri and choroid plexus have been reported in some cases of Papillon–Lefèvre syndrome (Corson 1939; Brunsting *et al.* 1964; Dosseva *et al.* 1972). In a review of 111 cases, it was reported that 26 showed an increased susceptibility to infection. This may be due to a cellular immune defect or a deficiency in the phagocytic function of PMNs (Djawari 1978; Haneke *et al.* 1975).

Aetiology

Although Papillon–Lefèvre syndrome is an inherited disorder, its aetiology remains obscure. An early investigation suggested that the syndrome was a combination of an ecto- and mesodermal malformation (Wannenmacher 1938). Later studies put forward the idea that the periodontal component was caused by cementum acting as an irritant (Smith and Rosenzweig 1967). In some patients, this tissue has been described as being glossy and thin (Hawes 1960). Other workers have suggested that the periodontal destruction may arise as a consequence of an epithelial defect at the dentogingival junction (Schroeder *et al.* 1983), or dyskeratosis of the gingival epithelium (Lyberg 1982). Gingival dyskeratosis would be analogous to the epithelial changes found in the palms and soles. It could bring about a continuous and perhaps increased exposure of the underlying connective tissue to the toxins and enzymes of bacterial plaque. The increased inflammatory response would lead to periodontal breakdown. Changes in gingival epithelium may be secondary to a local defect in vitamin A metabolism (Gorlin *et al.* 1964).

Biopsy material obtained from the gingival tissues of this syndrome is reported to have an imbalance of collagenolytic activity (Shoshan *et al.* 1970). Furthermore, the skin lesions may also be due to imbalance between mucoproteolytic and proteolytic enzyme systems, which will cause changes in the molecular integrity of the dermal collagen.

A subepithelial 'wall zone' in the pocket wall, free of neutrophilis, has been described in a person with Papillon–Lefèvre syndrome (Rateitschak-Pluss and Schroeder 1984). This finding may indicate that leukotoxin-producing bacteria are involved, possibly with the ability to invade the tissue.

Laboratory findings

People with Papillon–Lefèvre syndrome have been subjected to a variety of biochemical and immunological investigations in attempts to identify further the aetiological factors. Lyberg (1982) concluded that there was no defect in metabolism or immunological function in two siblings with the syndrome. However, two other affected children were shown to have a deficiency in their peripheral blood monocytes of Fc receptor-mediated phagocytosis (Preus and Morland 1987). It has been reported that people with Papillon–Lefèvre syndrome have a cellular immune defect, with a decreased phytohaemagglutinin stimulation of their lymphocytes (Haneke *et al.* 1975). Their PMNs show impaired chemotaxis and phagocytic function (Djawari 1978; van Dyke *et al.* 1984). These findings may account for the increased incidence of infection found in this syndrome. Not all studies support this view: Schroeder *et al.* (1983) reported that PMNs from a 10-year-old with Papillon–Lefèvre syndrome behaved normally. Some evidence suggests that the PMN (dys-) function may be more directly related to specific types of bacteria in the subgingival plaque (see below).

Microbiological findings

Examination of the subgingival microflora from subjects with Papillon–Lefèvre has produced mixed findings. Bacteriological and scanning electron microscopic studies have reported that Gram-negative, anaerobic rods, such as *Capnocytophaga* and *Bact. gingivalis* together with large numbers of spirochaetes are found in their subgingival plaque (Newman *et al.* 1977; Jung *et al.* 1981). Other studies have shown that subgingival plaque samples contain *Capnocytophaga*, *Fusobacterium nucleatum*, and *Eikenella corrodens* (Tinanoff *et al.* 1986). One case described by Preus (1988) showed an elevated serum antibody titre against *A. actinomycetemcomitans*. Investigations within the family suggested that the bacteria had been transmitted to the child from the family dog.

An ultrastructural investigation of the periodontal lesion in this syndrome showed that the composition at the apical border of subgingival plaque was restricted to Gram-negative cocci and rods (Vrahopoulos *et al.* 1988). There was no evidence of bacterial invasion of the gingival connective tissue.

Treatment

Attempts at treating the periodontal component of Papillon–Lefèvre syndrome have, up to fairly recently, been unsuccessful (Martinez-Lalis *et al.* 1965; Haneke 1979; Hathaway 1982; Schroeder *et al.* 1983; Glenwright and Rock 1990). Others have suggested early radical treatment of the primary dentition to avoid periodontal breakdown in the permanent dentition (Coccia *et al.* 1966; Baer and McDonald 1981; McDonald and Avery 1978). Recommended treatment includes extraction of the primary teeth at the age of 3 years, and systemic antimicrobial therapy (tetracycline 250–500 mg/day) for 10 days during the eruption of the permanent dentition or during a period of an acute exacerbation. Systemic tetracycline treatment does not appear to cause staining of the permanent dentition. A very high standard of oral hygiene is a prerequisite for treatment, and patients should be monitored regularly, i.e. every three months (Preus and Gjermo 1987; Tinanoff *et al.* 1986).

Oral retinoids have been reported to be of some value in the management of two cases of the syndrome (Driban and Jung 1982; Bravo-Piris *et al.* 1983). The vitamin A analogues improved both the periodontal and cutaneous lesions, but there is little long-term information on the value of these drugs in the management of this condition.

A significant problem for those with Papillon–Lefèvre syndrome is maintenance of the alveolar ridge after premature tooth loss. Vital root submersion is one procedure for maintaining ridge height and this has been attempted in one patient with the syndrome (Lu *et al.* 1987). After six months, the alveolar ridges appeared fibrotic and the patient was wearing dentures satisfactorily. New dentures will have to be made to accommodate growth.

Conclusions

The precise aetiology of the periodontal component of Papillon–Lefèvre syndrome is obscure. It may well be that the destruction arises as a result of a combination of several factors. These could include: (a) a defect in the gingival epithelium, or (b) a disorder in the host's immune response. As a consequence of both (a) and (b), periodontal destruction and pocket formation facilitates the growth of certain periodontopathogens (i.e. *Bacteriodes* and *Capnocytophaga* spp.).

Treatment must be radical if there is to be any chance of survival of the permanent dentition. The remaining deciduous teeth should be extracted and the patients periodically treated with antimicrobial therapy to control acute exacerbations. Excellent plaque control is essential for the prognosis of the permanent teeth.

3.4.5 EHLERS–DANLOS SYNDROME

Introduction

Ehlers–Danlos syndrome is an inherited disorder affecting connective tissue. The syndrome is named after two clinicians, who described excessive joint mobility, skin hyperextensibility (Plate 3), and easy bruising (Ehlers 1901), and peculiar scarring, which occurs after skin wounds (Plate 4) (Danlos 1908). Ten variants have now been identified and their features are described in Table 3.4 (Beighton *et al.* 1969). Types I, II, and III are the most common form and have an incidence of less than 1:150 000 (Beighton 1978). There are several case reports of the oral and dental problems of this syndrome (Barabas and Barabas 1967; Recant and Lipman 1969; Hughes 1970; Hoff 1977; Sadeghi *et al.* 1989).

The basic defect in Ehlers–Danlos syndrome is a disorder in collagen molecular biology, but the nature of the defect is unknown. In type IV, the defect in collagen is due to reduced lysyl hydroxylation on a low level of hydroxylysine in the collagen molecule. This is because of impaired activity of the enzyme lysyl hydroylase. Hydroxylation of lysine is not required for the secretion and polymerization of procollagen, but it does affect the ability to generate bone-specific collagen cross-links (Pinnell *et al.* 1972; Krane *et al.* 1972).

In type IV of the syndrome there is a deficiency in the synthesis, secretion, and structure of type III collagen. Cell culture studies show that skin fibroblasts from these subjects predominantly produce type I collagen (Pope *et al.* 1975; Gay *et al.* 1976). This may well be due to a defect in the fibroblast's endoplasmic reticulum.

Laboratory findings have shown that the syndrome type IV is characterized by a deficiency of the enzyme procollagen peptidase. This enzyme removes the non-helical terminal portions of the procollagen molecule (Penttinen *et al.* 1975).

Oral and periodontal manifestations

The oral mucosa, gingival tissues, teeth, and temporomandibular joint can all be affected by Ehlers–Danlos syndrome. Because of the collagen defect, the oral mucosa is fragile and susceptible to bruising. Post-extraction haemorrhage can be a problem (Recant and Lipman 1969), owing to fragility of blood vessels and defects in the supporting connective tissue. Furthermore, the oral tissues are very difficult to suture and large 'bites' of mucosa [$\frac{1}{4}$ inch (approx. 5 mm) or more] are necessary to approximate the flaps (Hughes 1970).

The gingival tissues are often fragile and bleed readily on toothbrushing. Patients with type VIII Ehlers–Danlos syndrome are reported to have advanced periodontal destruction (Stewart *et al.* 1977), but this does not appear to be a feature in other variants (Barabas and Barabas 1967).

The teeth in Ehlers–Danlos syndrome are fragile and fracture easily. Histological examination shows the following abnormalities (Barabas 1969):

(1) an abnormality in the enamel–dentine junction with an increased amount of argyrophilic material and lack of normal scalloping;
(2) an increase in 'vascular' inclusions in the dentine, especially in root dentine;
(3) fibrous degeneration of the pulp, which contains numerous pulp stones;
(4) disorganization of cementum, especially from the root surfaces of molar teeth, and an increase in the number of cementicles.

Recurrent subluxation of the temporomandibular joints has been reported in this syndrome (Thexton 1965; Goodman and Allison 1969), which may be related to the generalized joint hypermobility. However, it has been suggested that any instability in these joints is more likely to be related to muscle balance than restraint afforded by the joint ligament (Barabas and Barabas 1967).

Treatment

There is little information on the effectiveness of periodontal treatment in Ehlers–Danlos syndrome. Persons with the type VIII syndrome appear to be susceptible to periodontal breakdown and thus require a thorough preventative programme.

Conventional periodontal treatment is difficult in all types of this syndrome. The fragility of the oral mucosa and gingival tissue can present serious problems if root planing, scaling, or surgery are attempted. The tissues split under the slightest provocation. Furthermore, there is the risk of haemorrhage and the problem of suturing the oral mucosa. It is therefore important that periodontal therapy in those with Ehlers–Danlos syndrome should be as atraumatic as possible.

3.4.6 HEREDITARY GINGIVAL FIBROMATOSIS

This is a rare condition characterized by a benign enlargement of the gingival tissues. It is also known as elephantiasis gingivae, idiopathic hyperplasia of the gums, fibromatosis gingivae, and diffuse fibroma of the gums. Gingival fibromatosis can occur singularly, but is also associated with a variety of other syndromes, which are listed in Table 3.5. Hereditary gingival fibromatosis is usually inherited as an autosomal-dominant trait (Witkop 1971) with transmission through an affected parent. However, sporadic cases are said to occur (Rushton 1957; Buchner 1937). The frequency for the anomaly has been estimated to be

Table 3.4 Variants of Ehlers–Danlos syndrome

Type	Mode of inheritance	Skin hyperextensibility	Joint hypermobility	Skin fragility	Bruising	Major complications	Basic defect
Type I (severe)	AD[a]	Marked	Marked	Marked	Moderate	Musculoskeletal deformities common; varicose veins. Patient is usually born prematurely because of early rupture of fetal membranes	Unknown
Type II (mild)	AD	Moderate	Moderate	Moderate	Moderate	–	Unknown
Type III (benign hypermobile type)	AD	Variable, usually marked	Marked	Minimal	Minimal	–	Unknown
Type IV (ecchymotic type)	AR[b]	Minimal	Digits only	Marked	Marked	Thin skin with prominent veins; cardiovascular accidents are common. Death is usually from ruptured aorta or intestinal perforation	Type III collagen deficiency
Type V (X-linked)	X-linked	Marked	Digits only	Minimal	Minimal	Musculoskeletal disorders are common	Lysyloxidase deficiency
Type VI (ocular)	AR	Marked	Marked	Minimal	Minimal	Scarring with spheroid and mulluscoid tumours. Scleral and corneal fragility	Hydroxylysine deficiency
Type VII (procollagen peptidase deficiency)	AR	Moderate	Marked	Moderate	Moderate	Short stature, multiple joint dislocations	Procollagen peptidase deficiency
Type VIII (periodontitis)	AD	Minimal	Moderate (digits only)	Marked	Minimal	Similar to type II, but with excessive periodontal destruction	Unknown
Type IX (cutis laxa)	X-linked	–	–	–	–	Horn-like projections on the occipital bone	Unknown
Type X	X-linked	–	–	Marked	Marked	Bladder-neck obstruction	Unknown

[a]Autosomal dominant; [b]autosomal recessive.

Table 3.5 Syndromes containing gingival fibromatosis

Syndrome	Mode of inheritance	Features	Reference
Gingival fibromatosis with hypertrichosis	Autosomal dominant	Gingival fibromatosis, hypertrichosis, mental deficiency and/or epilepsy	Winter and Simpkiss (1974)
Leband syndrome	Autosomal dominant	Gingivial fibromatosis; ear, nose, bone and nail defects with splenomegaly Defects are related to a soft consistency in cartilage	Leband *et al.* (1964)
Cross syndrome	Autosomal dominant	Gingivial fibromatosis, microphthalmia, mental retardation, athelosis and hypopigmentation	Cross *et al.* (1967)
Gingivial fibromatosis with progressive deafness	Autosomal dominant	Gingivial fibromatosis with hearing loss, which becomes apparent in the late teenage years	Jones *et al.* (1967)
Murray–Puretic–Drescher syndrome	Autosomal recessive	Gingival fibromatosis; multiple hyaline fibrous tumours on scalp and back Joint changes with osteoporosis of terminal phalanges	Drescher *et al.* (1967) Puretic and Puretic (1971)
Rutherfurd's syndrome	Autosomal dominant	Gingival fibromatosis, mental deficiency, aggressive behaviour, corneal opacities, impaired tooth eruption, root resorption and dentigerous cysts	Rutherfurd (1931)

1:350 000, with a phenotype frequency of 1:175 000 (Fletcher 1966). Although this condition has a genetic basis, the underlying cellular and molecular mechanisms of gingival fibromatosis are poorly understood.

Clinical features

Details of the clinical features of hereditary gingival fibromatosis have been documented in numerous reports and reviews on series of patients (Rushton 1957; Araiche and Brode, 1959; Yokoya 1962; Winstock 1964; Emerson 1965; Becker *et al.* 1967; Jorgenson and Cocker 1974). The condition is not seen before the eruption of teeth, and is more commonly associated with the permanent teeth rather than the deciduous.

The gingival tissues are enlarged, pink, firm, and can show exaggerated stippling. Their overgrowth is usually slow. The excessive fibrous tissue often impedes tooth eruption and can completely cover the crowns. If this occurs, then mastication is painful and speech may be impaired. The enlargement of the gingival tissues may be localized or generalized. Local involvement is most common around the maxillary tuberosities (Plate 5) and on the lingual surfaces of the lower molars.

The histological features of hereditary gingival fibromatosis include hyperplasia of the subepithelial layer; the surface epithelium is parakeratotic and varies in thickness; the epithelial/connective tissue interface is characterized by prominent rete ridges, which extend deeply into the subjacent connective tissues. The main feature is the thick bundles of collagen in an avascular corium. The few fibroblasts are scattered throughout the collagen connective tissue in the vicinity of the gingival crevice. This area also shows an infiltration of plasma cells (Savara *et al.* 1954; Rushton 1957; Becker *et al.* 1967).

Treatment

The main treatment for the gingival enlargement is surgical excision (gingivectomy). However, recurrence is reported after surgery, but does not happen if teeth are extracted. This would suggest that the environment of the gingival crevice is important in the pathogenesis of this condition. Regardless of this speculation, there is little information on the rate of gingival growth and its relationship with plaque and inflammation.

Patients with hereditary gingival fibromatosis should be carefully monitored after gingival surgery. Despite the lack of evidence connecting overgrowth and plaque, it would seem sensible to advocate a thorough plaque-control programme in these patients, as gingival inflammation may be an exacerbating factor. The immediate family and relatives of the patient should be screened for gingival changes.

3.4.7 MUCOPOLYSACCHARIDOSES (MPS)

Introduction

These are a group of disorders that include Hurler's syndrome or gargoylism (MPS I), Hunter's syndrome (MPS II), and I-cell disease. Other variants include MPS III, IV, V, and VI. As their name suggests, these disorders are characterized by a disturbance in mucopolysaccharide metabolism, which results in the increased storage of these substances in various tissues. They are genetic in origin, whereby Hurler's syndrome is inherited as an autosomal-recessive trait, Hunter's syndrome is an X-linked recessive disorder, and I-cell disease probably represents the homozygous state of a recessive mutation (McKusick *et al.* 1965).

Hurler's syndrome becomes apparent in early childhood and children usually die before the age of 10 years. Death is usually due to respiratory infection or cardiac disease. The latter results from the deposition of mucopolysaccharides into heart valves and the tunica intima of the coronary arteries. The main clinical features of this syndrome include mental retardation, dwarfism, hernia, deformed head, typical facies, short neck, and spinal abnormalities (Gardner 1971).

Hunter's syndrome is considered to be a less severe form of Hurler's syndrome, hence the survival rate is much greater. In both conditions there are increased levels of two acid mucopolysaccharides in the urine—chondroitin sulphate B and heparatin sulphate.

I-cell disease has similar clinical features to Hurler's syndrome (Galili *et al.* 1974). The most significant differential aspect is observed in tissue culture of skin fibroblasts, which show peculiar cytoplasmic granular inclusions, hence the term inclusion body or I cell.

Oral manifestations

Although there are several types of MPS, the associated oral changes have been documented in case reports restricted to Hurler's syndrome (for review, see Cawson 1962; Gardner 1971). The mandible, teeth, and gingiva are mainly affected.

The mandible is enlarged and thickened, with marked gonial prominences and short rami (Worth 1966). The shape of the mandible may well be related to an enlarged tongue, which is also a feature of the mucopolysaccharidoses. Radiographs of the mandible from patients with Hurler's syndrome often show radiolucent areas associated with the permanent and deciduous molars, and resembling dentigerous cysts. At biopsy, these radiolucencies are found to be hyperplastic dental follicles that consist of dense, collagenous connective tissue interspersed with pools of a metachromatic ground substance (Gardner 1971).

The teeth in Hurler's syndrome are often small and widely spaced and show delayed eruption (Cawson 1962). Spacing may be due to hyperplasia of the alveolar ridges and/or the distoangular tilting of the molars. The shape of the teeth is essentially normal.

Gingival enlargement is a feature of the mucopolysaccharidoses, but the incidence of this problem is difficult to determine. In a review of 140 cases of Hurler's syndrome, gingival hyperplasia was mentioned in only 12 subjects (Cawson 1962). In a further series of 12 patients with the syndrome, two had gingival hyperplasia (Gardner 1971). Mouth breathing, poor oral hygiene, and hyperplasia of the underlying alveolar process may all be contributing factors to this problem. Mouth breathing is very common in these disorders, owing to abnormalities in the facial and nasal skeletons, and the large mass of adenoidal tissues.

The enlarged gingival tissues have been described as nodular, fibrotic, oedematous, and haemorrhagic (Caffey 1952; Cantor 1965). Gingival tissues from patients with Hurler's syndrome contain the characteristic 'Hurler cells' within the lamina propria. These cells were originally macrophages and have relatively large amounts of metachromatically staining cytoplasm, which is either agranular or finely granular. The number of 'Hurler cells' in the gingival tissues appears to increase with age (Gardner 1968).

Treatment

Gingival overgrowth associated with any of the mucopolysaccharidoses is removed by surgical excision to recreate the normal form. There is little information on the recurrence rate after gingivectomy or the predisposition of the patient to further periodontal destruction.

3.4.8 HYPEROXALURIA (OXALOSIS)

Introduction

Hyperoxaluria or oxalosis is the accumulation, or deposition, of calcium oxalate in various tissues throughout the body. Organs or structures most frequently involved include the heart, skeletal muscle, blood vessel walls, bone marrow, and skin. The disorder can occur as a primary defect or as a secondary or acquired defect (Williams and Smith 1973).

Primary hyperoxaluria is a rare, recessively inherited, autosomal disorder of glycoxalate metabolism. Its clinical features include nephrolithiasis, nephrocalcinosis, acute arthritis, heart block, and peripheral neuropathy. The life expectancy is poor and death is usually due to renal failure secondary to the generalized oxalosis. The basic defect in primary hyperoxaluria is thought to be an enzymic defect in oxalate metabolism.

The secondary or acquired form of hyperoxaluria is due to excessive consumption of oxalate ions or substances that are metabolized to oxalate. Such substances include rhubarb and ethylene glycol (Chaplin 1977). Secondary hyperoxaluria may also be associated with bowel disorders and malabsorption syndromes. In health, calcium binds with oxalate in the gastrointestinal tract to form insoluble calcium oxalate. When there is bowel disease, or malabsorption syndrome, calcium ions bind with fatty acids leaving the more soluble oxalate available for absorption (Canos *et al.* 1981). Secondary hyperoxaluria also occurs in chronic renal failure, where oxalate deposition occurs in the kidneys. It is thought that recurrent dialysis is partly responsible for the oxalosis, owing to ineffective removal of the calcium oxalate. Renal patients prone to this problem are those that synthesize excessive amounts of oxalate (Milgram and Salyer 1974).

Oral and periodontal manifestations

To date, there have been five case reports of the oral manifestations of hyperoxaluria (Glass 1973; von Bunte *et al.* 1977; Wysocki *et al.* 1982; Fantasia *et al.* 1982; Moskow 1989). These changes mainly involve the teeth and periodontal tissues.

Root resorption (both internal and external) is the main dental feature. Histologically, the areas of resorption show deposits of calcium oxalate crystals and a granulomatous foreign-body reaction. Calcium oxalate crystals are also found attached to cementum and project towards the periodontal ligament. Pain may arise from an inflammatory reaction elicited by oxalate deposition in the pulp and periodontal ligament (Wysocki *et al.* 1982).

Deposition of calcium oxalate crystals may occur in the gingival connective tissue and periodontal ligament (Fantasia *et al.* 1982; Moskow 1989). In the gingiva, the crystals are surrounded by multinucleated foreign-body giant cells and lymphocytes. Within the ligament, crystals can make up at least half of the structure and cause widening of the membrane (Moskow 1989). The crystals are contained in a stroma of fibrous connective tissue, interspersed with lymphocytes, plasma cells, and multinucleated giant cells. Crystals are also contained within islands of odontogenic epithelium (the cell rests of Malassez). It has also been shown that oxalate crystals within the periodontal ligament can promote or act as seeds for localized areas of calcification.

The various case reports suggest that the periodontal structures are susceptible to deposition of calcium oxalate crystals in hyperoxaluria. This may be related to inflammatory changes within the periodontal tissues and the subsequent increase in vascular permeability. The latter will facilitate the escape of plasma proteins and oxalate into the gingival connective tissue and periodontal ligament. Such deposition will intensify the inflammatory response and this intensification may lead to local root resorption (Fantasia *et al.* 1982).

Treatment

Extractions appear to be the only treatment provided for the patients. There is no mention in the case reports of any preventative measures to inhibit root or tooth resorption, or the periodontal changes. The systemic disorder of oxalate metabolism is treated by renal dialysis, which has improved the life expectancy of these patients. It is important to distinguish hyperoxaluria from other disorders of calcium metabolism, notably primary and secondary hyperparathyroidism and osteomalacia.

3.5 GRANULOMATOUS DISORDERS

Granulomatous disorders are a diverse group of diseases that have in common the presence of non-caseating granulomas. The disorders that can affect the periodontium include Crohn's disease, pyostomatitis vegetans, sarcoidosis, and orofacial granulomatosis. These disorders have many common features, especially their oral manifestations and their effect on the periodontal tissues.

Wegener's granulomatosis is a vasculitis and is characterized by granulomatous lesions. For the sake of convenience, this condition is also considered in this section.

3.5.1 CROHN'S DISEASE

Crohn's disease or regional enteritis was first described in 1932 as a granulomatous disorder of the terminal ileum (Crohn *et al.* 1932). The current definition of Crohn's disease is a non-specific, submucosal alteration of the gastrointestinal tract, which is accompanied by stenosis, necrotic breakdown, and scarring of the mucosa. All areas of the tract, including the mouth, can be affected by the disease, but the common site of the initial lesion is the terminal ileum. The incidence of Crohn's disease in the United States is 15/100 000; this figure is higher in Jews, siblings of patients with the disease, and patients with ankylosing spondylitis (Sandler and Golden 1986). Approximately 25 per cent of cases begin before the age of 20 years.

Symptoms of Crohn's disease include abdominal pain, pyrexia, intermittent diarrhoea, joint pains, and generalized malaise. These symptoms are usually of slow onset. The oral manifestations of Crohn's disease were first reported in 1969 (Dudeney and Todd 1969) and include a cobblestone appearance of the oral mucosa, aphthous-type ulceration, labial and buccal gingival swellings, mucosal tags, fissuring of the midline of the lower lip, and angular cheilitis.

The disease is diagnosed on the clinical symptoms and laboratory findings. The erythrocyte sedimentation rate (ESR) is raised and haemoglobin levels are depressed. Sigmoidoscopy and barium contrast radiography will identify bowel segments that are undergoing granulomatous changes.

The aetiology of Crohn's disease is uncertain. An intolerance to certain foods may be an important factor (Jones *et al.* 1985), as many individuals with the disease are atopic (Hammer *et al.* 1968). Alternatively, there may be a familial tendency, although no genetic pattern has been established.

Periodontal manifestations

There have been several case reports of the oral manifestations of Crohn's disease. Oral lesions may be the presenting signs of the disease. Twenty-two reports were reviewed in 1978 (Bernstein and MacDonald 1978); specific involvement of the gingival tissues was mentioned in six (Schiller *et al.* 1971; Bottomley *et al.* 1972; Croft and Wilkinson, 1972; Eisenbud *et al.* 1972; Simpson *et al.* 1974; van Steenberghe *et al.* 1976).

The incidence and severity of oral involvement secondary to Crohn's disease varies from study to study. Basu *et al.* (1975) reported a 9 per cent incidence of oral lesions in a population with Crohn's disease. Aphthous-type ulceration may be the most frequent oral lesion, with an incidence in the range of 4–20 per cent (Croft and Wilkinson 1972; Kyle 1972; Greenstein *et al.* 1976). The relationship between the oral lesions of Crohn's disease and lesions elsewhere in the gastrointestinal tract is again uncertain. Some studies have shown that oral lesions correlate with the exacerbations of intestinal symptoms, whilst others have failed to confirm this finding (for review see Bernstein and MacDonald 1978).

The characteristic gingival lesion in Crohn's disease is a diffuse erythematous, granular enlargement of the attached gingiva (Plate 6). The classic cobblestone appearance of the oral mucosa is mainly confined to the buccal mucosa and mucobuccal fold. The lesions are lobulated, hypertrophic, oedematous, and fissured. Ulceration may be present. The cobblestone effect is due to a combination of hypertrophy and oedema that produces an elevation of the mucosa. This soon becomes subdivided by linear fissures. Lesions in the mucobuccal fold are tags (Plate 7) that commonly resemble denture-induced granulomas.

Severe periodontal destruction has been reported in patients with Crohn's disease (Lamster *et al.* 1978; Engel *et al.* 1988). In one patient, a 28-year-old male, there was severe alveolar bone destruction, enhanced PMN phagocytosis and lysis to *E. coli* (Lamster *et al.* 1978). These findings were further evaluated in a group of patients with inflammatory bowel disease (Crohn's disease and ulcerative colitis) (Lamster *et al.* 1982). Thirty patients in this study were further subdivided into those with active and inactive bowel disease; their PMN function was compared with a group of otherwise healthy controls. The investigations included spontaneous and stimulated assessments of PMN metabolic activity and serum levels of circulating immune complexes. PMN metabolic activity was highest in the patients with active inflammatory bowel disease and lowest in the control group. Similarly, the patients with active inflammatory bowel disease had the highest levels of circulating immune complexes. This correlation between PMN metabolic activity and circulating immune complexes in patients with inflammatory bowel disease suggests that PMNs are not acting effectively at clearing circulating immune complexes from the serum. PMNs from patients with inflammatory bowel disease have elevated levels of alkaline phosphatase, which is indicative of the early release of these cells from the bone marrow (Keleman 1973; Koldjaer *et al.* 1977). Hence the altered function of PMNs in inflammatory bowel disease may be related to their maturity.

Further laboratory studies were made on a 60-year-old woman with Crohn's disease and severe generalized periodontitis (Engel *et al.* 1988). Haematological investigations revealed a paucity of B lymphocytes and an increase in the portion of T lymphocytes. Her B-cell function was 50 per cent less than in otherwise healthy controls. Furthermore, serum levels of leukotriene B_4 were 11 times higher than the mean for normal subjects. Engel suggests that the immunological and inflammatory changes arising from the Crohn's disease may have exacerbated or accelerated the periodontal breakdown, but were not the cause of it.

An investigation into the microflora of periodontal pockets of 10 patients with inflammatory bowel disease has shown a unique flora of small, Gram-negative rods, which were most consistent with the genus *Wolinella* (van Dyke *et al.* 1986). These patients also had a serum-mediated defect in neutrophil chemotaxis, but phagocytosis was normal. The investigators suggest that the colonization of the mouth by *Wolinella* in patients with inflammatory bowel disease may play a role in the pathogenesis of the disease, either as an infective agent or by modifying the host response. Periodontal findings in their patients suggest that the lesions show more inflammatory than destructive changes when compared with healthy controls.

Treatment

Few studies have reported on the periodontal management of patients with Crohn's disease. The case described by Engel *et al.* (1988) responded favourably to conventional periodontal treatment (oral hygiene, scaling, root planing, and flap surgery). Hence it would seem that the inflammatory changes in the periodontal tissues respond to local measures. However, there is no information on long-term prognosis and further vulnerability to periodontal breakdown.

Troublesome gingival enlargement can be removed surgically, although bleeding may be a problem because the overgrowth is granulomatous and inflamed.

Patients with Crohn's disease appear to have a high incidence of dental caries (Sundh and Hulten 1982). This may be related to unusual dietary habits ('food fads'), malabsorption, or a neglect of oral hygiene during an acute phase of the disease. It is therefore recommended that, in patients with Crohn's disease, oral hygiene is reinforced and regular fluoride treatment given.

3.5.2 PYOSTOMATITIS VEGETANS

This unusual condition is the oral manifestation of the rare skin condition pyodermatitis vegetans (McCarthy 1949). Pyostomatitis is often associated with inflammatory bowel disease and therefore may be regarded as an oral manifestation of Crohn's disease (see above) or ulcerative colitis (Cataldo *et al.* 1981). The skin disorder is a benign variant of pemphigus vegetans (see p. 52), and the characteristic lesion is of a vegetating, pustular nature. The skin disease is more common in men and occurs in middle age.

Mucosal lesions may affect any area of the mouth, although the common site is the labial attached gingiva. The gingival tissues have a pustular or cobblestone appearance, owing to intra- or subepithelial abscess formation. These abscesses usually begin as small, round or oval, raised areas (2–5 mm in diameter) on an inflamed, erythematous mucosa. The surface becomes necrotic and hence has a grey to yellowish appearance. Local areas of necrosis may coalesce. Surprisingly, pain and discomfort are not prominent features of this condition. Vegetating tissues are confined to the labial and buccal mucosa and lips, and rarely affect the gingival tissues.

Biopsy of the gingival tissues shows epithelial abscess formation and, in the early stages, the underlying connective tissue is infiltrated with eosinophils. These cells tend to disappear as the disease becomes established. Other cell types in the connective tissue include small lymphocytes and plasma cells (Cataldo *et al.* 1981).

The aetiology of pyostomatitis vegetans is uncertain. Although there is abscess formation, the condition does not appear to be of microbial origin. Furthermore, antimicrobial agents are of limited value in the management of this disorder. Drugs that are useful include sulphasalazine and systemic and topical corticosteroids (Cataldo *et al.* 1981; Wray 1984). The disease appears to follow a protracted course, and in most cases, the severity of the oral lesions relates to exacerbations of the inflammatory bowel disease (Forman 1965).

3.5.3 SARCOIDOSIS

This is another granulomatous disorder, which commonly involves the lymph nodes, lungs, liver, spleen, skin, eyes, phalangeal bones, and parotid glands. The disease has been regarded as an atypical form of tuberculosis, because of certain similar features; however, this idea has now been abandoned. Other variants of sarcoidosis include Lofgren's syndrome, which consists of erythema nodosum, bilateral hilar lymphadenopathy, cutaneous sarcoidosis, fever, and arthralgia (Lofgren and Lundbeck 1952), and Heerfordt's syndrome, which comprises of an inflammation of the uveal tracts and bilateral enlargement of the parotid glands.

Three stages of sarcoidosis are now recognized, based on the appearance of the chest radiograph. These are:

- Stage I: bilateral enlargement of the hilar nodes without pathological changes in the lung fields.

- Stage II: bilateral enlargement of the hilar nodes with pathological changes in the lung fields around the hila.

- Stage III: no enlargement of the lymph nodes, but extended and sometimes patchy or stripy changes in both lung fields. The patches can join together and bullae may form.

The incidence of sarcoidosis shows marked variation according to the population studied. The worldwide prevalence is 20/100 000; however, the disease is 10 times more common in negroid blacks than whites (Dunner and Williams 1961). Women are affected twice as often as men.

Clinical symptoms of sarcoidosis are dependent upon the site affected. There may be a persistent cough, malaise, or fever. The disease may present as an unexplained enlargement of the lymph nodes, spleen, or liver. Often sarcoidosis is discovered on routine chest radiography. Eye signs may be an important symptom of sarcoidosis, and include loss of lacrimation, iritis, and uveitis.

Diagnosis is confirmed by the chest radiograph, bronchoscopy, lymph node biopsy, and a positive Kveim test. This test is an intradermal injection of a reagent prepared from proven sarcoid lymphoid tissue. If the test is positive, a sarcoid granuloma develops at the site of innoculation after 6–8 weeks. The role of biopsy of the oral mucosa in the diagnosis of sarcoidosis is discussed later.

The aetiology of sarcoidosis is uncertain. The Third International Conference on Sarcoidosis suggested three possible hypotheses (Lofgren 1964):

1. Sarcoidosis is due to an unidentified specific agent, and the interaction between this agent and the host is the cause of the immunological peculiarities.

2. Sarcoidosis is related to the collagenoses or to the reticuloses, in which immunological changes are prominent.

3. Sarcoidosis occurs only in individuals who have a pre-existing immunological peculiarity, and in them develops a reaction to an agent, or one of several agents, which may or may not be known already as causing some well-known disease (e.g. tuberculosis).

The prognosis for sarcoidosis is good, with most cases showing spontaneous healing. Corticosteroids are the drugs of choice for this condition; they appear to accelerate the disappearance of lesions (Eule *et al.* 1980).

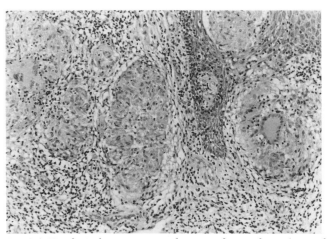

Fig. 3.4 Histological appearances of a sarcoid granuloma (original magnification × 150).

Oral and periodontal manifestations

Sarcoidosis is not an uncommon disease, but the incidence of oral involvement is rare. This may be related to the problem of identifying oral lesions, which therefore remain undiagnosed. In a review of the oral manifestations of sarcoidosis, the most common findings were asymptomatic swelling of the parotid glands and enlargement of the cervical lymph nodes (Gold and Sager 1976); involvement of the gingival tissues was cited in only two cases (Tillman 1964; Watts 1968).

Histopathological changes also occur in the minor salivary glands under an apparently healthy mucosa. It has been suggested that biopsy of normal oral mucosa from the palate or buccal surfaces is useful in the diagnosis of sarcoidosis (Cahn *et al.* 1964; Nessan and Jacoway 1979). Sarcoid granulomas (see later) were found in 38 and 58 per cent, respectively, of biopsy specimens in those studies. Hence the investigators advocate biopsy of oral mucosa, as oral involvement can be an early manifestation of the systemic disease. If a biopsy proves positive, then the patient should be referred to a chest physician.

The sarcoid granuloma is the characteristic histological feature (Fig. 3.4). The prominent feature of this lesion is a non-caseating, non-necrotizing, epithelioid tubercle. There is a focal collection of monocyte-derived epithelioid cells (giant cells), admixed with T lymphocytes, occasional plasma cells, and fibroblasts (Jones-Williams 1979). The granuloma may contain inclusion bodies referred to as the Schaumann or conchoid body, the asteroid body, and microcentrosomes (Tarpley *et al.* 1972).

Since the review by Gold and Sager in 1976, there have been several case reports of sarcoid gingivitis (Hogan 1983; Sloan *et al.* 1983; Tyldesley 1983; Altman and Robertson 1984; Zakrzewska and Nally 1985; Hayter and Robinson 1988). Clinically, the gingival tissues have a hyperplastic, granulomatous appearance. Superficial ulceration may be present, which could be due to toothbrush trauma. The tissues are invariably inflamed and bleed on probing. Histologically, they have a granulomatous appearance with a chronic inflammatory infiltrate and numerous giant cells.

Severe and rapid periodontal destruction has also been reported as an oral complication of sarcoidosis (van Swol 1973; Cohen *et al.* 1981; Makris and Stoller 1983). The onset of periodontal bone loss appears to coincide with the initiation of the systemic disease. In one case (Cohen *et al.* 1981), the alveolar bone showed areas of radiographic lysis; on biopsy, these were diagnosed as a non-specific osteomyelitis. No treatment was given to the patient, and 10 months after diagnosis, there was a clinical improvement with radiographic evidence of bone regeneration in previously lytic areas.

The severe periodontal destruction reported in the two other cases may be related to the systemic disease causing an alteration in the host response. A feature of sarcoidosis is a depression of T-cell function and a subsequent increase in B-cell activity. As discussed in Chapter 1, the B-cell lesion is related to bursts of periodontal disease activity. Laboratory investigations in the patient described by Makris and Stoller (1983) showed that the patient's serum inhibited the leukotoxic effect of *A. actinomycetemcomitans*. The same reaction is seen in patients with juvenile periodontitis (see Chapter 5). Although PMN activity was not assessed, it has been reported that impairment of PMN chemotaxis is associated with sarcoidosis. As discussed on p. 43, any disorder of PMN function will invariably predispose the patient to rapid periodontal breakdown. Thus, in patients with sarcoidosis, the following factors may render them susceptible to periodontal destruction:

(1) an increase in B-cell activity;

(2) secondary infection with *A. actinomycetemcomitans*;

(3) an impairment of PMN chemotaxis.

Treatment

There is little information on the management or treatment of the periodontal manifestations of sarcoidosis. Gingival hyperplasia can be removed surgically, but unless the systemic disease is treated or kept under control, then recurrence will occur (Sloan *et al.* 1983). The severe periodontal destruction that has been reported to be associated with sarcoidosis is a rare manifestation. This may take the form of a disease-mediated alteration in the host response or lytic lesions involving the alveolar bone.

As *A. actinomycetemcomitans* may be implicated in the periodontal destruction, then the antimicrobial agent tetracycline may be of benefit in these patients. However, such cases do emphasize the importance of monitoring patients with sarcoidosis, both clinically and radiographically.

3.5.4 OROFACIAL GRANULOMATOSIS

This is a chronic disorder characterized by the presence of non-caseating granulomatous lesions involving the tissues of the mouth and face (Wiesenfeld *et al.* 1985). Orofacial granulomatosis can be a localized entity, but may also represent the oral manifestations of sarcoidosis and Crohn's disease (see above). Closely related to orofacial granulomatosis is the Melkersson-Rosenthal syndrome, which consists of fissured tongue, facial oedema, and VIIth nerve paralysis.

The incidence of localized orofacial granulomatosis is very low, but may be slightly higher in Indians and Pakistanis than in other ethnic groups. There appears to be no sex predilection, and the disorder can occur at any age.

The clinical features include swelling of the lips, facial swelling, mucosal thickening, oral ulceration, hyperplastic gingiva, mucosal tags, and angular cheilitis. Lip swelling (Plate 8) is the most frequent complaint and the swelling may fluctuate. It does not pit on pressure and can cause splitting of the vermilion border.

The aetiology of the localized form of orofacial granulomatosis is uncertain. There is some evidence to suggest a familial tendency (Scott 1964; Carr 1966). Also, patients with this disorder have a higher incidence (60 per cent) of atopic conditions than in a control population (James *et al.* 1986). More recently, it has been shown that in orofacial granulomatosis there is an intolerance to toothpastes and certain foods (Patton *et al.* 1985). Foods implicated include chocolate, cinnamon, dairy products, wheat, eggs, and peanuts.

The management of orofacial granulomatosis is difficult. Obviously, patients should be screened for sarcoidosis and Crohn's disease and if positive referred to the appropriate specialist. The localized lesions may resolve of their own accord. Corticosteroids, antimicrobial agents, surgery, and radiotherapy have all been used in management (for review, see Ferguson and MacFadyen 1986). In some patients, food intolerance is important; therefore, switching to a low-allergen diet has produced marked improvement (Ferguson and MacFadyen 1986). Similarly, a non-allergenic toothpaste should be used.

Periodontal manifestations

A characteristic gingival appearance has been described in patients with orofacial granulomatosis. Indeed, the gingival lesions may be the only oral involvement (Ferguson and MacFadyen 1986). Clinically, the gingival tissues are thickened and inflamed, and this involves the entire width of attached gingiva. The surface may be shiny or have a granular appearance. The distribution of gingival involvement is irregular, with the upper anterior tissues most commonly affected. This may be related to mouth breathing or frequent exposure to the main bulk of toothpaste when brushing (i.e. people tend to brush their front teeth first). Histologically, the appearance of the gingival tissues is the same as in sarcoidosis and Crohn's disease.

3.5.5 WEGENER'S GRANULOMATOSIS

Introduction

Wegener's granulomatosis is a systemic disease or syndrome first described in 1936 (Wegener 1936). It is characterized by a necrotizing and granulomatous vasculitis of the respiratory tract and kidneys. A pathological triad has been described for this condition consisting of: (a) necrotizing granulomas in the nose, paranasal sinuses, and lungs, (b) vasculitis of small arteries and veins (especially in the lungs), and (c) glomerulitis characterized by necrosis of loops of the glomerular capillary tufts, capsular adhesions, and granulomatosis lesions (Goodman and Churg 1954). The clinical features that can accompany these pathological changes include an intractable rhinitis and sinusitis, cough and haemoptysis, and terminal uraemia (Fahey *et al.* 1954). Lesions that can resemble Wegener's granulomatosis are lethal midline granuloma (malignant granuloma) and/or unusual forms of periarteritis nodosa.

The aetiology of Wegener's granulomatosis is obscure. The disease may be an immunological disorder, as it responds to immunosuppressive therapy (Cassan *et al.* 1970; Israel and Patchefsky 1971). There is no evidence that microbial agents are involved in its pathogenesis.

The prognosis for Wegener's before chemotherapy was very poor. The condition is now treated with a combination of prednisolone and cyclophosphamide.

Oral and gingival manifestations

In an early review of this condition, which reported on 56 cases (Walton 1958), oropharyngeal lesions occurred in 21 patients. Seven of these were confined to the tongue and a further seven involved the gingival tissues. Other oral lesions include palatal ulceration and failure of tooth sockets to heal.

A characteristic hyperplastic gingivitis (plate 9) is the main periodontal feature of Wegener's granulomatosis. Apart from the seven cases reported by Walton, 11 further cases presenting as a specific hyperplastic gingivitis have now been reported. Their features are summarized in Table 3.6 (Appendix to this chapter).

Clinically, the hyperplastic gingival changes can have an ulcerative or granular appearance. Many petechiae are often present and the term 'strawberry gingivitis' aptly describes this condition. Gingival changes can be localized to one or two papillae or be generalized. In the cases described in Table 3.6, the gingival changes were the initial manifestations of the disease. However, it has not been determined if gingival changes reflect changes in the lungs and kidneys.

Histological examination of the gingiva often shows a non-specific, chronic histiocytic inflammation. The overlying epithelium invariably shows pseudoepitheliomatous hyperplasia and eosinophilia. Microabscesses, multinucleated giant cells, focal necrosis, fibrinoid degeneration, and vasculitis are variable findings described in some cases. Gingival vascular changes in Wegener's granulomatosis have been examined under the electron microscope (Raustia *et al.* 1985). Changes reported include swelling and necrosis of the endothelial cells, along with eosinophilic granulocytes and plasma cells around the capillary wall. Where more advanced destruction occurred, there was total necrosis of the endothelial lining and the lumen was filled with degranulating platelets and fragments of the contents of PMNs and endothelial cells.

Treatment

The institution of systemic drug therapy (prednisolone and cyclophosphamide) brings about an improvement in the gingival condition (Cohen and Meltzer 1981 Israelson *et al.* 1981). One case report (Raustia *et al.* 1985) showed that attention to plaque control had little effect on the gingival appearance. There is no evidence that Wegener's granulomatosis predisposes to an increased rate of periodontal destruction.

3.6 SCLERODERMA

3.6.1 INTRODUCTION

Scleroderma is a connective tissue disorder, which is also known as systemic sclerosis, progressive systemic sclerosis, and systemic scleroderma. The characteristic feature of the disease is an inflammatory, vascular, and fibrotic change in the skin and other structures. Three forms of scleroderma have been described:

1. Circumscribed scleroderma or morphea, where the changes outlined above are limited to the skin;
2. Generalized or progressive scleroderma, where in addition to skin involvement, there are changes in the lungs, heart, kidneys, gastrointestinal tract, and osteolytic changes in the skeleton.
3. Acrosclerosis, a combination of scleroderma of the extremities and Raynaud's disease. Scleroderma is also related to two syndromes, the Crest syndrome which is identified by the presence of calcinosis (C), Raynaud's disease (R), oesophageal structures (E), sclerodactyly (S), and skin telangiectasia (T) (Velayos *et al.* 1979), and the Thibierge–Weissenbach syndrome, which describes extensive subcutaneous tissue calcinosis. The incidence of scleroderma is three times higher in women than men.

The aetiology of scleroderma is uncertain. Although the disease results in an overproduction of collagen, the initial event may involve the endothelial cells of blood vessels. Disruption of these cells would lead to an increase in vascular permeability, oedema formation, fibroblast stimulation, and eventually fibrosis. A serum cytotoxic factor and/or an immunological abnormality may be important in the pathogenesis of this disease (Gilliland and Mannik 1984).

There are many signs and symptoms associated with the various types of scleroderma. The incidence and severity of these varies from patient to patient and the site predominantly involved. The common problems include skin changes (dermal fibrosis), sclerodactyly and bilateral basilar pulmonary fibrosis. The head and neck region is frequently the site for the manifestations of scleroderma. Features include microstomia, thinning of the lips, restricted mouth opening (due to skin changes around the mouth and in the cheeks), telangiectasia, and xerostomia (Traiger 1961; Hoggins and Hamilton 1969; Green 1972; Wood and Lee 1988). A relationship between scleroderma and Sjogren's disease has been reported which may account for the xerostomia (Alarcon-Segovia *et al.* 1974; Drosos *et al.* 1988). Osseous resorption of the mandibular rami can occur in scleroderma (Seifert *et al.* 1975) and this can be of sufficient severity to cause fracture (Weber *et al.* 1970). Resorption of the mandibular rami may be associated with atrophy of the masseter muscle (White *et al.* 1977). If the oral mucosa is involved, it is pale, thin, and tends to ulcerate (Smith 1958).

The prognosis for patients with scleroderma is poor, especially if there is involvement of the lungs, heart, and kidneys. D-penicillamine has been shown to be effective in the management of the skin problems, and non-steroidal anti-inflammatory drugs are used to treat musculo-skeletal complaints.

Periodontal manifestations

Scleroderma produces several changes in the periodontal tissues; some of these are directly related to the disease process whilst others are secondary. The characteristic periodontal finding of scleroderma is widening of the periodontal ligament. This condition was first reported in 1944 by Stafne and Austin, and they recorded 6 features as follows:

1. Widening of the periodontal ligament space occurs at the expense of alveolar bone. The lamina dura is obliterated.

2. The periodontal space of a posterior tooth is more likely to be involved than the corresponding space of an anterior tooth. The differences in widths may be due to the greater occlusal loading placed on the posterior teeth.

3. Of an involved tooth, the increase in width of the periodontal membrane is fairly uniform around the entire root.

4. The affected teeth are not in supraclusion.

5. Affected teeth are surprisingly firm in their pockets considering the increase in width of the ligament space.

6. Almost without exception, the gingival attachment of the affected teeth is unbroken and the gingival crevice is normal.

Since Stafne and Austin's original observations, there have been several studies reporting on the periodontal findings of patients with scleroderma (White *et al.* 1977; Rowell and Hopper 1977; Alexandridis and White 1984; Wood and Lee 1988). These studies report on incidence of widening of the periodontal ligament in the range of 10–65 per cent. However, it has been suggested that widening of the periodontal ligament space, provided it is measured meticulously, is always a feature of scleroderma (Mammary *et al.* 1981).

Histological investigations of the periodontal ligament from scleroderma patients has shown that there is loss of the normal arrangement of collagen fibres, and the blood vessel walls are thickened (Gores 1957). A more detailed analysis reports that affected periodontal ligaments show the following features.

1. Erratic bone resorption in the region of the alveolar bone approximating the membrane.

2. Thickening due to a proportionate increase of collagen and oxytalan fibres which contain areas of degradation.

3. Sclerosis and hyalinization of collagen, particularly adjacent to the teeth. There is the development of elastic fibres in this region.

4. The formation off coal areas of bone or irregular calcified deposits (Fulner and White 1962).

The incidence of periodontal disease is reported to be higher in patients with scleroderma than otherwise healthy controls (Mammary *et al.* 1981; Wood and Lee 1988). Plaque and calculus scores were similar in both groups which suggest that systemic factors are influencing the response of the periodontal tissues to plaque. Vascular changes (i.e. deposition of an adventital cuff of collagen plus mucoid thickening of the intima) are a feature of scleroderma (Norton and Nardo 1970). Such changes could lead to local tissue ischaemia and hence increase the susceptibility of the periodontal tissues to disease.

Specific changes in the gingival tissues in relation to scleroderma have been reported (Eversole *et al.* 1983). Crenations were found on the buccal mucosa and tongue, and there were severe mucogingival problems with localized recession. The latter was due to a fibrotic structure along the mandibular mucobuccal fold which reduced the width of attached gingiva.

Microstomia, limited mouth opening, and hand changes associated with scleroderma are going to impede routine mechanical plaque control (Uthman *et al.* 1978; Wardrop *et al.* 1987). Various means of overcoming this problem are discussed later.

Management

The management of the periodontal problems associated with scleroderma does not differ from those in the rest of the population. As previously outlined, mechanical plaque control is the main problem in these patients. Mouth stretching exercises can increase restricted opening and reduce the microstomia (Naylor 1982). Severe sclerodactyly will make it difficult to hold a conventional toothbrush. Handles may need augmenting to fit the patients hand or they may find an electric toothbrush easier to use. Chemical plaque control will certainly benefit these patients. Regular rinsing with 0.2 per cent chlorhexidine is probably the treatment of choice.

Localized gingival recession may require mucogingival surgical procedure to maintain the width of the attached gingiva (Eversole *et al.* 1984).

3.7 HAEMATOLOGICAL DISORDERS

3.7.1 INTRODUCTION

Disorders of the blood and blood-forming tissues can have a profound effect on the periodontal tissues and their response to bacterial plaque. The haematological disorders that can affect the periodontium can be considered under the headings of white blood-cell (WBC) disorders, red blood-cell disorders, and disturbances of haemostasis. The WBC disorders have the most pronounced effect on the periodontal tissues. Various types of anaemia can affect the periodontium, although iron-deficiency anaemia does not appear to predispose to an increased susceptibility to periodontal destruction (Wray and Dagg 1980).

Disorders of haemostasis can be classified according to the underlying defect. There can be a defect in vascular constriction, platelet adhesion and aggregation, coagulation, and fibrinolysis. Severe disturbances in haemostasis can affect the gingival tissues. Cases have been reported of patients with severe thrombocytopenic purpura experiencing gingival haemorrhage after toothbrushing and severe haemorrhage after scaling (Peltier and Oliver 1961). Gingival bleeding in such cases will be exacerbated by inflammation.

From the periodontal aspect, the main problem presented by patients with disorders of haemostasis is one of management during treatment. These patients are at risk from haemorrhage, even after simple scaling. If surgery is to be considered, then it is essential that this is undertaken only after consultation with the patient's physician. Additional medical treatment will be required and the type will depend upon the nature of the underlying defect. Treatments might include platelet transfusion, alteration in anticoagulant therapy, Factor VIII cover, and treatment with vitamin K or tranexamic acid.

3.7.2 THE WBC DISORDERS

The role of the various WBCs in the pathogenesis of periodontal disease has been discussed in Chapter 1. The WBC disorders that affect the periodontium can be categorized as either a disorder of numbers (i.e. an increase or decrease) or a defect in function. In the latter, the defect may be due to a failure of the WBC to respond to chemotaxis or a failure to phagocytose.

An alteration in the number of circulating WBCs has a profound effect on the periodontal tissues. The term granulocytopenia refers to an absolute reduction in the number of granulocytes (neutrophils, eosinophils, basophils, and monocytes in the peripheral blood). However, the term is usually synonymous with a reduced number of neutrophils (neutropenia). Agranulocytosis strictly means a reduction in all forms of granulocytes, but the term is often restricted to a syndrome characterized by an extremely severe neutropenia, accompanied by fever, malaise, ulceration, and necrosis of tissue around the mouth, throat, anus, and vulva.

The leukaemias are a group of conditions in which there is progressive, uncontrolled proliferation of white blood cells. They can be further classified as chronic or acute and also according to the cell type involved (i.e. lymphocytic, granulocytic or myeloid, and monocytic).

Neutropenias

These conditions are characterized by a decrease or absence of circulating PMNs. They are a heterogeneous group and several forms have been described in both adults and childhood. Neutropenias may be idiopathic, familial, secondary to viral, bacterial, or protozoal infection, secondary to a systemic disease (e.g. lupus erythematosus), or drug-induced. Because of the importance of PMNs in maintaining periodontal health, all types of neutropenia can have an effect on the periodontal tissues. Those types that have been reported to be associated with periodontal problems include cyclic neutropenia, chronic benign and severe familial neutropenia, and chronic idiopathic neutropenia.

Cyclic neutropenia

This is a rare condition that, as its name suggests, is characterized by a cyclical depression of the PMN count in peripheral blood. The cyclic intervals are usually between 19 and 21 days, but may vary from 15 to 35 days. Occasionally, periods of continuous neutropenia may last for one or two months (Page and Good 1957). There may be a familial feature of this condition, and it would appear that this form is transmitted as an autosomal-dominant trait. The onset of cyclical neutropenia is frequently during infancy or early childhood.

Clinical problems include pyrexia during the episode of neutropenia, oral ulceration (plate 10), and skin infections. The severity of these symptoms often directly relates to the degree of neutropenia. During the neutropenic phase, the PMNs may disappear completely from the blood and, in half of these patients, there is an accompanying monocytosis (Morley *et al.* 1967). Between cycles, the PMN count rises, but seldom does it exceed 50 per cent of the differential WBC count.

Bone marrow biopsies obtained during the periods of neutropenia show either myeloid hypoplasia or an apparent arrest in the maturation of cells at the myeloid stage.

The aetiology of cyclic neutropenia is uncertain. Experimental evidence suggests that the disorder is due to failure in the bone marrow, possibly as a result of periodic stem-cell failure (Guerry *et al.* 1972). The failure may be related to an exaggerated haematopoietic feedback control (Zucker-Franklin *et al.* 1977).

Many treatments have been used in the management of cyclic neutropenia, all with a varying degree of success. These include splenectomy, corticosteroids, oestrogen, progesterone, and testosterone.

Periodontal manifestations.
The oral mucosa and periodontal tissues are frequently affected by the cyclical decline in PMNs that is the main feature of this disease. Many case reports and reviews cite oral ulceration, inflamed gingiva, rapid periodontal breakdown, and alveolar bone loss as features of this disorder (Gorlin and Chaudhry 1960; Cohen and Morris 1961; Wade and Stafford 1963; Rylander and Ericsson 1981; Scully *et al.* 1982; Long *et al.* 1983; Prichard *et al.* 1984; Spencer and Fleming 1985). In most of the cases, the disorder was diagnosed before the age of 10 years. Bone loss is most obvious around the lower incisors and first permanent molars. The recurrent oral ulceration often makes mechanical plaque control difficult and therefore exacerbates the periodontal problem.

Management.
The management of the periodontal problems associated with cyclic neutropenia is no different from the management of a patient with normal periodontal disease. The emphasis must be placed on plaque control and other supportive measures. These would include the use of an antiseptic mouthwash and antimicrobial therapy to treat acute episodes. Periodontal surgery, if necessary, can be carried out on a patient with cyclic neutropenia, but it is advisable to arrange the operation when their WBC count is

high (Rylander and Ericsson 1981). Antibiotic cover should be given before surgery to reduce the risks of infection arising from the bacteriaemia (Spencer and Fleming 1985).

Long-term follow-up of the periodontal status of three patients with cyclic neutropenia has been reported in three studies (Wade and Stafford 1963; Binon and Dykema 1974; Rylander and Ericsson 1981). Further loss of teeth had occurred in these cases, but the dentition remained functional. The investigators emphasize the importance of a rigorous home-care programme and the placement of the margins of restorations above the gingival tissues. Regular use of fluoride gels and mouthrinses will reduce the risk of caries.

Chronic benign neutropenia of childhood

This type of neutropenia was first described in 1941 (Fanconi 1941). The onset is usually between 6–20 months of age and, in most patients, the condition is self-limiting. Haematological investigations usually show a WBC count of 2000–10 000/ml, with an absolute lymphocytosis. There is frequently an absolute monocytosis and an occasional eosinophilia. The bone marrow is essentially normal in chronic benign neutropenia, except for a slight degree of immaturity in the granulocyte series. It has been suggested that this type of neutropenia may be due to an increased peripheral destruction of WBCs with depletion of the marrow storage pool (Zuelzer and Bajochli 1964).

Pyogenic infections of the skin and mucous membranes are features of this condition. However, in some instances, the monocytes can compensate for the lack of neutrophils, thus providing a relative resistance to infections (Biggar *et al.* 1974). Splenectomy and corticosteroids are only of limited therapeutic value.

Periodontal manifestations.

There are several case reports of the periodontal manifestations of chronic benign neutropenia (Andrews *et al.* 1965; Hjortdal 1971; Lampert and Fesseler 1975; Reichart and Dornow 1978; Baehni *et al.* 1983). Most of these cases have usually occurred in young boys aged 4–12 years.

The main periodontal feature of this condition is a bright-red, hyperplastic, oedematous gingivitis confined to the width of attached gingiva. The gingival tissues bleed readily on probing and show occasional desquamation. Varying degrees of gingival recession and pocketing accompany the inflammation. There appears to be premature loss of the deciduous dentition owing to early bone loss. Some of the older children have the characteristic gingival appearance, and evidence of generalized bone loss and mobility of the permanent dentition. The severity of bone loss appears related to the age of tooth eruption.

Management.

It would appear from a review of the various case reports that the management of the periodontal components of chronic benign neutropenia is unsatisfactory. Progressive periodontitis with early loss of the deciduous and permanent dentition seems difficult to prevent (Reichart and Dornow 1978). Local treatment, i.e. plaque and calculus removal, mouthwashes (hydrogen peroxide and hexetidine) appears

to cause only a negligible improvement in the gingival condition (Lampert and Fesseler 1975). Periodontal and odontogenic infections should be treated with the appropriate antimicrobial agent (penicillin or erythromycin). Systemic, prophylactic administration of antibiotics for the treatment of gingivitis and periodontitis is not indicated.

With more vigorous periodontal therapy (i.e. surgery) there is the risk of creating an acute infection because of the lack of a normal defence mechanism. Corticosteroids are used to treat this type of neutropenia, albeit with limited success. These drugs have an adverse effect in children, causing growth disturbances and oesteoporosis (Seymour and Walton 1988). Furthermore, the presence of corticosteroids in association with an infectious disease tends to decrease the body's defence against infection.

Benign familial neutropenia

This condition is transmitted as an autosomal-dominant trait. The disease is characterized by a moderate neutropenia, and often an accompanying monocytosis. Bone marrow cultures have demonstrated excellent colony growth, which suggests that the neutropenia is due to an anomaly in the marrow release mechanism (Mintz and Sachs 1973).

The periodontal manifestations of benign familial neutropenia have been described in a single case report of a 14-year-old boy (Deasy *et al.* 1980). In this case, the gingival tissues were hyperplastic, oedematous, and had a bright-red appearance. There was marked bone loss around the first permanent molars. The gingival tissues bled profusely on probing, and biopsy showed all the features of chronic inflammation with a large plasma-cell infiltrate. The family history showed that the father and younger sister were also neutropenic, although the nature of the neutropenia and their periodontal status was not commented upon. The main emphasis of treatment was on plaque control and the use of antimicrobial mouthwashes. Long-term follow-up of the patient's periodontal condition was not reported.

Severe familial neutropenia

Again, this is an inherited disorder, but it is more severe than the benign form. The condition was first described in 1959 (Hitzig 1959), and is probably transmitted as an autosomal-dominant trait. Children are susceptible to repeated infections. There is often a reciprocal relationship between the number of neutrophils and monocytes, but some monocytosis occurs in virtually all patients.

Chronic idiopathic neutropenia

This condition was first described in 1968 (Kyle and Linman 1968) in a series of 15 adult patients, 14 of whom were females. The features of this condition include a persistent neutropenia from birth. The neutropenia is not cyclical and there is no familial history. Chronic idiopathic neutropenia differs from chronic benign neutropenia in that the former condition does not appear self-limiting. Clinical symptoms include persistent recurrent infections throughout the patient's lifetime. The pathogenesis of chronic idiopathic neutropenia is uncertain. Bone marrow biopsy shows a maturation abnormality of the granulocytes, which may be related to an autoimmune disorder.

Periodontal manifestations.

The periodontal manifestations of chronic idiopathic neutropenia have been the subject of two case reports (Kyle and Linman 1970; Kalkwarf and Gutz 1981). The first discussed two patients, aged 6 and 2 years, who were diagnosed as having chronic idiopathic neutropenia. Their clinical course was followed for 12 years. The most striking feature reported was the severe, persistent gingivitis. The gingiva were cherry-red, oedematous, and hypertrophic, with occasional desquamation. Conventional treatment had no apparent effect on the appearance. No information about the condition of the supporting alveolar bone was provided.

The second report was of a more aggressive periodontal manifestation of this type of neutropenia in a $3\frac{1}{2}$-year-old girl. The case was followed through for four years. Plaque control was poor and there was gingival recession, a granulomatous collar around the cervical margins of the teeth, and alveolar bone loss. The investigators emphasized that the management of these cases required a strict oral hygiene programme, scaling, and regular prophylaxis. Antiseptic irrigation and antibiotic prophylaxis is desirable before tissue manipulations that can result in a bacteriaemia.

Leukaemia

Introduction

Leukaemia is a malignant disease caused by the proliferation of the WBC-forming tissues, especially those in the bone marrow. It usually results in an increase in the number of leukocytes in the peripheral circulation, together with an infiltration of leukaemic cells into other tissues, e.g. lymph nodes. Leukaemic infiltration commonly occurs into the cervical and submandibular lymph nodes (Michaud *et al.* 1977; Stafford *et al.* 1980).

The condition may be acute or chronic and can affect any of the WBC—granulocytes (myeloid), lymphocytes, or monocytes. In the acute form, the cell type is commonly a primitive stem cell or blast cell. Some patients with many of the features of acute myeloblastic leukaemia have some cells with features similar to those of monocytes. This condition is referred to as acute myelomonoblastic leukaemia.

Acute types of leukaemia are more frequent in people under 20 years of age, but there is a further increase in incidence between 55 and 75 years. Acute lymphoblastic leukaemia mainly occurs in children under 10 years. The chronic leukaemias occur most commonly in the over-40 year age group. The incidence of chronic lymphatic leukaemia is twice that of the granulocytic form.

In many instances, the initial clinical signs and symptoms of acute leukaemia are similar to those of viral infections, especially infectious mononucleosis. These symptoms include lethargy, malaise, sore throat, and fever. More specific clinical features include oral ulceration, skin infections or skin lesions that fail to heal, purpura, cervical lymphadenopathy, splenomegaly, and hepatomegaly. Skin infiltration in the form of widespread pinkish plaques is a feature of acute monocytic leukaemia.

In chronic leukaemias, clinical features include tiredness, weight loss, fatigue, splenomegaly, abdominal discomfort, pyrexia, and skin infiltrations.

The aetiology of leukaemia is uncertain; however, certain factors have been implicated. These include radiation injury, chemical injury (i.e. benzene), genetic factors (i.e. Down's syndrome), immune deficiency, and viral infections.

Various types of treatment have evolved for the management of the different types of leukaemia. Generally, the main categories of treatment are chemotherapy, supportive radiotherapy, and bone marrow transplantation.

Periodontal manifestations

The periodontal tissues are markedly affected by leukaemia and also by the various therapies used in its management, i.e. chemotherapy and/or radiotherapy. The effect of these entities on the periodontium will be discussed later. The periodontal problems associated with leukaemia *per se* can be categorized as follows: gingival enlargement, gingival bleeding (Plate 11), and periodontal infections. The incidence and severity of these problems varies according to the type and nature of the leukaemia. They are more common in acute than chronic leukaemia (Stafford *et al.* 1980).

In addition to the periodontal problems, patients with leukaemia also suffer from other oral disorders including erosions and ulceration of the mucosa, punctate petechiae and ecchymoses, and fungal, bacterial, and viral infections (Michaud *et al.* 1977; Ferguson *et al.* 1978;). Bone pain is a characteristic complaint in acute leukaemia. Leukaemic cell infiltration into the dental pulp, which can cause pain, has been described (Sinrod 1957). Indeed, it has been suggested that these oral lesions, together with the periodontal manifestations, may be a useful diagnostic indicator of the disease (Lynch and Ship 1967; Stafford *et al.* 1980).

Gingival enlargement.

This is usually a feature of acute monocytic leukaemia, with an incidence of 20–34 per cent. The incidence of gingival enlargement is 10 per cent in acute myelomonocytic leukaemia, 4–8 per cent in acute myloid leukaemia, and 2 per cent in acute lymphocytic leukaemia (Presant *et al.* 1973).

The enlargement is primarily due to a massive leukaemic cell infiltration into the gingival connective tissue. This appears to coincide with the increase in the WBC count (Hou and Tsai 1988). Gingival tissues are susceptible to leukaemic cell infiltration, partly because of their microanatomy and also the inherent extravascular infiltrative properties of the leukaemic cell (Barrett 1986). The apparent acceleration in the mitotic rate and the absolute numbers of leukaemic cells are other key factors in initiating this infiltration (Dreizen *et al.* 1983).

The enlarged gingiva will hinder mechanical plaque removal, hence there will be an inflammatory component enhancing this enlargement. It has also been reported that the dense cellular infiltrate may cause gingival pain (Sydney and Serio 1981).

Gingival bleeding.

Blood oozing from the gingiva or more frank bleeding is a common oral manifestation of acute leukaemia (Plate 11). The bleeding is secondary to the thrombocytopenia that accompanies the leukaemia. It is especially marked when the platelet count drops below 10 000/ml, and is compounded by poor oral hygiene (Michaud *et al.* 1977; Stafford *et al.* 1980).

Periodontal infections.

Infections of the periodontal tissues secondary to leukaemia can be of two types, either an exacerbation of an existing periodontal disease, or through an increased susceptibility of the periodontium to fungal, viral, or bacterial infections. The latter group of infections are more likely to occur after chemotherapy or radiotherapy.

An existing periodontitis may be exacerbated by the onset of leukaemia or by chemotherapy. The effect of chemotherapy on the periodontal tissues has been investigated in 22 adult leukaemic patients over a two-year period (Overholser *et al.* 1982). Initially, their periodontal status was similar to that in the normal population. During the investigation, 47 acute infections developed in the 22 patients; 13 of these were of periodontal origin. Acute infections were accompanied by pain and invariably occurred during episodes of pronounced granulocytopenia.

Alveolar bone loss and an increase in tooth mobility are also periodontal features of leukaemia. Severe, rapid, periodontal destruction has been described in a patient with acute lymphocytic leukaemia during the period of bone marrow regeneration (Stansbury *et al.* 1988). This destruction may have been due either to impaired neutrophil function or to collagen synthesis secondary to the chemotherapeutic agents used to control the leukaemia.

A variety of oral infections can affect the periodontal tissues in leukaemia. These usually arise during periods of granulocytopenia after chemotherapy or radiotherapy. Acute herpetic gingivostomatitis is a common oral infection in the immunosuppressed leukaemic patient. The gingival tissues may be affected alone or as part of a widespread oral infection (Barrett 1984). Similarly, fungal infections are common in the immunosuppressed leukaemic patient and such infections can affect the gingival tissues (Barrett 1984). The common oral fungal infections in these patients are *C. albicans*, but infections due to *Cryptococcus neoformans* and *Histoplasma capsulatum* have been reported (Newman and Rosenbaum 1962; Miller *et al.* 1982).

The incidence of ANUG in leukaemic patients is reported to be high, especially during treatment (Shepard 1978). However, it is uncommon for this infection to be present as an initial complaint (Barrett 1984).

Management of the periodontal problems in leukaemic patients

The main problem is one of plaque control in the presence of hyperaemic, hyperplastic, and sometimes painful gingiva. Furthermore, during phases of chemotherapy or radiotherapy, the patient's bone marrow is suppressed and the peripheral WBC count may drop as low as 500 cells/ml. During these phases, patients are unable to mount an effective defence against any periodontal infection.

Mechanical plaque control may be difficult to achieve when there is gingival hyperplasia, bleeding, and pain. It has even been suggested that when the patient is immunosuppressed (i.e. during the granulocytopenic phase secondary to chemotherapy or radiotherapy), mechanical plaque control may increase the incidence of bacteraemias or even septicaemia (Peterson and Overholser 1979). However, the investigators did emphasize that the presence of oral disease may greatly contribute to illness and death in the leukaemic patient and should be treated vigorously.

It would seem that the initial periodontal management of patients with leukaemia should be mechanical plaque control, where possible backed up by the use of antiplaque agents (e.g. chlorhexidine, 0.2 per cent). Acute periodontal infections should be treated with the appropriate antimicrobial agent (penicillin, metronidazole, or tetracycline). A localized periodontal infection may well respond to drainage and the application of a topical antimicrobial agent into the pocket (e.g. tetracycline fibres).

Specific periodontal infections, which will invariably be part of an overall oral infection, should again be treated with the appropriate antimicrobial agent. Acute herpetic gingivostomatitis should be treated with systemic acyclovir at a dose of 200–400 mg, five times a day for five days. For children under 2 years of age, this dose should be halved. Fungal infections should be treated with amphotericin B lozenges or nystatin pastilles. Both drugs should be allowed to dissolve in the mouth, four times a day for up to 14 days. ANUG responds to systemic metronidazole; a dose of 200 mg, three times a day for three days, is usually sufficient.

Gingival haemorrhage after local debridement can usually be controlled by simple pressure. If the bleeding is severe, then the site should be injected (local infiltration) with lignocaine containing 1:80 000 adrenaline. The vasoconstrictive action of the adrenaline usually controls bleeding. Alternatively, topical adrenaline 1:1000 may be applied on a pledget of cotton wool. Bleeding from a periodontal pocket may require packing with small squares of ribbon gauze saturated with bismuth–iodoform paraffin paste (BIPP) or Whitehead's varnish. A Coe-Pack dressing to cover the area may aid haemostasis and prevent the area from being disturbed by eating.

Gingivectomy or any other form of periodontal surgery should only be contemplated during periods of remission. Even so, such procedures on leukaemic patients should only be done as a last resort. It is essential that the patient's physician be consulted before surgery; antibiotic cover will be necessary.

Preleukaemia

As the name implies, preleukaemia is the clinical designation for the haematological abnormalities that precede the development of overt leukaemia. However, the changes are not of sufficient magnitude or specificity to permit a diagnosis by the usual criteria. The proportion of cases of preleukaemia that develop into overt leukaemia varies from study to study, but is in the range of 5–32 per cent. Symptoms of this condition include weakness, malaise, weight loss, haemorrhage, and an increased susceptibility to infections (Saarni and Linman 1973).

Investigations can show a mixture of either an anaemia, thrombocytopenia, and/or neutropenia. The peripheral blood smear reveals aniso- and poikilocytosis. Bone marrow biopsy usually shows a normal or increased cellularity. The red blood-cell precursors are described as megaloblastoid, whilst the precursors of WBCs show a slight predominance of early forms.

The duration of preleukaemia before it develops into acute leukaemia varies between 6 months and 2 years. Most cases of preleukaemia develop into acute myelocytic or monocytic leukaemia.

The periodontal problems associated with preleukaemia have been described in a single case report (Deasy *et al.* 1976) involving a 13-year-old black girl. Excessive gingival bleeding, gingival inflammation, and extensive bone loss were the clinical features. The patient was treated with a strict oral hygiene regimen. No long-term follow-up has been reported.

Graft versus host reaction (GVHR)

Bone marrow transplantation is being extensively used in the treatment of various types of acute leukaemia. This transplantation procedure can produce a whole range of immunological phenomena, which are now categorized as the GVHR. About 70 per cent of patients who undergo bone marrow transplantation develop some form of GVHR. The disorder is probably caused by the T lymphocytes from the donor tissue. These lymphocytes give rise to a generation of effector cells that react with the host's tissues (Elkins 1971). The tissues mainly affected by GVHR are haematopoietic, epithelial, and the reticulo-endothelial system.

GVHR can exist as either an acute or chronic form. Acute GVHR occurs within 100 days of transplantation, whilst the chronic form has a more subtle presentation. The labial salivary glands can be affected by GVHR, and changes in these structures have been used in the diagnosis and the monitoring of this condition (Sale *et al.* 1981).

The oral findings in GVHR have been illustrated in two cases (Rodu and Gockerman 1983). The main feature appears to be a lichenoid keratosis of the buccal mucosa, which can involve the attached gingiva and tongue. Histologically, there was mildly hyperplastic, hyperkeratotic squamous cell epithelium with focal, vacuolar degeneration of the basal cell layer. The lamina propria contained scatterings of small lymphocytes that infiltrated the epithelium. Focal necrosis of epithelial cells was evident and associated with the areas of lymphocyte infiltration.

Both patients were treated with prednisolone and azathioprine for their GVHR and the medications reduced the oral lichenoid keratosis.

Disorders of WBC function

This section is primarily concerned with disorders of PMN function. Disorders of lymphocyte function will be considered in the section on immunological disorders (see p.49). The PMN has two basic functions, first to respond to chemotatic stimulation and secondly to phagocytose. Functional disturbance in PMN function can be a primary disease or secondary to a systemic disease. In the latter, disturbances in function occur in diabetes mellitus (see p.19) and in Down's syndrome (see p.22). Primary functional disturbances in PMNs, which have been reported to affect the periodontal tissues, occur in the Chediak–Higashi syndrome and the lazy leukocyte syndrome.

The Chediak–Higashi syndrome

This is a rare familial and often fatal disease, which is transmitted as an autosomal-recessive trait. The syndrome was described by Chediak (1952) and Higashi (1954). The clinical features of the syndrome include partial oculocutaneous albinism with photophobia and nystagmus, frequent pyogenic infections, and intermittent febrile episodes. An accelerated (lymphoma-like) phase develops in the majority of cases of the syndrome, with an accompanying neutropenia, anaemia, and thrombocytopenia. Death usually results from infection, haemorrhage, or dense lymphohistiocytic infiltration. Various chemotherapeutic drugs may be of value in the management of this phase (Blume and Wolff 1972).

The haematological hallmark of Chediak–Higashi syndrome is the presence of giant, abnormal granules in the peripheral circulating leukocytes, their marrow precursors, and many other cells in the body. These giant granules appear to be abnormal lysosomes, but their relationship to the disease process is uncertain. PMNs from patients with this syndrome show defective migration *in vivo*, defective *in vitro* chemotaxis, failure of postphagocytic degranulation, and diminished intracellular bactericidal capacity (Dale *et al.* 1972). Some or all of these defects in leukocyte function may account for the increased susceptibility to infection and the periodontal findings in this condition.

Periodontal features.

Severe gingival inflammation appears to be a common finding in Chediak–Higashi syndrome (Gillig and Caldwell 1970; Hamilton and Giansanti 1974). The nature of the inflammatory changes has not been recorded—it may be plaque-induced, secondary to infection, or related to the underlying PMN defect. Excessive and early periodontal destruction resulting in premature loss of the permanent dentition seems to be the usual outcome of the syndrome (Hamilton and Giansanti 1974). There appears to be no information on the long-term periodontal management of patients with this syndrome.

The Chediak–Higashi syndrome also occurs in cattle, mink, and mice. A study has been made of the clinical and histopathological features of inflammatory periodontal disease in normal mink and mice and those carrying the syndrome trait (Lavine *et al.* 1976). Severe periodontal destruction and advanced periodontal disease were found in the minks with the trait. The investigators suggest that the periodontal destruction is likely to be related to the PMN defect. Two mechanisms are possible: first, that the defect in the PMNs directly alters the matrix of epithelium and connective tissue by release of lysosomal enzymes and other neutral proteases such as collagenase; secondly, that the impaired PMN function fails to protect the host tissues from bacterial plaque or products produced by bacteria. Animals that have the Chediak–Higashi trait provide information on the pathogenesis of periodontal disease.

Lazy leukocyte syndrome

This syndrome of neutrophil function was first reported in 1971 (Miller *et al.* 1971). As the name suggests, the feature of the syndrome is a defect in leukocyte chemotaxis and random mobility. This may be due to a defect in the leukocyte cell membrane. The number of neutrophils in the peripheral blood and bone marrow appear normal. Two children with lazy leukocyte syndrome have been described (Miller *et al.* 1971) and both had marked gingivitis. No further information on the periodontal status and prognosis was provided.

Chronic granulomatous disease

This is a rare, genetically transmitted disorder characterized by the inability of phagocytic cells to destroy certain infecting micro-organisms. The condition was first described in 1957 (Berendes *et al.* 1957) and is transmitted as an autosomal-recessive trait in females and as an X-linked recessive trait in males. Clinically, chronic granulomatous disease is associated with a granulomatous response to inflammation that involves lymph nodes, skin, spleen, liver, and lungs. Hence affected people will have a generalized lymphadenopathy, hepatosplenomegaly, and parenchymatous granulomas. Patients with this disease are very prone to infection and are susceptible to osteomyelitis, liver abscesses, and pneumonia. The prognosis is poor and survival into adulthood is rare.

Laboratory findings.

The essential defect in chronic granulomatous disease is an inability of WBCs to carry out phagocytosis. This is due to a metabolic defect within these cells, arising from an inability to generate hydrogen peroxide. Production of hydrogen peroxide is an essential part of phagocytosis as it enables a local increase in oxygen for cellular requirements. Also, hydrogen peroxide stimulates the pentose shunt, which is essential if bacteria are to be destroyed. Therefore, in this disease, WBCs do not have the oxidative potential for normal phagocytosis. The nature of the defect in hydrogen peroxide generation is perhaps related to a deficiency in NADPH oxidase activity. In normal circumstances, NADPH combines with oxygen to form hydrogen peroxide in a reaction catalysed by NADPH oxidase.

Patients with chronic granulomatous disease are very susceptible to infections from catalase positive micro-organisms (e.g. *staphylococci*, *E. coli*, and *Candida*), which destroy any locally produced hydrogen peroxide.

The disease is diagnosed by the nitroblue-tetrazolium test. Normal leukocytes reduce nitroblue-tetrazolium to purple formazon, whereas leukocytes in chronic granulomatous disease fail to do this (Johnson 1969).

Periodontal manifestations.

The periodontal manifestations of chronic granulomatous disease have been described in two case reports (Wolf and Ebel 1978; Allan and Straton 1983). In both there was a marked, diffuse, severe gingivitis with an accompanying ulceration of the buccal mucosa. The gingival ulceration appears to respond to oral hygiene measures and regular use of chlorhexidine mouthwashes.

Treatment.

The prognosis for patients with this disease is poor. Treatment of the underlying condition is unsatisfactoy. Sulphonamides, corticosteroids, and bone marrow transplantation have been attempted with limited success. The periodontal manifestations may respond to systemic antimicrobial therapy.

3.7.3 RED BLOOD-CELL DISORDERS

Introduction

The main function of red blood cells is to supply, via their haemaglobin molecules, oxygen to the tissues and to remove carbon dioxide. There are many types of red blood-cell disorders but only a few appear to have any effect on the periodontal tissues. The aplastic anaemias have been reported to be associated with severe periodontal destruction, but in these conditions a generalized pancytopenia contributes to this finding. Other types of red blood-cell disorders that have been investigated for their effects on the periodontal tissues include the sickling disorders and acatalasia.

Aplastic anaemia

This is a bone marrow disorder characterized by a reduction in haematopoietic tissue, replacement of the bone marrow with fat, and a pancytopenia. Aplastic anaemia can be caused by drugs, chemicals, radiation, infections, immunological injuries, and neoplasia. Drugs that have been implicated in this condition include chloramphenicol and phenylbutazone. The disease has been reported to occur as a sequel to hepatitis and tuberculosis.

All the haematopoietic cells are affected in aplastic anaemia. Therefore, the signs and symptoms of the disease will be those that accompany anaemia, neutropenia, and thrombocytopenia. These include weakness, fatigue, recurrent infections, pyrexia, epistaxis, and retinal haemorrhage.

Periodontal manifestations

There are a few case reports of the effect of aplastic anaemia on the periodontal tissues (Alty 1962; Stamps 1974). Bleeding from the gingival margins appears to be a feature in these cases, and in the patient described by Alty, this was the initial complaint—the outcome of the disease was fatal, the patient died one month after the initial consultation.

In Stamps' report, severe periodontal destruction occurred in a 16-year-old girl with idiopathic aplastic anaemia. The periodontal disease responded to regular prophylaxis, but the periodontal status and gingival bleeding during treatment related to the changes in platelet count. Scaling was done under antibiotic cover and after platelet transfusion.

Fanconi's anaemia

This is a rare type of aplastic anaemia characterized by a familial bone-marrow hypoplasia that becomes manifest in the first decade of life. The disease appears to be transmitted by an autosomal-recessive gene of variable penetrance. Apart from the signs of anaemia, the other features of this condition include brown pigmentation of the skin, hypoplasia of the kidney and spleen, absent or hypoplastic thumb or radius, microcephaly, and mental and sexual retardation (Meme *et al.* 1980). The prognosis for this type of aplastic anaemia is poor; death is usually caused by haemorrhage, infectious leukaemia, or some other type of malignancy.

The periodontal manifestations of Fanconi's anaemia have been described in a case report (Opinya *et al.* 1988) of a 24-year-old man who was the product of consanguineous marriage. Several teeth had been lost and those remaining showed severe bone loss with pocketing in excess of 10 mm. The gingiva were bluish-red, bled on probing, and showed suppuration on gentle pressure. No follow-up or details of further periodontal management were reported.

Sickling disorders

Sickling disorders are those states in which the red blood cell undergoes sickling when subjected to hypoxia. The sickle cell diseases in which this phenomenon can occur are sickle cell haemoglobin C disease, sickle cell haemoglobin D disease, thalassaemia, and sickle cell anaemia. These diseases all contain abnormal haemoglobin genes, which in sickle cell anaemia are homozygous.

Patients with sickle cell anaemia are susceptible to infections. This may be due to a local vascular factor, i.e. a vaso-occlusive phenomena leading to infarction or a defect in the reticulo-endothelial system (Onwubalili 1983). In view of this finding, the periodontal status of patients with sickling disorders has been investigated (Crawford 1988). Radiographic and clinical evidence suggested that patients with sickling disorders did not have more gingival inflammation or periodontal destruction than otherwise healthy, age-matched controls. However, it was stressed that in some patients with sickle cell anaemia, periodontal disease may provide a sufficient inflammatory response to precipitate a sickling crisis.

Acatalasia

This rare inherited condition is caused by a lack of the enzyme catalase in many cells, especially the red blood cells and leukocytes. Within these cells, catalase converts hydrogen peroxide to oxygen and water. The enzymic activity protects the haemoglobin and red blood-cell membrane against oxidizing agents. Bacteria in plaque (especially haemolytic streptococci and pneumococci) can produce hydrogen peroxide, which will oxidize haemoglobin if the red blood cell is deficient in catalase. This will cause local hypoxia and necrosis of the gingival tissues.

The periodontal problems associated with acatalasia have been reported in two Peruvian siblings aged 10 and 11 years (Delgado and Calderon 1979). Severe periodontal destruction and gingival necrosis were present in both children. Subgingival plaque samples and bacteriological smears taken from the necrotic gingival tissue produced a predominant growth of pneumococci. The investigators suggest that the periodontal findings are related to the lack of catalase activity in the gingival tissues, which facilitates the colonization of hydrogen peroxide-producing bacteria. The periodontal condition of both children improved when oral hygiene measures were instituted.

3.8 DISORDERS OF THE RETICULO-ENDOTHELIAL SYSTEM

3.8.1 INTRODUCTION

Peripheral blood monocytes produced in the bone marrow from myeloid stem cells are the precursors of tissue macrophages. Macrophages have a predilection for lymph nodes, the spleen, liver, and bone marrow, where some are fixed to the endothelial structures lining the sinusoids of these organs. This fixed phagocytic capacity is known as the reticulo-endothelial system and is an integral part of the body's defence mechanisms. Other macrophages roam freely through tissues and respond to chemotactic stimuli produced at sites of inflammation or infection (see Chapter 1). Disorders of the reticulo-endothelial system may be divided into infections, neoplastic, lipid and non-lipid reticulo-endothelioses. The lipid reticulo-endothelioses include Gaucher's disease, which is a familial disease characterized by a derangement of lipid metabolism in which kerasin (a galactoside) is deposited throughout the entire reticulo-endothelial system, and Niemann–Pick disease, which is characterized by abnormal storage of phospholipids.

Histiocytosis X is the principal non-lipid reticulo-endotheliosis, and this group of diseases has the most pronounced effect on the periodontium.

3.8.2 HISTIOCYTOSIS X

Three clinical disorders (Letterer–Siwe disease, Hand–Schuller–Christian disease, and eosinophilic granuloma) constitute the condition known as histiocytosis X. All three conditions are characterized histologically by an abnormal proliferation of histiocytes and a collection of eosinophilic leukocytes. The eosinophils destroy tissue locally and invade the area of destruction. The essential features of the three are:

- *Letterer–Siwe disease*: this disease occurs mainly in children. It is a very aggressive and destructive form of histiocytosis X and has a very poor prognosis.

- *Hand–Schuller–Christian disease*: also known as chronic disseminated histiocytosis X, consists of multiple eosinophilic granuloma mainly involving the skeleton. As a consequence of bony involvement, the following symptoms can be found; diabetes insipidus, due to granulomatous destruction of the sella turcica and invasion of the pituitary gland, and exopthalmus arising from retro-orbital pressure, due to granulomatous involvement of the orbital wall, frontal bone, and sphenoid bone.

- *Eosinophilic granuloma*: this is a benign osteolytic lesion that can be solitary or polyostotic. It is usually seen in young adults. Lesions may occur in the alveolar bone and involve the overlying mucosa.

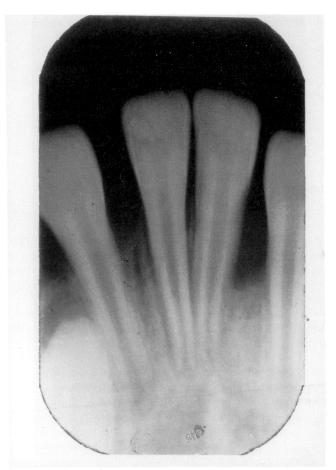

Fig. 3.5 Periapical radiograph of lower incisor teeth in the patient with histiocytosis X shown in Plate 8; there is advanced bone loss.

Periodontal manifestations

The periodontal manifestations of histiocytosis X have recently been reviewed by Artzi *et al.* (1989). A synopsis of the cases that have cited oral involvement is given in Table 3.7 (Appendix to this chapter). Oral manifestations of histiocytosis X are common and have an incidence ranging from 10 to 36 per cent (Sigala *et al.* 1972; Hartman 1980). Oral lesions are more common in the mandible, especially the posterior region. Mandibular lesions occur in 50–82 per cent of cases where there is oral involvement (Hartman 1980; Smith and Evans 1984; Artzi *et al.* 1989).

Periodontal manifestations of histiocytosis X are perhaps one of the earliest signs. Necrosis and oedema of the gingiva have been reported (Sweet *et al.* 1979; McCarthy and Shklar 1980). Other common findings include gingival bleeding, pocketing, bone loss, and abscess formation (Plate 12) (see Table 3.7). In the series reported by Artzi *et al.* (1989), oral pain followed by tooth mobility were the patients' main complaints. The radiographic appearances can show extensive destruction of the alveolar bone (Fig.3.5), lytic lesions, and the appearance of teeth floating in a sea of radiolucency.

Histologically, the lesions associated with histiocytosis X are dominated by eosinophilic leukocytes and large monocytes (histiocytes). The histiocytes may coalesce and form multinucleated giant cells. Early lesions contain large numbers of eosinophils, which in time are replaced by fibrous tissue.

Treatment

If histiocytosis X is suspected of causing periodontal breakdown, then a full screening should be carried out to determine whether the lesion is localized (eosinophilic granuloma) or part of the more generalized condition (Hand–Schuller–Christian disease). Biopsy of the local lesion is essential, followed by a full-body, computed tomographic scan (Mitnick and Pinto 1980).

A single, localized lesion just involving alveolar bone responds to curettage and excision. More disseminated lesions are treated by radiation and chemotherapy.

The prognosis is excellent if the localized lesion is confined to bone. If both bone and soft tissue are involved, then the mortality rate is approximately 4 per cent. For multiple lesions, especially if soft tissue is involved, the mortality rate is in excess of 50 per cent (Lahey 1975).

Other findings that can affect the prognosis in histiocytosis X include the age of the patient, with younger age groups having a poor prognosis, and the number of organs involved (Lahey 1975; Daneshbod and Kissane 1976).

3.9 INFECTIONS

3.9.1 INTRODUCTION

Infections involving the periodontal tissues can be localized or generalized. The localized lesion can be specific to the gingival tissues, and the two common examples are ANUG and acute herpetic gingivostomatitis. Localized infections affecting other parts of the mouth can spread to or involve the gingival tissues. An obvious example of such an infection is candidiasis.

However, this section is primarily concerned with the effect of systemic infection on the periodontal tissues and their response to plaque. Acute systemic infections tend to be of short duration and self-limiting. Hence, they would have only a transient effect on the periodontium. An example is infectious mononucleosis, which can be associated with an episode of gingival inflammation.

The chronic infections tend to have a more profound effect on the periodontal tissues, and the main condition that will be discussed in this section is the acquired immune deficiency syndrome (AIDS). Periodontal manifestations have also been reported in patients with tuberculosis, leprosy, and histoplasmosis. In tuberculosis and histoplasmosis, the gingival tissues have become involved because of contact with infected sputum.

3.9.2. AIDS

The AIDS epidemic is now evolving into one of the major challenges facing modern medicine and science. The disease is due to an RNA retrovirus known as the human immuno-

Table 3.8 Opportunist infections and neoplasms associated with AIDS

Infections
Oral and oesophageal candidiasis
Mucocutaneous herpes simplex
Pneumocystis carinii pneumonia
Mycobacterium tuberculosis
Salmonellosis
Cryptococcal meningitis
Toxoplasma encephalitis
Cytomegalovirus disease
Cryptosporidiosis
Atypical mycobacterial infection

Neoplasms
Kaposi's sarcoma
B-cell lymphoma
Hodgkin's disease

Table 3.9 Classification of the oral lesions associated with AIDS (after Pindborg 1989)

Fungal infections
Candidiasis
Histoplasmosis
Cryptococcosis
Goetrichosis

Bacterial infections
Acute necrotizing ulcerative gingivitis (ANUG)
Rapid periodontal destruction
Mycobacterium avium intracellulare
Actinomycosis
Cat-scratch disease
Klebsiella pneumoniae
Enterobacteriacea
Escherichia coli
Exacerbation of periapical abscess
Sinusitis
Submandibular cellulitis

Viral infections
Herpetic stomatitis
Cytomegalovirus
Epstein–Barr virus
Varicella–zoster virus
Papillomavirus

Neoplasms
Kaposi's sarcoma
Non-Hodgkin's lymphoma
Squamous cell carcinoma

Neurological disturbances
Trigeminal neuropathy
Facial palsy

Unknown causes
Recurrent aphthous ulceration
Progressive necrotizing ulceration
Toxic epidermolysis (Lyell's syndrome)
Delayed wound healing
Idiopathic thrombocytopenia
Salivary gland enlargement
Xerostomia
Oral mucosal hypopigmentation

deficiency virus (HIV). This virus occurs in most of the body's fluids, but is only present in significant amounts in blood and semen. The infection is therefore spread by sexual transmission, through blood and blood products, and from an infected mother to her fetus. Hence, those most at risk from AIDS are homosexuals, prostitutes, intravenous drug abusers, and patients receiving blood products on a regular basis (e.g. haemophiliacs). All blood products are now screened for HIV.

When the virus gains access to the body it seeks out its target cell, the CD4-bearing, T4-helper lymphocyte, and becomes incorporated into the lymphocyte's chromosomal make-up. Once incorporated within the cell's nucleus, it can remain for a short (active) or prolonged (latent) period of time. Cellular infection with HIV is for the life of that cell. The lymphocyte is the main target cell for HIV, but other cells can become infected, and examples include macrophages, endothelial cells, and glial cells in the central nervous system.

Infection is usually accompanied by a viraemia with antigen and virus present in the blood. Antibodies are produced against the virus and these act as markers of the disease and are important in the identification of a patient exposed to HIV. Autoantibodies may also be produced against the infected CD4-helper cell, which may account for the profound immunosuppression that accompanies AIDS.

At varying time intervals up to two years, the effect of HIV on the immune system will increase the susceptibility of the host to opportunist infections and neoplasia. A list of AIDS-related infections and neoplasms is shown in Table 3.8.

The clinical features of AIDS are many and varied, but none is diagnostic. Features include lymphadenopathy, weight loss, oral candidiasis, unexplained diarrhoea, dermatitis, shingles, and hairy oral leukoplakia. Laboratory investigations will show a leukopenia, anaemia, raised ESR and T4-lymphocyte depletion. Biopsy of lymph nodes will show follicular involution and destruction of follicular dendritic cells.

Oral manifestations

AIDS can have a variety of oral manifestations and these have recently been classified (Pindborg 1989); a list is shown in Table 3.9. There is increasing evidence that the oral lesions associated with AIDS, especially candidiasis, hairy leukoplakia, periodontal disease, and Kaposi's sarcoma, are more likely to be associated with HIV seropositivity (Melnick *et al.* 1989). If a subject had one or more of these oral lesions, they were 5.7 times more likely to have serum antibodies to HIV. Many of the oral manifestations associated with AIDS can affect the periodontal tissues.

Periodontal manifestations

Two distinct types of periodontal disease have been described in HIV-infected patients. These have been designated HIV-associated gingivitis (HIV-G) and HIV-associated periodontitis (HIV-P) (Winkler and Murray 1987).

HIV gingivitis.

This has been defined as a lesion confined to the soft tissue, which shows distinctive erythema of the free gingiva, attached gingiva (Plate 13), and alveolar mucosa. There is often extensive bleeding on both toothbrushing and gentle probing. The gingival margins often show a well-circumscribed erythematous band. HIV-G frequently involves all the gingival tissues. An important feature is the lack of response of this type of gingivitis to conventional periodontal treatment (plaque control and scaling). It would seem that HIV-G is not a reversible condition (Winkler *et al.* 1988).

HIV periodontitis.

HIV-P has been defined as sites with the signs described for HIV-G, with, in addition, extensive soft tissue necrosis and severe loss of periodontal attachment. Soft tissue destruction can be rapid and is often accompanied by interproximal cratering, necrosis, and ulceration (Plate 14). Unlike chronic adult periodontitis, there is not deep pocket formation. The ulceration and necrosis which is a feature of HIV-P can cause exposure and sequestration of alveolar bone. Pain is a prominent feature of HIV-P; it is localized to the alveolar bone. This differs from the pain associated with ANUG, which is usually confined to the gingiva (Winkler *et al.* 1988).

Microbiology of HIV-G and HIV-P lesions.   The microflora of subgingival plaque associated with HIV-G and HIV-P has been investigated with indirect immunofluorescence and direct culturing techniques (Murray *et al.* 1988). Findings were compared with those from a group of HIV-seropositive patients and HIV-seronegative controls. The HIV-G and HIV-P sites contained significantly more *C. albicans* than control sites. Detailed microbial analysis showed that the following species were more prevalent in HIV-G and HIV-P sites than controls; *Bact. gingivalis*; *Bact. intermedius*; *F. nucleatum*; *A. actinomycetemcomitans*; *Eik. corrodens* and *Wolinella*. Apart from *Candida* spp., the distribution of other bacterial types in HIV-G and HIV-P is similar to adult periodontitis. Serum antibodies to *Bact. gingivalis*; *Bact. intermedius*; *F. nucleatum* and *A. actinomycetemcomitans* were significantly higher in HIV-seropositive than in HIV-seronegative patients.

Pathogenesis of HIV-associated periodontal disease

The role of the immune system in the pathogenesis of periodontal disease has been discussed in Chapter 1. Thus, it is not surprising that a disorder which significantly affects this system is associated with severe periodontal destruction. There is uncertainty as to whether HIV-P is preceded by HIV-G or whether HIV-G is a mild variant of HIV-P. It has been shown that levels of CD4 lymphocytes may be an important factor in the progression of HIV-G to HIV-P (Winkler and Murray 1987).

The microflora associated with both HIV-G and HIV-P is similar to that found in patients with periodontal disease. However, the disruption of the immune system that accompanies HIV infection may increase the pathogenicity of the virulence factors associated with these bacterial species.

The role and function of PMNs in periodontal disease has similarly been discussed elsewhere (see Chapter 1). When there is a defect in PMN numbers or function, there is often an accompanying severe form of periodontal destruction (see p. 39). PMNs harvested from HIV-positive patients have been shown to have increased phagocytosis, oxidative bursts, and F-actin formation (Ryder *et al.* 1988). This finding would suggest that PMNs from HIV-infected patients appear to show an increase in activity, which is in contrast to the decrease in activity typical of these cells in most destructive forms of periodontal disease.

In chronic adult periodontitis, the PMNs form the first line of defence against plaque toxins and antigens. When there is an increase in plaque antigens, the PMNs are replaced by macrophages and lymphocytes. In HIV-infected patients, this replacement is unlikely to occur, therefore PMNs have a more important role in 'protecting' the periodontal tissues in these patients.

PMNs from patients with AIDS are 'primed', possibly because of their prolonged exposure to fungal and bacterial infections and/or the failure of the CD4-lymphocyte and macrophage response. 'Priming' may also be caused by the transient bacteraemia (from periodontal pockets) that results from chewing. These 'primed' or hyperactive PMNs may have the capacity to produce local tissue damage.

It would seem that many factors contribute to the severe periodontal destruction seen in certain HIV-positive patients. These would include: (a) the 'primed' or hyperactive PMNs; (b) the failure of the CD4-lymphocyte and macrophage response; (c) the increased pathogenicity of the specific subgingival microflora.

Treatment

Three treatment approaches have been evaluated in the management of HIV-associated periodontal disease (Grassi *et al.* 1988). These are: (a) conventional therapy (i.e. plaque control, scaling, and root planing); (b) conventional therapy supplemented with local irrigation of a 10 per cent povidone–iodine solution (Betadine); (c) conventional therapy plus rinsing twice a day with a 0.12 per cent chlorhexidine solution. All patients were assessed at one and three months after scaling and root planing.

Patients treated with conventional therapy and chlorhexidine mouthwashes showed a significant improvement in all clinical measures (plaque index, gingival index, and pocket depth) and complete resolution of spontaneous bleeding. There was no further loss of attachment in this group. Patients using the 10 per cent povidone–iodine irrigation appeared to benefit from the topical anaesthetic and haemostatic effects of this compound.

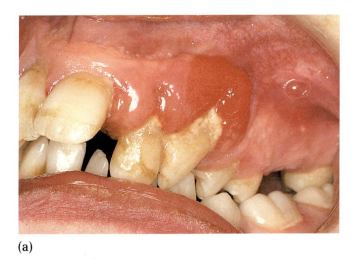
(a)

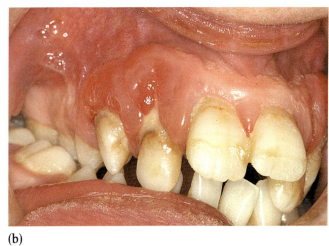
(b)

Plate 1 (a) Extensive periodontal disease and (b) a typical malocclusion in patient with Down's syndrome.

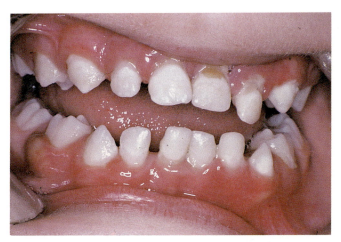

Plate 2 Papillon–Lefèvre syndrome in a 3-year-old child with spacing and mobility of the upper and lower incisors.

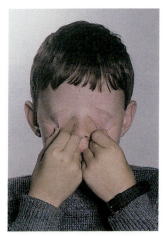

Plate 3 Cutaneous hyperextensibility of the upper eyelids in a 9-year-old child with Ehlers–Danlos syndrome.

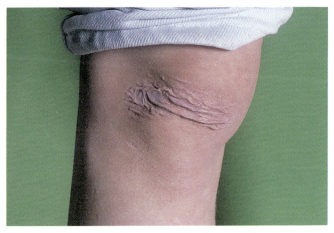

Plate 4 Papyraceous scarring of the left knee in the patient shown in 3.6.

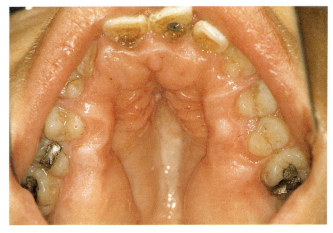

Plate 5 Enlargement of the maxillary tuberosities in an adult with hereditary gingival fibromatosis.

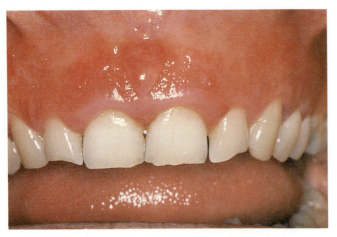

Plate 6 Diffuse erythematous attached gingiva in the upper anterior region in a patient with Crohn's disease.

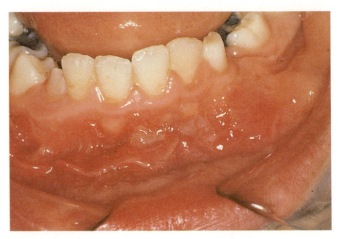

Plate 7 Mucosal tags in the lower labial sulcus in a patient with Crohn's disease.

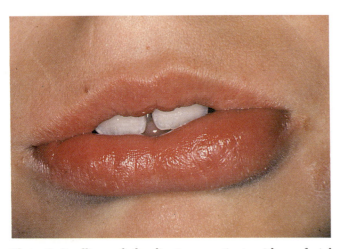

Plate 8 Swelling of the lip in a patient with orofacial granulomatosis.

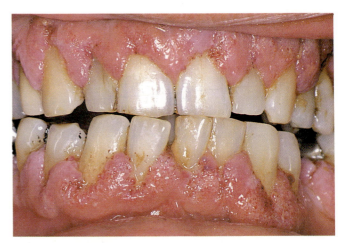

Plate 9 Hyperplastic gingivitis in a 65-year-old male suffering from Wegener's granulomatosis.

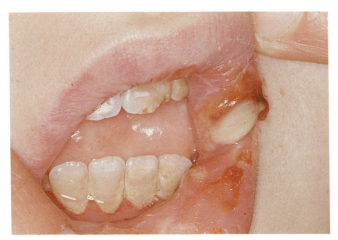

Plate 10 Oral ulceration associated with cyclic neutropenia.

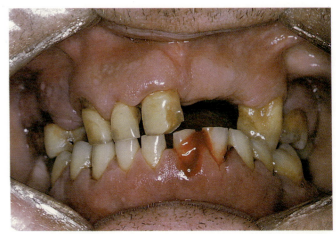

Plate 11 Spontaneous gingival bleeding associated with acute leukaemia.

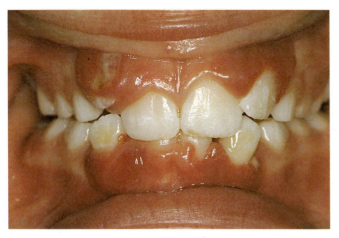

Plate 12 Clinical condition of periodontal tissues in a 6½-year-old child with histiocytosis X.

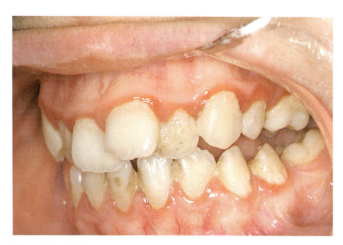

Plate 13 HIV gingivitis.

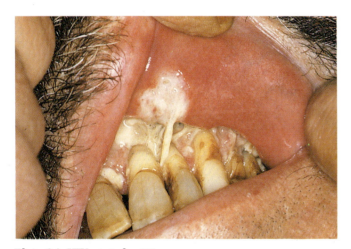

Plate 14 HIV periodontitis.

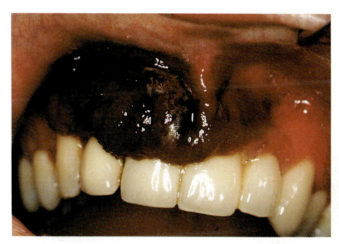

Plate 15 Kaposi's sarcoma of the palatal tissues in an HIV-positive patient.

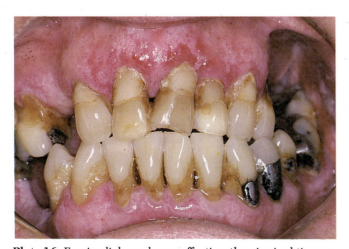

Plate 16 Erosive lichen planus affecting the gingival tissues.

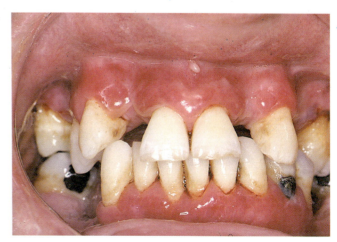

Plate 17 Benign mucous membrane pemphigoid appearing as 'desquamative gingivitis'.

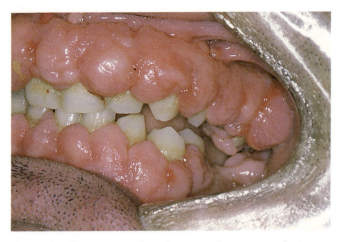

Plate 18 Phenytoin-induced gingival overgrowth in an adult epileptic patient.

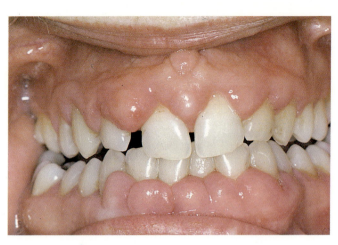

Plate 19 Cyclosporin-induced gingival overgrowth in a heart transplant patient.

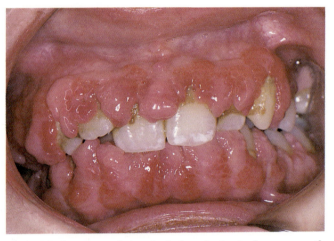

Plate 20 Severe cyclosporin-induced gingival overgrowth in a renal transplant patient.

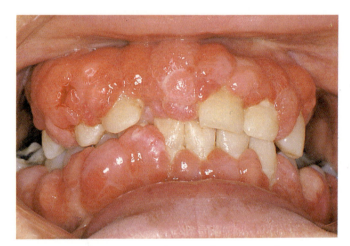

Plate 21 Nifedipine-induced gingival overgrowth.

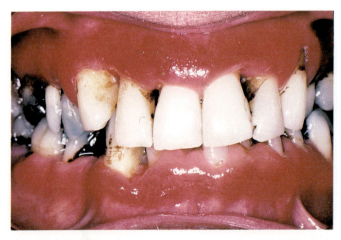

Plate 22 Plasma cell gingivitis related to the use of a herbal toothpaste.

Other AIDS-related disorders that can affect the periodontal tissues

The incidence of ANUG is higher in HIV patients than the rest of the population (Pinborg and Holmstrup 1987). The microbiology of HIV-associated ANUG is similar to that of non-infected individuals; thus the increased incidence is perhaps a reflection of the decreased immunocompetence found in AIDS patients.

The various oral infections listed in Table 3.8 can all involve the gingival tissues—in particular, herpetic gingivostomatitis, candidiasis, and human papillomavirus causing multiple condylomas of the gingival margin. Gingival ulceration due to *Mycobacterium avium intracellulare* has been reported in an AIDS patient (Volpe *et al.* 1985).

Kaposi's sarcoma (Plate 15) is the most common oral tumour affecting HIV-positive patients (Lozada *et al.* 1983). The gingival tissues are a frequent site. The sarcoma is thought to be of vascular origin arising from the endothelial cells of either blood vessels or lymphatics. Kaposi's sarcoma of the gingival tissues can start as a diffuse swelling of a single dental papilla. The gingival enlargement can have a red, blue, or purplish colour. Kaposi's sarcoma can also be generalized, giving rise to extensive bony destruction and the radiographic appearance of floating teeth. Such lesions need to be distinguished from eosinophilic granuloma (see p. 45). Localized Kaposi's sarcoma affecting a solitary gingival papilla can be treated by excision. The more generalized lesions require a combined approach of surgery, radiotherapy, and chemotherapy.

Non-Hodgkin's lymphoma has been found in a small number of AIDS patients and this lesion can manifest as a diffuse gingival swelling, epulis, or nodule (Phelan *et al.* 1987).

3.10 DISORDERS OF THE IMMUNE SYSTEM

3.10.1 INTRODUCTION

A fully functional and effective immune system is essential to protect the body against infection, to recognize and eliminate foreign protein, and destroy tumour cells. This system involves lymphocytes (both T and B cells), macrophages, PMNs, immunoglobulins, and the complement proteins. The role of the immune system in the pathogenesis of periodontal disease is discussed in Chapter 1. Any disorder of this system has the potential to have a profound effect on the periodontium and its response to plaque. Furthermore, patients with a defined immunodeficiency can provide some insight into the role of the immune system in the development of periodontal disease.

Disorders of the immune system can be considered as either primary or secondary. The primary disorders are usually genetically determined and rare. These include hypogammaglobulinaemia, Di George syndrome, IgA deficiency, and deficiencies in the complement proteins. Involvement of the periodontal tissues appears only to be reported in cases of hypogammaglobulinaemia.

Secondary disorders of the immune system can be caused by a disease or drug therapy. Many of the diseases that have an immunological disorder have previously been discussed (e.g. AIDS, diabetes mellitus, sarcoidosis, sickle cell disease). Conditions to be discussed here include renal disease, renal transplantation and immunosuppression, and the plasma cell dyscrasias.

3.10.2 HYPOGAMMAGLOBULINAEMIA

Primary hypogammaglobulinaemia is a rare condition characterized by very low or undetectable levels of the serum immunoglobulins. These rare diseases are usually non-familial, although there is an X-linked type that starts in early childhood. A secondary form of hypogammaglobulinaemia is associated with chronic lymphocytic leukaemia and myeloma. Patients with hypogammaglobulinaemia are susceptible to infections, especially those of the respiratory tract.

Periodontal manifestations

Severe periodontal disease has been reported in a 17-year-old patient with a profound immunodeficiency disorder (Roberts and Walker 1976). Although its precise nature was not elucidated, the family history and the patient's low serum IgA levels suggested that hypogammaglobulinaemia may have been the underlying cause. Furthermore, the patient's PMNs showed impaired phagocytosis, which contributed to the poor host resistance. Surgical intervention was avoided in the patient and the mobile teeth were left to exfoliate of their own accord.

The nature of the gingival response to plaque has been investigated in three patients suffering from hypogammaglobulinaemia (Barrickman *et al.* 1973). Essentially, these patients have no immunoglobulins or plasma cells in their gingival tissues. Thus the aim of this investigation was to try and identify the role of these immunological components in gingivitis. Gingival biopsies from these patients showed that PMNs, lymphocytes, macrophages, and mast cells are the inflammatory cells present in the connective tissue. None of the patients' tissues showed evidence of an immediate hypersensitivity reaction. It was also suggested that the absence of plasma cells in the gingival tissues may be useful in identifying cases of hypogammaglobulinaemia.

Another study has shown that patients with primary immunodeficiencies experience less caries and gingival inflammation than healthy controls (Robertson *et al.* 1978). The low caries incidence may be related to the extensive use of antibiotics in these patients. The differences in gingival inflammation between the two groups may be attributable to the interaction between the inflammatory and immune responses. In the healthy subjects, this interaction would lead to more overt clinical signs of inflammation, whereas this reaction would not be so extensive in the immunodeficient patient.

3.10.3 RENAL DISEASE

Renal failure can be due to many factors; these are beyond the scope of this book. Such failure can lead to uraemia, the need for dialysis, and transplantation. Patients with renal disease are of interest to the periodontologist and have been the subject of many investigations. This is, in part, due to the finding that uraemic patients have a reduced immunocapacity (Birkeland 1976). Furthermore, renal transplant patients are treated with immunosuppressive drugs to prevent graft rejection. Hence these patients provide a further opportunity to investigate the effect of a reduced immunocapacity on the response of the periodontal tissues to bacterial plaque.

Immunosuppressant drugs

These drugs act on various components of the immune system causing selective inhibition and suppression. Those used for this purpose include corticosteroids (mainly prednisone and prednisolone) azathioprine, and, more recently, cyclosporin. The actions of cyclosporin and corticosteroids on the periodontal tissues are discussed in Chapters 4 and 11, respectively.

Azathioprine is a derivative of the antimetabolite mercaptopurine. On absorption, azathioprine is metabolized to 6-mercaptopurine, which is then further converted to the active metabolite 6-mercaptopurine riboside. The active metabolite inhibits nucleic acid and protein synthesis by competing with isonic acid for enzymes involved in the synthesis of guanylic and adrenylic acid. The latter two are purine bases that are essential for the biosynthesis of nucleic acid (Berenbaum 1967). The drug also suppresses the cell-mediated immune response by inhibiting the migration of T lymphocytes, but has little or no action on antibody production (Fournier *et al.* 1973).

Periodontal findings in renal and immunosuppressed patients

As discussed previously, patients with uraemia are immunosuppressed. Similarly, renal transplant patients are treated with immunosuppressive drugs to prevent graft rejection. Thus, it is not surprising that renal patients, either before or after transplantation, have been the subjects of many periodontal investigations (Schuller *et al.* 1973; Tollefsen *et al.* 1978, 1982; Kardachi and Newcomb 1978; Oshrain *et al.* 1979; Been and Engel 1982; Sutton and Smales 1983; Tollefsen and Johansen, 1985a,b). These studies have two main objectives. First, to see if the drugs or the disease state alter the response of the periodontal tissues to plaque, and secondly, to determine the role of the various components of the immune system in the progression of periodontal disease.

Immunosuppressant drugs (azathioprine and prednisone), when given to renal transplant patients, reduce the inflammatory response of the periodontal tissues to plaque (Schuller *et al.* 1973; Kardachi and Newcomb 1978). In some of the subsequent studies (Tollefsen *et al.* 1978; Oshrain *et al.* 1979; Been and Engel 1982), comparisons of various periodontal measures were made between renal transplant patients taking immunosuppressants, patients on haemodialysis, and healthy controls. Oshrain *et al.* reported

that gingival inflammation, periodontal destruction, and plaque accumulation were similar in all three groups, but in the transplant group there was again a lack of correlation between plaque levels and both gingival inflammation and periodontal destruction.

The use of immunosuppressants in renal transplant patients has been associated with significantly lower scores for connective tissue inflammation in gingiva than those of patients on haemodialysis or healthy controls (Tollefsen *et al.* 1978, 1982). Although the drugs did not abolish the reaction of the gingival tissues to plaque, the reaction that did occur was less marked than in the other groups. Histologically, the gingival tissues in the immunosuppressed group showed a greater response to treatment, with resolution and an absence of inflammatory cells in the connective tissues.

In one of the few longitudinal studies (Been and Engel 1982), the effects of azathioprine and prednisone on gingival health were evaluated in four renal transplant patients; the control group comprised three patients undergoing haemodialysis and six healthy controls. All subjects in each group were matched for age and sex and were investigated over a period of 9 months. The findings were that patients on immunosuppressive therapy had significantly reduced levels of gingival inflammation in the presence of high levels of bacterial plaque. A further longitudinal study (Tollefsen and Johansen, 1985 *a, b*), which monitored renal transplant patients before and after transplantation, found significantly less bone loss in patients with an immunocapacity than in healthy controls or diabetics.

It can be concluded that the immunosuppressed patient (either drug-induced or secondary to uraemia) is afforded some degree of protection against periodontal destruction. The findings from these studies confirm the role of the immune system in the pathogenesis of periodontal disease, in particular the activation of this system with regard to bone loss.

Treatment

The main problem with periodontal treatment in the immunosuppressed patient is the risk of infection arising after operative procedures. Most renal physicians advocate antibiotic cover in the immunosuppressed renal-transplant patient before any periodontal procedure that results in a significant bacteriaemia. Subgingival scaling, root planing, and any form of periodontal surgery should be covered. Amoxycillin, 3 g orally, is the antimicrobial of choice; if the patient is allergic to penicillin, then they should receive erythromycin, 1.5 g, one hour before the procedure. Repeated antibiotic dosages should be avoided in the renal transplant patient because impaired renal function will affect the excretion of the drug. Thus it is often advisable to carry out as much treatment as possible under the single antibiotic cover.

Renal transplant patients will also be receiving prednisolone concurrently with their other immunosuppressant drugs. They will therefore require steroid cover if the periodontal procedures are likely to cause any degree of stress.

Cyclosporin is a relatively new immunosuppressant drug and in certain centres is the agent of choice to prevent graft rejection. An unfortunate side-effect of cyclosporin is gingival hyperplasia. This topic is discussed in chapter 4.

Before renal transplantation, it is essential that the patient is rendered free of any dental infections because, in immunosuppression, such foci could lead to a systemic infection and graft failure.

Patients on peritoneal dialysis will not present a problem for conventional periodontal treatment, although haemostasis is poor, owing to impaired platelet function. Renal patients on haemodialysis do present a problem because their blood is heparinized during dialysis. If periodontal surgical procedures are necessary they should be carried out the day after dialysis, and haemostasis should be achieved before packs are placed. It is always advisable to consult with the patient's physician before any periodontal procedures or changes in the patient's drug regimen. This will ensure that the patient receives the best management.

3.10.4 PLASMA CELL DYSCRASIAS

The plasma cell dyscrasias are a rare group of B-lymphocyte disorders where there is overproduction of specific immunoglobulins. Six types of these dyscrasias have been recognized and these include multiple myeloma, solitary myeloma, Waldenström's macroglobulinaemia, heavy-chain disease, and primary amyloidosis. Of these conditions, periodontal manifestations only appear to have been reported in cases of multiple myeloma.

Multiple myeloma

This is the most common of the plasma cell dyscrasias and is characterized by a neoplastic proliferation of multifocal, tumorous masses of plasma cells. These are widespread throughout the skeleton and occasionally involve soft tissue. The mandible, especially the ramus and angle region, are common sites of bony lesions. Bence–Jones proteinuria is a diagnostic feature of multiple myeloma. This abnormal protein is a light-chain immunoglobulin.

The prognosis for multiple myeloma is poor, and patients are treated with a combination of chemotherapy and radiotherapy.

Multiple myelomatous lesions involving the periodontium and gingival tissues have recently been reported (Petit and Ripamonti 1990). Oral lesions included gingival bleeding, ulceration, a rapidly growing, retromolar, myelomatous mass, multiple foci of alveolar bone destruction, and expansion of the buccal cortical plates. The patient was treated with both radiotherapy and chemotherapy but died 22 months after the initial diagnosis was made.

3.11 MUCOCUTANEOUS DISORDERS

3.11.1 INTRODUCTION

Many skin disorders have oral manifestations and likewise affect the gingival tissues. Clinically, the gingival manifestations of skin diseases are often referred to as 'desquamative gingivitis'. However, it should be emphasized that this term is a clinical description only. Desquamative gingivitis may also be caused by drug hypersensitivity (see Chapter 4) and related to the menopause (see Chapter 7).

The dermatoses that can manifest as desquamative gingivitis are lichen planus, pemphigus vulgaris, benign mucous membrane pemphigoid, and perhaps psoriasis.

3.11.2 LICHEN PLANUS

This is a chronic disease of unknown aetiology. It affects about 2 per cent of the population and is more common in the over-40s. The disease has a higher incidence in women and acute exacerbations appear to be related to stress and emotional upsets. It has been reported that oral lesions occur in 70 per cent of patients who present with skin lesions (Laufer and Kuffer 1971). However, studies that have solely concentrated on oral lesions have shown that the incidence of skin lesions is in the range of 28–44 per cent (Silverman and Griffith 1974).

Skin lesions usually occur on the flexor surfaces of the wrist, shins, and around the umbilicus. They present as purplish or violaceous itchy plaques, which may show the characteristic, lacy, white network of striae (Wickham's striae).

Oral and gingival lesions

Oral lesions of lichen planus have either a keratotic, erosive, or atrophic appearance (Plate 16). In any one patient all three types may be present in different parts of the mouth. Wickham's striae may be present, especially if the lesion involves the buccal mucosa. All parts of the mouth can be affected, but the common sites include the posterior part of the buccal mucosa, the lateral borders of the tongue, and the gingiva.

Lichenoid eruptions can be drug-induced and drugs commonly implicated include chlorpropamide, methyldopa, propanalol, and gold salts (Seymour and Walton 1988).

Gingival involvement with lichen planus occurs in approximately 20 per cent of cases, and in 15 per cent of patients the lesion is confined solely to the gingival tissues. Four categories of gingival lesions have been described (Jandinski and Shklar 1976). These include: (a) white papular keratotic lesions, (b) vesiculobullous lesions, (c) erosive or ulcerative lesions, and (d) atrophic lesions.

Keratotic lesions

These occur on the attached gingiva and rarely involve the gingival margin. Keratotic lesions are probably the easiest to diagnose. The clinical appearance can be further categorized into discrete papular, plaque-like linear lesions, and reticulate lesions. Keratotic lesions are white in appearance, and the linear and 'reticulate lesions are usually seen on an erythematous background.

Vesiculobullous lesions

This is an uncommon form of gingival and oral lichen planus, and can present a problem with diagnosis. Small vesicles may appear within the width of the attached gingiva and burst leaving an ulcerative area. Similarly, large bullae may form and burst, which gives the appearance of sloughing epithelium.

Erosive or ulcerative lesions

These are frequently seen in acute exacerbations of lichen planus, and often occur with the keratotic form. Ulceration and erosions are confined to the width of the attached gingiva.

Atrophic lesions

When atrophic lesions are present, the gingival tissues appear red and shiny. The term 'desquamative gingivitis' is most applicable to atrophic lichen planus. This type of gingival lichen planus is often difficult to diagnose from the clinical appearance, especially if there are no other oral manifestations of the disease.

Histopathology

Biopsy of the gingival tissues is useful when trying to arrive at a diagnosis of lichen planus. Usual microscopic features include epithelial hyperkeratosis or parakeratosis, infiltration of the upper corium with a dense band of lymphocytic cells, and hydropic or liquefaction degeneration of the stratum germinativum. Although 'saw-tooth' rete pegs are a diagnostic feature of the skin lesion, they are rarely seen in oral or gingival specimens.

The different gingival lesions of lichen planus show histopathological changes that are commensurate with their clinical appearance. In the erosive form, there is thinning of the epithelium, necrosis, ulceration, and sometimes evidence of haemorrhage. In the vesiculobullous form, vesicles or bullae appear beneath the epithelium. They form as a consequence of extensive oedema collecting at the epithelial–connective tissue interface after hydropic degeneration of the stratum germinativum. Vesicular or bullous fluid may be blood-stained.

In the atrophic form, the epithelium is thin, poorly keratinized, and shows an absence of rete pegs. It is difficult to distinguish the stratum corneum from the stratum spinosum. There are often areas of ulceration and desquamation of the surface epithelium. The underlying connective tissue is usually very vascular and contains a dense infiltrate of lymphocytes, plasma cells, PMNs, and histiocytes.

Skin lesions from patients with lichen planus have been subjected to direct immunofluorescent techniques. Biopsies have revealed IgG, IgM, C3, and fibrin in cytoid bodies. In the later stages of skin lesions, fibrin bodies are observed along the basement membrane (Shousha and Svirbely 1977). The value of direct immunofluorescence in the diagnosis of oral lichen planus is limited. In two studies (Rogers and Jordan 1977; Daniels and Quadra-White 1980), cytoid bodies were found in 27 per cent of biopsy specimens of oral lesions, whereas fibrin deposits along the basement membrane were found in between 70 and 97 per cent of the specimens. These indifferent findings may be related to the different types of lichen planus found in the mouth or the age of the lesion (Nisengard and Neiders 1981).

Management

Most cases of lichen planus are usually asymptomatic and require little treatment apart from reassurance. One study has shown that oral lichen planus is associated with a higher incidence of squamous cell carcinoma (Silverman and Griffiths 1974). Although oral lichen planus cannot be considered a premalignant condition, the erosive and atrophic forms lack the normal epithelial protective barrier. Thus, the tissues may be more vulnerable to carcinogens. Patients with these types of lichen planus should be advised to stop smoking and be monitored on a regular basis (every 6 months) for any clinical signs of dysplastic changes.

The erosive and atrophic forms are particularly troublesome for the patient. Topical corticosteroids are the treatment of choice, and hydrocortisone hemisuccinate pellets, 2.5 mg, are useful in the management of localized lesions. The pellets are allowed to dissolve against the lesion and applied 3–4 times a day. For more widespread cases of lichen planus, the patient would find a solution of sodium betamethasone, 500 µg/20 ml, easy to use and efficacious. Severe lichen planus will require treatment with systemic corticosteroids (prednisolone).

Plaque control is going to be an inevitable problem where lichen planus involves the gingival tissues. During acute phases, mechanical plaque control is difficult and patients may find a chlorhexidine mouthwash (0.2 per cent) useful. Some patients may find that this concentration 'irritates' the already inflamed tissues and should therefore dilute the solution with water. A soft toothbrush should be used when the lesions start to resolve. Other proprietary mouthwashes such as Diflan may be useful in the management of oral and gingival lichen planus.

3.11.3 Pemphigus

Pemphigus is a chronic, acantholytic, vesiculobullous, autoimmune disease that exists in four forms depending upon where the acantholysis occurs. In pemiphigus erythematosus or foliaceous, acantholysis occurs in the upper layer of the epidermis. These two variants of pemphigus rarely involve the mouth. In pemphigus vulgaris and vegetans, acantholysis occurs above the basal cell layer within the spinous cell layer. Both types have oral and gingival lesions; however, some consider that the vegetans form is a milder version of pemphigus vulgaris (Lever and Schaumburg-Lever 1977; McCarthy and Shklar, 1980). Immunological and immunofluorescent investigations show that patients with active pemphigus have both tissue-bound and circulating autoantibodies to the intercellular substance of stratified squamous epithelium (Jordan et al. 1971; Nisengard et al. 1978).

Pemphigus vulgaris

This variant of pemphigus is seen in the older patient and is more common in patients of Mediterranean and Jewish origin (Pisanty et al. 1974). Women appear to be more susceptible to this type of pemphigus than men (Laskaris et al. 1982). Most patients develop oral lesions and these are usually the initial presenting symptoms (Zegarelli and Zegarelli 1977; Laskaris *et al.* 1982).

Skin lesions appear as crops of fluid-filled bullae that burst, ulcerate, and heal slowly. A positive Nikolsky sign is a useful diagnostic test of pemphigus. This test consists of applying lateral pressure to the skin. If there is dislodgement of the epidermis, the test is positive. However, a positive Nikolsky test can also be elicited in pemphigoid (Polifka and Krusinski 1980).

Apart from the mouth, lesions in pemphigus vulgaris can occur on the conjunctiva and the mucosal surfaces of the larynx, nose, and genitals.

Oral and gingival lesions

The oral mucosa is nearly always affected in cases of pemphigus vulgaris, and lesions frequently involve the gingival tissues. Occasionally, the gingival involvement is the sole presenting symptom (Shklar *et al.* 1978; Markitziu and Pisanty 1983; Orlowski *et al.* 1983; Barnett 1988).

Bullae can affect any part of the oral mucosa, but the soft palate seems to be a common site (Laskaris *et al.* 1982). The bullae quickly burst, ulcerate, and are covered with a necrotic mass. Ulcers are painful and slow to heal, with no scarring.

The gingival involvement has the clinical appearance of a severe desquamative or erosive gingivitis. Vesicles or bullae may be seen, but these quickly rupture leaving large, ulcerative areas. The periphery of the ulcer may show flaps of peeling tissue. Denuded areas are very painful and bleed readily. Lesions involve the width of attached gingiva and the gingival margins show the most marked inflammatory changes. This may be related to plaque, as oral hygiene in these patients is usually very poor. Healing of the ulcerative areas is slow, but there is no scarring. A positive Nikolsky sign can be elicited from the gingival tissues.

Histopathology.

Gingival lesions of pemphigus vulgaris are similar to the oral mucosal lesions. Biopsy specimens from properly selected sites show extensive acantholysis, with the basal cell layer of the epithelium remaining attached to the underlying corium. Cells in the upper layers of epithelium show separation from each other. This separation is preceded by oedema within the cells of the stratum spinosum. As the process proceeds, a space is formed above the basal cell layer that contains fluid. The fully developed lesion is characterized by the presence of an intra-epithelial bulla. Epithelial cells within the bulla become rounded. These are referred to as Tzanck cells, and they can sometimes be found on exfoliative cytology. The underlying connective tissue is infiltrated with PMNs and lymphocytes.

At an ultrastructural level, there is widening of the intercellular spaces of the stratum spinosum, a gradual disintegration of desmosomes, and clumping of tonofilaments. As the desmosomal attachments disappear, the cells separate and cell surfaces develop numerous microvilli (Hashimoto 1972).

Direct immunofluorescent techniques are useful in the diagnosis of pemphigus vulgaris. Intercellular deposits of IgG are present in the skin and mucous membranes of virtually all patients with pemphigus vulgaris (Jordan *et al.* 1971; Daniels and Quadra-White 1980). Patients with pemphigus vulgaris have a raised serum antibody titre to epithelial intercellular substance. This finding provides a further useful diagnostic test.

Management

Before the advent of corticosteroid therapy, most cases of pemphigus were fatal. Systemic prednisolone is the treatment of choice and, for very severe forms of the disease, dosages of up to 180 mg day can be given. These high dosages are not without their own complications and such patients will need to be carefully monitored. Immunosuppressive agents such as azathioprine, methotrexate, and cyclophosphamide are also used in the management of pemphigus. These immunosuppressant agents reduce the need for high doses of prednisolone (Lever 1972). Gold salts have also been used in conjunction with corticosteroids in the management of pemphigus vulgaris. Although the prognosis for pemphigus is much improved with the use of combined corticosteroid and immunosuppressant therapy, the mortality rate is still about 8 per cent (Lever and Schaumburg-Lever 1977).

Local corticosteroids are also useful in the management of pemphigus vulgaris. Triamcinolone acetonide and fluocinolone acetenonide have both been shown to be useful topical preparations (Orlowski *et al.* 1983).

A further management problem where lesions involve the gingiva is that of plaque control. Pain, soreness, and bleeding prohibit mechanical plaque control. Furthermore, the build up of plaque exacerbates the gingival inflammatory changes. Where possible, toothbrushing with a soft brush should be encouraged. As with all these desquamative and erosive lesions, chlorhexidine mouthwash (0.2%) will inhibit plaque build-up and reduce secondary infection of ulcerative areas.

3.11.4 Benign mucous membrane pemphigoid (BMMP)

This chronic vesiculobullous condition is sometimes referred to as cicatrical pemphigoid or mucous membrane pemphigus. BMMP occurs most often after 40 years of age and is more 'common' in women (Laskaris *et al.* 1982). Lesions are nearly always found on the oral mucosa. Other commonly affected sites include the eyes, genitals, oesophagus, nasal and rectal mucosa; the skin is rarely involved.

In BMMP, bullae or vesicles appear below the epidermis at the level of the basement membrane. Oral lesions heal without scarring, but ocular lesions cause conjunctivitis, shallowing of the fornix, and entropion with trichiasis. In severe cases the lesions can cause blindness. Oesophageal involvement can lead to dysphagia.

Although BMMP has distinct clinical and histological features, evidence from skin and mucosal biopsies suggest that this condition may comprise a heterogeneous group of diseases that include bullous pemphigoid and linear IgA disease (Williams *et al.* 1984).

Oral and gingival lesions

Although bullae do appear in the mouth in cases of BMMP, they do not persist for long, and the typical lesion is an area of ulceration. However, the most characteristic oral lesion is desquamative gingivitis (Shklar and McCarthy 1971). The entire width of the attached gingiva is affected and may appear as a diffuse or patchy zone of erythema with varying degrees of redness (Plate 17). Some desquamation may be visible, and it can usually be elicited when the gingival tissues are gently scraped. Edentulous areas are not as frequently involved as dentate. If a denture is being worn and is causing trauma to the underlying mucosa, then erosions and ulcers may be seen. Healing of erosive or ulcerative areas in BMMP is very slow and can take months or even years. Healing of the gingival lesions occurs without scarring. Also, scarring of the oral mucosa is not a prominant feature of BMMP (Fine and Weathers 1980).

Histopathology

The histopathological features of oral BMMP include subepithelial vesiculation and a chronic inflammatory infiltrate into the underlying corium (Shklar and McCarthy 1971). This infiltrate consists of lymphocytes, plasma cells, and histiocytes. If the vesicle has ruptured, then these changes can be observed at the margins of the lesion. Acantholysis is never observed in BMMP, which helps to distinguish the lesion from pemphigus vulgaris.

Electron microscopical studies have shown the following changes in the tissue adjacent to a developing vesicle: increased cellularity in the connective tissue, increased amounts of basal lamina material, evidence of increased activity of basal cells, projections of basal cells through the basal lamina, and decreased numbers of anchoring fibrils (Susi and Shklar 1971).

Immunofluorescent techniques are very useful in the diagnosis of BMMP. IgG, IgA, C3 and C4 have been found along the basement membrane zone (Bean *et al.* 1972; Holubar *et al.* 1973). In a small proportion of cases, circulating antibodies to basement membrane are found. This supports the view that BMMP is closely related to the skin condition of bullous pemphigoid (Williams *et al.* 1984).

Management

Combinations of topical, systemic corticosteroids, and immunosuppressent drugs (azathioprine and cyclophosphamide) have been used in the management of BMMP. However, it is, in general, less responsive to corticosteroid than the other vesiculobullous disorders and treatment is often aimed at controlling the disease rather than complete resolution (Person and Rogers 1977).

Topical corticosteroids remain the treatment of choice and alleviate symptoms without causing serious systemic effects. Skin grafting has been used to treat a denture-bearing area affected by BMMP (O'Hara *et al.* 1980). A 12-month follow-up showed satisfactory healing and no recurrence of the lesion.

Eye changes are the most important lesions of BMMP. These patients should be regularly seen by an ophthalmologist.

The problems of plaque control in patients with desquamative gingivitis have previously been discussed and equally apply to patients with BMMP.

3.11.5 Psoriasis

Psoriasis is a common skin disorder characterized by well-circumscribed papules covered with scales. Biopsy of skin lesions shows hyperkeratosis with parakeratosis, acanthosis, elongation of the rete ridges and dermal papillae, epidermal microabscess formation, and oedema. Psoriasis may be associated with arthritis.

Oral and gingival lesions

It is still uncertain whether psoriasis has any oral manifestations; certainly oral lesions are rare. Pindborg (1980) described three oral lesions that may be related to this skin disorder. These are: (a) minute, well-defined, grey to yellowish-white, raised oral plaques; (b) geographic tongue; (c) diffuse erythema of the oral mucosa that coincides with acute skin exacerbations.

Desquamative gingivitis has also been described in cases of psoriasis (Degregori *et al.* 1971; Jones and Dolby 1972). Such lesions are managed with topical corticosteroids.

3.11.6 Differential diagnosis

Many of the mucocutaneous disorders present as desquamative gingivitis and therefore pose a problem of differential diagnosis. A thorough clinical examination of the mouth and skin may reveal a characteristic feature of a particular disease and thus facilitate diagnosis. In most cases, biopsy and immunofluorescent techniques are required to establish a definitive diagnosis. Desquamative gingivitis can also be drug-induced and related to the menopause. These factors should be considered if laboratory investigations are inconclusive.

APPENDIX

Table 3.2 Synopsis of the various findings from epidemiological studies investigating the relationship between diabetes mellitus and periodontal disease

Study	No. of diabetic patients (ages in years)	No. of control patients (ages in years)	Type of diabetes	Periodontal measures	Diabetic measures	Findings
Mackenzie and Millard (1963)	60 confirmed diabetics (32–78) 64 suspected diabetics	54 arteriosclerotic patients	Mixed	Tooth loss Calculus index Bone loss	Retinal change Blood glucose	Calculus scores did not differ significantly between groups A high positive correlation between levels of calculus and bone loss Diabetes mellitus is not associated with increased alveolar bone loss
Belting et al. (1964)*	78 males (20–89)	79 males (20–89)	Mixed	Periodontal index Brushing frequency Calculus index Bruxism	Age of patient Hypoglycaemic therapy	Severity of periodontal disease was greater among diabetics Age of patient played a more important role in the severity of periodontal disease than the degree of diabetes as determined by the method of control
Finestone and Boorujy (1967)**	189	64	Mixed	Periodontal index	Age of patient Method of control Duration of diabetes Blood sugar Systemic complications	Prevalence and severity of periodontal disease is increased in diabetics Periodontal index was related to age, duration of diabetes, the presence of diabetic complications, and variation in blood sugar
Benveniste et al.(1967)	53 (5–72)	71 (5–72)	Mixed	Gingival inflammation Calculus formation Pocket depth	Age of patient	No significant differences between diabetics and non-diabetics for gingival inflammation, calculus formation, and pocket depth
Hove and Stallard (1970)	28 (20–40, 40+)	16 (20–40, 40+)	Mixed	Oral debris index Calculus index Gingival index Pocket depth Bone loss Gingival biopsy	Age of patient Severity of diabetes	No significant differences between diabetics and non-diabetics for any of the periodontal measures Vascular changes in the gingival connective tissue were more frequent in the diabetic (71%) than in the non-diabetic Periodontal disease increased with age in both groups and was directly related to the accumulation of plaque and calculus
Cohen* et al. (1970)* 2-year longitudinal study	21 females (18–35)	18 females (18–35)	Not stated	Gingival index Attachment loss Plaque score Calculus score Tooth mobility	–	Diabetic group had a significantly greater gingival index and greater loss of attachment at each visit than the non-diabetic group. Plaque scores were significantly less in the diabetics Calculus scores were the same in each group

Table 3.2 continued

Study	No. of diabetic patients (ages in years)	No. of control patients (ages in years)	Type of diabetes	Periodontal measures	Diabetic measures	Findings
Nichols et al. (1978)	54 (30–73)	–	Mixed	Periodontal disease index (PDI)	Age of patient Diabetic control Duration Systemic complications Blood glucose	No significant relationship between PDI and duration of diabetes, type of treatment, frequency of systemic complications Periodontal disease in the diabetic appears to be affected by the same aetiological agents as would be expected in the non-diabetic
Sznajder et al. (1978)**	83 (5–50)	65 (9–50)	Mixed	Plaque index Gingival index Calculus index Attachment loss	Age of patient (<30, >30 years)	Loss of attachment was higher in the diabetic group age >30 Gingival index was greater in the diabetic group, but plaque and calculus indices were similar In both groups, periodontal destruction increased with age
Ervasti et al. (1985)*	50 (<30, 30–40, >40)	53 (<30, 30–40, >40)	Mixed	Plaque index Plaque retention areas Presence of supra- and gingival calculus Gingival bleeding	Control of diabetes Duration Systemic complications Treatment Age of patient	Overall, no significant differences between diabetics and controls for periodontal measures Poorly controlled diabetics suffered significantly more gingival bleeding than other diabetics Gingival changes in diabetics did not relate to complications, medication, or duration of disease
Tervonen and Knuuttila, (1986)	50 (<30, 30–40, >40)	53 (<30, 30–40, >40)	Mixed	Plaque retention Calculus score Gingival bleeding Probing depth Bone loss	Age of patient Control of diabetes	Alveolar bone loss and frequency of periodontal pockets were not significantly different between controls and diabetics Well-controlled diabetics had better periodontal health than controls. Within the diabetic group, the prevalence of pockets declined as the control of diabetes improved
Glavind* et al. (1968)*	51 males (20–40)	51 males (20–40)	IDDM†	Plaque score Gingival index Attachment loss Pocket depth	Age of patient Duration of diabetes Dosage of insulin Retinal changes	No significant difference in gingival index, pocket depth, and plaque scores between diabetics and controls Attachment loss was similar in both groups up to the age of 30. Between the age of 30–40, greater attachment loss occurred in the diabetics No correlation between periodontal destruction and insulin dosages Diabetics with retinal changes showed greater loss of attachment

Study	No. (age range)	No. (age range)	Type	Indices	Factors considered	Results
Bernick et al. (1975)*	50 (3–16)	36 (3–16)	IDDM	Plaque scores, Calculus scores, Gingival inflammation, Attachment loss	Age of patient, Duration of diabetes	Greater incidence of gingival inflammation in diabetic group. Plaque scores, calculus scores, and attachment loss were similar in both groups
Ringelberg et al. (1977)*	56 (10–16)	41 (10–12)	IDDM	Modified Gingival Index (MGI), Flow of gingival crevicular fluid (GCF)	Age of patient	Children with diabetes had significantly more gingival inflammation than control children. A small but significant correlation between GCF and MGI in the diabetics
Gislen et al. (1980)*	43 (7–17)	43 (7–17)	IDDM	Plaque Index, Gingival Index (GI)	Degree of metabolic control	For children with high plaque scores, the diabetic patients showed a significantly higher GI than controls. Diabetic children with poor metabolic control showed a clear tendency towards higher GI scores than non-diabetics
Cianciola et al. (1982)**	263 (<10, >19)	208 (<10, >19)	IDMM	Plaque Index, Gingival inflammation, Probing depths, Bone loss, Tooth mobility	Age of patient, Duration of diabetes	Diabetic patients had a higher prevalence of severe gingivitis and periodontitis than controls, and this prevalence increased with age. The plaque indices were similar in both groups. Alveolar bone loss in diabetics occurs most frequently around the first molars and incisors
Gusberti et al. (1983)*	77 (6–17)	64 (6–15)	IDDM	Papillary Bleeding Score (PBS), Microbial investigation	Age of patient, Sexual maturity, Blood glucose, Diabetic control	Diabetic children exhibited an increase in gingivitis as a function of both age and puberty. Diabetic measures did not relate to gingival changes except in prepubertal children. A significant increase in Capnocytophaga spp. occurred at the onset of puberty and then declined
Barnett et al. (1984)	45 (10–18)	–	IDDM	Plaque Index, Gingival Index, Bone loss	Age of patient, Duration of diabetes, Diabetic control	Gingival index did not relate to age of patient or duration of disease. Degree of diabetic control, as assessed by HbA_1 levels, did not correlate with gingival index, plaque index, or duration of disease. There was no radiographic evidence of interproximal bone loss
Goteiner et al. (1986)	169 (5–18)	80 (mean 12)	IDDM	Plaque Index, Gingival Index, Periodontal Disease Index (PDI)	Family history of diabetes	Diabetic group had a significantly higher plaque score than the control group. However, the gingival index and PDI were practically identical for both groups

Table 3.2 *continued*

Study	No. of diabetic patients (ages in years)	No. of control patients (ages in years)	Type of diabetes	Periodontal measures	Diabetic measures	Findings
Rylander *et al.* (1986)**	46 (19–25)	41 (18–26)	IDDM	Plaque Index Gingival Index Probing depth Attachment loss Gingival recession Bone loss	Duration of diabetes Insulin dosage Metabolic control Presence of retinopathy/ nephropathy	No significant difference between the 2 groups in their oral hygiene status, probing depths > 3 mm, and bone loss. Diabetics had a higher frequency of inflamed gingival units, sites with attachment loss > 2 mm, and more gingival recession No correlations were found between periodontal variables and the duration of diabetes, insulin dosage, and HbA$_1$ levels Diabetics with retinopathy and nephropathy had significantly more gingival inflammation than diabetics without these complications
Rosenthal *et al.* (1988)	52 (11–22)	Diabetics were assigned to a periodontitis/ non-periodontitis group	IDDM	Plaque Index Gingival Index Sulcular Bleeding Index (SBI) Pocket depth Bone loss	Age of patient Duration of diabetes Insulin dose Serum glucose Systemic complications	Moderate to advanced periodontitis was found in 5.8 per cent of subjects GI and SBI were significantly higher in periodontitis group There was a greater % of ketoacidosis, retinopathy and neuropathy in the periodontitis group
Hugoson *et al.* (1989)*	82 diabetics of long duration 72 diabetics of short duration	77	IDDM	2-point plaque score Presence/absence of supra- and subgingival calculus Gingival bleeding Probing pocket depth Bone loss	–	No significant difference in plaque scores and the presence of both types of calculus between the diabetics and controls. Diabetics had more gingival inflammation than non-diabetics Diabetics of long duration had greater probing depths and more bone loss than those of short duration
Sastrowijoto *et al.* (1989)	22 divided into normal and poor metabolic control (18–60)	–	IDDM	Plaque Index Sulcus bleeding index Periodontal pocket bleeding index Microbiology of subgingival plaque	Diabetic control Age of patient Duration of diabetes	No significant differences between groups for any of the periodontal measures Neither the age of the patient nor duration of diabetes influenced the periodontal measures Proportionally higher percentages of *A. actinomycetemcomitans*, *Bact. gingivalis* and *Bact. intermedius* were isolated from diseased periodontal pockets in both groups of patients. Findings suggest that the degree of metabolic control does not appear to have a direct effect on the periodontium

* Study showing that diabetics are slightly susceptible to increased periodontal breakdown.
** Study showing that diabetics are markedly susceptible to increased periodontal breakdown.
† Insulin-dependent diabetes mellitus.

Table 3.3 Synopsis of periodontal findings from epidemiological studies on periodontal disease in Down's syndrome

Study	No. of patients (sex, age in years)	Control group (age in years)	Periodontal measures	Findings
Brown and Cunningham (1961)	80 (50M,30F; 1.5–39) Institutionalized	–	Pocket depth Tooth mobility Gingival ulceration Microbiology Gingival colour Severity of periodontal disease	The incidence of periodontal disease was approx. 90%. The disease appears to commence at an early age, affect the lower incisor region, and bear little relation to local factors Severity of periodontal disease increased with age of sample 36% of children below 6 years of age had pocket formation
Cohen et al. (1961)	100 (1–30)	–	Gingival inflammation and no. of teeth involved Bone loss Pocket formation Tooth migration Gingival biopsy (20 patients only)	Severe periodontal disease was found in 96% of the subjects ANUG was found in 29 Down's patients Although local factors were present in abundance the severe alveolar bone loss and inflammatory changes suggest that systemic factors may influence the response of the periodontal tissues to plaque
Kisling and Krebs (1963)	71 M (19–25) 57 institutionalized; 14 non-institutionalized	–	Plaque score Gingival inflammation Calculus score Ramfjord's Periodontal Score Mobility	All patients suffered from periodontal disease with the upper first molars and lower central incisors frequently involved A high correlation between Ramfjord's index and the calculus scores No significant correlation between plaque scores and gingival findings
Johnson and Young (1963)	70 (mean 10.8)	40 (mean 11.8) Non-mongoloid, mentally defective	Periodontal condition was assessed on a 4-point scale: 0 = healthy 3 = obvious destruction of periodontal tissues Bone loss	Both groups had a high prevalence of periodontal disease, but the severity in Down's syndrome was twice that of the mentally defective patients The severity and pattern of periodontal destruction in Down's syndrome is suggestive of a systemic aetiological factor
Cohen and Winer (1965)	123 (3–30) Institutionalized	94 Institutionalized, mentally retarded	Gingival condition was assessed by the PMA index Periodontal disease assessed by Russell Index	The PMA index in the mentally retarded group was slightly higher than in the Down's group Russell Index was considerably higher in the Down's group than in the mentally retarded patients
Sznajder et al. (1968)	123 (4–21) Non-institutionalized	–	Ramfjord's indices for: (a) gingivitis (b) calculus (c) mobility (d) plaque Ramfjord's Periodontal Disease Index	A high incidence of severe periodontal disease with pocket formation was found associated with heavy plaque formation The most severe changes were in the lower anterior region

Table 3.3 *continued*

Study	No. of patients (sex, age in years)	Control group (age in years)	Periodontal measures	Findings
Shapiro et al. (1969)	14 (10–27) Institution-alized	–	Oral Hygiene index (Green and Vermillion) Bone loss Plasma levels of citrate	Poor oral hygiene, severe bone loss, and elevated blood citrate levels (means = 2.47 mg/%) were observed in the Down's patients Suggestion that macroglossia and systemic hormonal disturbances may be additional contributory factors to the early occurrence of periodontitis
Cutress (1971)	106 (10–24) Institution-alized 117 (10–24) Non-institutionalized	130 (10–24) Institution-alized, mentally retarded 127 (10–24) Non-institutionalized mentally retarded 464 (10–24) Normal	Oral Hygiene Index (Green and Vermillion) Periodontal Index (Russell)	All groups had similar correlations between oral hygiene and periodontal scores The Periodontal Index was highest in the institutionalized Down's patients and lowest in the normal controls No significant difference in Periodontal Index scores were found between institutionalized Down's and institutionalized mentally retarded patients An institutionalized environment increases the susceptibility of Down's patients to periodontal disease
Orner (1976)	212 (5–19)	124 (5–20) Siblings of Down's patients	Russell Periodontal Index	The prevalence of periodontal disease was 89% in the Down's group and 58% in their siblings
Miller and Ship (1977)	12 (mean age 18.1) Institutionalized	18 (mean age 18.9) Institutionalized epileptics 18 (mean age 19) Institutionalized spastics	Russell Periodontal Index at 1-yearly intervals	47 of the 48 subjects had some form of periodontal disease 31% of the sample had atrophic periodontal disease characterized by gingivitis, pocket formation, bone loss, and mobility Periodontal disease progressed at the rate of 0.9 P.I. per year in Down's children and this rate of loss was highest in the youngest age group
Saxen et al. (1977)	35 (9–39) Institutionalized	35 (9–39) Institutionalized; 9 mentally retarded	Bone loss Radiographic presence of calculus	69% of patients with Down's syndrome showed advanced bone loss (>5 mm) as compared to 29% in the control group Bone loss was detected around the lower first molars in 17.8% of Down's and 3% of controls Levels of radiographically detectable calculus were similar for both groups
Brown (1978)	32 (2–16) Institutionalized	Longitudinal study:	Oral Hygiene Index	In each age group, gingival, periodontal, and oral hygiene scores increased at successive examinations (yearly intervals). The greatest increase was in the youngest group
	3 groups: <6, 6–10, 11–16	Patients assessed over 2 years	Ramfjord's Periodontal Disease Index	Advanced periodontal disease could develop very rapidly and was associated with crowding of the teeth and episodes of ANUG

Reference	Subjects (n, age range)	Indices	Findings
Saxen and Aula (1982) [5-yr. follow-up study on Saxen et al. (1977)]	24 (14–43) Institutionalized 28 (17–40) Institutionalized, mentally retarded	As Saxen et al. (1977)	The prevalence rate of bone loss >5mm showed little or no increase in Down's patients (69–75%), whereas in the controls, the rate of increase was greater (20–43%) Percentage of affected teeth with bone loss >5mm had increased in the Down's patients from 25 to 47%; for control patients, the increase was 1.8 to 6.8% Around mandibular first molars, the progress in bone loss was more rapid in controls (28.3%) than Down's patients (12.7%)
Vigild (1985)	19 (6–19) Institutionalized, mentally retarded 38 (6–19) Non-institutionalized, mentally retarded	Gingival Index Plaque Index Presence of supra gingival calculus	Patients with Down's syndrome have a tendency for a more severe gingivitis, despite the finding that they had lower plaque and calculus scores than the controls Socio-economic status was a more important determinant of periodontal condition than whether the subjects were residential or otherwise
Izmui et al. (1989)	14 (12–34) 14 (23–26) Healthy subjects	Oral hygiene (O'Leary) Gingival Index Pocket depth Bone loss Neutrophil chemotaxis	Down's patients showed significantly lower neutrophil chemotaxis than healthy controls. However, random neutrophil migration was the same for both groups Down's patients had various prevalences of bone loss, which was inversely proportional to the neutrophil chemotactic index. Thus, defective neutrophil may influence the progression of periodontal disease in these patients

Table 3.6 Synopsis of dental reports of Wegener's granulomatosis

Reference	Age	Sex	Initial symptoms	Duration of illness	Ginvigal involvement	Gingival pathology	Other oral lesions	Extraoral involvement	ESR	Treatment	Outcome
Milner (1955)	41	F	Painful enlargement of gingiva	8½ weeks	Enlarged, painful nodular gingival tissues; bluish-grey colour. Changes confined to the upper and lower anterior teeth	Epithelial hyperplasia with microabscesses, granuloma formation. Multinucleated giant cells throughout gingival connective tissues	Failure of extraction sites to heal	Paranasal sinuses, kidney, eyes and skin	–	Antimicrobials	Fatal
Morgan and O'Neil (1956)	26	M	Recurring neck ulcer and gingivitis	7 months	Generalized, hyperplastic, granular gingivitis	Non-specific chronic inflammation; no vascular changes	Alveolar bone loss and an unhealed extraction site	Lung, kidney, and an ulcer on forehead	33	Antimicrobials	Death within 4 months
Walton (1958)	39	M	Painful gums and limb pains	6 weeks	–	–	–	Skin	–	–	–
Levan (1960)	29	F	–	4 months	Enlarged, painful, friable, granular gingiva	–	Tooth mobility, alveolar bone loss and necrosis	Paranasal sinuses, skin, and lung	–	–	Fatal
Cawson (1965)	17	F	Gingivitis, together with a painless, progressive swelling of lymph nodes	4 weeks	Bleeding from interdental papillae; granular gingival appearance with several petechiae	Non-specific chronic inflammation with giant cells; no vascular changes	Periodontal pocketing	Severe and persistent rhinitis; spleen enlargement	–	Corticosteroids	Fatal in 4 months
Kakehashi et al. (1965)	37	M	Persistent swollen and painful gingiva. Headache, sinus pain, rhinitis, and weight loss	2 months	Gingival tissues friable, enlarged; changes on both the free and attached gingiva	Non-specific inflammation, no vascular changes; giant cells in connective tissue. Epithelium showed pseudo-epitheliomatous hyperplasia with microabscess formation	Gross alveolar bone loss in retromolar area; slow healing of an extraction site	Nose, right antrum, cervical lymph nodes, thyroid gland, kidney	–	Antimicrobials and prednisolone	Fatal within 16 weeks
Brooke (1969)	44	M	Bleeding and a painless swelling of the gums; patient felt 'run down'	6 weeks	Enlarged gingiva around most of the standing teeth; gingival tissues had a purplish-red, granular appearance	Non-specific inflammation with giant cells; no vascular changes seen	Marked alveolar bone loss around lower incisors	Liver, nose antrum, lungs, and kidneys	59	Prednisolone	Fatal within 1 month
Scott and Finch (1972)	23	F	Swelling, bleeding and painful gums; progressively enlarging skin ulcers	4 months	Pale hyperplastic gingiva with multiple, dark-red petechiae; tissues had a granular and spongy consistency	Intense, acute and chronic, granulomatous infiltration of connective tissue with occasional giant cells; no vascular changes; pseudo-epitheliomatous hyperplasia with abscess formation	Severe bone loss, especially around molars	Lungs, sinuses, middle ear, and skin	104	Prednisone, azathioprine, cyclophosphamide, methotrexate	Alive at 21 months

Reference	Age	Sex	Presenting complaint	Duration	Oral findings	Histology	Other findings	Organs involved	ESR	Treatment	Outcome
Edwards and Buckerfiled (1976)	31	M	Non-healing extraction site	4 months	Gingiva red, friable, granulomatous; changes confined to extraction quadrant	Acute and chronic inflammatory changes with localized granulomas, which contained giant-cell necrotic tissue and showed fibrinoid degeneration and microabscess formation	Loss of alveolar bone, oroantral fistula at extraction site, mobile teeth	Nose, antrum, skin, myocardium, pancreas, spleen, and kidneys	35	Prednisone penicillin, nasal drops, and cyclophosphamide	Fatal after 5 weeks
Israelson et al. (1981)	49	F	Painful, bleeding, and swollen gums; rhinitis and sinusitis	6 weeks	Gingiva had an exophytic, red-purple appearance (strawberry gingiva)	Pseudo-epitheliomatous hyperplasia, connective tissue showed acute and chronic inflammatory changes with multinucleated giant cells and eosinophils	—	Nasal septum, antrum, and skin	85	Prednisone and cyclophosphamide	Alive
Cohen and Meltzer (1981)	57	M	Swelling of the gums, shortness of breath, polyarthralgia, haemoptysis, and fever	4 months	Hyperplastic granular gingiva, with petechiae on the inderdental papillae	Acute necrotizing vasculitisa; pseudo-epitheliomatous hyperplasia	—	Lung, nose, kidney, and skin	126	Prednisone and cyclophosphamide	Alive
Handlers et al. (1985)	11	M	Swelling of the gums and otitis media	24 months	Hyperplastic gingivitis, especially in the interdental areas; petechiae on attached gingiva	Pseudo-epitheliomatous hyperplasia; connective tissues showed haemorrhagic changes, acute and chronic inflammation with giant cells and eosinophils	—	Ear, nose, sinuses, lung, and kidney	High	Prednisone and cyclophosphamide	Alive after 14 months
Raustia et al. (1985)	36	M	Sinusitus, otitis, bleeding and swollen gums, pyrexia, and weight loss	3 months	Hyperplastic, bleeding gingiva with strawberry appearance	Non-specific, intense inflammation characterized by acute necrotizing vasculitis and giant cells	Enlargement of the right maxillary tuberosity	Lungs, eyes, nose, larynx, and kidney	—	Prednisone and azathioprine	Alive
Horan et al. (1986)	36	F	Gingival enlargement, night sweats	1 month	Marked gingival hyperplasia with a spongy, bluish-red appearance; changes more obvious in the mandible	Pseudo-epitheliomatous hyperplasia with marked inflammatory changes in the connective tissues; blood vessels engulfed by inflammatory changes and contained fibrinous thrombi	—	Skin and lungs	112	Prednisone and cyclophosphamide	Alive
Parsons et al. (1991)	63	M	Spreading, swollen gums	1 month	Generalized hyperplastic gingivitis with petechiae	Irregular hyperplastic epithelium; connective tissue was grossly inflamed with multiple foci of chronic suppuration; no vascular changes	—	Left antrum	48	Steroid mouthwash	Alive

Table 3.7 Synopsis of the case reports of oral involvement in histiocytosis X

Study	Sex	Age (years)	First complaint	Oral involvement	Intraoral radiographic appearance	Extraoral involvement	Extraoral radiographic appearance	Treatment
Moskow et al. (1971)	M	37	Mobile teeth; gingival bleeding	Mobile teeth; gingival bleeding	Marked vertical alveolar destruction			Excision and radiation
	F	25	Soreness and ulceration on the right palate; discomfort on left mandibular region	Deep pockets, suprabony and intrabony, in right palatal region and lower left molars; exposure of roots; crater-like ulcers on right side of palate	Marked destruction of alveolar bone			
Cararo et al. (1972)	M	24	Pain in gum; tooth mobility for several months	Pain in mandibular right molar area; attached gingival alveolar mucosa of the central incisors showed circumscribed area of periodontal destruction and ulceration without gingival margin	Resorption of alveolar crest in area of maxillary left molars and mandibular central incisors; osteolytic areas in edentulous mandibular right posterior region			Radiation
Whitehead (1972)	M	24	Discomfort and intermittent pain	Discomfort and pain in lower incisors	Periapical lesion in lower incisors		Translucency in neck of left femur	Radiation
	M	25	Pain from lower left incisor	Lateral periodontal abscess from lower incisor	Translucency around $\overline{1}$		Translucency of ileum, pelvis, humerus, skull, neck of femur, and one rib	Radiation
McKelvy et al. (1975)	F	37	Persistent left mandibular swelling	Erythematous gingiva; persistent fistula tract; several nodules in left mandibular buccal vestibule	Radiolucency in left body of mandible with diffuse border	Diabetes insipidus; enlargement in lower facial area, axilla, vulva, left leg	Skull	
Kaufman et al. (1976)	F	54	Mobile teeth	Mobile teeth	Numerous lytic defects of alveolar bone	Polyuria; polydipsia		ACTH
Soskolne et al. (1977)	F	28	Acute pain and swelling on lower right jaw	Swelling around $\overline{2}$	Radiolucency and alveolar destruction between $\overline{2}$ and $\overline{3}$			Excision
Lin et al. (1979)	F	17	Pain and discomfort from lower left jaw	Mobile teeth $\overline{6\ 7}$	Periapical radiolucency $\overline{6}$			Radiation
Cranin and Rockman (1981)	M	21	Severe thirst; tooth mobility	Mobile teeth	Radiolucency in maxillary molar region and lower incisors	Occipital cyst; upper respiratory infection; urination		Radiation; pitressin
	F	24	Pain in lower right jaw	Mobile teeth	Alveolar bone destruction	Ileum; anaemia; diabetes insipidus	Left pelvis	Radiation; prednisone
Fitzpatrick et al. (1981)	F	19	Tenderness on right side of jaw; frequent headaches; chronic itching and drainage from ear canals	Chronic inflammation and ulceration of gingiva	Multiple osteolytic defect in the mandible	Diabetes insipidus; cervical adenopathy; drainage from ear canals; amenorrhea; discharge from nipples		Radiation to the pituitary gland; chlorpropamide; prednisone; vasopressin
Cohn et al. (1982)	M	16		Palate, right maxilla		Diabetes insipidus; exophthalmos; skull—sella turcica	Skull	
Jensen et al. (1982)	M	27	Mobile, painful teeth in lower jaw	Mobile teeth of lower right molars and tenderness	Cystic radiolucent area in the mandible			Radiation; prednisone; methotrexate; aminopterin; vincristine

Reference	Sex	Age						Treatment
Gorsky et al. (1983)	M	13	Pelvic pain	Periodontal lesions	Radiolucency in the mandible		Pelvic; pituitary gland: lymphadenopathy; diabetes insipidus	Radiation and chemotherapy (Velban and prednisone)
	F	16	Pain and mobility on the lower right of the mandible	Precocious periodontitis	Severe alveolar bone loss		Hip; lung; clavicle	Radiation followed by chemotherapy (Velban and prednisone)
	M	30	Painful ulcer	Erythematous gingival lesion	Multiple mandibular lesions	Hip and knee	Diabetes insipidus; polyuria	Radiation
	F	31	Pain in lower left jaw	Gingival necrosis; mobile teeth	Radiolucency in mandible			Radiation and chemotherapy
	M	36	Acute pain of the right upper jaw	Swelling and pain of the right maxillary molar area	Radiolucency in the maxilla	Radiolucency of the frontal skull	Lump on the frontal skull; diabetes insipidus	Radiation
	M	40	Painful swelling	Swelling in lower right jaw	Radiolucency in right ramus of the mandible			Radiation
Krutchkoff and Jones (1984)	F	21	Painful gums	Erythematous and tender gingival margins	Extensive destruction; lytic area in left mandible			Radiation; prednisone; methotrexate
Zuendel et al. (1984)	M	19	Mobile and sore teeth	Mobile teeth, painful to percussion	Multiple bony lesions in the mandible	Multiple lesions in skull and two ribs		Extractions; radiation; methotrexate; mercaptopurine
Hashimoto et al. (1985)	M	63	Painful oral lesions	Ulcerations: xerostomia			Polyuria; polydipsia malaise; fatigue	Radiation
Macintyre et al. (1985)	M	31	Generalized malaise; gum abscess	Recurrent acute periodontal abscesses	Extensive radiolucent areas related to mandibular teeth—'floating in space'	Radiolucency in the right ileum	Cervical lymphadenopathy; diabetes insipidus	Radiation and chemotheraphy
Pareek and Hawass (1985)	M	20	Gum enlargement	Destructive periodontal disease			Ulcers in groin and axilla; discharge from right ear; nails; upper left eyelid; pneumothorax; perianal ulceration	Chemotherapy
Urbano-Marquez et al. (1985)	F	48	Mobile teeth	Mobile teeth			Diabetes insipidus; ulcerative vulval lesions; severe pain in humoral region	Etoposiole epipadophyllatoxin
Moorthy (1986)	M	31	Localized abscess: mobile teeth in upper and lower quadrants	Severe periodontal disease; enlarged submaxillary lymph node, tender to palpation	Marked foci of bone destruction			Curettage
Whitcher and Webb (1986)	M	28	Pain in right jaw	Right mandibular swelling	Multiple radiolucent lesions in right mandibular ramus and body regions	Lytic lesions with well-defined borders in the 6th rib and left acetabulum	Left rib, flank pain	Radiation; curettage; autogenous bone graft
Artzi et al. (1989)	M	32	Painful gums	Gingival inflammation; erosions and ulceration			Enlargement of submaxillary salivary glands and right lobe of the thyroid gland; severe bilateral otitis externa	Excision and chemotherapy

REFERENCES

Diabetes mellitus

Asplund, K. (1981). Diabetes, mumps and HLA antigens. *Lancet*, **ii**, 807.

Barnett, M. L., Baker, R. L., and Yancey, J. M. (1984). Absence of periodontitis in a population of insulin-dependent diabetes mellitus patients. *Journal of Periodontology*, **55**, 402–5.

Bay, I., Ainamo, J., and Gad, I. (1974). The response of young diabetics to periodontal treatment. *Journal of Periodontology*, **45**, 806–16.

Belting, C. M., Hiniker, J. J., and Dummett, C. O. (1964). Influence of diabetes mellitus on the severity of periodontal disease. *Journal of Periodontology*, **35**, 476–80.

Beneviste, R., Bixler, D., and Conneally, P. M. (1967). Periodontal disease in diabetes. *Journal of Periodontology*, **38**, 271–9.

Bernick, S. M., Cohen, D. W., Baker, L., and Laster, L. (1975). Dental diseases in children with diabetes mellitus. *Journal of Periodontology*, **46**, 241–5.

Bunn, H. F., Hanney, D. N., Kamin, S., Gabbay, K. H., and Gallop, P. M. (1976). The biosynthesis of human hemoglobin A^{Ic}: slow glycosylation of hemoglobin *in vivo*. *Journal of Clinical Investigation*, **57**, 1652–9.

Burkjett, L. and Sindoni, A. (1959). Diabetes and the dental patient. *Journal of the American Dental Association*, **58**, 81–5.

Chavers, B., Etzwiler, D., and Michael, A. (1981). Albumin deposition in dermal capillary basement membrane in insulin-dependent diabetes mellitus. *Diabetes*, **30**, 275–8.

Cianciola, L. J., Park, B. H., Bruck, E., Mosovich, L., and Genco, R. J. (1982). Prevalence of periodontal disease in insulin-dependent diabetes mellitus (juvenile diabetes). *Journal of the American Dental Association*, **104**, 653–60.

Clark, R. (1978). Disorders of granulocyte chemotaxis. In *Leukocyte chemotaxis* (ed. J. Gallin and P. Quie), pp. 329–52. Raven Press, New York.

Cohen, D. W., Friedman, L. A., Shapiro, J., Kyle, G., and Frankin, S. (1970). Diabetes mellitus and periodontal disease: two-year longitudinal observations. Part I. *Journal of Periodontology*, **41**, 709–12.

Ervasti, T., Knuttila, M., Phjamo, L., and Haukipuro, K. (1985). Relation between control of diabetes and gingival bleeding. *Journal of Periodontology*, **56**, 154–7.

Ficara, A., Leven, M., Grower, M., and Fraker, G. (1975). A comparison of the glucose and protein content of gingival fluid from diabetics and non-diabetics. *Journal of Periodontal Research*, **10**, 171–5.

Finestone, A. and Boojury, S. (1967). Diabetes mellitus and periodontal disease. *Diabetes*, **16**, 336–40.

Frantzis, T. G., Reeve, C. M., and Brown, A. L. (1971). The ultrastructure of capillary basement membranes in the attached gingiva of diabetic and non-diabetic patients with periodontal disease. *Journal of Periodontology*, **42**, 406–11.

Gabbay, K. H., Hasty, K., Breslow, J. L., Ellison, R. C., Bunn, H. F., and Gallop, P. M. (1977). Glycosylated hemoglobins and long-term blood glucose control in diabetes mellitus. *Journal of Clinical Endocrinology and Metabolism*, **44**, 859–64.

Gislen, G., Nilsson, K. O., and Matsson, L. (1980). Gingival inflammation in diabetic children related to degree of metabolic control. *Acta Odontologica Scandinavica*, **38**, 241–6.

Glavind, L., Lund, B., and Loe, H. (1968). The relationship between periodontal status and diabetes duration, insulin dosage and retinal changes. *Journal of Periodontology*, **39**, 341–7.

Glickman, I. (1946). The periodontal structures in experimental diabetes. *New York Journal of Dentistry*, **16**, 226.

Golub, L. *et al.* (1983). Minocycline reduces gingival collagenolytic activity during diabetes. *Journal of Periodontal Research*, **18**, 516–26.

Goteiner, D., Vogel, R., Deasy, M., and Goteiner, C. (1986). Periodontal and caries experience in insulin-dependent diabetes mellitus. *Journal of the American Dental Association*, **113**, 277–9.

Grower, M., Ficara, A., Chandler, D., and Kramer, G. (1975). Differences in cAMP levels in the gingival fluid of diabetics and non-diabetics. *Journal of Periodontology*, **46**, 669–72.

Gusberti, F. A., Syed, S. A., Brown, G., Grossman, N., and Loesche, W. J. (1983). Puberty gingivitis in insulin-dependent diabetic children. *Journal of Periodontology*, **54**, 715–20.

Handwerger, B., Gernandes, G., and Brown, D. (1980). Immune and autoimmune aspects of diabetes mellitus. *Human Pathology*, **11**, 338–52.

Hove, K. A. and Stallard, R. E. (1970). Diabetes and the periodontal patient. *Journal of Periodontology*, **41**, 713–18.

Hugoson, A., Thorstensson, H., Falk, H., and Kuylenstierna, J. (1989). Periodontal conditions in insulin-dependent diabetics. *Journal of Clinical Periodontology*, **16**, 215–23.

Keene, J. (1969). Observations of small blood vessels in human non-diabetic and diabetic gingiva. *Journal of Dental Research*, **48**, 968.

Ketcham, B., Coff, C., and Denys, F. (1975). Comparison of the capillary basal lamina width in marginal gingiva of diabetic and non-diabetic patients. *Alabama Journal of Medical Sciences*, **12**, 295–301.

Kjellman, O., Henriksson, C-O., Berghagen, N., and Anderson, B. (1970). Oral conditions in 105 subjects with insulin-treated diabetes mellitus. *Swedish Dental Journal*, **63**, 99–110.

Lin, J., Duffy, J., and Roginsky, M. (1975). Microcirculation in diabetes mellitus: a study of gingival biopsies. *Human Pathology*, **6**, 77–97.

Listgarten, M., Ricker, E., Laster, L., Shapiro, J., and Cohen, D. (1974). Vascular basement lamina thickness in the normal and inflamed gingiva of diabetics and non-diabetics. *Journal of Periodontology*, **45**, 676–84.

MacKenzie, R. S. and Millard, H. D. (1963). Interrelated effects of diabetes, arteriosclerosis and calculus on alveolar bone loss. *Journal of the American Dental Association*, **66**, 191–8.

McMullen, J., Legg, M., Gottsegen, R., and Camerini-Davalos, R. (1967). Microangiopathy within the gingival tissues of diabetic subjects with special reference to the pre-diabetic state. *Periodontics*, **5**, 61–9.

McMullen, J. A., van Dyke, T. E., Horoszewicz, H. U., and Genco, R. J. (1981). Neutrophil chemotaxis in individuals with advanced periodontal disease and a genetic predisposition to diabetes mellitus. *Journal of Periodontology*, **52**, 167–73.

McNamara, T., Rammamurthy, N., Mulvihill, J., and Golub, L. (1982). The development of an altered gingival crevicular microflora in the alloxan-diabetic rat. *Archives of Oral Biology*, **27**, 217–23.

Manouchehr-Pour, M., Spagnuolo, P. J., Rodman, H. M., and Bissada, N. F. (1981). Comparison of neutrophil chemotactic response in diabetic patients with mild and severe periodontal disease. *Journal of Periodontology*, **52**, 410–15.

Mashimo, P. A., Yamamoto, Y., and Slots, J. (1983). The periodontal microflora of juvenile diabetics. Culture, immunofluorescence and serum antibody studies. *Journal of Periodontology*, **54**, 420–9.

Miller, K. and Michael, A. (1976). Immunopathology of renal extracellular membranes in diabetes mellitus. *Diabetes*, **25**, 701–8.

Nerup, J., Ortved-Anderson, O., and Bendixen, G. (1971). Antipancreatic cellular hypersensitivity in diabetes mellitus. *Diabetes*, **20**, 424–7.

Nichols, C., Laster, L., and Bodak-Gyova, L. (1978). Diabetes mellitus and periodontal disease. *Journal of Periodontology*, **49**, 85.

Nord, C., Kjellman, O., and Soder, P. O. (1969). Proteolytic activity of dental plaque material from patients with diabetes mellitus. *Svensk Tandlak*, **62**, 795–9.

Rammamurthy, N. and Golub, L. (1983). Diabetes increases collagenase activity in extracts of rat gingiva and skin. *Journal of Periodontal Research*, **18**, 23–30.

Ray, H. (1948). Study of the histopathology of the gingiva in patients with diabetes mellitus. *Diabetes*, **25**, 701–8.

Ringelberg, M. L., Dixon, D. O., Francis, A. O., and Plummer, R. W. (1977). Comparison of gingival health and gingival crevicular fluid flow in children with and without diabetes. *Journal of Dental Research*, **56**, 108–11.

Rohrbach, D. and Martin, G. (1982). Structure of basement membrane in normal and diabetic tissue. *Annals of the New York Academy of Science*, **401**, 203–11.

Rosenthal, I. M., Abrams, H., and Kopczyk, R. A. (1988). The relationship of inflammatory periodontal disease to diabetic status in insulin-dependent diabetes mellitus patients. *Journal of Clinical Periodontology*, **15**, 425–9.

Russell, B. (1966). Gingival changes in diabetes mellitus. *Acta Pathologica, Microbiologica et Immunologica Scandinavica*, **68**, 161–8.

Rutledge, C. E. (1940). Oral and roentgenographic aspects of the teeth and jaws of juvenile diabetics. *Journal of the American Dental Association*, **27**, 1740–50.

Rylander, H., Ramberg, P., Blohme, G., and Lindhe, J. (1986). Prevalence of periodontal disease in young diabetics. *Journal of Clinical Periodontology*, **14**, 38–43.

Saadoun, A. (1980). Diabetes and periodontal disease: a review and update. *Journal of the Western Society of Periodontology*, **28**, 116–39.

Sastrowijoto, S. H., Hillemans, P., van Steenbergen, T. J. M., Abraham-Inpijin, L., and de Graff, J. (1989). Periodontal condition and microbiology of healthy and diseased periodontal pockets in type I diabetes mellitus patients. *Journal of Clinical Periodontology*, **16**, 316–22.

Scully, C. and Cawson, R. A. (ed.) (1987). Endocrine diseases and metabolic disease. In *Medical problems in dentistry*, (2nd edn), pp. 234–85. Wright, Bristol.

Swenson, H. (1954). Alveolar bone resorption associated with diabetes. *Journal of Periodontology*, **25**, 52–3.

Sznajder, N., Carraro, J. J., Rugna, S., and Sereday, M. (1978). Periodontal findings in diabetic and nondiabetic patients. *Journal of Periodontology*, **49**, 445–8.

Tervonen, T. and Knuuttila, M. (1986). Relation of diabetes control to periodontal pocketing and alveolar bone level. *Oral Surgery, Oral Medicine, Oral Pathology*, **61**, 346–9.

Zambon, J. J., Reynolds, H., Fisher, J. G., Shlossman, M., Dunford, R., and Genco, R. J. (1988). Microbiological and immunological studies of adult periodontitis in patients with non-insulin-dependent diabetes mellitus. *Journal of Periodontology*, **59**, 23–31.

Down's Syndrome

Barkin, R. M., Weston, W. L., Humbert, J. R., and Maire, F. (1980a). Phagocytic function in Down's syndrome I. Chemotaxis. *Journal of Mental Deficiency Research*, **24**, 243–9.

Barkin, R. M., Weston, W. L., Humbert, J. R., and Sunada, K. (1980b). Phagocytic function in Down's syndrome II. Bactericidal activity and phagocytosis. *Journal of Mental Deficiency Research*, **24**, 251–6.

Brown, R. H. (1971). Crown and root lengths, and root–crown ratios of lower incisor teeth of mongoloid, non-mongoloid retarded and normal individuals. *Journal of Periodontal Research*, **6**, 140–5.

Brown, R. H. (1973). Necrotising ulcerative gingivitis in mongoloid and non-mongoloid retarded individuals. *Journal of Periodontal Research*, **8**, 290–5.

Brown, R. H. (1978). A longitudinal study of periodontal disease in Down's syndrome. *New Zealand Dental Journal*, **74**, 137–44.

Brown, R. H. and Cunningham, W. M. (1961). Some dental manifestations of mongolism. *Oral Surgery, Oral Medicine, Oral Pathology*, **14**, 664–76.

Claycomb, C. K., Summers, G. W., Hall, W. B., and Hart, R. W. (1970). Gingival collagen biosynthesis in mongolism. *Journal of Periodontal Research*, **5**, 30–5.

Cohen, M. M. (1958). *Proceedings of the workshop on dentistry for the handicapped*, (ed. M. Manuel), p. 34. Album

Cohen, M. M. and Winer, R. A. (1965). Dental and facial characteristics in Down's syndrome. *Journal of Dental Research*, **44**, 197–208.

Cohen, M. M., Winer, R. A., Schwartz, S., and Shklar, G. (1961). Oral aspects of mongolism. Part 1. Periodontal disease in mongolism. *Oral Surgery, Oral Medicine, Oral Pathology*, **14**, 92–107.

Costello, G. and Webber, A. (1976). White cell function in Down's syndrome. *Clinical Genetics*, **9**, 603–5.

Cutress, T. W. (1971). Periodontal disease and oral hygiene in trisomy 21. *Archives of Oral Biology*, **16**, 1345–55.

Cutress, T. W., Brown, R. H., and Guy, E. M. (1970). Occurrence of some bacterial species in the dental plaque of trisomy 21 (mongoloid), and other mentally retarded, and normal subjects. *New Zealand Dental Journal*, **66**, 153–61.

Cutress, T. W., Mickelson, K. N. P., and Brown, R. H. (1976). Vitamin A absorption and periodontal disease in trisomy G. *Journal of Mental Deficiency Research*, **20**, 17–23.

Dallapiccola, B., Alboni, P., and Ballerini, G. (1971). Capillary fragility in Down's syndrome. *Coagulation*, **4**, 217–20.

Dow, R. S. (1951). A preliminary study of periodontoclasia in mongolian children at Polk State School. *American Journal of Mental Deficiency*, **55**, 535–8.

Eastcott, A. D. and Loutit, M. W. (1968). Aerobic bacteria in saliva of mongols. *New Zealand Dental Journal*, **64**, 11–17.

Epstein, L. B., Lee, S. H. S., and Epstein, C. J. (1980). Enhanced sensitivity of trisomy 21 monocytes to the maturation-inhibiting effect of interferon. *Cellular Immunology*, **50**, 191–4.

Eschenbach, C. and Budenbender, B., (1976). Ingestions-und NBT-Reduktronskapazitat neutophiler Granulocyten bei Trisomie 21. *Klinische Wochenschrift*, **54**, 1147–51.

Gullikson, J. S. (1973). Oral findings in children with Down's syndrome. *Journal of Dentistry for Children*, **40**, 293–7.

Hall, B. (1962). Down's syndrome (mongolism) with normal chromosomes. *Lancet*, **ii**, 1026–7.

Izumi, Y., Sugiyama, S., Shinozuka, O., Yamazaki, T., Ohyama, T., and Ishikawa, I. (1989). Defective neutrophil chemotaxis in Down's syndrome patients and its relationship to periodontal destruction. *Journal of Periodontology*, **60**, 238–42.

Johnson, N. P. and Young, M. A. (1963). Periodontal disease in mongols. *Journal of Periodontology*, **34**, 41–7.

Kahn, A. J., Evans, H. E., Glass, L., Shin, Y. H., and Almonte, D. (1975). Defective neutrophil chemotaxis in patients with Down's syndrome. *Journal of Pediatrics*, **87**, 87–9.

Keyes, P. H., Bellack, S., and Jordan, H. V. (1971). Studies on the pathogenesis of destructive lesions of the gums and teeth in mentally retarded children. I. Dentobacterial plaque infection in children with Down's syndrome. *Clinical Pediatrics*, **10**, 711–18.

Kisling, E. and Krebs, G. (1963). Periodontal conditions in adult patients with mongolism (Down's syndrome). *Acta Odontologica Scandinavica*, **21**, 391–405.

Kretschmer, R. R., Lopez-Osuna, M., de la Rosa, L., and Armendares, S. (1974). Leukocyte function in Down's syndrome: quantitative N.B.T. reduction and bactericidal capacity. *Clinical Immunology and Immunopathology*, **2**, 449–55.

Kroll, R. G., Budnici, J., and Kobren, A. (1970). Incidence of dental caries and periodontal disease in Down's syndrome. *New York State Dental Journal*, **36**, 151–6.

Levin, S. et al. (1979). Thymic deficiency in Down's syndrome. *Pediatrics*, **63**, 80–7.

Mellman, W. J., Raab, S. O., and Oski, F. A. (1967). Abnormal granulocyte kinetics: an explanation of the atypical granulocyte enzymic activities observed in trisomy 21. In *Mongolism*, Ciba Foundation Study Group No. 25, pp. 77. Churchill Livingstone, London.

Meskin, L. H., Farsht, E. M., and Anderson, D. L. (1968). Prevalence of *Bacteroides melaninogenicus* in the gingival crevice area of institutionalised trisomy 21 and cerebral palsy patients and normal children. *Journal of Periodontology*, **39**, 326–8.

Miller, M. F. and Ship, I. I. (1977). Periodontal disease in the institutionalised mongoloid. *Journal of Oral Medicine*, **32**, 9–12.

Naeim, F. and Walford, R. L. (1980). Disturbance of redistribution of surface membrane receptors on peripheral mononuclear cells of patients with Down's and of aged individuals. *Journal of Gerontology*, **35**, 650–5.

Nishida, Y., Akaoka, I., Suzuki, T., Kobayashi, M., and Maruki, K. (1981). Serum lymphocytotoxins and lymphocyte responses to mitogens of Down syndrome persons. *American Journal of Mental Deficiency*, **85**, 596–600.

Orner, G. (1976). Periodontal disease among children with Down's syndrome and their siblings. *Journal of Dental Research*, **55**, 778–82.

Penrose, L. S., Ellis, J. R., and Delhanty, J. D. A. (1960). Chromosomal translocation in mongolism in normal relatives. *Lancet*, **ii**, 409–10.

Polson, A. M. (1986). The relative importance of plaque and occlusion in periodontal disease. *Journal of Clinical Periodontology*, **13**, 923–7.

Rappoport, S. and Kaplan, W. D. (1961). Chromosomal aberrations in man. *Journal of Pediatrics*, **59**, 415–38.

Reuland-Bosma, W. and van Dijk, J. (1986). Periodontal disease in Down's syndrome: a review. *Journal of Clinical Periodontology*, **13**, 64–73.

Reuland-Bosma, W., van Dijk, L. and van der Weele, L. (1986). Experimental gingivitis around deciduous teeth in children with Down's syndrome. *Journal of Clinical Periodontology*, **13**, 294–300.

Reuland-Bosma, W., van den Barselaar, M. T., van de Gevel, J. S., Leijh, P. C. J., Vries-Huiges, H., and The, H. T. (1988a). Nonspecific and specific immune responses in a child with Down's syndrome and her sibling. *Journal of Periodontology*, **59**, 249–53.

Reuland-Bosma, W., Liem, R. S. B., Jansen, H. W. B., van Dijk, L. J., and van der Weele, L. T. (1988b). Morphological aspects of the gingiva in children with Down's syndrome during experimental gingivitis. *Journal of Clinical Periodontology*, **15**, 293–302.

Reuland-Bosma, W., Liem, R. S. B., Jansen, H. W. B., van Dijk, L. J., and van der Weele, L. T. (1988c). Cellular aspects of and effects on the gingiva in children with Down's syndrome during experimental gingivitis. *Journal of Clinical Periodontology*, **15**, 303–11.

Rigas, D., Elsasser, P., and Hecht, F. (1970). Impairment of *in vitro* response of circulating lymphocytes to phytohemagglutinin in Down's syndrome: dose and time response curves and relation to cellular immunity. *International Archives of Allergy and Applied Immunology*, **39**, 587–92.

Rosner, F., Kozinn, P. J., and Jervis, G. A. (1973). Leukocyte function and serum immunoglobulins in Down's syndrome. *New York State Journal of Medicine*, **73**, 672–5.

Saxen, L. and Aula, S. (1982). Periodontal bone loss in patients with Down's syndrome: a follow up study. *Journal of Periodontology*, **53**, 158–62.

Saxen, L., Aula, S., and Westermarck, T. (1977). Periodontal disease associated with Down's syndrome, an orthopantomographic evaluation. *Journal of Periodontology*, **48**, 337–40.

Scully, C. and Cawson, R. (ed.) (1987). The handicapped patient and the elderly. In *Medical problems in dentistry*, pp. 406–28. Wright, Bristol.

Seger, R. *et al.* (1976). Defects in granulocyte function in various chromosome abnormalities (Down's, Edwards, cri-du-chat syndrome). *Klinische Wochenschrift*, **54**, 177–9.

Seger, R., Buchinger, G., and Stroder, J. (1977). On the influence of age on immunity in Down's syndrome. *European Journal of Pediatrics*, **124**, 77–87.

Shapiro, S., Gedalia, I., Hoffman, A., and Miller, M. (1969). Periodontal disease and blood citrate levels in patients with trisomy 21. *Journal of Dental Research*, **48**, 1231–3.

Silimbani, C. (1962). Contribution to the study of dental anomalies in mongolian idiocy. *Panminerva Medica*, **4**, 432–545.

Swallow, J. N. (1964). Dental disease in children with Down's syndrome. *Journal of Mental Deficiency Research*, **8**, 102–18.

Sznajder, N., Carraro, J. J., Otero, E., and Carranza, F. A. (1968). Clinical periodontal findings in trisomy 21 (mongolism). *Journal of Periodontal Research*, **3**, 1–5.

Tsunemitsu, A., Honjo, K., Kani, M., and Matsumura, T. (1963). Blood citrates in severe early destructive periodontal disease. *Journal of Dental Research*, **42**, 783–5.

Vigild, M. (1985). Periodontal conditions in mentally retarded children. *Community Dentistry and Oral Epidemiology*, **13**, 180–2.

Whittingham, S., Sharm, D. L. B., Pitt, D. B., and Mackay, I. R. (1977). Stress deficiency of the T-lymphocyte system exemplified by Down's syndrome. *Lancet*, **i**, 163.

Winer, R. A. and Feller, R. P. (1972). Composition of parotid and submandibular saliva and serum in Down's syndrome. *Journal of Dental Research*, **51**, 449–54.

Winer, R. A., Cohen, M. M., Feller, R. P., and Chauncey, H. (1965). Composition of human saliva, parotid gland secretory rate, and electrolyte concentration in mentally subnormal persons. *Journal of Dental Research*, **44**, 632–4.

HYPOPHOSPHATASIA

Baab, D. A., Page, R. C., and Morton, T. H. (1985). Studies of a family manifesting premature exfoliation of deciduous teeth. *Journal of Periodontology*, **56**, 403.

Baab, D. A., Page, R. C., Ebersole, J. L., Williams, B. L., and Scott, C. R. (1986). Laboratory studies of a family manifesting premature exfoliation of deciduous teeth. *Journal of Clinical Periodontology*, **13**, 677–83.

Baer, P. N., Brown, N. C., and Hammer, J. E. (1964). Hypophosphatasia: report of two cases with dental findings. *Periodontics*, **2**, 209–15.

Baysal, C. M. (1965). Premature loss of deciduous teeth in identical twins with congentital hypophosphatasia. *Dental Digest*, **71**, 516–39.

Beumer, J., Trowbridge, H. O., Silverman, S., and Eisenberg, E. (1973). Childhood hypophosphatasia and the premature loss of teeth. *Oral Surgery, Oral Medicine, Oral Pathology*, **35**, 631–40.

Brittain, J. M., Oldenburg, T. R., and Burkes, E. J. (1976). Odontohypophosphatasia: report of 2 cases. *Journal of Dentistry for Children*, **43**, 106–11.

Bruckner, R. J., Rickles, N. H., and Porter, D. R. (1962). Hypophosphatasia with premature shedding of teeth and aplasia of cementum. *Oral Surgery, Oral Medicine, Oral Pathology*, **15**, 1352–69.

Casson, M. H. (1969). Oral manifestations of primary hypophosphatasia. *British Dental Journal*, **127**, 561–6.

Fraser, D. (1957). Hypophosphatasia. *American Journal of Medicine*, **22**, 730–46.

Fung, D. (1983). Hypophosphatasia. *British Dental Journal*, **154**, 49–50.

Harris, H. and Robson, E. B. (1959). A genetical study of ethanolamine phosphate excretion in hypophosphatasia. *American Journal of Human Genetics*, **23**, 421–41.

Houpt, M. I., Kenny, F. M., and Listgarten, M. A. (1970). Hypophosphatasia: case reports. *Journal of Dentistry for Children*, **37**, 126–37.

Jedrychowski, J. R. and Duperon, D. (1979). Childhood hypophosphatasia with oral manifestations. *Journal of Oral Medicine*, **34**, 18–22.

Listgarten, M. A. and Houpt, M. I. (1969). Ultrastructural features of the root surface of deciduous teeth in patients with hypophosphatasia. *Journal of Periodontal Research*, **4** (Suppl.), 34–5.

McCormick, J. and Ripa, L. W. (1968). Hypophosphatasia: review and report of case. *Journal of the American Dental Association*, **77**, 618–25.

Page, R. C. and Baab, D. A. (1985). A new look at the etiology and pathogenesis of early onset periodontitis. *Journal of Periodontology*, **56**, 748–51.

Pimstone, B., Eisenberg, E., and Silverman, S. (1966). Hypophosphatasia: genetic and dental studies. *Annals of Internal Medicine*, **65**, 722–9.

Rathbun, J. C. (1948). Hypophosphatasia. *American Journal of Diseases of Children*, **75**, 822–31.

Scriver, C. E. and Cameron, D. (1969). Pseudohypophosphatasia. *New England Journal of Medicine*, **381**, 604–6.

Williams, B. L., Ebersole, J. L., Spector, M. D., and Page, R. C. (1985). Assessment of serum antibody patterns and analysis of subgingival microflora of members of a family with a high prevalence of early-onset periodontitis. *Infection and Immunity*, **49**, 742–50.

PAPILLON–LEFÈVRE SYNDROME

Baer, P. N. and Benjamin, S. D. (1974). *Periodontal disease in children and adolescents*, pp.206–9. Lippincott, Philadelphia.

Baer, P. N. and McDonald, R. E. (1981). Suggested mode of periodontal therapy for patients with Papillon–Lefevre syndrome. *Periodontal Case Reports*, **8**, 40–41.

Bravo-Piris, J., Aparicio, M., Moran, M., and Armijo, M. (1983). Papillon–Lefevre syndrome. Report on a case treated with oral retinoid RO 10–9359. *Dermatologia*, **166**, 97–103.

Brunsting, L. A., Kierland, R. R., Perry, H. O., Winkelmann, R. R., and Muller, S. A. (1964). Palmar plantar hyperkeratosis with periodontitis (Papillon–Lefevre syndrome). *Archives of Dermatology*, **90**, 330–4.

Coccia, C. T., McDonald, R. E., and Mitchell, D. F. (1966). Papillon–Lefevre syndrome: precocious periodontosis with palmar–plantar hyperkeratosis. *Journal of Periodontology*, **37**, 408–14.

Corson, E. F. (1939). Keratosis palmaris et plantaris with dental alteration. *Archives of Dermatology*, **40**, 639–43.

Djawari, D. (1978). Deficient phagocytic function in Papillon–Lefevre syndrome. *Dermatologia*, **156**, 184–92.

Dosseva, D., Balcheva, E., and Konstantinova, B. (1972). Clinical, genetic and cytogenetic investigation in the Papillon–Lefevre syndrome. *Stomatologie* (Sofia), **54**, 2–8.

Driban, E. and Jung, J. R. (1982). Papillon–Lefevre syndrome. A clinical and therapeutical contribution. *Dermatologia*, **165**, 653–9.

Garant, P. R. and Mulvihill, J. E. (1972). The fine structure of gingivitis in the beagle. III. Plasma cell infiltration of the subepithelial connective tissue. *Journal of Periodontal Research*, **7**, 161–72.

Glenwright, H. D. and Rock, W. P. (1990). Papillon–Lefevre syndrome. A discussion of aetiology and a case report. *British Dental Journal*, **168**, 27–9.

Gorlin, R. J., Sedano, H., and Anderson, V. E. (1964). The syndrome of palmar–plantar hyperkeratosis and premature periodontal destruction of the teeth. *Journal of Pediatrics*, **65**, 895–908.

Haneke, E. (1979). The Papillon–Lefevre syndrome. Keratosis palmoplantaris with periodontopathy. *Human Genetics*, **51**, 1–35.

Haneke, E., Hornstein, O. P., and Lex, C. (1975). Increased susceptibility to infection in the Papillon–Lefevre syndrome. *Dermatologia*, **150**, 283.

Hathaway, R. (1982). Papillon–Lefevre syndrome. *British Dental Journal*, **153**, 370–1.

Hawes, R. R. (1960). Report of three patients experiencing juvenile periodontitis and early loss of teeth. *Journal of Dentistry for Children*, **27**, 169–77.

Jung, J., Carranza, F. A., and Newman, M. G. (1981). Scanning electron-microscopy of plaque in Papillon–Lefevre syndrome. *Journal of Periodontology*, **52**, 442–6.

Lu, H-K.J., Lin, C-T. and Kwan, H-W. (1987). Treatment of a patient with Papillon–Lefevre syndrome. A case report. *Journal of Periodontology*, **58**, 789–93.

Lyberg, T. (1982). Immunological and metabolic studies in 2 siblings with Papillon–Lefevre syndrome. *Journal of Periodontal Research*, **17**, 563–8.

McDonald, R. E. and Avery, D. R. (1978). *Dentistry for the child and adolescent*, (3rd edn) p.249. C.V. Mosby, St. Louis,

Martinez-Lalis, R. R., Lopez-Otero, R., and Carranza, F. A. (1965). A case of Papillon–Lefevre syndrome. *Periodontics*, **3**, 292–5.

Newman, M., Angel, I., Karge, H., Weiner, M., Grinenco, V., and Schusterman, L. (1977). Bacterial studies of the Papillon–Lefevre syndrome. *Journal of Dental Research*, **56**, 545.

Papillon, M. M. and Lefèvre, P. (1924). Deux cas de keratodermie palmaire et plantaire symétrique familiale (maladie de Meleda) chez le frere et la soeur. Coexistence dan les deux cas d'alterations dentaire graves. *Bulletin de la Société Française de Dermatologie et de Syphiligraphie*, **31**, 82–7.

Preus, H. R. (1988). Treatment of rapidly destructive periodontitis in Papillon–Lefevre syndrome. Laboratory and clinical observations. *Journal of Clinical Periodontology*, **15**, 639–43.

Preus, H. and Gjermo, P. (1987). Clinical management of prepubertal periodontitis in 2 siblings with Papillon–Lefevre syndrome. *Journal of Clinical Periodontology*, **14**, 156–60.

Preus, H. R. and Morland, B. (1987). *In vitro* studies of monocyte function in 2 siblings with Papillon–Lefevre syndrome. *Scandinavian Journal of Dental Research*, **95**, 59–64.

Rateitschak-Pluss, E. M. and Schroeder, H. E. (1984). History of periodontitis with a child with Papillon–Lefevre syndrome. *Journal of Periodontology*, **55**, 35–46.

Schroeder, H. E., Seger, R. A., Keller, H. U. and Rateitschak-Pluss, E. M. (1983). Behaviour of neutrophilic granulocytes in a case of Papillon–Lefevre syndrome. *Journal of Clinical Periodontology*, **10**, 618–35.

Shoshan, S., Finkelstein, S., and Rosenzweig, K. A. (1970). Disc electrophoretic pattern of gingival collagen isolated from a patient with palmoplantar hyperkeratosis. *Journal of Periodontal Research*, **5**, 255–8.

Sloan, P., Soames, J. V., Murray, J. J., and Jenkins, W. M. M. (1984). Histopathological and ultrastructural findings in a case of Papillon–Lefevre syndrome. *Journal of Periodontology*, **55**, 482–5.

Smith, P. and Rosenzweig, K. A. (1967). Seven cases of Papillon–Lefevre syndrome. *Periodontics*, **5**, 42–6.

Tinanoff, N., Tanzer, J. M., Kornman, K. S., and Maderazo, E. G. (1986). Treatment of the periodontal component of Papillon–Lefevre syndrome. *Journal of Clinical Periodontology*, **13**, 6–10.

Van Dyke, T. E. *et al.* (1984). The Papillon–Lefevre syndrome. Neutrophil dysfunction with severe periodontal disease. *Clinical Immunology and Immunopathology*, **31**, 419–29.

Vrahopoulos, T. P. Barber, P., Liakoni, H. and Newman, H. N. (1988). Ultrastructure of the periodontal lesion in a case of Papillon–Lefevre syndrome (PLS). *Journal of Clinical Periodontology*, **15**, 17–26.

Wannenmacher, E. (1938). Ursachen auf dem Gebiet der Papadentoses. *zbl. Gesamt.Zahn-Mund, Kieferheilkd*, **7**, 1–15.

EHLERS–DANLOS SYNDROME

Barabas, G. M. (1969). The Ehlers–Danlos syndrome: abnormalities of the enamel, dentine, cementum and the dental pulp: a histological examination of 13 teeth from 6 patients. *British Dental Journal*, **126**, 509–15.

Barabas, G. M. and Barabas, A. P. (1967). The Ehlers–Danlos syndrome. A report of the oral and haematological findings in nine cases. *British Dental Journal*, **123**, 473–9.

Beighton, P. (1978). *Inherited disorders of the skeleton*. Churchill Livingstone, New York.

Beighton, P., Price, A., Lord, J., and Dickson, E. (1969). Variants of the Ehlers–Danlos syndrome: clinical, biochemical, haematological and chromosomal features of 100 patients. *Annals of Rheumatic Diseases*, **28**, 228–45.

Danlos, H. (1908). Un cas de cutis laxa avec tumerus par contusion chronique des coudes et des genoux. *Bulletin de Société Français de Dermatologie*, **19**, 70–2.

Ehlers, E. (1901). Cutis laxa; Neiging su Hemorrhagien in der Haut, Lockerung Mehrere Artikulalionen. *Dermatologica*, **2**, 173–4.

Gay, S., Martin, G. R. and Muller, P. K. (1976). Simultaneous synthesis of types I and III collagen by fibroblasts in culture. *Proceedings of the National Academy of Science (USA)*, **72**, 4037–41.

Goodman, R. M. and Allinson, M. L. (1969). Chronic temporomandibular joint subluxation in Ehlers–Danlos syndrome: report of a case. *Journal of Oral Surgery*, **27**, 659–61.

Hoff, M. (1977). Dental manifestation in Ehlers–Danlos syndrome. *Oral Surgery, Oral Medicine, Oral Pathology*, **44**, 864–71.

Hughes, C. L. (1970). Odontectomy in the treatment of Ehlers–Danlos syndrome: report of a case. *Journal of Oral Surgery*, **28**, 612–14.

Krane, S. M., Pinnell, S. R. and Erbe, J. (1972). Lysyl–protocollagen deficiency to fibroblast in siblings with hydroxylysine-deficient collagen. *Proceedings of the National Academy of Science (USA)*, **69**, 2899–903.

Penttinen, R. P., Lichtenstein, J. R., and Martin, G. R. (1975). Abnormal collagen metabolism in cultured cells in osteogenesis imperfecta. *Proceedings of the National Academy of Science (USA)*, **72**, 586–9.

Pinnell, S. R. Krane, S. M., Kenzora, J. E., and Glimcher, M. J. (1972). A hereditable disorder of connective tissue: hydroxylysine deficient collagen disease. *New England Journal of Medicine*, **286**, 1013–20.

Pope, F. M., Martin, G. R., and Lichtenstein, J. R. (1975). Patients with Ehlers–Danlos syndrome. Type IV lack type III collagen. *Proceedings of the National Academy of Science (USA)*, **72**, 1314.

Recant, B. S. and Lipman, J. S. (1969). The Ehlers–Danlos syndrome. *Oral Surgery, Oral Medicine, Oral Pathology*, **28**, 460–3.

Sadeghi, E. M., Ostertag, P. R., and Esumi, A. (1989). Oral manifestations of Ehlers–Danlos syndrome: report of a case. *Journal of the American Dental Association*, **118**, 187–91.

Stewart, R. E., Hollister, D. W., and Rimoin, D. L. (1977). A new variant of Ehlers–Danlos syndrome: an autosomal dominant disorder of fragile skin, abnormal scarring and generalised periodontitis. *Birth Defects*, **13**, 85–93.

Thexton, A. (1965). A case of Ehlers–Danlos syndrome presenting with recurrent dislocation of the temporomandibular joint. *British Journal of Oral Surgery*, **2**, 190–3.

HEREDITARY GINGIVAL FIBROMATOSIS

Araiche, M. and Brode, H. (1959). A case of fibromatosis gingivae. *Oral Surgery, Oral Medicine, Oral Pathology*, **12**, 1307–10.

Becker, W., Collings, C. K., Zimmerman, E. R., De la Rosa, M., and Singdahlsen, D. (1967). Hereditary gingival fibromatosis. *Oral Surgery, Oral Medicine, Oral Pathology*, **24**, 313–18.

Buchner, H. J. (1937). Diffuse fibroma of the gums. Report of two cases. *Journal of the American Dental Association*, **24**, 2003–7.

Cross, H. E., McKusick, V. A., and Been, W. A. (1967). A new oculocerebral syndrome with hypopigmentation. *Journal of Pediatrics*, **70**, 398–406.

Drescher, E., Woyke, S., Markiewicz, C., and Tegi, S. (1967). Juvenile fibromatosis in siblings (fibromatosis hyatinica multiplex juvenitis). *Journal of Pediatric Surgery*, **2**, 427–30.

Emerson, T. G. (1965). Hereditary gingival hyperplasia. *Oral Surgery, Oral Medicine, Oral Pathology*, **19**, 1–9.

Fletcher, J. P. (1966). Gingival abnormalities of genetic origin: preliminary communication with special reference to hereditary generalised gingival fibromatosis. *Journal of Dental Research*, **45**, 597–612.

Jones, G., Willroy, R. S., and McHaney, V. (1977). Familial gingival fibromatosis associated with progressive deafness in five generations of a family. *Birth Defects*, **13**, 195–201.

Jorgensen, R. J. and Cocker, M. E. (1974). Variation in the inheritance and expression of gingival fibromatosis. *Journal of Periodontology*, **45**, 472–7.

Leband, P. F., Habib, G., and Humphreys, G. S. (1964). Hereditary gingival fibromatosis. Report of an affected family with associated splenomegaly, and skeletal and soft tissue abnormalities. *Oral Surgery, Oral Medicine, Oral Pathology*, **17**, 339–51.

Puretic, S. and Puretic, B. (1971). Clinical and histopathological observations on systemic familial mesenchymatosis. In *Proceedings of the 13th International Congress on Pediatrics*, **5**, pp. 373–81.

Rushton, M. A. (1957). Hereditary or idiopathic hyperplasia of the gums. *Dental Practitioner*, **7**, 136–46.

Rutherfurd, M. E. (1931). Three generations of inherited dental defect. *British Medical Journal*, **II**, 9–11.

Savara, B. S., Suher, T., Everett, F. G. and Burns, A. G. (1954). Hereditary gingival fibrosis. Study of a family. *Journal of Periodontology*, **25**, 12–21.

Winstock, D. (1964). Hereditary gingivo-fibromatosis. *British Journal of Oral Surgery*, **2**, 59–64.

Winter, G. B. and Simpkiss, M. J. (1974). Hypertrichosis with hereditary gingival hyperplasia. *Archives of Disease in Childhood*, **49**, 349–99.

Witkop, C. J. (1971). Heterogeneity in gingival fibromatosis. *Birth Defects*, **7**, 210–21.

Yokoya, M. M. (1962). Fibromatous gingival hypertrophy: report of two cases. *Oral Surgery, Oral Medicine, Oral Pathology*, **15**, 904–7.

MUCOPOLYSACCHARIDOSES

Caffey, J. (1952). Gargoylism: prenatal and neonatal bone lesions and their early postnatal evaluation. *American Journal of Roentgenography*, **67**, 715–31.

Cantor, H. (1965). Macrogingivae of Hurler's syndrome. *Journal of Clinical Stomatology*, **6**, 27–30.

Cawson, R. A. (1962). The oral changes in gargoylism. *Proceedings of the Royal Society of Medicine*, **55**, 1066–70.

Galili, D., Yatziv, S., and Russell, A. (1974). Massive gingival hyperplasia preceding dental eruption in I-cell disease. *Oral Surgery, Oral Medicine, Oral Pathology*, **37**, 533–9.

Gardner, D. G. (1968). Metachromatic cells in the gingiva in Hurler's syndrome. *Oral Surgery, Oral Medicine, Oral Pathology*, **26**, 782–9.

Gardner, D. G. (1971). The oral manifestations of Hurler's syndrome. *Oral Surgery, Oral Medicine, Oral Pathology*, **32**, 46–57.

McKusick, V. A. *et al.* (1965). The genetic mucopolysaccharidoses. *Medicine*, **44**, 445–83.

Worth, H. M. (1966). Hurler's syndrome: a study of radiologic appearances in the jaws. *Oral Surgery, Oral Medicine, Oral Pathology*, **22**, 21–35.

HYPEROXALURIA

Canos, H. J., Hogg, G. A., and Jeffrey, J. R. (1981). Oxalate nephropathy due to gastrointestinal disorders. *Canadian Medical Association Journal*, **124**, 729–33.

Chaplin, A. J. (1977). Histopathological occurrence and characterisation of calcium oxalate: a review. *Journal of Clinical Pathology*, **30**, 800–11.

Fantasia, J. E., Miller, A. S., Chen, S-Y., and Foster, W. B. (1982). Calcium oxalate deposition in the periodontium secondary to chronic renal failure. *Oral Surgery, Oral Medicine, Oral Pathology*, **53**, 273–9.

Glass, R. T. (1973). Oral manifestations in primary hyperoxaluria and oxalosis. *Oral Surgery, Oral Medicine, Oral Pathology*, **35**, 502–9.

Milgram, J. W. and Salyer, W. R. (1974). Secondary oxalosis of bone in chronic renal failure. A histopathologic study of 3 cases. *Journal of Bone and Joint Surgery*, **56A**, 373–95.

Moskow, B. S. (1989). Periodontal manifestations of hyperoxaluria and oxalosis. *Journal of Periodontology*, **60**, 271–8.

Von Bunte, M., Bitter, K., and Gross, U. M. (1977). Dentomaxillare Deestruktionen bei Oxalose. *Deutche Zahnaerztliche Zeitschrift*, **32**, 617.

Williams, H. E. and Smith, L. H. (1973). Disorders of oxalate metabolism. *American Journal of Medicine*, **54**, 673–81.

Wysocki, G. P., Fay, W. P., Ulrichsen, R. F., and Ulan, R. A. (1982). Oral findings in primary hyperoxaluria and oxalosis. *Oral Surgery, Oral Medicine, Oral Pathology*, **53**, 267–72.

CROHN'S DISEASE AND PYOSTOMATITIS VEGETANS

Basu, M. K., Asquith, P. Thompson, R. A., and Cooke, W. T. (1975). Oral manifestations of Crohn's disease. *Gut*, **16**, 259–64.

Bernstein, M. L. and MacDonald, J. S. (1978). Oral lesions in Crohn's disease: report of 2 cases and update of the literature. *Oral Surgery, Oral Medicine, Oral Pathology*, **46**, 234–45.

Bottomley, W. K., Giorgini, G. L., and Julienne, C. H. (1972). Oral extension of regional enteritis (Crohn's disease). *Oral Surgery, Oral Medicine, Oral Pathology*, **34**, 417–20.

Cataldo, E., Covino, M. C., and Tesone, P. E. (1981). Pyostomatitis vegetans. *Oral Surgery, Oral Medicine, Oral Pathology*, **52**, 172–7.

Croft, C. B. and Wilkinson, A. R. (1972). Ulceration of the mouth, pharynx and larynx in Crohn's disease of the intestines. *British Journal of Surgery*, **59**, 249–52.

Crohn, B. B., Ginzburg, L., and Oppenheimer, G. D. (1932). Regional ileitis, a pathologic and clinical entity. *Journal of the American Medical Association*, **99**, 1323–9.

Dudeney, T. P. and Todd, I. P. (1969). Crohn's disease of the mouth. *Proceedings of the Royal Society of Medicine*, **62**, 1237.

Eisenbud, L., Katzka, I., and Platt, N. (1972). Oral manifestations of Crohn's disease: report of a case. *Oral Surgery, Oral Medicine, Oral Pathology*, **34**, 770–3.

Engel, L. D., Pasquinelli, K. L., Leone, S. A., Moncla, B. J., Nielson, K. D., and Rabinovitch, P. S. (1988). Abnormal lymphocyte profiles and leukotriene B₄ status in a patient with Crohn's disease and severe periodontitis. *Journal of Periodontology*, **59**, 841–7.

Forman, L. (1965). Two cases of pyodermatite vegetante (hallopean): An eosinophilic pustular and vegetating dermatitis with conjunctival, oral and colonic involvement. *Proceedings of the Royal Society of Medicine*, **58**, 244–9.

Greenstein, A. J., Janowitz, H. D., and Sachar, D. B. (1976). The extraintestinal complications of Crohn's disease and ulcerative colitis: a study of 700 patients. *Medicine*, **55**, 401–12.

Hammer, B., Achlirst, P., and Naish, J. (1968). Diseases associated with ulcerative colitis and Crohn's disease. *Gut*, **9**, 17–21.

Jones, V. A., Shorthouse, M., McLaughlan, P., Workman, E., and Hunter, J. O. (1985). Food intolerance a major factor in the pathogenesis of irritable bowel syndrome. *Lancet*, **ii**, 1115–17.

Keleman, E. (1973). Granulocyte alkaline phosphatase activity: a measure of the emergence time of mature marrow neutrophils. *Acta Haematologica*, **50**, 19–24.

Koldjaer, O., Klitgaard, N. A., and Schmidt, K. G. (1977). Indices of granulocyte activity in ulcerative colitis and Crohn's disease. *Danish Medical Bulletin*, **24**, 72–6.

Kyle, J. (1972). *Crohn's disease*, p. 78. Appleton-Century-Crofts, New York.

Lamster, I. B., Sonis, S. T., Hannigan, A., and Koldkin, A. (1978). An association between Crohn's disease, periodontal disease and enhanced neutrophil function. *Journal of Periodontology*, **49**, 475–9.

Lamster, I. B., Rodrick, M. L., Sonis, S. T., and Falchuk, Z. M. (1982). An analysis of peripheral blood and salivary polymorphonuclear leukocyte function, circulating immune complex levels and oral status in patients with inflammatory bowel disease. *Journal of Periodontology*, **53**, 231–8.

McCarthy, F. P. (1949). Pyostomatitis vegetans: report of 3 cases. *Archives of Dermatology and Syphilis*, **60**, 750–64.

Sandler, R. S. and Golden, A. L. (1986). Epidemiology of Crohn's disease. *Journal of Clinical Gastroenterology*, **8**, 160–5.

Schiller, K. F. R., Goldring, P. L., Peebles, R. A., and Whitehead, R. (1971). Crohn's disease of the mouth and lips. *Gut*, **12**, 864–5.

Simpson, H. E., Howell, R. A., and Summersgill, G. B. 1974). Oral manifestations of Crohn's disease. *Journal of Oral Medicine*, **29**, 49–52.

Sundh, B. and Hulten, L. (1982). Oral status in patients with Crohn's disease. *Acta Chirurgica Scandinavica*, **148**, 531–4.

Van Dyke, T. E., Dowell, V. R., Offenbacher, S., Snyder, W., and Hersh, T. (1986). Potential role of micro-organisms isolated from periodontal lesions in the pathogenesis of inflammatory bowel disease. *Infection and Immunity*, **53**, 671–7.

Van Steenberghe, D., Vanherle, G., and Fossion, E. (1976). Crohn's disease of the mouth. Report of a case. *Journal of Oral Surgery*, **34**, 635–8.

Wray, D. (1984). Pyostomatitis vegetans. *British Dental Journal*, **157**, 316–18.

SARCOIDOSIS

Altman, K. and Robinson, P. D. (1984). Sarcoidosis with oral involvement. *British Dental Journal*, **157**, 310–11.

Cahn, L. R., Eisenbud, L., Blake, M. N., and Stern, D. (1964). Biopsies of normal-appearing palates of patients with known sarcoidosis: a preliminary report. *Oral Surgery, Oral Medicine, Oral Pathology*, **18**, 342–5.

Cohen, C., Krutchkoff, D., and Eisenberg, E. (1981). Systemic sarcoidosis: report of 2 cases with oral lesions. *Journal of Oral Surgery*, **39**, 613–18.

Dunner, E. and Williams, J. H. (1961). Epidemiology of sarcoidosis in the United States. *American Review of Respiratory Disease*, **84**, 163–8.

Eule, H., Roth, I., and Weide, W. (1980). Clinical and functional results of a controlled clinical trial of the value of prednisolone therapy in sarcoidosis, stages I and II. In *Proceedings 8th International Conference on Sarcoidosis and Other Granulomatous Diseases* (ed. W.W. Jones and B. H. Davies). New York pp. 624–8. Alpha Omega Publications.

Gold, R. S. and Sager, E. (1976). Oral sarcoidosis: review of the literature. *Journal of Oral Surgery*, **34**, 237–44.

Hayter, J. P. and Robertson, J. M. (1988). Sarcoidosis presenting as gingivitis. *British Medical Journal* (Clinical Research), **296**, 1504.

Hogan, J. J. (1983). Sarcoid gingivitis. *British Dental Journal*, **154**, 109–10.

Jones-Williams, W. (1979). The nature and significance of granulomas in sarcoidosis. In *Abstracts of the International Siena Sarcoidosis Symposium*, Siena, Italy.

Lofgren, S. L. (1964). Proceedings of the Third International Conference on Sarcoidosis. *Acta Medica Scandinavica*, **425** (Suppl.), 11–14.

Lofgren, W. and Lundbeck, H. (1952). The bilateral hilar lymphoma syndrome. A study of the relation to tuberculosis and sarcoidosis in 212 cases. *Acta Medica Scandinavia*, **174**, 265–73.

Makris, G. P. and Stoller, N. H. (1983). Rapidly advancing periodontitis in a patient with sarcoidosis. A case report. *Journal of Periodontology*, **54**, 690–3.

Nessan, V. J. and Jacoway, J. R. (1979). Biopsy of minor salivary glands in the diagnosis of sarcoidosis. *New England Journal of Medicine*, **301**, 922–4.

Sloan, P. J., O'Neil, T. C., Smith, C. J., and Holdsworth, C. D. (1983). Multisystem sarcoid presenting with gingival hyperplasia. *British Journal of Oral Surgery*, **21**, 31–5.

Tarpley, T. M., Anderson, L., Lightbody, P., and Sheagren, J. N. (1972). Minor salivary gland involvement in sarcoidosis: report of 3 cases. *Oral Surgery, Oral Medicine, Oral Pathology*, **33**, 755–62.

Tillman, H. H. (1964). Sarcoidosis with unsuspected oral manifestations: report of a case. *Oral Surgery, Oral Medicine, Oral Pathology*, **18**, 130–5.

Tyldesley, W. R. (1983). Sarcoid gingivitis. *British Dental Journal*, **154**, 235.

Van Swol, R. L. (1973). Periodontosis in a patient with previously diagnosed sarcoidosis. *Journal of Periodontology*, **44**, 697–704.

Watts, K. D. (1968). Sarcoid of the gingiva: a case report. *British Journal of Oral Surgery*, **6**, 108–13.

Zakrzewska, J. and Nally, F. F. (1985). Sarcoid with oral involvement. *British Dental Journal*, **158**, 3–4.

OROFACIAL GRANULOMATOSIS

Carr, D. R. (1966). Is Melkersson–Rosenthal syndrome hereditary? *Archives of Dermatology*, **93**, 426–7.

Ferguson, M. M. and MacFadyen, E. E. (1986). Orofacial granulomatosis—a 10 year review. *Annals of the Academy of Medicine*, **15**, 370–7.

James, J., Patton, D. W., Lewis, C. J., Kirkwood, E. M., and Ferguson, M. M. (1986). Orofacial granulomatosis and clinical atrophy. *Journal of Oral Medicine*, **41**, 29–30.

Patton, D. W., Ferguson, M. M., Forsyth, A., and James, J. (1985). Orofacial granulomatosis—a possible allergic basis. *British Journal of Oral and Maxillofacial Surgery*, **23**, 235–42.

Scott, G. A. (1964). Melkersson's syndrome. *British Journal of Clinical Practice*, **18**, 415–18.

Wiesenfeld, D., Ferguson, M. M., and Mitchell, D. N. (1985). Orofacial granulomatosis—a clinical and pathological analysis. *Quarterly Journal of Medicine*, **54**, 101–13.

WEGENER'S GRANULOMATOSIS

Brooke, R. I. (1969). Wegener's granulomatosis involving the gingivae. *British Dental Journal*, **127**, 34–6.

Cassan, S. M., Coles, D. T., and Harrison, E. G. (1970). The concept of limited forms of Wegener's granulomatosis. *American Journal of Medicine*, **49**, 366–79.

Cawson, R. A. (1965). Gingival changes in Wegener's granulomatosis. *British Dental Journal*, **118**, 30–2.

Cohen, P. S. and Meltzer, J. A. (1981). Strawberry gums. A sign of Wegener's granulomatosis. *Journal of the American Medical Association*, **246**, 2610–11.

Edwards, M. B. and Buckerfield, J. P. (1978). Wegener's granulomatosis: a case with primary mucocutaneous lesions. *Oral Surgery, Oral Medicine, Oral Pathology*, **46**, 53–63.

Fahey, J., Leonard, E., Churg, J., and Goodman, G. (1954). Wegener's granulomatosis. *American Journal of Medicine*, **17**, 168–79.

Goodman, G. C. and Churg, J. (1954). Wegener's granulomatosis. *Archives of Pathology*, **58**, 533–53.

Handlers, J. P., Waterman, J., Abrams, A. M., and Melrose, R. J. (1985). Oral features of Wegener's granulomatosis. *Archives of Otolaryngology*, **111**, 267–70.

Horan, R. F., Kerdel, F. A., Maschella, S. L., and Haynes, H. A. (1986). Recent onset of gingival enlargement. *Archives of Dermatology*, **122**, 1436–9.

Israel, H. L. and Patchefsky, A. S. (1971). Wegener's granulomatosis of lung: diagnosis and treatment. *Annals of Internal Medicine*, **74**, 881–91.

Israelson, H., Binnie, W. H., and Hurt, W. C. (1981). The hyperplastic gingivitis of Wegener's granulomatosis. *Journal of Periodontology*, **52**, 81–7.

Kakehashi, S., Hammer, J. E., Baer, P. N., and McIntyre, J. A. (1965). Wegener's granulomatosis: report of a case involving the gingiva. *Oral Surgery, Oral Medicine, Oral Pathology*, **19**, 120–7.

Levan, N. E. (1960). Progressive gingival hyperplasia associated with deep abscess of buttock and arm (? monocytic leukaemia). *Archives of Dermatology*, **81**, 149–51.

Milner, P. F. (1955). Nasal granuloma and periarteritis nodosa. *British Medical Journal*, **2**, 1597–9.

Morgan, A. D. and O'Neil, R. (1956). The oral complications of polyarteritis and giant cell granulomatosis (Wegener's granulomatosis). *Oral Surgery, Oral Medicine, Oral Pathology*, **9**, 845–57.

Parsons, E., Seymour, R. A., Macleod, R. I., Nand, N., and Ward, M. K. (1991). Wegener's granulomatosis—a distinct gingival lesion. *Journal of Clinical Periodontology* (in press).

Raustia, A. M., Autio-Harmainen, H. I., Knuuttila, M. L. E., and Raustia, J. M. (1985). Ultrastructural findings and clinical follow-up of 'strawberry gums' in Wegener's granulomatosis. *Journal of Oral Pathology*, **14**, 581–7.

Scott, J. and Finch, L. D. (1972). Wegener's granulomatosis presenting as gingivitis. Review of the clinical and pathologic features and report of a case. *Oral Surgery, Oral Medicine, Oral Pathology*, **34**, 920–32.

Walton, E. W. (1958). Giant-cell granuloma of the respiratory tract (Wegener's granulomatosis). *British Medical Journal*, **2**, 265–70.

Wegener, F. (1936). Über generalisierte, septische Gefasserkrankungen. *Verhandlungen des Deutschen Gesellschaft für Pathologie*, **29**, 202–10.

SCLERODERMA

Alarcon-Segovia, D., Ibanez, G., and Hernandex-Ortiz, J. (1974). Sjogren's syndrome in progressive systemic sclerosis (scleroderma). *American Journal of Medicine*, **57**, 78–85.

Alexandridis, C. and White, S. C. (1984). Periodontal ligament changes in patients with progressive systemic sclerosis. *Oral Surgery, Oral Medicine, Oral Pathology*, **58**, 113–18.

Drosos, A. A., Andonopoulos, A. P., Costopoulos, J. S., Stavropoulos, E. D., Papadimitriou, C. S., and Moutsopoulos, H. M. (1988). Sjogren's syndrome in progressive systemic sclerosis. *Journal of Rheumatology*, **15**, 965–8.

Eversole, L. R., Jacobsen, P. L., and Stone, C. E. (1984). Oral and gingival changes in systemic sclerosis (scleroderma). *Journal of Periodontology*, **55**, 175–8.

Fullmer, H. M. and Witte, W. E. (1962). Periodontal membrane affected by scleroderma. (A histochemical study). *Archives of Pathology*, **73**, 184–9.

Gilliland, B. C. and Mannik, M. (1984). Progressive systemic sclerosis (diffuse scleroderma). In *Harrison's principles of internal medicine*, (10th edn), pp. 2002–996. McGraw Hill, New York.

Gores, R. J. (1957). Dental characteristics associated with acrosclerosis and diffuse scleroderma. *Journal of the American Dental Association*, **54**, 755–9.

Green, D. (1972). Scleroderma and its oral manifestations. *Oral Surgery, Oral Medicine, Oral Pathology*, **15**, 1312–24.

Hoggins, G. S. and Hamilton, M. (1969). Dentoalveolar defects associated with scleroderma. *Oral Surgery, Oral Medicine, Oral Pathology*, **27**, 734.

Mammary, Y., Glaiss, R., and Pisanty, S. (1981). Scleroderma: oral manifestations. *Oral Surgery, Oral Medicine, Oral Pathology*, **52**, 32–7.

Naylor, W. P. (1982). Oral management of the scleroderma patient. *Journal of the American Dental Association*, **105**, 814–17.

Norton, W. L. and Nardo, J. M. (1970). Vascular disease in progressive systemic sclerosis. *Annals of Internal Medicine*, **73**, 317–24.

Rowell, N. R. and Hopper, F. E. H. (1977). The periodontal membrane in systemic sclerosis. *British Journal of Dermatology*, **96**, 15–20.

Seifert, M. H., Steigerwald, J. C., and Cliff, M. M. (1975). Bone resorption of the mandible in progressive systemic sclerosis. *Arthritis and Rheumatology*, **18**, 507–17.

Smith, D. B. (1958). Scleroderma, its oral manifestations. *Oral Surgery, Oral Medicine, Oral Pathology*, **18**, 865–73.

Stafne, E. C. and Austin, L. T. (1944). Characteristic dental findings in acrosclerosis and diffuse scleroderma. *American Journal of Orthodontics*, **30**, 25–9.

Traiger, J. (1961). Scleroderma, its oral manifestations. *Oral Surgery, Oral Medicine, Oral Pathology*, **14**, 117–21.

Uthman, A. A., Winkler, S., and Scott, S. (1978). The scleroderma patient. *Journal of Oral Medicine*, **33**, 65–7.

Velayos, E. E., Masi, A. T., Stevens, M. B., and Schulman, L. E. (1979). The 'crest' syndrome: comparison with systemic sclerosis (scleroderma). *Archives of Internal Medicine*, **139**, 1240–4.

Wardrop, R. W. and Heggie, A. A. (1987). Progressive systemic sclerosis: oro-facial manifestations. Case report. *Australian Dental Journal*, **32**, 258–82.

Weber, D. D., Blunt, M. H., and Caldwell, J. B. (1970). Fracture of mandibular rami complicated by scleroderma. Report of a case. *Journal of Oral Surgery*, **28**, 860–2.

White, S. C., Frey, N. W., and Blaschke, D. D. (1977). Oral radiographic changes in patients with progressive systemic sclerosis (scleroderma). *Journal of the American Dental Association*, **94**, 1178–82.

Wood, R. E. and Lee, P. (1988). Analysis of the oral manifestations of systemic sclerosis (scleroderma). *Oral Surgery, Oral Medicine, Oral Pathology*, **65**, 172–8.

HAEMATOLOGICAL DISORDERS

Allan, D. and Straton, A. G. (1983). Chronic granulomatous disease with associated oral lesions. *British Dental Journal*, **154**, 110–12.

Alty, H. M. (1962). Aplastic anaemia due to chloramphenicol presenting as gingivitis. *British Dental Journal*, **112**, 498–500.

Andrews, R. G., Benjamin, S., Shore, N., and Canter, S. (1965). Chronic benign neutropenia of childhood with associated oral manifestations. *Oral Surgery, Oral Medicine, Oral Pathology*, **20**, 719–25.

Baehni, P. C., Payot, P., Tsai, G. C., and Cimasoni, G. (1983). Periodontal status associated with chronic neutropenia. *Journal of Clinical Periodontology*, **10**, 222–30.

Barrett, A. P. (1984). Gingival lesions in leukaemia: a classification. *Journal of Periodontology*, **55**, 585–8.

Barrett, A. P. (1986). Leukaemic cell infiltration of the gingiva. *Journal of Periodontology*, **57**, 579–81.

Berendes, H., Bridges, R. A., and Good, R. A. (1957). A fatal granulomatosis of childhood: the clinical study of a new syndrome. *Minnesota Medicine*, **40**, 309.

Biggar, W. D., Holmes, B., Page, A. R., Deinard, A. S., L'Esperance, P., and Good, R. A. (1974). Metabolic and functional studies of monocytes in congenital neutropenia. *British Journal of Haematology*, **28**, 233–4.

Binon, P. P. and Dykema, R. W. (1974). Rehabilitative management of cyclic neutropenia. *Journal of Prosthetic Dentistry*, **31**, 52–60.

Blume, R. S. and Wolff, S. M. (1972). The Chediak–Higashi syndrome: studies in 4 patients and a review of the literature. *Medicine*, **51**, 247–80.

Chediak, M. (1952). Nouvelle anomalie leucocytaire de caractère conditutionnel et familial. *Revue Hematologie*, **7**, 362–73.

Cohen, D. W. and Morris, A. L. (1961). Periodontal manifestations of cyclic neutropenia. *Journal of Periodontology*, **32**, 159–68.

Crawford, J. (1988). Periodontal disease in sickle cell disease subjects. *Journal of Periodontology*, **59**, 164–9.

Dale, D. C., Clark, R. A., Root, R. K., and Kimball, H. R. (1972). The Chediak–Higashi Syndrome: Studies of Host Defenses, NIH Conference. *Annals of Internal Medicine*, **76**, 293–306.

Deasey, M. J., Vogel, R., Annes, I., and Simon, B. (1976). Periodontal disease associated with preleukaemic syndrome. *Journal of Periodontology*, **47**, 41–5.

Deasey, M. J., Vogel, R. I., Macedo-Sobrinho, B., Gertzman, G., and Simon, B. (1980). Familial benign chronic neutropenia associated with periodontal disease—case report. *Journal of Periodontology*, **51**, 206–10.

Delgado, W. and Calderon, R. (1979). Acatalasia in two Peruvian siblings. *Journal of Oral Pathology*, **8**, 358–68.

Dreizen, S., McCredie, K. B., Keating, M. J., and Luna, M. A. (1983). Malignant gingival and skin 'infiltrates' in adult leukaemia. *Oral Surgery, Oral Medicine, Oral Pathology*, **55**, 572–9.

Elkins, W. L. (1971). Cellular immunology and the pathogenesis of graft versus host reactions. *Progress in Allergy*, **15**, 78–187.

Fanconi, G. (1941). Klinische Demonstrationen. *Annals of Paediatrics*, **157**, 308.

Ferguson, M. M., Stephen, K. W., Dagg, J. H., and Hunter, I. R. (1978). The presentation and management of oral lesions in leukaemia. *Journal of Dentistry*, **6**, 201–6.

Gillig, J. L. and Caldwell, C. M. (1970). The Chediak–Higashi syndrome: case report. *Journal of Dentistry for Children*, **37**, 527–9.

Gorlin, R. J. and Chaudry, A. P. (1960). The oral manifestations of cyclic (periodic) neutropenia. *Archives of Dermatology*, **82**, 344–8.

Guerry, D., Dalo, D. C., Omine, M., Perry, S., and Wolff, S. M. (1972). Studies on the mechanism of human cyclic neutropenia. *Blood*, **40**, 951.

Hamilton, R. E. and Giansanti, J. S. (1974). The Chediak–Higashi syndrome. *Oral Surgery, Oral Medicine, Oral Pathology*, **37**, 754–61.

Higashi, O. (1954). Congenital gigantism of peroxidase granules. The first case ever reported of qualitative abnormality of peroxidase. *Tohoku Journal of Experimental Medicine*, **59**, 315–22.

Hitzig, W. M. (1959). Familiare neutropenia mit dominanten Erbang und Hypergammaglobulinaimie. *Helvetica Medica Acta*, **26**, 779.

Hjortdal, O. (1971). Orale manifestasjoner ved agranulocytoses. *Den Norske Tannlaegeforenings Tidende*, **81**, 335–44.

Hou, G. L. and Tsai, C. C. (1988). Primary gingival enlargement as a diagnostic indicator in acute myelomonocytic leukaemia. *Journal of Periodontology*, **59**, 852–5.

Johnson, R. B. (1969). Screening test for the diagnosis of chronic granulomatous disease. *Pediatrics*, **43**, 122–3.

Kalkwarf, K. L. and Gutz, D. P. (1981). Periodontal changes associated with chronic idiopathic neutropenia. *Pediatric Dentistry*, **3**, 189–95.

Kyle, R. A. and Linman, J. W. (1968). Chronic idiopathic neutropenia: a newly recognised entity. *New England Journal of Medicine*, **279**, 1015–19.

Kyle, R. A. and Linman, J. W. (1970). Gingivitis and chronic idiopathic neutropenia: a report of 2 cases. *Mayo Clinic Proceedings*, **45**, 494–504.

Lampert, F. and Fesseler, A. (1975). Periodontal changes during chronic benign granulocytopenia in childhood. A case report. *Journal of Clinical Periodontology*, **2**, 105–10.

Lavine, W. S., Page, R. A., and Padgett, G. A. (1976). Host response in chronic periodontal disease. The dental and periodontal status of mink and mice affected by Chediak–Higashi syndrome. *Journal of Periodontology*, **47**, 621–35.

Long, L. M., Jacoway, J. R., and Bawden, J. W. (1983). Cyclic neutropenia: case report of two siblings. *Pediatric Dentistry*, **5**, 142–4.

Lynch, M. A. and Ship, I. I. (1967). Initial oral manifestations of leukaemia. *Journal of the American Dental Association*, **75**, 932–40.

Meme, J. S, Gripenberg, U., and Kahknonem, M. (1980). Fanconi's anaemia: chromosome breakage in a large African family. *Hereditas*, **93**, 255–61.

Michaud, M., Baehner, R. L., Bixler, D., and Kafrawy, A. H. (1977). Oral manifestations of acute leukemia in children. *Journal of the American Dental Association*, **95**, 1145–50.

Miller, M. E., Oski, F. A., and Harris, M. B. (1971). Lazy-leukocyte syndrome: a new disorder of neutrophil function. *Lancet*, **i**, 665–9.

Miller, R. L., Gould, A. R., Skolnick, J. L., and Epstein, W. M. (1982). Localized oral histoplasmosis. A regional manifestation of mild chronic disseminated histoplasmosis. *Oral Surgery, Oral Medicine, Oral Pathology*, **53**, 367–74.

Mintz, U. and Sachs, L. (1973). Normal granulocyte colony forming cells in the bone marrow of Yemenite Jews with genetic neutropenia. *Blood*, **41**, 745–51.

Morley, A. A., Carew, J. P., and Baikie, A. G. (1967). Familial cyclical neutropenia. *British Journal of Haematology*, **13**, 719–38.

Newman, C. W. and Rosenbaum, D. (1962). Oral cryptococcus. *Journal of Periodontology*, **33**, 266–9.

Onwubalili, J. K. (1983). Sickle cell disease and infection. *Journal of Infection and Immunity*, **7**, 2–9.

Opinya, G. N., Kaimenyi, J. T., and Meme, J. S. (1988). Oral findings in Fanconi's anaemia. *Journal of Periodontology*, **59**, 461–3.

Overholser, C. D., Peterson, D. E., Williams, L. T., and Schimpff, S. C. (1982). Periodontal infection in patients with acute nonlymphocytic leukaemia. *Archives of Internal Medicine*, **142**, 551–4.

Page, A. R. and Good, R. A. (1957). Studies on cyclic neutropenia. A clinical and experimental investigation. *Journal of Disease in Children*, **94**, 623–61.

Peltier, J. R. and Olivier, R. M. (1961). Oral manifestations of idiopathic thrombocytopenic purpura. *Journal of Oral Surgery*, **19**, 130–5.

Peterson, D. E. and Overholser, C. D. (1979). Dental management of leukemic patients. *Oral Surgery, Oral Medicine, Oral Pathology*, **47**, 40–2.

Presant, C. A., Safdar, S. H., and Cherrick, H. (1973). Gingival leukemic infiltration in chronic lymphocytic leukaemia. *Oral Surgery, Oral Medicine, Oral Pathology*, **36**, 672–4.

Prichard, J. F., Ferguson, D. M., Windmiller, J., and Hart, W. C. (1984). Prepubertal periodontitis affecting the deciduous dentition and permanent dentition in a patient with cyclic neutropenia: a case report and discussion. *Journal of Periodontology*, **55**, 114–22.

Reichart, P. A. and Dornow, H. (1978). Gingivo-periodontal manifestations in chronic benign neutropenia. *Journal of Clinical Periodontology*, **5**, 74–80.

Rodu, B. and Gockerman, J. P. (1983). Oral manifestations of the chronic graft-v-host reaction. *Journal of the American Medical Association*, **249**, 504–7.

Rylander, H. and Ericsson, I. (1981). Manifestations and treatment of periodontal disease in a patient suffering from cyclic neutropenia. *Journal of Clinical Periodontology*, **8**, 77–87.

Saarni, M. and Linman, J. W. (1973). Pre-leukemia—the hematological syndrome preceding acute leukemia. *American Journal of Medicine*, **55**, 38–48.

Sale, G. E., Strob, R., and Clift, R. A. (1981). Oral and ophthalmic pathology of graft versus host disease in man. Predictive value of the lip biopsy. *Human Pathology*, **12**, 1022–30.

Scully, C., MacFadyen, E., and Campbell, A. (1982). Oral manifestations in cyclic neutropenia. *British Journal of Oral Surgery*, **20**, 96–101.

Seymour, R. A. and Walton, J. G. (1988). *Adverse drug reactions in dentistry*. Oxford University Press.

Shepard, J. P. (1978). The management of the oral complications of leukaemia. *Oral Surgery, Oral Medicine, Oral Pathology*, **45**, 543–8.

Sinrod, H. S. (1957). Leukemia as a dental problem. *Journal of the American Dental Association*, **55**, 809–18.

Spencer, P. and Fleming, J. E. (1985). Cyclic neutropenia: a literature review and report of a case. *Journal of Dentistry for Children*, **52**, 108–13.

Stafford, R., Sonis, S., Lockhart, P., and Sonis, A. (1980). Oral pathoses as diagnostic indicators in leukemia. *Oral Surgery, Oral Medicine, Oral Pathology*, **50**, 134–9.

Stamps, J. T. (1974). The role of oral hygiene in a patient with idiopathic aplastic anaemia. *Journal of the American Dental Association*, **88**, 1025–7.

Stansbury, D. M., Peterson, D. E., and Suzuki, J. B. (1988). Rapidly progressive acute periodontal infection in a patient with acute leukemia. *Journal of Periodontology*, **59**, 544–7.

Sydney, S. B. and Serio, F. (1981). Acute monocytic leukemia diagnosed in a patient referred because of gingival pain. *Journal of the American Dental Association*, **103**, 886–7.

Wade, A. B. and Stafford, J. L. (1963). Cyclic neutropenia. *Oral Surgery, Oral Medicine, Oral Pathology*, **16**, 1443–8.

Wolf, J. E. and Ebel, L. K. (1978). Chronic granulomatous disease. Report of a case and review of the literature. *Journal of the American Dental Association*, **96**, 292–5.

Wray, D. and Dagg, J. H. (1980). Diseases of the blood and blood-forming organs. In *Oral manifestations of systemic disease* (ed. J.H. Jones and D.K. Mason), pp. 262–96. Saunders, London.

Zucker-Franklin, D., L'Esperance, P., and Good, R. A. (1977). Congenital neutropenia: an intrinsic cell defect demonstrated by electron microscopy of soft agar colonies. *Blood*, **49**, 425–36.

Zuelzer, W. W. and Bajochli, M. (1964). Chronic granulocytopenia in childhood. *Blood*, **23**, 359–74.

RETICULO-ENDOTHELIAL SYSTEM

Artzi, Z., Gorsky, M., and Raviv, M. (1989). Periodontal manifestations of adult onset of histiocytosis X. *Journal of Periodontology*, **60**, 57–66.

Cararo, J. J., Sznajder, N., Barros, R., and Martinez-Lalis, R. (1972). Periodontal involvement in eosinophilic granuloma. *Journal of Periodontology*, **43**, 427–32.

Cohn, E. R., Grover, K. L., and Metz, H. C. (1982). Ventropharyngeal incompetence in a patient with multiple eosinophilic granuloma (Hand–Schuller–Christian disease). *Journal of Speech and Hearing Disorders*, **47**, 320–6.

Cranin, A. N. and Rockman, R. (1981). Oral symptoms in histiocytosis X. *Journal of the American Dental Association*, **103**, 412–16.

Daneshbod, K. and Kissane, J. M. (1976). Histiocytosis X—the progress of polyostotic eosinophilic granuloma. *American Journal of Clinical Pathology*, **65**, 601–11.

Fitzpatrick, R., Rappaport, M. G., and Silva, D. G. (1981). Histiocytosis X. *Archives of Dermatology*, **117**, 253–7.

Gorsky, M., Silverman, S., Lozada, F., and Kushner, J. (1983). Histiocytosis X: occurrence and oral involvement in six adolescent and adult patients. *Oral Surgery, Oral Medicine, Oral Pathology*, **55**, 24–8.

Hartman, K. S. (1980). Histiocytosis X: a review of 114 cases with oral involvement. *Oral Surgery, Oral Medicine, Oral Pathology*, **49**, 38–54.

Hashimoto, K., Takahashi, S., Fligiel, A., and Savoy, B. (1985). Eosinophilic granuloma: presence of OKTG-positive cells and good response to intralesional steriod. *Archives of Dermatology*, **121**, 770–4.

Jensen, J. L., Carrell, R. W., and Bloom, C. Y. (1982). Painful mandibular and maxillary bone lesions in a young adult. *Journal of the American Dental Association*, **105**, 673–4.

Kaufman, A., Bukberg, P. R., Werlin, S., and Young, I. S. (1976). Multifocal eosinophilic granuloma (Hand–Schuller–Christian disease). *American Journal of Medicine*, **60**, 541–8.

Krutchkoff, D. J. and Jones, C. R. (1984). Multifocal eosinophilic granuloma. A clinical pathologic conference. *Journal of Oral Pathology*, **13**, 472–88.

Lahey, M. E. (1975). Histiocytosis X—an analysis of prognostic factors. *Journal of Pediatrics*, **87**, 179–84.

Lin, L. M., Wyman, T. P., Bushell, A., and Langeland, K. (1979). Eosinophilic granuloma of the jawbone. *Journal of Endodontics*, **5**, 25–9.

McCarthy, P. L. and Shklar, G. (1980). *Textbook of diseases of the oral mucosa*, (2nd edn.) Lea & Febiger, Philadelphia.

Macintyre, D. R., Canty, A. J., and Pell, G. M. (1985). Multifocal eosinophilic granuloma presenting in the mandible. *British Dental Journal*, **159**, 338–40.

McKelvy, B. D., Sanders, B., Cox, R. L., and Arnett, G. W. (1975). Chronic disseminated histiocytosis X of adulthood clinically mimicking subacute osteomyelitis. *Journal of Oral Medicine*, **30**, 73–5.

Mitnick, J. S. and Pinto, R. S. (1980). Computed tomography in the diagnosis of eosinophilic granuloma. *Journal of Computer Assisted Tomography*, **4**, 791–6.

Moorthy, A. P. (1986). Eosinophilic granuloma manifesting as a periodontal problem. *British Dental Journal*, **161**, 66–7.

Moskow, R., Levine, L. J., and Marin, A. (1971). Multifocal eosinophilic granuloma stimulating periodontal disease. *New York State Dental Journal*, **37**, 607–10.

Pareek, S. S. and Hawass, N. E. D. (1985). An unusual presentation of histiocytosis X. *International Journal of Dermatology*, **24**, 126–31.

Sigala, J. L., Silverman, S., Brody, H. A., and Kushner, J. H. (1972). Dental involvement in histiocytosis. *Oral Surgery, Oral Medicine, Oral Pathology*, **33**, 42–8.

Smith, R. J. H. and Evans, J. N. G. (1984). Head and neck manifestations of histiocytosis X. *Laryngoscope*, **94**, 395–9.

Soskolne, W. A., Lustmann, J., and Azaz, B. 1977). Histiocytosis X: report of six cases initially in the jaws. *Journal of Oral Surgery*, **35**, 30–3.

Sweet, R. M., Kornblut, A. D., and Hayms, V. J. (1979). Eosinophilic granuloma in the temporal bone. *Laryngoscope*, **89**, 1545–52.

Urbano-Marquez, A., Estruch, R., and Fernandez-Huerta, S (1985). Etoposide in the treatment of multifocal eosinophilic granuloma. Cancer Treatment Reports, 69, 238–239.

Whitcher, B. L. and Webb, J. (1986). Treatment of recurrent eosinophilic granuloma of the mandible following radiation therapy. *Journal of Oral and Maxillofacial Surgery*, **44**, 565–70.

Whitehead, F. I. H. (1972). Histiocytosis X. *British Journal of Oral Surgery*, **10**, 199–204.

Zuendel, M. T., Bowers, D. F., and Kramer, R. N. (1984). Recurrent histiocytosis X with mandibular lesions. *Oral Surgery, Oral Medicine, Oral Pathology*, **58**, 420–3.

INFECTIONS (INCLUDING AIDS)

Grassi, M., Williams, C. A., Winkler, J. R., and Murray, P. A. (1988). Management of HIV-associated periodontal diseases. In *Oral manifestations of AIDS* (ed. P. B. Robertson and J. S. Greenspan), pp.119–30. PSG Publishing Company, Littleton MA

Lozada, F., Silverman, S., Migliorati, C. A., Conant, M. A., and Volberding, P. A. (1983). Oral manifestations of tumour and opportunistic infections in the acquired immunodeficiency syndrome (AIDS): findings in 53 homosexual men with Kaposi's sarcoma. *Oral Surgery, Oral Medicine, Oral Pathology*, **56**, 491–4.

Melnick, S. L. *et al.* (1989). Oral mucosal lesions: association with the presence of antibodies to the human immunodeficiency virus. *Oral Surgery, Oral Medicine, Oral Pathology*, **68**, 37–43.

Murray, P. A. *et al.* (1988). Microbiology of HIV-associated gingivitis and periodontitis. In *Oral manifestations of AIDS* (ed. P. B. Robertson and J. S. Greenspan), pp.105–18. PSG Publishing Company, Littleton, MA.

Phelan, J. S., Saltzman, B. R., Friedland, G. H., and Klein, R. S. (1987). Oral findings in patients with acquired immunodeficiency syndrome. *Oral Surgery, Oral Medicine, Oral Pathology*, **64**, 50–6.

Pindborg, J. J. (1989). Classification of oral lesions associated with HIV infection. *Oral Surgery, Oral Medicine, Oral Pathology*, **67**, 292–5.

Pindborg, J. J. and Holmstrup, P. (1987). Necrotizing gingivitis related to human immunodeficiency virus (HIV) infection. *African Dental Journal*, **1**, 5–8.

Ryder, M. I., Winkler, J. R., and Weintrub, P. S. (1988). Elevated phagocytosis, oxidative bursts and F-actin formation in PMNs from individuals with intra-oral manifestations of HIV-infection. *Journal of Acquired Immune Deficiency Syndrome*, **1**, 346–56.

Volpe, F., Schwimmer, A., and Barr, C (1985). Oral manifestations of disseminated Mycobacterium avium intracellulare in a patient with AIDS. *Oral Surgery, Oral Medicine & Oral Pathology*, **60**, 567–570.

Winkler, J. R., and Murray, P. A. (1987). Periodontal disease—a potential intra-oral expression of AIDS may be a rapidly progressive periodontitis. *Journal of the Californian Dental Association*, **15**, 20–4.

Winkler, J. R. Grassi, M., and Murray, P. A. (1988). Clinical description and aetiology of HIV-associated periodontal diseases. In *Oral manifestations of AIDS* (ed. P. B. Robertson and J. S. Greenspan), pp.49–70. PSG Publishing Company, Littleton, MA.

DISORDERS OF THE IMMUNE SYSTEM

Barrickman, R. W., Callerame, M. L., and Condemi, J. J. (1973). Gingivitis in hypogammaglobulinemia. *Journal of Periodontology*, **44**, 171–4.

Been, V. and Engel, D. (1982). The effects of immunosuppressive drugs on periodontal inflammation in human renal allograft patients. *Journal of Periodontology*, **53**, 245–8.

Berenbaum, M. C. (1967). Immunosuppressive agents and allogenic transplantation. *Journal of Clinical Pathology*, **20**, 471–98.

Birkeland, S. A. (1976). Uraemia as a state of immune deficiency. *Scandinavian Journal of Immunology*, **5**, 107–15.

Fournier, C., de Tand, M. F., and Bach, J. F. (1973). Activities of immunosuppressive agents *in vitro*. *Annals of Immunology*, **124C**, 209.

Kardachi, B. J. R. and Newcomb, G. M. (1978). A clinical study of gingival inflammation in renal transplant recipients taking immunosuppressive drugs. *Journal of Periodontology*, **49**, 307–9.

Oshrain, H. I., Menders, S., and Mandel, I. D. (1979). Periodontal status of patients with reduced immunocapacity. *Journal of Periodontology*, **50**, 185–8.

Petit, J. C. and Ripamonti, U. (1990). Multiple myeloma of the periodontium. A case report. *Journal of Periodontology*, **61**, 132–7.

Roberts, W. R. and Walker, D. M. (1976). The periodontal management of a patient with a profound immunodeficiency disorder. *Journal of Clinical Periodontology*, **3**, 186–92.

Robertson, P. B., Wright, T. E., Mackler, B. F., Lenertz, D. M., and Levy, B. M. (1978). Periodontal status of patients with abnormalities of the immune system. *Journal of Periodontal Research*, **13**, 37–45.

Schuller, P. D., Freedman, H. L., and Lewis, D. W. (1973). Periodontal status of renal transplant patients receiving immunosuppressive therapy. *Journal of Periodontology*, **44**, 166–70.

Sutton, R. B. O. and Smales, F. C. (1983). Cross-sectional study of the effects of immunosuppressive drugs on chronic periodontal disease in man. *Journal of Clinical Periodontology*, **10**, 317–26.

Tollefsen, T. and Johansen, J. R. (1985*a*). The periodontal status of prospective and renal transplant patients. *Journal of Periodontal Research*, **20**, 220–6.

Tollefsen, T. and Johansen, J. R. (1985*b*). Periodontal status in patients before and after renal allotransplantation. *Journal of Periodontal Research*, **20**, 227–36.

Tollefsen, T., Saltved, E., and Koppang, H. S. (1978). The effect of immunosuppressive agents on periodontal disease in man. *Journal of Periodontal Research*, **13**, 240–50.

Tollefsen, T., Koppang, H. S., and Messelt, E. (1982). Immunosuppression and periodontal disease in man. Histological and ultrastructural observations. *Journal of Periodontal Research*, **17**, 329–44.

MUCOCUTANEOUS DISORDERS

Barnett, M. L. (1988). Pemphigus vulgaris presenting as a gingival lesion—a case report. *Journal of Periodontology*, **59**, 611–14.

Bean, S. F., Weisman, M., Michal, B., Thomas, C. I., Knox, J. M., and Levine, M. (1972). Cicatricial pemphigoid: immunofluorescent studies. *Archives of Dermatology*, **106**, 195–9.

Daniels, T. E. and Quadra-White, C. (1980). Direct immunofluores-cence in oral mucosal diseases: a diagnostic analysis of 130 cases. *Oral Surgery, Oral Medicine, Oral Pathology*, **51**, 38–47.

Degregori, G., Pippen, R., and Davies, E. (1971). Psoriasis of the gingiva and the tongue. *Journal of Periodontology*, **42**, 97–100.

Fine, R. M. and Weathers, D. R. (1980). Desquamative gingivitis. A form of cicatricial pemphigoid? *British Journal of Dermatology*, **102**, 393–9.

Hashimoto, K. (1972). Electron microscopy and histochemistry of pemphigus and pemphigoid. *Oral Surgery, Oral Medicine, Oral Patho-logy*, **33**, 206–19.

Holubar, K., Honigsmann, H., and Wolff, K. (1973). Cicatricial pem-phigoid, immunofluorescent investigations. *Archives of Dermatology*, **108**, 50–2.

Jandiski, J. and Shklar, G. (1976). Lichen planus of gingiva. *Journal of Periodontology*, **47**, 724–33.

Jones, L. E. and Dolby, A. E. (1972). Desquamative gingivitis associated with psoriasis. *Journal of Periodontology*, **43**, 35–7.

Jordan, R. E., Triftshauser, C. T., and Schroeder, A. L. (1971). Direct immunofluorescent studies of pemphigus and bullous pemphigoid. *Archives of Dermatology*, **103**, 486–91.

Laskaris, G., Sklavounou, A., and Stratigos, J. (1982). Bullous pemphi-goid, ciciatricial pemphigoid and pemphigus vulgaris. *Oral Surgery, Oral Medicine, Oral Pathology*, **54**, 656–62.

Laufer, J. and Kuffer, R. (1971). Oral lichen planus. *Revue de Stomatolo-gie Chirurgie Maxillo Faciale*, **72**, 214–24.

Lever, W. F. (1972). Methotrexate and prednisone in pemphigus vulgaris. *Archives of Dermatology*, **106**, 491–7.

Lever, W. and Schaumburg-Lever, G. (1977). Immunosuppressants and prednisolone in pemphigus vulgaris. *Archives of Dermatology*, **113**, 1236–41.

McCarthy, P. L. and Shklar, G. (1980). *Diseases of the oral mucosa*. Lea & Febiger, Philadelphia.

Markitziu, A. and Pisanty, S. (1983). Gingival pemphigus vulgaris: report of a case. *Oral Surgery, Oral Medicine, Oral Pathology*, **55**, 250.

Nisengard, R. J. and Neiders, M. (1981). Desquamative lesions of the gingiva. *Journal of Periodontology*, **52**, 500–10.

Nisengard, R. J., Alpert, A. M., and Krestow, V. (1978). Desquamative gingivitis: immunologic findings. *Journal of Periodontology*, **40**, 27–32.

O'Hara, D. B., Goldberg, M. H., and Galbraith, D. A. (1980). Split thickness skin graft for the treatment of benign mucous membrane pemphigoid. *Oral Surgery, Oral Medicine, Oral Pathology*, **49**, 487–91.

Orlowski, W. A., Bressman, E., Doyle, J. L., and Chasens, A. I. (1983). Chronic pemphigus vulgaris of the gingiva. A case report with a 6-year follow-up. *Journal of Periodontology*, **54**, 685–9.

Person, J. R. and Rogers, R. S. (1977). Bullous and cicatricial pemphi-goid, clinical histopathologic and immunopathologic considerations. *Proceedings of the Mayo Clinic*, **52**, 54–66.

Pindborg, J. J. (1980). Diseases of the skin. In *Oral manifestations of systemic disease* (ed. J. H. Jones and D. K. Mason), pp.318–70. Saunders, London.

Pisanty, S., Sharav, Y., Kaufman, E., and Posner, L. N. (1974). Pemphigus vulgaris: incidence in Jews of different ethnic groups according to age, sex and initial lesion. *Oral Surgery, Oral Medicine, Oral Pathology*, **38**, 382–7.

Polifka, M. and Krusinski, P. A. (1980). The Nikolsky sign. *Cutis*, **26**, 521–6.

Rogers, R. S. and Jordan, R. E. (1977). Immunopathology of oral mucosal inflammatory diseases. *Clinical and Experimental Dermato-logy*, **2**, 1–7.

Seymour, R. A. and Walton, J. G. (1988). *Adverse drug reactions in dentistry*. Oxford University Press.

Shklar, G. and McCarthy, P. L. (1971). Oral lesions of mucous membrane pemphigoid. A study of 85 cases. *Archives of Otolaryng-ology*, **39**, 354–64.

Shklar, G., Frim, S., and Flynn, E. (1978). Gingival lesions of pemphi-gus. *Journal of Periodontology*, **49**, 428–35.

Shousa, S. and Svirbely, J. (1977). Immunohistochemical study of lichen planus. *Journal of Clinical Pathology*, **30**, 569–74.

Silverman, S. and Griffith, M. (1974). Studies on oral lichen planus. *Oral Surgery, Oral Medicine, Oral Pathology*, **37**, 705–10.

Susi, F. R. and Shklar, G. (1971). Histochemistry and fine structure of oral lesions of mucous membrane pemphigoid. *Archives of Dermato-logy*, **104**, 244–53.

Williams, D. M. *et al.* (1984). Benign mucous membrane (cicatricial) pemphigoid revisited. *British Dental Journal*, **157**, 313–16.

Zegarelli, D. J. and Zegarelli, E. V. (1977). Intraoral pemphigus vulgaris. *Oral Surgery, Oral Medicine, Oral Pathology*, **44**, 384–93.

4. Adverse drug reactions and the periodontal tissues

4.1 INTRODUCTION

Systemic drug therapy and, in certain instances, local therapy can have an adverse effect that can manifest itself in the periodontal tissues. The two main drug-induced problems of concern to the periodontologist are drug-induced gingival overgrowth and hypersensitivity reactions or the so-called plasma cell gingivitis.

Adverse drug reactions can be classified as type A and B (Rawlins and Thompson 1985). Type A reactions are the result of an exaggerated but otherwise normal pharmacological action of a drug given in the usual therapeutic doses. These reactions are more likely to develop in individuals lying at the extreme of the dose–response curve for pharmacological effects. They are largely predictable on the basis of a drug's known pharmacological properties; examples include xerostomia with anticholinergics, an increase in bleeding time with aspirin, and drowsiness from the benzodiazepines. Type A reactions are usually dose-dependent, and although their incidence and morbidity in the community is high, their mortality is low.

Type B reactions are totally aberrant effects that are not to be expected from the known pharmacological actions of the drug when given in the usual therapeutic doses to a patient whose body handles the drug in the usual way. Many of these reactions have an immunological basis. For example, contact stomatitis or plasma cell gingivitis is a Type IV delayed hypersensitivity reaction. Drug-induced gingival overgrowth does not appear to be mediated via the immune system. However, this adverse effect is not predictable from the known pharmacological properties of the implicated drugs, and therefore must be considered a type B reaction.

4.2 DRUG-INDUCED GINGIVAL OVERGROWTH

4.2.1 INTRODUCTION

Phenytoin, cyclosporin, and the calcium-channel blocking agents are all associated with the unwanted effect of gingival overgrowth. Although there are many theories about the pathogenesis of this condition, a common, unifying link between the three drugs has not been established. Clinically and histologically these three gingival overgrowths are similar. The target cell is the gingival fibroblast, as all lesions are characterized by an increase in the connective tissue component. Gingival inflammation also appears to be an important predisposing factor to this unwanted effect. This suggests that the lesion is a consequence of the interaction between gingival fibroblasts, the cellular and biochemical mediators of inflammation, and the drug or its metabolites.

4.2.2 PHENYTOIN

Phenytoin is an anticonvulsant drug widely used in the control of epilepsy and other convulsive disorders. It is also used in the management of trigeminal, glossopharyngeal, and postherpetic neuralgia, and occasionally to treat ventricular arrhythmias. Phenytoin is a weak acid with poor solubility. When given orally, it is slowly absorbed from the gastrointestinal tract. Absorption shows marked interindividual variation. The drug is extensively bound to plasma protein (90 per cent) and is metabolized in the liver by microsomal enzymes. The major metabolite of phenytoin is 5-(parahydroxyphenyl)-5-phenylhydantoin (5-p-HPPH). The metabolites, together with 5 per cent unchanged phenytoin, are excreted in the urine (Richens 1979).

The anticonvulsant properties of phenytoin are due its action on the neuronal cell membrane. The drug stabilizes the membrane to the action of sodium, potassium, and calcium ions (see later).

Apart from gingival overgrowth, other unwanted effects of phenytoin include cardiac arrhythmias, depression of the central nervous system, drowsiness, hirsutism, and osteomalacia.

Phenytoin-induced gingival overgrowth

It is now well established that phenytoin therapy is associated with gingival overgrowth. Many studies of this unwanted effect have been reviewed by Hassell (1981). The incidence of this overgrowth is approximately 50 per cent (Angelopoulos and Goaz 1972), but is higher in both teenagers (Kapur et al. 1973) and institutionalized epileptics (Hassell et al. 1984). Phenytoin-induced gingival overgrowth does not appear to be related to the patient's age, sex, or race (Hassell 1981).

The overgrowth usually becomes apparent in the first three months after phenytoin dosage (Dummett 1954) and is most rapid in the first year (Aas 1963). Clinically it starts as a diffuse swelling of the interdental papillae, which may then coalesce (Angelopoulos 1975). The gingiva may have a nodular appearance, but their colour (which ranges from coral pink to a deep bluish-red) depends upon the amount of inflammatory infiltrate present (Esterberg and White 1945). In severe overgrowth, the clinical crowns may be covered (plate 18) (Dolin 1951). The incidence and severity of phenytoin-induced gingival overgrowth is greatest on the labial aspects of the upper and lower anterior teeth (Esterberg and White 1945; Angelopoulos and Goaz 1972).

There have been a few cases reported of hyperplasia developing in edentulous ridges (Dallas 1963; Dreyer and Thomas, 1978; Darling *et al.* 1988). In such cases, the hyperplasia may be initiated and exacerbated by irritation from the denture, denture plaque, and/or food debris.

The relationship between the dose of phenytoin and the incidence and severity of gingival overgrowth is uncertain. A few studies have found a correlation between these variables (Panuska *et al.* 1961; Klar 1973), but most reports do not support this finding (Glickman and Lewitus 1941; Esterberg and White 1945; Dolin 1951; Angelopoulos and Goaz 1972; Conrad *et al.* 1974). However, there does appear to be a significant relationship between serum levels of phenytoin and the severity of the overgrowth (Kapur *et al.* 1973; Little *et al.* 1975). There is marked interindividual variation between the dose of phenytoin and serum concentrations (Partington *et al.* 1974). Thus serum concentrations of the drug, as opposed to its dose, may provide more pertinent information on the incidence and severity of gingival overgrowth.

Many studies have shown a clear relationship between the patient's oral hygiene status and the incidence and magnitude of phenytoin-induced gingival overgrowth, although some reports have contested this finding (for review, see Hassell 1981). Mouth-breathing and other local factors such as crowding significantly relate to the occurrence of the overgrowth (Glickman and Lewitus 1941).

It has been reported that patients receiving phenytoin have less periodontal bone loss than those taking sodium valproate (Seymour *et al.* 1985). Thus patients on phenytoin appear to have a degree of 'resistance' to further periodontal destruction. This finding may also be attributable to the action of phenytoin on the immune system (see later).

Histopathology

Several changes have been observed in both epithelium and connective tissue in phenytoin-induced gingival overgrowth. The epithelium shows varying degrees of acanthosis, with elongated, thin rete ridges that tend to be divided at their ends. This can give rise to an increased incidence of epithelial pearls. The degree of inflammation in the biopsy specimen will determine the presence and extent of polymorphonuclear leukocytes (PMNs) in the gingival epithelium.

The main change in the lamina propria is a proliferation of fibroblasts and an increase in collagen production. Other changes depend upon the level of inflammation and the stage of development of the overgrowth. In normal circumstances, collagen production from fibroblasts is controlled by the coordination of transcriptional and post-translation collagen regulatory mechanisms, including intracellular degradation. Exposure of gingival fibroblasts to phenytoin increases the levels of translatable collagen RNA (Benvineste and Bitar 1980). Overproduction of collagen by gingival fibroblasts in phenytoin-induced gingival enlargement involves an increased steady-state level of collagen

mRNA and not a decrease in collagen degradation (Narayanan *et al.* 1988). Such fibroblasts may be selected during the development of the overgrowth.

When normal gingival fibroblasts are grown in culture there is an age-related decrease in collagen and protein synthesis; fibroblasts from patients taking phenytoin do not appear to show this (Johnson *et al.* 1990). This difference may, in part, contribute to the overgrowth and it suggests that these cells are of a unique phenotype.

There has been much interest in the non-collagenous protein content in phenytoin-induced gingival overgrowth. It is estimated that these proteins comprise 20 per cent of the dry weight in gingival tissue from phenytoin patients and only 7 per cent in normal tissue (Ballard and Butler 1974). Patients on prolonged phenytoin therapy have significantly raised levels of hexosamine, uronic acid, and total protein per wet weight of tissue when compared to controls (Goultschin *et al.* 1983). It has also been shown that the connective tissue in phenytoin overgrowth has a significantly higher volume of density of the non-collagenous matrix than of the collagenous matrix (Dahllof *et al.* 1984). Studies on the tissue contents of proteoglycans and glycosaminoglycans have confirmed this finding (Dahllof *et al.* 1986). It is uncertain whether the increased amount of glycosaminoglycans in phenytoin-induced gingival overgrowth is due to increased synthesis or reduced degradation. It has been reported that cultures of gingival fibroblasts from patients with this overgrowth synthesize increased amounts of sulphated glycosaminoglycans (Kantor and Hassell 1983).

Other histochemical studies have shown an increase in tissue alkaline phosphatase activity in association with phenytoin-induced gingival overgrowth (Staple 1953) and depolymerization of the ground substance (Masi 1953). Under the electron microscope, the collagen fibres appear thinner and shorter compared with those in gingiva from normal individuals (Haim 1955). The significance of the various histological and histochemical changes in relationship to the pathogenesis of phenytoin-induced gingival overgrowth remains uncertain.

Pathogenesis

There are many theories as to why phenytoin causes gingival overgrowth. The most attractive at present is the direct effect of the drug or metabolites on the gingival tissues (Conrad *et al.* 1972; Hassell 1981; Modeer *et al.* 1982). Although it would seem straightforward to confirm this hypothesis by tissue culture experiments, the results of such studies have shown marked variation. This is probably due to differences in culture technique, concentration of drug used, and the degree of inflammation in the harvested gingival tissues (Hassell 1981).

It is suggested that there are in the gingival tissues different subpopulations of fibroblasts, some of which can synthesize large amounts of protein and collagen (high-activity fibroblasts), and others which are only capable of low protein synthesis (low-activity fibroblasts). The proportion of high- to low-activity fibroblasts appears to be genetically determined (Hassell and Gilbert 1983). Hassell (1981) has suggested that high-activity fibroblasts, in the presence of certain predisposing factors (e.g. inflammation), become sensitive to phenytoin, with a subsequent increase in collagen production; phenytoin or its metabolites will have no effect on other (low-activity) fibroblasts. Alternatively, phenytoin or its metabolites may be cytotoxic to low-activity fibroblasts, thus facilitating an increase in the population of high-activity fibroblasts.

For the drug or its metabolites to act on the different subpopulations of fibroblasts, the substances have to be present in the gingival tissues at greater concentrations than in the systemic or peripheral circulation. It has been demonstrated that certain gingival fibroblasts can metabolize phenytoin. This metabolic activity may determine the susceptibility of a patient to phenytoin-induced gingival overgrowth (Fine *et al.* 1974; Hassell and Cooper 1980).

Other unwanted effects of phenytoin that may relate to gingival overgrowth

Immunosuppression.

Long-term phenytoin therapy is reported to cause immunosuppression (Sorrell *et al.* 1971; Seager *et al.* 1975; Fontana *et al.* 1976). Abnormalities in immune function include deficiency of circulating IgA; inability to develop antibody to various types of antigen challenge, e.g. staphyloccoci; depression of the capacity to manifest delayed hypersensitivity reactions; depression of lymphocyte transformation.

Attempts have been made to link the immunosuppressant properties of phenytoin with gingival overgrowth (Aarli 1976). In the gingival tissues, secretory IgA is one of the first 'lines of defence' against bacterial plaque; a reduction in secretory IgA will render the tissues more susceptible to inflammation. Aarli has suggested that it is the body's attempts to deal with this inflammation via the repair processes that cause gingival enlargement. The demonstration of a clear correlation between phenytoin-induced gingival overgrowth and levels of IgA in crevicular fluid would add support to this hypothesis.

The immunosuppressant properties of phenytoin may in part explain the lack of alveolar bone loss in patients on this drug (Seymour *et al.* 1985). Suppression of both the humoral and cell-mediated immune responses will result in a reduction of lymphokine production, formation of antibody–antigen complexes, and complement activation (MacKinney and Booker 1972; Church and Dolby 1978). All of these factors, acting either directly or indirectly, are responsible for activating osteoclasts and hence bone resorption.

The action of phenytoin on the immune system may be a contributing (or predisposing) factor to gingival overgrowth, but it is unlikely to be the only cause. Other antiepileptic drugs (e.g. phenobarbitone and carbamazepine) also cause immunosuppression. Neither drug has been associated with gingival overgrowth.

Folic acid depletion.

Approximately half of patients taking phenytoin have a low serum level of folic acid (Waxman *et al.* 1970). In these patients, the incidence of megaloblastic anaemia is in the order of 0.75 per cent (Flexner and Hartman 1960). The mechanism of phenytoin-induced folic acid depletion is uncertain. The drug may reduce absorption of folic acid from the gastro intestinal tract or block its transport across intestinal epithelium. Alternatively, it may inhibit folate reductase, an enzyme found in the upper small intestine that hydrolyses dietary folate in the polyglutamate form to the monoglutamate form, thus facilitating absorption (Mallek and Nakamoto 1981).

It has been suggested that phenytoin-induced overgrowth is related to folic acid deficiency (Vogel 1977). Folic acid is essential for DNA synthesis, thus a deficiency will affect those cells with a high rate of turnover (i.e. bone marrow and also oral epithelium). A deficiency of folic acid may result in an impaired maturation of the gingival sulcular epithelium, thus rendering the underlying connective tissue more susceptible to inflammation (Dreizen *et al.* 1970). It has also been shown in animal studies that folic acid supplements reduce the incidence and severity of phenytoin-induced gingival overgrowth (Vogel 1980). However, in epileptics taking phenytoin, Mallek and Nakamato (1981) were unable to demonstrate that folic acid supplementation reduces or eliminates gingival overgrowth. Subsequent studies (see below) have contested this finding and show that folic acid supplementation may be of value.

Phenytoin and the adrenal glands.

Phenytoin therapy is reported to cause an alteration in the metabolism of the adrenal glands (Staple 1951, 1952) that results in a degree of adrenocortical unresponsiveness. This action may be due to suppression of ACTH production and consequent alteration in pituitary–adrenal activity. Suppression of adrenocortical function results in a reduction of glucocorticoid synthesis and this has been suggested as an explanation for the gingival overgrowth (Korff and Mutschelknauss 1963). When ACTH production is suppressed by phenytoin, there is a compensatory increase in the production of somatotrophic hormone (Nenning 1972), a hormone that may cause fibroblast proliferation.

Phenytoin also stimulates the sodium pump (Bihler and Sawh 1971), which acts as a stimulus to fibroblasts.

Although these ideas are attractive, there is little experimental evidence to support the possibility of interaction between phenytoin and the adrenal glands as a mechanism of gingival overgrowth. It may well be that suppression of adrenocortical function is yet another predisposing factor that contributes to the sensitivity of gingival fibroblasts to phenytoin (Hassell 1981).

Phenytoin and epidermal growth factor (EGF).

EGF is a polypeptide that takes part in tissue repair and regeneration. It also promotes glycosaminoglycan synthesis and stimulates the influx of calcium ions into mammalian fibroblasts (Turley *et al.* 1985; Pandiella *et al.* 1987). These biological actions are mediated by activation of specific receptors on the plasma membrane (Carpenter 1987). In a recent study (Modeer *et al.* 1990), human gingival fibroblasts were obtained from two patients, before and nine months after phenytoin therapy. One of the patients developed gingival overgrowth during that nine months whilst the other did not. The fibroblasts were studied for the effect of EGF on the incorporation of ^{3}H-thymidine into DNA, the binding of EGF to its cell-surface receptor, the internalization of EGF receptor–ligand complexes, and receptor mRNA levels to EGF. Fibroblasts from the two patients showed no difference in the affinity of the receptor for EGF. However, those from the patient that developed overgrowth showed an increase in the internalization of EGF receptor–ligand after phenytoin therapy whereas in those from the patient who showed no gingival changes, a decrease was observed. The steady-state level of EGF receptor mRNA increased significantly in fibroblasts derived from the patient with overgrowth, but decreased in the non-responder. Affinity cross-linking studies of the ligands showed that all gingival fibroblasts had one major component of EGF receptor with a molecular weight of 170 kDa. These findings suggest that phenytoin causes a down-regulation of EGF receptor metabolism in gingival fibroblasts from a patient who is to develop gingival overgrowth, whereas in non-responders there is an up-regulation.

Phenytoin and calcium metabolism.
Phenytoin exerts its anticonvulsant properties by stabilizing neuronal cell membranes to the action of sodium, potassium, and calcium. In addition the drug affects the transport of calcium ions across cell membranes and decreases the influx of calcium ions across membranes by decreasing membrane permeability and blocking intracellular uptake (Pincus 1972). This action of phenytoin on calcium transport could reduce or inhibit the secretory function of all affected cells.

Changes in the calcium metabolism of gingival fibroblasts may be important in the pathogenesis of the overgrowth. EGF is another factor that can affect the influx of calcium into fibroblasts (Pandiella *et al.* 1987). Brunius and Modeer (1989) have compared the effect of phenytoin alone or in combination with EGF on the intracellular accumulation of calcium in gingival fibroblasts *in vitro*. When normal fibroblasts were subjected to either phenytoin or EGF there was an increase in the intracellular accumulation of calcium, whereas fibroblasts obtained from a patient taking phenytoin showed no increase in intracellular calcium. However, when normal gingival fibroblasts were exposed to the combination of phenytoin and EGF, the EGF-induced increase in intracellular calcium was abolished. These findings suggest that phenytion influences the intracellular calcium metabolism of gingival fibroblasts, and that these drug-induced changes may be important in the activity of these cells and the subsequent development of overgrowth.

Conclusion

The precise pathogenesis of phenytoin-induced gingival overgrowth is unclear. Several factors, both systemic and local, contribute towards this condition. The fundamental disturbance is in the gingival fibroblast and protein synthesis. This cell is subjected to a variety of chemical messengers that are enhanced when the tissues are inflamed. Phenytoin or its metabolites act on these chemical messengers, either directly or via blocking receptors. How important these various actions are in the pathogenesis of gingival overgrowth remains uncertain.

4.2.3 CYCLOSPORIN

Cyclosporin is a hydrophobic, cyclic endecapeptide derived from the metabolic products of two fungal species, *Trichoderma polysporum* and *Cylindrocarpon lucidium*. The drug was initially produced as an antimicrobial agent, but early investigations showed that it had an inhibitory effect on lymphocyte proliferation (Borel *et al.* 1976). Since the discovery of these immunosuppressant properties, several studies have shown that the drug selectively acts on the T-lymphocyte response, with little or no action on B lymphocytes.

Cyclosporin can be given orally, intramuscularly, or intravenously. After oral administration, the drug is absorbed from the gastrointestinal tract and absorption shows marked interindividual variation. Peak plasma concentrations occur 3–4 h after dosage, and the drug has a serum half-life of between 17 and 40 h (Beveridge *et al.* 1981). Cyclosporin is extensively metabolized in the liver and metabolism is mediated through the cytochrome P450 mono-oxygenase system (Maurer 1985). Some of the metabolites of cyclosporin have been identified. In humans, the primary metabolites are 1, 17, and 21.

To maintain immunosuppression, an oral therapeutic dose of between 10 and 20 mg/kg body weight/day is required. Such a dose would result in a serum concentration of between 100 and 400 ng/ml.

The main use of cyclosporin is to prevent graft rejection in organ transplantation. The drug is also used in the treatment of a variety of autoimmune disorders such as type I diabetes, rheumatoid arthritis, psoriasis, and other skin disorders.

Cyclosporin and gingival overgrowth

The association between cyclosporin therapy and gingival overgrowth was first noticed in the early 1980s when the drug was undergoing initial evaluation in transplant surgery (Starzl *et al.* 1980; Calne *et al.* 1981). Subsequent animal experiments confirmed this unwanted effect. Both dogs and cats dosed with cyclosporin at 15–45 mg/kg and 45–95 mg/kg, respectively, developed gingival overgrowth (Ryffel *et al.* 1983). The changes were reversible on cessation of the drug. The first cases of cyclosporin-induced gingival overgrowth were reported in the dental literature in 1983 (Rateitschak-Pluss *et al.* 1983). There have subsequently been several case reports and studies of the various factors that can influence the incidence and severity of this problem. The findings are summarized in Table 4.1.

Cyclosporin-induced gingival overgrowth commences as a papillary swelling that is more pronounced on the labial aspects of the gingiva than on the palatal or lingual (Tyldesley and Rotter 1984). The swelling enlarges and adjacent papillae appear to coalesce. This gives the gingiva a lobulated appearance (Plate 19). Overgrowth is restricted to the width of the attached gingiva, but can extend coronally and interfere with the occlusion, mastication, and speech (Plate

20). Cyclosporin-induced gingival overgrowth has not been reported in edentulous subjects (Friskop and Klintmalm 1986).

The hyperplastic gingiva often show marked inflammatory changes. They bleed readily on probing and are generally more hyperaemic than the gingiva from phenytoin-induced overgrowth. This impression is confirmed by those who have found marked haemorrhage when the tissues are removed surgically.

If a patient is 'at risk' from developing gingival overgrowth, then it usually occurs within three months of cyclosporin dosage (Seymour *et al.* 1987). However, changes have been reported to occur as early as one month after starting therapy (Tyldesley and Rotter 1984). The incidence of gingival overgrowth varies from study to study, with a range of between 25–81 per cent (see Table 4.1). These differences may be related to drug dosage, plasma concentration of cyclosporin, duration of therapy, method of assessing gingival overgrowth, the underlying periodontal status, and the medical condition for which the drug is being used.

Thus it would seem that some patients are more susceptible to gingival changes from cyclosporin therapy than others. The relationship between cyclosporin dosage, plasma concentration, and gingival overgrowth is a contentious issue. Obviously some baseline concentration of cyclosporin is required to stimulate the hyperplastic changes. Some have shown that gingival overgrowth is related to high doses of cyclosporin (Adams and Davies 1984; Rostock *et al.* 1986), whilst others have shown significant correlations between plasma and salivary concentration of the drug and the severity of gingival overgrowth (McGaw *et al.* 1987; Seymour *et al.* 1987). Many of the other studies in Table 4.1 suggest that plaque scores are more important determinants of the gingival changes in cyclosporin treated patients. Recently, it has been shown, in a controlled study, that an intensive course of plaque control and removal of gingival irritants does not inhibit the development of cyclosporin-induced gingival overgrowth (Seymour and Smith 1990). However, such measures improved the gingival health of the patients.

It may be that susceptibility to cyclosporin-induced gingival changes is related to an interaction between the drug and local inflammation. This possible relationship is discussed later.

Renal transplantation is the most common organ-grafting procedure and hence one where cyclosporin is most widely used. There is some evidence that when the drug is used in bone-marrow grafting the incidence of gingival overgrowth is very low (2 per cent) (Beveridge 1983). As mentioned above, cyclosporin is used in a variety of medical conditions (e.g. type I diabetes, psoriasis, rheumatoid arthritis) and in most organ transplants. These various patients provide an opportunity to determine whether the underlying medical problem is an important determinant of the overgrowth.

Age of the patient may be a further factor that can influence the incidence and severity of this overgrowth. Children and adolescents suffering from type I diabetes were more affected by the overgrowth than were adults (Daley *et al.* 1986). This suggests a possible interaction between cyclosporin, sex hormones, and gingival fibroblasts, or alternatively, fibroblasts from young patients may be more susceptible to the drug.

Histology

The histological appearance of cyclosporin-induced gingival overgrowth is similar to that resulting from phenytoin. It consists primarily of connective tissue with an overlying irregular, multilayered, parakeratinized epithelium of variable thickness. In some areas, epithelial ridges penetrate deeply into the subepithelial connective tissue, and irregularly arranged collagen fibre bundles are associated with them. The connective tissue is highly vascularized and focal accumulations of infiltrating inflammatory cells have been seen (Rateitschak-Pluss *et al.* 1983).

These findings have been confirmed in numerous studies, but with considerable variation in the reported intensity of the inflammatory cell infiltrate. The predominant type in the infiltrate is the plasma cell, with smaller numbers of lymphocytes. They are often located adjacent to bundles of connective tissue fibres and may be present in sufficient quantity to appear neoplastic, although no nuclear or cytoplasmic abnormalities have been found (Deliliers *et al.* 1986). Detailed characterization of mononuclear cell infiltrates has shown T lymphocytes and monocytes adjacent to the junctional epithelium with virtually no B lymphocytes (Friskopp *et al.* 1986). It is unclear whether this mononuclear cell infiltrate is related to the cyclosporin-induced enlargement, the presence of gingivitis, or both.

Others have described acanthosis and parakeratinization of the epithelium, with pseudoepitheliomatous proliferation and oedema. Immunohistological investigation has demonstrated an increase in the number of Langerhans cells intraepithelially and immediately subjacent, in inflamed sites (Savage *et al.* 1987). Focal areas of myxomatous change alternating with zones of dense collagen have been reported, especially in the tissue immediately beneath the epithelium (Rostock *et al.* 1986). These changes have been seen in conjunction with conspicuous epithelial enlargement. This finding, together with the presence of foci of PAS-positive material within the epithelium and stroma, has led to the view that cyclosporin-induced gingival enlargement may result from an accumulation of non-collagenous extracellular material and a thickening of the epithelium (Pisanty *et al.* 1990).

A degree of fibroplasia, characterized by the presence of increased numbers of fibroblasts (often with enlarged, ovoid, vesicular nuclei) has been described within the gingival connective tissue (Wysoki *et al.* 1983). Other studies, however, have failed to demonstrate an increase in the numerical density of fibroblasts, and a volume density of extracellular collagen similar to that of normal gingiva has also been found (McGaw and Porter 1988). It has been suggested that these contrasting findings may be due to differences in the evolutionary stage of the overgrowth, with changes in fibroblast density occurring as the lesion progresses. The disagreement over fibroblast numbers indicates that cyclosporin-induced gingival enlargement may not be a true hyperplasia and hence the term gingival overgrowth or enlargement is more appropriate.

Table 4.1 Synopsis of the findings from case reports and studies that have investigated cyclosporin-induced gingival hyperplasia

Study	Number of patients	Medical condition	Periodontal measures	Cyclosporin dosage/measures	Treatment	Findings
Adams and Davies (1984)	2	Heart transplants	—	500 mg/day	Gingivectomy scaling and intensive oral hygiene instructions	Gingival hyperplasia may be dose related. However, attention should be placed on rigorous plaque control and intensive oral hygiene.
Bartold (1987)	1	Renal transplant	—	Initial dosage of 12.5 mg/kg. Reduced over a 2 year period to 1.9 mg/kg	Gingivectomy. Patient was monitored for 6/12, no recurrence	Patient presented with localised gingival enlargement on labial aspects of anterior teeth. Oral hygiene was poor. Fibroblasts from normal and overgrown sites were studied *in vitro*. Those from overgrown tissue proliferated at a slower rate and produced slightly less protein than cells from healthy sites.
Bennett and Christian (1985)	1	Renal transplant	—	450 mg/day	Gingivectomy followed by 2 months maintenance with attention to oral hygiene	Gingival hyperplasia occurred within 2 months of cyclosporin therapy. In the post gingivectomy maintenance period, there was no recurrence.
Daley et al. (1986)	100	18 Renal transplants 78 Type I diabetics	Hyperplasia score Plaque score Presence of local irritants	Dose of cyclosporin. Serum trough levels	—	70% of patients exhibited some degree of gingival hyperplasia, which was not related to the dose of cyclosporin. However, a threshold serum concentration is necessary for hyperplastic concentrations to occur. The severity of hyperplasia was not directly related to serum levels of the drug, but weakly related to the abundance of dental plaque. Children and adolescents are more susceptible to cyclosporin-induced gingival changes.
Friskopp and Klintmalm (1986)	30 + 19 controls	Renal transplants	Pocket depths Plaque score CPITN Gingival enlargement	Average dose of cyclosporin = 6.8 mg/kg/day Trough cyclosporin plasma levels	Scaling and oral hygiene instruction	81% of the cyclosporin treated patients showed gingival enlargement. There was no difference in periodontal status and cyclosporin measures between the patients who experienced gingival enlargement and those who did not. Gingival condition improved with oral hygiene.
McGaw et al. (1987)	30	Renal transplants	Gingival overgrowth index Plaque score Gingival inflammation	Serum and salivary levels of cyclosporin	—	Eight patients [27%] were classified as 'responders', i.e. showed signs of gingival hyperplasia. A positive correlation was found between gingival overgrowth scores and both plaque and gingival inflammation scores. Similarly, a significant correlation was found between whole saliva levels of cyclosporin and gingival overgrowth scores.
Rateitschak-Pluss et al. (1983)	3	Renal transplants	Probing depths Bone loss	Average dose of cyclosporin was 10 mg/kg body wt	In one case, extraction of teeth and gingivectomy Others gingivoplasty	Seven patients out of 50 developed gingival problems attributable to cyclosporin. 3 were reported in the paper. Gingival enlargement began 4–6 weeks after transplant. Gingival condition improved after initial debridment. Rigorous plaque control is of utmost importance in preventing recurrence.

Reference	Number of patients	Transplant type	Clinical measures	Cyclosporin measurement	Treatment	Findings
Ross et al. 1989	21 + 21 age and sex matched controls	Liver transplants	Plaque index, Gingival index, Pocket depths, Width of free gingiva	Serum cyclosporin levels assessed 24 hours after dental examination	—	No significant correlations were found between serum concentrations of cyclosporin and any of the periodontal measures. Plaques scores were more important determinants of gingival changes. The authors recommended strict oral hygiene in liver transplant patients treated with cyclosporin.
Rostock et al. (1986)	1	Liver transplant	—	Initial dose 500 mg b.i.d. reduced to 200 mg b.i.d. then increased to 500 mg b.i.d.	Combined gingivectomy and flap procedure to remove hyperplastic tissue	Recurrence of hyperplasia occurred when cyclosporin dosage was increased to 500 mg b.i.d. Findings from this case report suggest that cyclosporin-induced gingival hyperplasia is a result of an interrelationship between local factors [i.e. plaque and calculus] and the dose of cyclosporin.
Seymour et al. (1987)	12 + 12 controls	Renal transplants	Plaque index, Gingival index, Probing depths, % Gingival Hyperplasia scores	Mean plasma concentrations of cyclosporin over a 6 month investigation period	—	Patients treated with cyclosporin had significantly more gingival hyperplasia and probing sites > 3 mm than those treated with azathioprine. Gingival hyperplasia scores and the number of probing sites > 3 mm were significantly higher in the cyclosporin group at 3 and 6 months post transplant. A significant correlation was observed between mean plasma concentrations of cyclosporin throughout the 6 month investigation period and percentage change in gingival hyperplasia scores from baseline. There was no significant correlation between gingival hyperplasia and plaque scores.
Seymour and Smith (1990)	27	Renal transplants	Plaque index, Gingival index, Probing depths, % Gingival Hyperplasia score	Mean dose of cyclosporin and whole blood concentrations throughout 6 month investigation period	After baseline 12 patients entered an oral hygiene programme. The remaining 15 received no treatment for 6 months	In both treatment groups there was a significant increase [$p < 0.05$] in gingival hyperplasia scores. Dosages of cyclosporin, whole blood concentrations of the drug, gingival index and plaque scores were not important determinants for the increase in gingival overgrowth. However, plaque control and the removal of local irritants is of some benefit for the gingival health of cyclosporin treated renal transplant patients.
Tyldesley and Rotter (1984)	36	Renal transplants	Presence or absence of gingival hyperplasia observed over a 2 year period	—	Gingival surgery where necessary, plaque control and maintenance	Nine patients [25%] developed gingival hyperplasia. Emphasis was placed on the early attainment of a high standard of oral hygiene to prevent gingival hyperplasia.
Wysocki et al. (1983)	18 (4 showed slight gingival changes, 2 showed severe gingival changes)	Renal transplants	—	Pre- and 2 hour post-dosage serum levels of cyclosporin	Two cases with severe gingival hyperplasia underwent gingivectomy	The degree of gingival hyperplasia induced by cyclosporin was in part related to gingival irritants, but hyperplasia may also be related to the individual patients sensitivity to the drug or its metabolite. The severity of gingival hyperplasia may follow a cyclical course.

Electron microscopic examination of gingival fibroblasts in patients taking cyclosporin has revealed ultrastructural characteristics of active protein synthesis and secretion, with reduced cytotoxic or degenerative changes. An increased proportion of cells containing microfilament bands with semiperiodic dense nodes, nuclear indentations, and basal lamina associated cell-to-stromal junctions has also been found (Yamasaki *et al.* 1987). The term myofibroblast has been applied to such cells (Gabbiani 1977).

Laboratory studies

Functionally heterogeneous subpopulations of fibroblasts have been found within normal human gingival tissue (Hassell and Stanek 1983). These discrete and phenotypically stable subpopulations are characterized by differences in a number of functional measures including the rate of cell proliferation, protein synthesis, collagen production, and response to various chemical agents. There is evidence that the gingival overgrowth which occurs in some patients receiving phenytoin may be due to the presence of genetically determined, phenytoin-sensitive fibroblast subpopulations (Hassell and Gilbert 1983), as discussed in the preceding section. A similar mechanism has been suggested to account for the effect of cyclosporin on the gingival tissues of some individuals and it has been shown that the drug does have differential effects on fibroblast subpopulations (Tipton and Dabbous 1986).

A number of studies have examined the direct effect of cyclosporin on fibroblasts in cell culture and it has been shown that the drug can enhance cell proliferation at a concentration of 400 ng/ml. The effect of cyclosporin on the synthetic activity of fibroblasts is variable, with both stimulation and inhibition found in different individual cell strains and at different drug concentrations (Coley *et al.* 1986). This variability of response may be attributable to the heterogeneity of gingival fibroblast subpopulations described above. Other investigators have reported a stimulatory effect of cyclosporin on fibroblast proliferation, protein synthesis, and collagen production. The responses were dose-dependent and significant at a drug concentration of 500 ng/ml (Zebrowski *et al.* 1986).

Fibroblast cultures derived from normal and enlarged gingiva of a patient receiving cyclosporin showed no morphological differences by phase-contrast microscopy. There was a significant reduction in the proliferative activity of cells from overgrown tissue when compared with normal gingival fibroblasts. Protein synthesis was also reduced in the fibroblast cultures from the enlarged gingiva although this was not statistically significant (Bartold 1987). Bartold later reported a stimulatory effect of cyclosporin on fibroblast DNA synthesis and cell proliferation. The effect on DNA synthesis was greater in cells derived from overgrown gingival tissue. Stimulation of protein synthesis was found, although this was not statistically significant. Cyclosporin also negated the inhibitory effect of lipopolysaccharide on fibroblast cultures, indicating a possible reason for the observed relationship between areas of prominent gingival overgrowth and dental plaque (Bartold 1989).

Animal studies have included an investigation into the synthetic activity of cultured gingival fibroblasts from normal and cyclosporin-treated beagle dogs (W. Seibel, personal communication). The majority of fibroblast cultures obtained after cyclosporin was given showed increased protein synthesis and collagen production when compared with cells obtained before administration of the drug. However, two out of seven cultures had reduced synthetic activity after cyclosporin treatment, again raising the question of individual susceptibility to the drug. Cyclosporin had no *in vitro* effect on protein and collagen formation by the fibroblast cultures.

Fluorescence-activated, vital cell-sorting of human fibroblast subpopulations has been attempted using a fluorescent (dansylated) form of cyclosporin (Hassell *et al.* 1988). Two separate cell populations could be identified: 35 per cent of cells did not bind with the dansylated cyclosporin whereas 41 per cent avidly bound the drug and were more responsive to cyclosporin in culture medium in terms of proliferation and synthetic activity.

The interrelationships of cells mediating the effects of cyclosporin have also been investigated. It was shown that gingival fibroblasts from different patients do not react in the same way to cyclosporin *in vitro*. At different drug concentrations, a variety of effects on fibroblast synthetic activity were found. These were modified by the addition of supernatants from lymphocyte cultures, indicating the possibility of an interaction between lymphocyte products and gingival fibroblasts (Hassell *et al.* 1988).

More recently, attention has been drawn to the role of cyclosporin metabolites in the aetiology of the various side-effects of the drug. The major cyclosporin metabolite, OL-17, has been shown to stimulate significantly fibroblast proliferation and it produces both stimulatory and inhibitory effects in the fibroblast subpopulations identified by fluorescence-activated cell-sorting (Jacobs *et al.* 1990).

4.2.4 CALCIUM-CHANNEL BLOCKERS

As their name suggests, these drugs block the inward displacement of calcium ions through the slow channels of active cell membranes. Three groups of calcium-channel blockers are in clinical use: verapamil, a benzeneacetonitrile; diltiazem, a benzothiazepine; and the dihydropyridines—nifedipine, nicardipine, nitrendipine, and oxodipine.

These drugs affect myocardial cells, the conducting system to the heart, and vascular smooth muscle. Hence they are used in the management of angina, arrhythmias, and hypotension. The various calcium-channel blockers differ in their predeliction for the various sites of action; therefore their therapeutic effects and clinical indications are variable. For example, verapamil decreases myocardial contractility and acts on the sinus and atrioventricular node. The drug is mainly used in the treatment of supraventricular arrhythmias, angina, and hypertension. Nifedipine relaxes vascular smooth muscle and dilates the coronary arteries. Hence this drug is mainly used in the prophylaxis and treatment of angina and in the control of mild to moderate hypertension.

Gingival overgrowth is an unwanted effect mainly associated with nifedipine. However, further case reports suggest that this is an unwanted effect common to all calcium-channel blockers.

Nifedipine

Gingival overgrowth associated with nifedipine therapy was first reported in 1984 (Lederman *et al.* 1984). Since then several case reports have documented this unwanted effect (Ramon *et al.* 1984; Van der Wall *et al.* 1985; Lucas *et al.* 1985; Bencini *et al.* 1985; Jones 1986; Puolijoki *et al.* 1988; Yusof 1989).

Clinically, nifedipine-associated gingival hyperplasia resembles phenytoin-induced gingival overgrowth. The hyperplasia appears shortly after the start of therapy and decreases on withdrawal of the drug (Lederman *et al.* 1984). It is most pronounced on the labial gingiva of the upper and lower anterior teeth (Plate 21), but does not occur in edentulous areas. The incidence of this problem may be in the order of 15 per cent, and the severity of the hyperplasia shows a weak correlation with dose (Barak *et al.* 1987).

Histologically, the gingival epithelium is parakeratinized and has elongated rete pegs ('test tubes'). The underlying connective tissue comprises a diffuse mixture of dense collagen with a varying amount of ground substance. Inflammatory cells are present in the connective tissue, mainly plasma cells and lymphocytes. Nifedipine-induced gingival hyperplasia also resembles phenytoin-induced gingival overgrowth histochemically. Gingival fibroblasts from both conditions contain strongly sulphated mucopolysaccharides and numerous secretory granules. Electron microscopy has shown that nifedipine-induced hyperplasia is due to an increase in ground substance (Lucas *et al.* 1985).

Animal studies have shown that gingival overgrowth is associated with two further dihydropyridines—oxodipine (Waner *et al.* 1988; Nyska *et al.* 1990) and nitrendipine (Heijl and Sundin 1988). In the oxodipine studies, gingival changes in both dogs and rats were dose-related. There was a purely fibroblastic proliferation without any infiltrate of inflammatory cells.

Nitrendipine administered to nine beagle dogs with established plaque and gingivitis caused the development of overgrowth as early as 10 weeks after dosage (Heijl and Sundin 1988). The principal histological change was that areas of non-infiltrated connective tissue in test specimens showed an increase in vascularity and appeared less dense. These vascular changes may be related to the vasodilatory properties of the drug.

Diltiazem

There have been fewer cases of gingival overgrowth associated with diltiazem therapy (Giustiniani *et al.* 1987; Bowman *et al.* 1988). The histological appearance is similar to that of nifedipine-induced gingival overgrowth.

Verapamil

Again, only a few cases of gingival overgrowth associated with verapamil have been reported (Cucchi *et al.* 1985;

Smith and Glenert 1987; Pernu *et al.* 1989). One series of tissue culture studies has shown that the proliferation rate, protein and collagen production of fibroblasts harvested from an overgrowth were markedly lower than in control cells cultured from healthy gingiva. Incubation of fibroblasts in the presence of verapamil reduced protein and collagen synthesis (Pernu *et al.* 1989).

Pathogenesis of gingival overgrowth induced by calcium-channel blockers

Calcium-channel blockers are extensively prescribed in medical practice, yet there is little information on the incidence and severity of gingival overgrowth associated with this group of drugs. The problem of overgrowth appears to be more often associated with nifedipine that the others. This may be related to drug usage; that is, nifedipine is more often prescribed than diltiazen or verapamil.

Factors that influence gingival overgrowth in patients taking calcium-channel blockers have yet to be elucidated. Much interest has focused on the action of these drugs on intracellular calcium metabolism and the possible relationship with gingival overgrowth. Both phenytoin and the calcium-channel blockers inhibit intracellular uptake of calcium (see p. 80). This inhibitory effect may affect the secretory properties of gingival fibroblasts or the production of collagenases. Nifedipine also inhibits T-cell proliferation and interleukin-2 production by preventing a change in intracellular uptake of calcium ions (Gelfand *et al.* 1986). Gingival overgrowth caused by nifedipine (and perhaps other calcium-channel blockers) and cyclosporin may be related to the calcium-dependent inhibitory effect on T cells and subsequent immunosuppression.

Although the pathogenesis of this gingival overgrowth is uncertain, the pharmacodynamics of calcium-channel blockers and their effect on cellular calcium has provided a possible unifying mechanism for drug-induced gingival overgrowth.

4.2.5 MANAGEMENT OF DRUG-INDUCED GINGIVAL OVERGROWTH

The management of drug-induced gingival overgrowth can be considered under two categories: surgical excision, and prevention and maintenance.

Surgical management

Excessive gingival tissue needs to be removed to restore contour and the knife-edge gingiva. This in turn will facilitate mechanical plaque control. The gingival incision will depend upon the extent of overgrowth and whether it is associated with underlying bone loss. Excessive tissue, with little or no accompanying bone loss, can be excised by a 45° gingivectomy incision. This procedure is usually done under local anaesthesia, and if the whole mouth is affected, one quadrant is treated at a time. Some patients may prefer such 'whole mouth' surgery to be carried out under general anaesthesia. Indeed, for patients with severe cyclosporin-induced gingival overgrowth this may be the most appropriate method of dealing with the problem. The organ-transplant patient on cyclosporin will also be taking prednisolone. Thus, before surgery they will require corticosteroid cover (100 mg hydrocortisone hemisuccinate, intramuscularly, half-an-hour before surgery) and antibiotic cover. The advantage of treating these patients under general anaesthesia is that the procedure can be completed under one antibiotic and corticosteroid cover. If the gingival surgery is done under local anaesthesia, they will require multiple visits and several covers.

Cyclosporin and nifedipine-induced gingival overgrowths tend to be very hyperaemic and the surgeon should be prepared for marked bleeding. If the gingivectomy is to be done under general anaesthesia, then the patient's blood should be cross-matched and transfused if necessary. Where possible, an infiltration of the tissues with local anaesthetic containing a vasoconstrictor just before surgery will facilitate haemostasis.

Where gingival overgrowth occurs with bone loss, then gingival recontouring should be done together with a mucopereosteal flap to facilitate root-surface debridement. A proprietary dressing material (Coe-Pack) is placed over the wound. Analgesics are rarely required after periodontal surgery because the incidence and severity of pain is usually slight (Seymour *et al.* 1983). In the event of postoperative pain, the patient should take aspirin or paracetamol. Pack and sutures are removed after one week and proper oral hygiene technique reinforced. After pack removal, patients should be prescribed chlorhexidine mouthrinse, 0.2 per cent (10 ml twice daily), as toothbrushing may be uncomfortable in the early postoperative period.

Prevention

The precise aetiology and pathogenesis of drug-induced gingival overgrowth is uncertain. Therefore, methods of controlling or preventing this problem are empirical. The various techniques that can be used are now discussed under the headings of the appropriate drugs.

Phenytoin

It appears that some patients on phenytoin therapy are more susceptible to gingival overgrowth than others (see p. 78). The pathogenesis suggests that certain susceptibility factors can be identified or determined. These include the magnitude of inflammation present in the gingival tissues, the proportion of high-activity to low-activity fibroblasts, the ability of the gingival fibroblast to concentrate and metabolize phenytoin, and the serum concentration of the drug and its metabolites. Variation in these factors may account for the variable gingival responses in patients taking phenytoin.

Gingival inflammation is one of the factors that can be readily changed by attention to plaque control and the removal of other predisposing factors, (e.g. ill-fitting partial dentures, overhanging restorations, and supra- and subgingival calculus). However, the precise role of gingival inflammation and hence plaque control in the pathogenesis of phenytoin-induced gingival hyperplasia is uncertain.

Some reports (Kerr 1952; King 1954; Panuska *et al.* 1962) have shown an association between poor oral hygiene and the most advanced stages of gingival overgrowth. However, earlier work was not in accord with this finding (Millhon and Esterberg 1942; Stern *et al.* 1943; Esterberg and White 1945).

Later investigations have considered the effect of a plaque-control programme on the incidence and severity of phenytoin-induced gingival overgrowth. King *et al.* (1976) examined the efficacy of good oral hygiene measures in 13 young male epileptics who had gingival overgrowth resulting from their phenytoin therapy. The excess gingiva was excised and the patients received 'operator assisted oral hygiene' around half of their teeth. Less inflammation and less regrowth of gingival tissue occurred around the teeth subjected to good oral hygiene. It was concluded that gingival overgrowth can be significantly reduced after excision, provided good oral hygiene is maintained. However, the impact of the surgical procedure on the gingival tissues was not considered and the investigators point out that surgery itself may modify the gingival response to any therapeutic measures.

The efficacy of plaque control measures in preventing gingival overgrowth has also been investigated in a group of patients starting medication with phenytoin (Philstrom *et al.* 1980). In spite of good oral hygiene, gingival enlargement still occurred, especially around the anterior teeth, during the first six months of medication; no further enlargement developed during the subsequent nine months. The investigator recommended that a comprehensive plaque-control programme be instituted as soon as patients are treated with phenytoin.

More recent work in children has shown that the development of phenytoin-induced gingival overgrowth could not be prevented by a specific plaque-control programme (Dahllof and Modeer, 1986). However, in a further study (Modeer and Dahllof 1987), it was shown that the effectiveness of a plaque-control programme in preventing the development of the overgrowth was dependent upon the intensity of the instructions and their timing prior to phenytoin therapy. For optimal efficacy the plaque-control programme should be instituted before the start of the medication.

Chlorhexidine mouthrinse may also be of value in preventing phenytoin-induced gingival overgrowth, especially after gingival surgery (O'Neil and Figures 1982). Use of chlorhexidine is associated with taste disturbances, and staining of the teeth and oral mucosa (see Chapter 9). These unwanted effects may deter patients from using this plaque inhibitory agent long-term.

The evidence from the various studies suggests that excellent plaque control alone does not completely prevent the occurrence of gingival overgrowth in patients on phenytoin. However, good plaque control will reduce gingival inflammation, which in turn may reduce the incidence and severity of the gingival response to the drug.

The relationship between phenytoin-induced gingival overgrowth and folic acid deficiency has been discussed (see p.79). Animal studies have shown that folic acid supplements reduced the incidence and severity of this problem. In a controlled study (Drew *et al.* 1987), the effect of topical and systemic folate was evaluated in a group of patients taking phenytoin. Topical folate significantly inhibited gingival overgrowth to a greater extent than either systemic folate or placebo. It has been suggested that topical folate may reduce gingival inflammation by binding to plaque-derived endotoxin (George and Pack 1983). This action may, in turn, reduce gingival overgrowth. The value of topical folate in reducing phenytoin-induced gingival overgrowth requires further appraisal.

The effect of systemic folic acid on the incidence and severity of this gingival overgrowth appears to be dependent upon baseline plasma, and red blood-cell levels of folate, and serum levels of phenytoin (Backman *et al.* 1989). In a controlled study, 31 epileptic children receiving phenytoin were randomly assigned to groups with or without daily supplementation of folic acid (5 mg). Their phenytoin serum levels were below the lower reference range and, before folic acid supplementation, their red blood-cell and plasma folate levels were normal. After one year, the systemic folic acid produced no significant changes in the size of the gingival tissues. A further nine mentally retarded adult epileptics taking phenytoin were similarly treated with folic acid. Before treatment their phenytoin levels were above the higher reference range and their plasma and red blood-cell folic acid levels were below normal. In this second group of patients, folic acid supplementation significantly reduced the phenytoin-induced gingival overgrowth. Thus it would appear that this supplementation is only of benefit in preventing that overgrowth if plasma and red blood-cell levels of folate are low in the first instance.

A fortuitous finding in a single case is that phenytoin-induced gingival overgrowth significantly improved when an epileptic patient was treated with isotretinoin to resolve her facial acne (Norris and Cunliffe 1987). Isotretinoin inhibits the proliferation and collagen synthesis of fibroblasts (Hein *et al.* 1984).The drug has a modulatory effect on cyclic adenosine 3′, 5′-monophosphate, which is an important factor in the inhibition of fibroblast growth; it also has an inhibitory effect on ornithine decarboxylase, which is the rate-limiting enzyme in the production of the polyamines. Polyamines are intimately associated with cellular growth and division.

It is difficult to draw firm conclusions from one case report. However, the marked improvement in the gingiva and the underlying theoretical basis would suggest that the use of isotretinoin as a means of preventing or treating phenytoin-induced overgrowth is worthy of further appraisal.

Cyclosporin

The incidence of cyclosporin-induced gingival overgrowth is approximately 30 per cent; it can be assumed from this that some patients on cyclosporin are more susceptible to this problem than others. However, susceptibility factors have not been clearly identified. Similarly, the role of plaque has not been fully elucidated. Early case reports advocated effective plaque control and the removal of other local predisposing factors (Rateitschak-Pluss *et al.* 1983). In a more extensive study (McGaw *et al.* 1987) of renal transplant patients taking cyclosporin, a significant correlation

was found between gingival overgrowth and both dental plaque and gingivitis scores, and between gingival overgrowth scores and concentrations of cyclosporin in whole saliva. Others have failed to find a correlation between the incidence and severity of cyclosporin-induced gingival overgrowth and plaque scores (Daley *et al.* 1986; Seymour *et al.* 1987).

The efficacy of a plaque-control programme in preventing cyclosporin-induced gingival overgrowth has been evaluated in a group of renal transplant patients (Seymour and Smith 1990). Those subjected to an intensive course of plaque control and removal of local irritants showed better gingival health than the controls. However, the oral hygiene measures did not prevent the development of gingival overgrowth.

Serum concentrations of cyclosporin may be a more important determinant for the development of gingival overgrowth (Adams and Davies 1984; McGaw *et al.* 1987 Seymour *et al.* 1987). After transplant surgery, the dose of cyclosporin is high in the early postoperative period and is then gradually reduced. In renal transplant patients this dose reduction is imperative because cyclosporin is nephrotoxic. Thus an early reduction in cyclosporin dosage may reduce the gingival problems. However, cyclosporin is an important immunosuppressive drug in preventing graft rejection. A too early or too rapid reduction in dosage cannot be contemplated if such a measure increases the risk of graft rejection. Furthermore, an alteration to the dose of cyclosporin can only be considered by the patient's physician, who may regard the problem of gingival overgrowth as insignificant when compared to the risk of graft rejection. Thus, until the mechanisms of cyclosporin-induced gingival overgrowth are discovered, the periodontologist should be concerned with reducing the problem of gingival inflammation in these patients.

Calcium-channel blockers

As with cyclosporin, the pathogenesis of this condition in relationship to plaque and gingival inflammation has not been established. Again, the periodontologist should be aware that this group of drugs can cause gingival problems, and try to ensure that such patients are regularly monitored and maintained as plaque-free as possible. If gingival hyperplasia is a persistent problem, then the patient's physician may consider changing the medication, if appropriate, to another drug that does not block calcium channels. As all calcium-channel blockers can cause gingival hyperplasia, there is little advantage in changing from one of these to another.

4.3 DRUG-INDUCED GINGIVAL HYPERSENSITIVITY REACTIONS

Introduction

This condition is frequently referred to as plasma cell gingivitis and is invariably due to a contact hypersensitivity reaction from a flavouring substance in toothpaste, chewing gum, or sucking mints. The condition has previously been described under a variety of names including atypical gingivostomatitis (Owings 1969), idiopathic gingivostomatitis (Kerr, *et al.* 1971*a*), and allergic gingivostomatitis (Kerr *et al.* 1971*b*). Plasma cell gingivitis should be distinguished from the rare extramedullary gingival plasmacytoma (plasmacytosis of the gingiva) (Poswillo 1968) and the plasma cell granuloma (Bhaskar *et al.* 1968).

Most of the early cases of plasma cell gingivitis implicated mint or cinnamon-flavoured chewing gum as the aetiological agent (Miller 1941; Sugarman 1950). Subsequently the condition has been caused by sucking mints (Lubow *et al.* 1984), toothpaste containing cinnamonaldehyde (Thyne *et al.* 1989; Lamey *et al.* 1990), mint-flavoured toothpaste (Perry *et al.* 1973) and a herbal toothpaste (Macleod and Ellis 1989). Two further cases of plasma cell gingivitis have been described where no obvious aetiological agent could be identified (Palmer and Eveson 1981). However, one of the patients was atopic and the other had a history of psoriasis.

Clinical features

The main complaint from patients with plasma gingivitis is 'a sore mouth and lips' of sudden onset. This condition is usually intensified by toothpastes or spicy foods. The lips, tongue, and attached gingiva are the structures commonly involved in these hypersensitivity reactions. The lips are often dry, atrophic, and shiny, with varying degrees of fissuring; an angular cheilitis is often present. The tongue is usually erythematous and may be swollen. The gingival lesion affects the free and attached tissues. They are usually bright red in appearance (Plate 22), oedematous, and enlarged. The redness may extend on to the palatal mucosa; edentulous areas are less severely involved.

Symptoms can involve the upper respiratory tract, and some patients may complain of a burning sore throat and hoarseness of the voice.

Laboratory findings

Biopsy of the gingiva invariably shows acanthosis with elongation of the rete pegs. Microvesicles can occur in the epithelium, owing to cell liquefaction; the microvesicles contain PMNs. The main histopathological feature is the heavy infiltration of plasma cells into the submucosa, which is so intense that many of the normal structures are obliterated (Kerr *et al.* 1971*a*; Perry *et al.* 1973).

Immunofluorescent studies show that most of the mononuclear inflammatory cells have an antibody halo on the cell membrane surface (Paul *et al.* 1978). This indicates that plasma cell gingivitis is the result of a hypersensitivity reaction. Furthermore, the serum of patients with this form of gingivitis does not contain autoantibodies for normal gingiva. This is one indication that it is not an autoimmune disease.

Treatment

In many instances, plasma cell gingivitis resolves on removal of the suspect allergen. Most of the current cases are due to flavouring agents in toothpastes. The patients should be told to discontinue their current toothpaste and symptoms usually resolve in 2–3 weeks (Lamey *et al.* 1990). Patch testing may help to confirm the diagnosis or identify the suspect allergen. In the standard test, the reagents are applied to the skin on the upper back. The skin is examined after 48 h for inflammatory reactions. If positive, then the results can be interpreted as either a delayed hypersensitivity or local irritant response. A further patch test for the reagent is applied to the scratched surface of the inner aspect of the forearm and left in place for 20 min. A positive response results in a wheal and a burning sensation at the site of application lasting for more than two hours.

If patch-testing facilities are not available, the patient can be rechallenged with the suspected allergen. However, this raises ethical questions, and although it will confirm the diagnosis, it will subject the patient to unnecessary discomfort.

Plasma cell gingivitis is usually a self-limiting condition once the suspected allergen has been identified and removed. During the period of resolution, the gingival tissues will be sore and the patient reluctant to carry out normal oral hygiene measures. Topical corticosteroids may facilitate resolution of the inflammation. Alternatively, chlorhexidine mouthrinse will prevent plaque accumulation.

REFERENCES

Aarli, J. A. (1976). Phenytoin-induced depression of salivary IgA and gingival hyperplasia. *Epilepsia*, **17**, 283–91.

Aas, E. (1963). Hyperplasia gingivae diphenylhydantoinea. *Acta Odontologica Scandinavica*, **21** (Suppl. 34).

Adams, D. and Davies, G. (1984). Gingival hyperplasia associated with cyclosporin A: a case report. *British Dental Journal*, **157**, 89–90.

Angelopoulos, A. P. (1975). Diphenylhydantoin gingival hyperplasia: a clinicopathological review. I. Incidence, clinical features and histopathology. *Journal of the Canadian Dental Association*, **41**, 103–6.

Angelopoulos, A. P. and Goaz, P. W. (1972). Incidence of diphenylhydantoin gingival hyperplasia. *Oral Surgery, Oral Medicine, Oral Pathology*, **34**, 898–906.

Backman, N., Holm, A-K., Hanstrom, L. Blomquist, H. K. S., Heijbel, J., and Safstrom, G. (1989). Folate treatment of diphenylhydantoin-induced gingival hyperplasia. *Scandinavian Journal of Dental Research*, **97**, 222–32.

Ballard, J. B. and Butler, W. T. (1974). Proteins of the periodontium. Biochemical studies on the collagen and noncollagenous proteins of human gingiva. *Journal of Oral Pathology*, **3**, 176–84.

Barak, S., Engelberg, I. S., and Hiss, J. (1987). Gingival hyperplasia caused by nifedipine: histopathologic findings. *Journal of Periodontology*, **58**, 639–42.

Bartold, P. M. (1987). Cyclosporine and gingival overgrowth. *Journal of Oral Pathology*, **16**, 464–8.

Bartold, P. M. (1989). Regulation of human gingival fibroblast growth and synthetic activity by cyclosporin-A *in vitro*. *Journal of Periodontal Research*, **24**, 314–21.

Bencini, P. L. *et al.* (1985). Gingival hyperplasia by nifedipine: report of a case. *Acta Dermatologica et Venereologica*, **65**, 362–5.

Bennett, J. A. and Christian, J. M. (1985). Cyclosporine-induced gingival hyperplasia: case report and literature review. *Journal of the American Dental Association*, **111**, 272–3.

Benveniste, K. and Bitar, M. (1980). Effects of phenytoin on cultured human gingival fibroblasts. In *Phenytoin-induced teratology and gingival pathology*, (eds. T. M. Hassell, M. C. Johnston, and K. M. Dudley), pp.199–213. Raven Press, New York.

Beveridge, T. (1983). Cyclosporin A: clinical results. *Transplantation Proceedings*, **15**, 433–7.

Beveridge, T., Gratwohl, A. and Michot, F. (1981). Cyclosporin A: pharmacokinetics after a single dose in man and serum levels after multiple dosing in recipients of allogenic bone marrow grafts. *Current Therapeutics Research*, **30**, 5–20.

Bhaskar, S. N. Levin, M., and Frisch, J. (1968). Plasma cell granuloma of periodontal tissues: report of 45 cases. *Periodontics*, **6**, 272–6.

Bihler, I. and Sawh, P. C. (1971). Effects of diphenylhydantoin on the transport of Na^+ and K^+ and the regulation of sugar transport in muscle in vitro. *Biochemica et Biophysica Acta*, **249**, 240–51.

Borel, J. F., Feurer, C. and Gubler, H. U. (1976). Biological effects of cyclosporin A: a new antilymphocytic agent. *Agents & Actions*, **6**, 468–75.

Bowman, J. M., Levy, B. A., and Grubb, R. V. (1988). Gingival overgrowth induced by diltiazem. *Oral Surgery, Oral Medicine & Oral Pathology*, **65**, 183–5.

Brunius, G. and Modeer, T. (1989). Effect of phenytoin on intracellular $^{45}Ca^{2+}$ accumulation in gingival fibroblasts *in vitro*. *Journal of Oral Pathology and Medicine*, **18**, 485–9.

Calne, R. Y., *et al.* (1981). Cyclosporin A in clinical organ grafting. *Transplantation Proceedings*, **13**, 349–58.

Carpenter, G. (1987). Receptors for epidermal growth factor and other polypeptide mitogens. *Annual Review of Biochemistry*, **56**, 881–914.

Church, H. A. and Dolby, A.E. (1978). The effect of Dilantin on the cellular immune responses to dento-gingival plaque extract. *Journal of Periodontology*, **49**, 373–7.

Coley, C., Jarvis, K. and Hassell, T. (1986). Effects of cyclosporin-A on human gingival fibroblasts in vitro. *Journal of Dental Research*, **65**, 353.

Conrad, G. J., Haavik, C. O., and Finger, K. F. (1972). The relationship of 5,5-diphenylhydantoin metabolism to the species specific induction of gingival hyperplasia in the rat. *Archives of Oral Biology*, **17**, 311–21.

Conrad, G. J., Jeffay, H., Boshes, J., and Steinberg, A. D. (1974). Levels of 5,5-diphenylhydantoin and its major metabolite in human serum, saliva and hyperplastic gingiva. *Journal of Dental Research*, **53**, 1323–9.

Cucchi, G., Giustiniani, S., and Robustelli, F. (1985). Gingival hyperplasia caused by verapamil. *International Journal of Cardiology*, **15**, 556–7.

Dahllof, G. and Modeer, T. (1986). The effect of a plaque control programme on the development of phenytoin-induced gingival overgrowth. *Journal of Clinical Periodontology*, **13**, 845–9.

Dahllof, G., Reinholt, F. P., Hjerpe, A., and Modeer, T. (1984). A quantitative analysis of connective tissue components in phenytoin-induced gingival overgrowth in children: a stereological study. *Journal of Periodontal Research*, **19**, 401–7.

Dahllof, G., Modeer, T., Reinholt, F. P., Wikstrom, B., and Hjerpe, A. (1986). Proteoglycans and glycosaminoglycans in phenytoin-induced gingival overgrowth. *Journal of Periodontal Research*, **21**, 13–21.

Daley, T. D., Wysocki, G. P., and May, C. (1986). Clinical and pharmacological correlations in cyclosporin-induced gingival hyperplasia. *Oral Surgery, Oral Medicine, Oral Pathology*, **62**, 417–21.

Dallas, B. M. (1963). Hyperplasia of the oral mucosa in an edentulous epileptic. *New Zealand Dental Journal*, **59**, 54–5.

Darling, M. R., Arendorf, T. M., Shaikh, A. B., and Stephen, L. X. G. (1988). Gingival hyperplasia of an edentulous alveolar ridge in an epileptic—a case report. *New Zealand Dental Journal*, **84**, 114–15.

Deliliers, G. L., Santoro, F., Polli, N., Bruno, E., Fumagalli, L., and Risciotti, E. (1986). Light and electron microscopic study of cyclosporin A-induced gingival hyperplasia. *Journal of Periodontology*, **57**, 771–5.

Dolin, H. (1951). Dilantin hyperplasia. *Military Surgery*, **109**, 134–7.

Dreizen, S., Levy, B. M., and Bernick, S. (1970). Studies on the biology of the periodontium of marmosets. VIII. The effect of folic acid deficiency on the marmoset oral mucosa. *Journal of Dental Research*, **49**, 616–20.

Drew, H. J., Vogen, R. I., Molofsky, W., Baker, H., and Frank, O. (1987). Effect of folate on phenytoin hyperplasia. *Journal of Clinical Periodontology*, **14**, 350–6.

Dreyer, W. P. and Thomas, C. J. (1978). Diphenylhydantoinate-induced hyperplasia of the masticatory mucosa in an edentulous epileptic patient. *Oral Surgery, Oral Medicine, Oral Pathology*, **45**, 701–6.

Dummett, C. O. (1954). Oral tissue reactions from Dilantin medication in the control of epileptic seizures. *Journal of Periodontology*, **25**, 112–22.

Esterberg, H. L. and White, P. H. (1945). Sodium dilantin gingival hyperplasia. *Journal of the American Dental Association*, **32**, 16–24.

Fine, A. S., Scopp, I. W., Egnor, R., Froum, S., Thaler, R., and Stahl, S. S. (1974). Subcellular distribution of oxidative enzymes in human, inflamed and Dilantin hyperplastic gingivae. *Archives of Oral Biology*, **19**, 565–71.

Flexner, J. M. and Hartman, R. C. (1960). Megaloblastic anaemia associated with anticonvulsant drugs. *American Journal of Medicine*, **28**, 386–96.

Fontana, A., Grob, P. J., Sauter, R., and Joller, N. (1976). IgA deficiency, epilepsy and hydantoin medication. *Lancet*, **ii**, 228–31.

Friskopp, J., and Klintmalm, G. (1986). Gingival enlargement: a comparison between cyclosporine and azathioprine treated renal allograft recipients. *Swedish Dental Journal*, **10**, 85–92.

Friskopp, J., Engstrom, P-E., and Sundqvist, K-G. (1986). Characterisation of mononuclear cells in cyclosporin A induced gingival enlargement. *Scandinavian Journal of Dental Research*, **94**, 443–7.

Gabbiani, G. (1977). Reparative processes in mammalian wound healing: the role of contractile phenomena. *International Review of Cytology*, **48**, 187–96.

Gelfand, E. W., Cheung, R. K., Grinstein, S., and Mills, G. (1986). Characterisation of the role for calcium influx in mitogen-induced triggering of human T-cell. Identification of calcium-dependent and calcium-independent signals. *European Journal of Immunology*, **16**, 907–12.

George, R. and Pack, A. R. C. (1983). Inhibition of mitogen-induced lymphoblastic transformation by folate. *Journal of Dental Research*, **62**, 404.

Giustiniani, S., Robustelli Della Cuna, F., and Marieni, M. (1987). Hyperplastic gingivitis during diltiazem therapy. *International Journal of Cardiology*, **15**, 247–9.

Glickman, I. and Lewitus, M. (1941). Hyperplasia of the gingivae associated with Dilantin (sodium diphenylhydantoinate) therapy. *Journal of the American Dental Association*, **26**, 199–207.

Goultschin, J., Sofer, B., and Shoshan, S. (1983). The effect of prolonged phenytoin administration on non-collagenous components of gingival tissue. *International Journal of Tissue Reactions*, **5**, 227–30.

Haim, G. (1955). Elektronenmikrokipische Untersuchungen über die Hydantoin-Hyperplasie der Gingiva bei Epileptikern. In *Les parodontopathies, rapports et communications du XIVeme Congrès de l'Association pour Recherches sur les Parodontopathies* (ARPA Internationale). Tipografia Luigi Salvangno, Venice.

Hassell, T. M. (1981). *Epilepsy and the oral maniufestations of phenytoin therapy*. Karger, Basel.

Hassell, T. M. and Cooper, C. G. (1980). Phenytoin gingival overgrowth: rate of drug metabolism by fibroblasts. *Journal of Dental Research*, **59**, 920.

Hassell, T. M. and Gilbert, G. M. (1983). Phenytoin sensitivity of fibroblasts as the basis for susceptibility to gingival enlargement. *American Journal of Pathology*, **112**, 218–23.

Hassell, T. M. and Stanek, E. J. (1983). Evidence that healthy human gingiva contains functionally heterogeneous fibroblast subpopulations. *Archives of Oral Biology*, **28**, 617–25.

Hassell, T. M., O'Donnell, J., Pearlman, J., Tesini, D., Murphy, T., and Best, H. (1984). Phenytoin-induced gingival overgrowth in institutionalised epileptics. *Journal of Clinical Periodontology*, **11**, 242–53.

Hassell, T. M. Buchanan, J., Cuchens, M., and Douglas, R. (1988). Fluorescence activated vital cell sorting of human fibroblast subpopulations that bind cyclosporin-A. *Journal of Dental Research*, **67**, 273.

Heijl, L. and Sundin, Y. (1988). Nitrendipine-induced gingival overgrowth in dogs. *Journal of Periodontology*, **60**, 104–12.

Hein, R., Mensing, M., and Muller, P. K. (1984). Effect of vitamin A and its derivatives on collagen production and chemotactic response of fibroblasts. *British Journal of Dermatology*, **111**, 37–44.

Jacobs, D., Buchanan, J., Cuchens, M., and Hassell, T. (1990). The effect of cyclosporin metabolite OL-17 on gingival fibroblast subpopulations. *Journal of Dental Research*, **69**, 221.

Johnson, B. D., Narayanan, A. S., Pieters, H. P., and Page, R. C. (1990). Effect of cell donor age on the synthetic properties of fibroblasts obtained from phenytoin-induced gingival hyperplasia. *Journal of Periodontal Research*, **25**, 74–80.

Jones, C. M. (1986). Gingival hyperplasia associated with nifedipine. *British Dental Journal*, **160**, 416–17.

Kantor, M. L. and Hassell, T. M. (1983). Increased accumulation of sulphated glycosaminoglycans in cultures of human fibroblasts from phenytoin-induced gingival overgrowth. *Journal of Dental Research*, **62**, 383–7.

Kapur, R. N., Girgis, S., Little, T. M., and Mosotti, R. E. (1973). Diphenylhydantoin-induced gingival hyperplasia: its relationship to dose and serum level. *Developmental Medicine and Child Neurology*, **15**, 483–7.

Kerr, D. A. (1952). Stomatitis and gingivitis in the adolescent and preadolescent. *Journal of the American Dental Association*, **44**, 27–36.

Kerr, D. A., McClatchey, K. D., and Regezi, J. A. (1971a). Idiopathic gingivostomatitis. *Oral Surgery, Oral Medicine, Oral Pathology*, **32**, 402–23.

Kerr, D. A., McClatchey, K. D., and Regezi, J. A. (1971b). Allergic gingivostomatitis (due to chewing gum). *Journal of Periodontology*, **42**, 709–12.

King, J. D. (1954). Experimental and clinical observations on gingival hyperplasia due to diphenylhydantoin. *British Dental Journal*, **90**, 237–48.

King, D. A., Hawes, R. R., and Bibby, B. G. (1976). The effect of oral physiology on dilantin gingival hyperplasia. *Journal of Oral Pathology*, **5**, 1–7.

Klar, L. A. (1973). Gingival hyperplasia during Dilantin therapy: a survey of 312 patients. *Journal of Public Health Dentistry*, **33**, 180–5.

Korff, M. and Mutschelknauss, R. (1963). Die Hydantoin-Hyperplasie. *Deutsche Zahnaerztliche Zeitschrift*, **28**, 1157–63.

Lamey, P-J., Rees, T. D., and Forsyth, A. (1990). Sensitivity reaction to the cinnamonaldehyde component of toothpaste. *British Dental Journal*, **168**, 115–18.

Lederman, D., Lumermanm, M., Reuben, S., and Freedman, P. D. (1984). Gingival hyperplasia associated with nifedipine therapy. *Oral Surgery, Oral Medicine, Oral Pathology*, **57**, 620–2.

Little, T. M., Girgis, S. S., and Masotti, R. E. (1975). Diphenylhydantoin-induced gingival hyperplasia: its response to changes in drug dosage. *Developmental Medicine and Child Neurology*, **17**, 421–4.

Lubow, R. M., Cooley, R. L., Hartman, K. S., and McDaniel, R. K. (1984). Plasma-cell gingivitis—report of a case. *Journal of Periodontology*, **55**, 235–41.

Lucas, R. M., Howell, L. P., and Wall, B. A. (1985). Nifedipine-induced gingival hyperplasia: a histochemical and ultrastructural study. *Journal of Periodontology*, **56**, 211–15.

McGaw, T., Lam, S., and Coates, J. (1987). Cyclosporin-induced gingival overgrowth: correlation with dental plaque scores, gingivitis scores and cyclosporin levels in serum and saliva. *Oral Surgery, Oral Medicine, Oral Pathology*, **48**, 293–7.

McGaw, T. and Porter, H. (1988). Cyclosporin-induced gingival overgrowth: an ultrastructural stereologic study. *Oral Surgery, Oral Medicine, Oral Pathology*, **65**, 186–90.

MacKinney, A. A. and Booker, H. E. (1972). Diphenylhydantoin effects on human lymphocytes *in vitro* and *in vivo*. *Archives of Internal Medicine*, **129**, 983–92.

Macleod, R. I. and Ellis, J. E. (1989). Plasma cell gingivitis related to the use of herbal toothpaste. *British Dental Journal*, **166**, 375–6.

Mallek, H. M. and Nakamoto, T. (1981). Dilantin and folic acid status: clinical implications for the periodontist. *Journal of Periodontology*, **52**, 225–9.

Masi, P. (1953). Ulterione contribuito alla conoscenze delle alterazioni paradentali da difenilidantoinato sodico. *Rivista Italiana Dt Stomatologia*, **11**, 1409–13.

Maurer, G. (1985). Metabolism of cyclosporine. *Transplantation Proceedings*, **17**, 19–25.

Miller, J. (1941). Cheilitis from sensitivity to oil of cinnamon present in bubble gum. *Journal of the American Medical Association*, **116**, 131–2.

Millhon, J. A. and Esterberg, A. E. (1942). Relationship between gingival hyperplasia and ascorbic acid in the blood and urine of epileptic patients undergoing treatment with sodium 5–5 diphenyl-hydantoin. *Journal of the American Dental Association*, **29**, 207–13.

Modeer, T. and Dahllof, G. (1987). Development of phenytoin-induced gingival overgrowth in non-institutionalized epileptic children subjected to different plaque control programs. *Acta Odontologica Scandinavica*, **45**, 81–5.

Modeer, T., Dahllof, G., and Otteskog, P. (1982). The effects of the phenytoin metabolite p-HPPH on proliferation of gingival fibroblasts *in vitro*. *Act Odontologica Scandinavica*, **40**, 353–7.

Modeer, T., Mendez, C., Dahllof, G., Anduren, I. and Andersson, G. (1990). Effect of phenytoin medication on the metabolism of epidermal growth factor receptor in cultured gingival fibroblasts. *Journal of Periodontal Research*, **25**, 120–7.

Narayanan, A. S., Meyers, D. F., and Page, R. C. (1988). Regulation of collagen production in fibroblasts cultured from normal and phenytoin-induced hyperplastic human gingiva. *Journal of Periodontal Research*, **23**, 118–21.

Nenning, K. (1972). Erkrankungen durch Arzneimittel im Mund-und Kieferbereich. *Deutsche Stomatology*, **22**, 897–903.

Norris, J. F. and Cunliffe, W. J. (1987). Phenytoin-induced gum hypertrophy improved by isotretinoin. *International Journal of Dermatology*, **26**, 602–3.

Nyska, A., Waner, T., Pirak, M., Galiano, A., and Zlotogorski, A. (1990). Gingival hyperplasia in rats induced by oxopidine—a calcium channel blocker. *Journal of Periodontal Research*, **25**, 65–8.

O'Neil, T. C. A. and Figures, K. H. (1982). The effects of chlorhexidine and mechanical methods of plaque control on the recurrence of gingival hyperplasia in young adults taking phenytoin. *British Dental Journal*, **152**, 130–3.

Owings, J. R. (1969). An atypical gingivostomatitis: a report of four cases. *Journal of Periodontology*, **40**, 538–42.

Palmer, R. M. and Eveson, J. W. (1981). Plasma cell gingivitis. *Oral Surgery, Oral Medicine, Oral Pathology*, **51**, 187–9.

Pandiella, A., Malgaroli, A., Meldolesi, J., and Vinventini, L. M. (1987). EGF raises cytolic Ca^{2+} in A-431 and Swiss 3T3 cells by dual mechanisms. *Experimental Cell Research*, **170**, 175–85.

Panuska, H. J., Gorlin, R. J., Bearman, J. E., and Mitchell, D. F. (1961). The effect of anticonvulsant drugs upon the gingiva—a series of analysis of 1048 patients. *Journal of Periodontology*, **31**, 15–28.

Panuska, H. J., Gorlin, R. J., Bearman, J. E., and Mitchell, D. F. (1962). Anticonvulsant combined therapy and gingival hyperplasia. *Journal of Periodontology*, **32**, 15–21.

Partington, M. W., Reilly, D. M., Stewart, J. H., and Vickery, S. K. (1974). Serum diphenylhydantoin levels following a change in drug brand. *Canadian Journal of Pharmacological Science*, **9**, 31.

Paul, R. E., Hoover, D., Dunlap, C., Gier, R., and Alms, T. (1978). An immunological investigation of atypical gingivostomatitis. *Journal of Periodontology*, **49**, 301–6.

Pernu, H. E., Oikarinen, K., Heitanen, J., and Knuuttila, M. (1989). Verapamil-induced gingival overgrowth: a clinical, histologic and biochemic approach. *Journal of Oral Pathology and Medicine*, **18**, 422–5.

Perry, H. O., Deffner, N. F., and Sheridan, P. J. (1973). Atypical gingivostomatitis. *Archives of Dermatology*, **107**, 872–8.

Philstrom, B. L., Carlson, J. F., Smith, Q. T., Bastien, S. A., and Keenan, K. M. (1980). Prevention of phenytoin associated gingival enlargement—a 15 month longitudinal study. *Journal of Periodontology*, **51**, 311–17.

Pincus, H. H. (1972). Diphenylhydantoin and ion flux in lobster nerve. *Archives of Neurology* (Chicago), **26**, 4–10.

Pisanty, S., Rahamim, E., Ben-Ezra, D., and Shoshan, S. (1990). Prolonged systemic administration of cyclosporin A affects gingival epithelium. *Journal of Periodontology*, **61**, 138–41.

Poswillo, D. (1968). Plasmacytosis of the gingiva. *British Journal of Oral Surgery*, **5**, 194–202.

Puolijoki, H., Siitonen, L., Saha, H., and Suojanen, I. (1988). Gingival hyperplasia caused by nifedipine. *Proceedings of the Finnish Dental Society*, **84**, 311–14.

Ramon, Y., Behar, S., Kishon, Y., and Engelberg, I. S. (1984). Gingival hyperplasia caused by nifedipine: a preliminary report. *International Journal of Cardiology*, **5**, 195–204.

Rateitschak-Pluss, E-M., Hefti, A., Lortscher, R., and Thiel, G. (1983). Initial observations that cyclosporin A induces gingival enlargement in man. *Journal of Clinical Periodontology*, **10**, 237–46.

Rawlins, M. D. and Thompson, J. W. (1985). Pathogenesis of adverse drug reactions In *Textbook of adverse drug reactions* (ed. D. M. Davies), pp. 12–38. Oxford University Press.

Richens, A. (1979). Clinical pharmacokinetics of phenytoin. *Clinical Pharmacokinetics*, **4**, 153–69.

Ross, P. J., Nazif, M. M., Zullo, T., Zitelli, B., and Guevara, P. (1989). Effects of cyclosporin A on gingival status following liver transplantation. *Journal of Dentistry for Children*, January–February, 56–9.

Rostock, M. H., Fry, H. R., and Turner, J. E. (1986). Severe gingival overgrowth associated with cyclosporine therapy. *Journal of Periodontology*, **57**, 294–9.

Ryffel, B., Donatsch, P., and Mandorin, M. (1983). Toxocological evaluation of cyclosporin A. *Archives of Toxicology*, **53**, 107–41.

Savage, N. W., Seymour, G. J., and Robinson, M. F. (1987). Cyclosporin-A-induced gingival enlargement: a case report. *Journal of Periodontology*, **58**, 475–80.

Seager, J., Jamison, D. L., Wilson, J., Hayward, A. R., and Soothill, J. F. (1975). IgA deficiency, epilepsy and phenytoin treatment. *Lancet*, **ii**, 632–5.

Seymour, R. A. and Smith, D. G. (1990). The effect of a plaque control programme on the incidence and severity of cyclosporin-induced gingival changes. *Journal of Clinical Periodontology*, **17** (in press).

Seymour, R. A., Blair, G. S., and Wyatt, F. A. R. (1983). Postoperative dental pain and analgesic efficacy. Part I. *British Journal of Oral Surgery*, **21**, 290–7.

Seymour, R. A., Smith, D. G., and Turnbull, D. N. (1985). The effects of phenytoin and sodium valproate on the periodontal health of adult epileptic patients. *Journal of Clinical Periodontology*, **12**, 413–19.

Seymour, R. A., Smith, D. G., and Rogers, S. R. (1987). The comparative effects of azathioprine and cyclosporin on some gingival health parameters of renal transplant patients. *Journal of Clinical Periodontology*, **14**, 610–13.

Smith, M. and Glenert, U. (1987). Gingival hyperplasi forarsaget of behandling med verapamil. *Tandlaegebladet*, **91**, 849.

Sorrell, T. R., Forbes, I. J., Burness, F. R., and Rischbieth, R. H. C. (1971). Depression of immunological function in patients treated with phenytoin sodium (sodium diphenylhydantoin). *Lancet*, **ii**, 1233–5.

Staple, P. H. (1951). Action of diphenylhydantoin sodium on the adrenal gland. *Lancet*, **260**, 1074.

Staple, P. H. (1952). Diphenylhydantoin, adrenal function and epilepsy. *Journal of Endocrinology*, **9**, 18–25.

Staple, P. H. (1953). Some tissue reactions associated with 5:5-diphenylhydantoin ('Dilantin') sodium therapy. *British Dental Journal*, **95**, 289–92.

Starzl, T. E. *et al.* (1980). The use of cyclosporin A and prednisone in cadaver kidney transplantation. *Surgery, Gynecology and Obstetrics*, **151**, 17–26.

Stern, L., Eisenbud, I., and Klatell, J. S. (1943). Analysis of oral reactions to dilantin sodium. *Journal of Dental Research*, **22**, 157–61.

Sugarman, M. M. (1950). Contact allergy due to chewing gum. *Oral Surgery, Oral Medicine, Oral Pathology*, **3**, 1145–7.

Thyne, G., Young, D. W., and Ferguson, M. M. (1989). Contact stomatitis caused by toothpaste. *New Zealand Dental Journal*, **85**, 124–6.

Tipton, D. A. and Dabbous, M. K. (1986). Heterogeneity of gingival fibroblast response to cyclosporine. *Journal of Dental Research*, **65**, 331.

Turley, E. A., Mollenberg, M. D., and Pratt, R. M. (1985). Effect of epidermal growth factor/urogastrone on glycosaminoglycan synthesis and accumulation *in vitro* in the developing mouse palate. *Differentiation*, **28**, 279–85.

Tyldesley, W. R. and Rotter, E. (1984). Gingival hyperplasia induced by cyclosporin-A. *British Dental Journal*, **157**, 305–9.

Van der Wall, E. E., Tuinzing, D. B., and Hess, J. (1985). Gingival hyperplasia induced by nifedipine, an arterial vasodilating drug. *Oral Surgery, Oral Medicine, Oral Pathology*, **60**, 38–41.

Vogel, R. I. (1977). Gingival hyperplasia and folic acid deficiency from anticonvulsive drug therapy: a theoretical relationship. *Journal of Theoretical Biology*, **67**, 269–78.

Vogel, R. I. (1980). Relationship of folic acid to phenytoin-induced gingival overgrowth. In *Phenytoin-induced teratology and gingival pathology* (ed. T. M. Hassell, M. C. Johnston and K. H. Dudley). Raven Press, New York.

Waner, T., Nyska, A., Nyska, M., Sela, M., Pirak, M., and Galiono, A. (1988). Gingival hyperplasia in dogs induced by oxodipine, a calcium channel blocker. *Toxicology and Pathology*, **16**, 327–32.

Waxman, S., Corcino, J. J., and Herbert, V. (1970). Drugs, toxins and dietary amino acids affecting B$_{12}$ and folic acid absorption or utilization. *American Journal of Medicine*, **48**, 559.

Wysocki, G. P., Gretzinger, H. A., Laupacis, A., Ulan, R. A., and Stiller, C. R. (1983). Fibrous hyperplasia of the gingiva: a side effect of cyclosporin A therapy. *Oral Surgery, Oral Medicine, Oral Pathology*, **55**, 274–8.

Yamasaki, A., Rose, G. G., Pinero, G. J., and Mahan, C. J. (1987). Ultrastructure of fibroblast in cyclosporin A-induced gingival hyperplasia. *Journal of Oral Pathology*, **16**, 129–34.

Yusof, W. Z. W. (1989). Nifedipine-induced gingival hyperplasia. *Journal of the Canadian Dental Association*, **55**, 389–91.

Zebrowski, E. J., Singer, D. L., and Brunka, J. R. (1986). Cyclosporin-A, nifedipine and phenytoin: comparative effects on gingival fibroblast metabolism. *Journal of Dental Research*, **65**, 331.

5. The effect of age on the periodontal tissues

5.1 INTRODUCTION

This chapter is concerned with the influence of age on the periodontal tissues and how such changes can affect the response of these tissues to bacterial plaque. Also, there are specific types of periodontal disease that are age-linked, for example, prepubertal and juvenile periodontitis. Certain age-related events in life can have a significant effect on the periodontal tissues, and such examples include puberty and pregnancy. As these are essentially hormonal-induced changes, they will be discussed in Chapter 7. Topics covered in this chapter include periodontal disease in children, prepubertal periodontitis, juvenile periodontitis, and age changes and their clinical significance in the periodontium. The references to this chapters are listed under their major topic headings.

5.2 PERIODONTAL DISEASES IN CHILDREN

5.2.1 INTRODUCTION

Children are susceptible to plaque-induced gingival and periodontal changes, and these changes appear to be age-related (for review, see Waite and Furniss 1987). There are also certain systemic diseases and congenital conditions that primarily or predominantly occur in children and have a marked effect on the periodontium. Such conditions include the white blood-cell disorders, hypophosphatasia, Papillon–Lefèvre syndrome, Down's syndrome, and Ehlers–Danlos syndrome. These are discussed in Chapter 3; the periodontal disorders described in this section refer to the otherwise healthy child.

The subject of periodontal disease in children is controversial. Early studies suggested that virtually all adult periodontal disease was initiated in childhood (McCall 1938; Baer 1957; Parfitt 1963). Subsequent investigations show that this does not appear to be the case (Ruben et al. 1971).

Periodontal disease in children has been the subject of many studies from anatomical, epidemiological, clinical, and cellular aspects.

5.2.2 ANATOMICAL CONSIDERATIONS

There are certain significant differences in the periodontal structures between childhood and adult life (Zappler 1948; Bradley 1961); these include the following. In children, the gingival tissues are more reddish, owing to a thinner epithelium, a lesser degree of cornification, and greater vascularity. The gingiva lack the stippling found in adults, owing to the shorter and flatter papillae from the lamina propria. The gingival margins in children may be rounded and rolled because of the hyperaemia and oedema that accompanies eruption. Changes in gingival contour and the relative ease of gingival retraction may lead to a greater sulcular depth. The gingiva in children may appear flabbier, owing to the lower density of the connective tissue in the lamina propria.

The cementum of children is often thinner and less dense than that of adults; it shows a tendency to hyperplasia of cementoid apical to the epithelial attachment. The periodontal ligament in children is wider, has fewer and less dense fibres per unit area, and has increased hydration with a greater blood and lymph supply than in adults. These changes apply to both deciduous and permanent teeth. There are marked differences in the alveolar bone between adults and children: in children, the lamina dura is thinner, there are fewer trabeculae, and larger marrow spaces. There is also a smaller amount of calcification, greater blood and lymph supply, and the alveolar crest associated with the deciduous teeth appears flatter.

The significance of these anatomical differences to the pathogenesis of periodontal disease during childhood remains to be determined.

A further area of controversy in the pathogenesis of periodontal disease in children is the role of the interdental 'col'. The col was described by Cohen (1959) as an irregular depression, bounded labially and lingually by the interdental papilla. The surface of the col was said to be covered by an odontogenically derived epithelium that is atrophic (four cell-layers thick), and has a diminished proliferative activity. The structure of this epithelium implied that the col would be very susceptible to inflammatory changes and ulceration (Fish 1961). The replacement of the odontogenically derived epithelium by ingrowing oral epithelium was considered essential for a healthy periodontium (Cohen 1959).

Although the approximal area is often the site of initial periodontal breakdown, it is now thought unlikely that 'developmental factors' are important here (Stallard 1967). In addition, the contact points between deciduous teeth are not as tight as those between the permanent dentition. Thus, the increased susceptibility of this area is more likely to be due to the favourable location provided by the shape of the interdental region for bacterial growth.

5.2.3 EPIDEMIOLOGY

There have been many studies of the incidence and severity of periodontal disease in children. Their findings show marked variations. Factors that influence this variability include sample population, the age of the children, and methods of assessing gingival and periodontal changes.

Gingivitis

In children under the age of 10 years the prevalence of gingivitis in developed countries (e.g. the United States and

United Kingdom) appears to be in the order of 40 per cent (Schour and Massler 1947). In the United Kingdom, this prevalence seems age-related, with 27 per cent of 6-year-olds showing some signs of gingivitis, compared with 51 per cent in children aged 10 years (Todd and Dodd 1983).

A higher prevalence of gingival changes has been reported in children from developing countries. For example, in Malaysia, the prevalence of gingivitis in 6-year-olds was 55 per cent in urban children and 67 per cent in children from rural areas; for 10-year-olds, the figures were 65 and 72 per cent, respectively (Majid 1983).

Several studies have shown that the prevalence of gingivitis increases markedly during puberty (Muhlemann 1958; Sutcliffe 1968; 1972; Biswas *et al.* 1977). The gingival changes are undoubtedly influenced by the increase in sex hormones, and the pathogenesis of these changes is discussed in Chapter 7.

During adolescence, there appears to be an increase in the prevalence of gingivitis, but figures vary from study to study and are in the range of 50–99 per cent (McHugh *et al.* 1964; Todd and Dodd 1983). The prevalence of gingivitis is less in girls than boys, which is probably related to the levels of oral hygiene (McHugh *et al.* 1964; Sutcliffe 1968).

Periodontitis

Most of the epidemiological studies investigating periodontitis in children have concentrated on adolescents. Periodontal destruction has been assessed by radiographs, probing depths, or attachment loss. As with the gingivitis studies, the findings on the prevalence and severity of periodontitis in adolescent children appear to be related to the population studied, and the method and criteria used for assessing periodontal destruction.

Attachment loss of up to 1 mm at one or more tooth surfaces has been reported in approximately 45 per cent of 15-year-old adolescent children (Bowden *et al.* 1973; Lennon and Davies 1974). Some 7.4 per cent of these subjects had loss of attachment of 2 mm or more (Lennon and Davies 1974). A comparative study of Norwegian and Sri Lankan 17-year-olds found attachment loss of 50 and 96.5 per cent, respectively (Loe *et al.* 1978). In the Norwegians, the main sites of attachment loss were the buccal aspects of the first premolar and molar teeth, whereas in the Sri Lankans, the main sites affected were the approximal and buccal surfaces of the mandibular incisors and first molar teeth in both jaws. When considering these findings, it should be pointed out that probing measurements are subject to many variables. These include the probing force, the thickness of the probe, and the extent of inflammation present in the gingival tissues (Listgarten 1980; Fowler *et al.* 1982; Freed *et al.* 1983). Probing depth measures must be interpreted with caution because they cannot be directly related to the true histological level of connective tissue attachment loss from the cementum–enamel junction (CEJ).

Radiographs are extensively used to assess the level of periodontal support. However, much controversy surrounds their interpretation in evaluating the status of the periodontium. The radiographic features of periodontitis have been described as irregularity of the alveolar crest, widening of the ligament space, and/or a distance greater than 3 mm between the CEJ and bone crest (Hull *et al.* 1975). This view is not shared by all workers, and these reservations may explain the different findings obtained from the various studies. Also, in some studies, radiographs were principally taken to detect caries. The views taken, the exposure time, and the processing of the films are not ideal for detecting alveolar bone loss.

Radiographic evidence of bone loss has been found in 51.5 per cent of 14-year-old British children (Hull *et al.* 1975), 28 per cent of 15-year-old Brazilian children (Gjermo *et al.* 1984), and 11 per cent of 15-year-old Norwegian children (Hansen *et al.* 1984). In the primary dentition, radiographic signs of bone loss were found in less than 1 per cent of 5-year-olds (Sweeney *et al.* 1987). By contrast, a study on 13 to 15-year-old English and Danish children showed radiographic evidence of bone loss in only 0.06 per cent of the sample (Blankenstein *et al.* 1978).

Longitudinal radiographic studies provide more pertinent information on the rate of bone loss in any given population. Over a 3-year period, the number of sites showing a distance greater than 1.5 mm from the CEJ to crestal bone increased from 18.5 per cent at baseline (when the children were aged 11–12 years) to 36.7 per cent (Davies *et al.* 1978). In a similar study (Clerehugh and Lennon 1986), changes in bone height and attachment level were assessed over an 18-month period; 175 sites were examined—7.5 per cent showed bone loss of 0.5 mm or more, 21 showed loss of attachment of 1 mm or more, and 11 had both features over this short period.

Although there is disagreement on the extent of periodontal disease in children, it is important to identify those at risk and institute appropriate treatment.

5.2.4 EXPERIMENTAL GINGIVITIS IN CHILDREN

The model of experimental gingivitis developed by Loe *et al.* (1965) has been used to investigate gingivitis in children. Longitudinal and cross-over studies in children of different ages have shown that the prevalence and severity of gingivitis increases with age (Pedersen 1944; Massler *et al.* 1950; Parfitt 1957; Massler 1958; Mieler and Reimann 1968; Hugosson *et al.* 1981). Similar findings have been reported in work with the beagle dog (Matsson and Attstrom 1979). More detailed studies have investigated the development of experimental gingivitis in preschool children (Mackler and Crawford 1973; Matsson 1978), children of different ages (Matsson and Goldberg 1985), and children with mixed dentitions (Matsson and Goldberg, 1986). A synopsis of the clinical findings from these studies is given in Table 5.1. In general, the younger the child, the less the severity of the gingival changes. Furthermore, the response of children's gingival tissue to plaque is different from that of adults.

Some studies have investigated changes in the plaque microflora during experimental gingivitis (Mackler and Crawford 1973; Moore *et al.* 1984); whilst others have concentrated on the host's cellular response (see below).

Table 5.1 Synopsis of gingivitis studies in children

Study	No. of subjects	Age range	Indices	Investigative procedures	Findings
Cox et al. (1974)	50	29–80 months	Plaque index Gingival index Orogranulocytic migration rate (OMR)	Rate of migration of leukocytes into the mouth was determined from the last 3 of 10 consecutive 30 s oral rinses	A minimal amount of localized marginal gingivitis in the presence of rather large plaque accumulations No significant correlation between OMR and Gingival Index OMR was low when compared with the rate in adults
Mackler and Crawford (1973)	13	36–66 months	Plaque index Gingival index Microbial sampling	Experimental gingivitis was induced for 26 days. Indices and sampling for 5 consecutive days in the first week, and alternate days in the subsequent 3 weeks	Generalized marginal gingivitis not found in any of the 13 children during the study; localized gingivitis occured in only 2 children Morphologically, plaque development in preschool children was similar to adults; *B. melaninogenicus* was found in many children, and spirochaetes were found in the 16-day plaque sample There was greater plaque accumulation on the mandibular than on the maxillary teeth, but there was no difference in plaque accumulation between anterior and posterior teeth The lack of development of gingivitis in this group may be attributed to dietary factors, preceding gingival health, the short duration of the investigation period and/or the host response
Matsson (1978)	6 children 6 adults	4–5 years 23–29 years	Plaque index Gingival exudate Crevicular leukocytes Gingival bleeding tendency	Experimental gingivitis was induced for 21 days. Monitoring visits were carried out at 0, 7, 14, and 21 days	Plaque growth increased continously in both groups In the children, the tendency to gingival bleeding, and the production of crevicular fluid and leukocytes was less than in the adults A marked difference between preschool children and adults in the propensity to develop gingivitis

Table 5.1 *continued*

Study	No. of subjects	Age range	Indices	Investigative procedures	Findings
Matsson and Goldberg (1985)	4 groups	4–6 years 7–9 years 14–16 years 20–22 years	Plaque index Gingival index	Patients were examined on two occasions about 2 weeks apart	With a given plaque score, the % of high gingivitis scores was less in 4–6-year-old children than in the older children and adults At all levels of plaque accumulation, the highest degree of gingival inflammation was in the 14–16-year-olds
Matsson and Goldberg (1986)	30	7–9 years (with mixed dentition)	Plaque index Gingival index		Mean distribution of Gingival Index scores did not differ significantly between deciduous and permanent dentition, but a higher % of plaque score was found in the permanent dentition The tendency towards a higher degree of gingivitis occurred around the deciduous teeth Structural differences between the gingiva of deciduous and permanent teeth have no impact on the gingival reaction to plaque in children with mixed dentition

5.2.5 HISTOPATHOLOGY OF GINGIVITIS IN CHILDREN

The plaque-induced inflammatory lesion in the child is usually confined to the more marginal aspects of the gingiva. With time, the lesion progresses to involve other tissues of the periodontium (Ruben et al. 1971).

Much interest has focused on the inflammatory infiltrate associated with gingivitis in children. In a preliminary study, this infiltrate was compared in gingival biopsy material from children and adults (Longhurst et al. 1977). The adult material was from patients undergoing surgical management for chronic periodontitis. Cell types were identified by their morphology and staining properties. Adult tissues had a greater density of plasma cells than those obtained from children. The numbers of plasma cells and lymphocytes in the adult samples were approximately the same, whereas in children, there were seven times as many lymphocytes as plasma cells. The investigators suggest that these differences in the cellular infiltrate may account for the differences observed in the natural history of periodontal disease with age.

In a further study (Longhurst et al. 1980), gingival connective tissue obtained from around deciduous teeth was subjected to electron microscopic quantitation. The main features were the large numbers of small and medium lymphocytes and an increase in vascularity. Other changes included a distinct population of peripherally distributed plasma cells, pathologically altered fibroblasts, and small numbers of macrophages and polymorphonuclear neutrophils (PMNs). Very few transforming T lymphocytes (T blasts) were found. Initial observations therefore suggest that the appearance of the gingival tissues in children is similar to the early lesion of adult gingivitis. However, the lack of T blasts and the rather large proportion of plasma cells place the childhood lesion between the early and established phases of the adult gingival lesion.

In contrast to the findings of Longhurst et al., others have shown that in childhood gingivitis, the predominant cell type is the T lymphocyte (Seymour et al. 1981, 1982). Using T- and B-cell markers, it was found that the lesion of childhood gingivitis consists of 70 per cent lymphocytes and between 11 and 26 per cent macrophages. Marker studies showed that the majority of the lymphocytes were T cells and that the childhood lesion is essentially a T-cell lesion. This investigation was repeated using monoclonal antibodies against lymphocyte differentiated antigens (Seymour et al. 1982). Again, the results confirmed that gingivitis associated with the deciduous dentition is a T-cell lesion.

Another marker study (Gillett et al. 1986) investigated the gingival infiltrate in childhood gingivitis using monoclonal antiHLADR antibodies. In these biopsy specimens, most of the cells were small lymphocytes, with over half being HLADR-positive. These investigators concluded that the lesion in childhood gingivitis is dominated by inactivated B lymphocytes.

The variable results obtained from these immunocytochemical studies on the infiltrate in childhood gingivitis may be due to the following factors: age and number of children in the studies; method of immunocytochemical staining; the preparation, staining, and orientation of the tissues; and the number of cells counted per specimen.

It would appear that the initial lesion in childhood gingivitis is composed mainly of untransformed B lymphocytes. Clinically, this lesion does not progress, and does not mediate tissue destruction. With increasing age and further exposure of the gingival tissues to plaque antigens, activation of a small population of T-helper cells may occur. This will cause many of the B cells to differentiate into plasma cells (i.e. a burst of activity). It is a matter of debate whether the plasma cell lesion results in effective protection of the periodontium and terminates the burst of activity, or causes further tissue destruction by activating various biochemical mediators (see Chapter 1).

5.2.6 MICROBIOLOGY OF PERIODONTAL DISEASE IN CHILDREN

There have been many studies comparing the microbiology of dental plaque from children of different ages with that from adults (Manganiello and Socransky 1971; Kleinberg et al. 1971). Early studies showed that in preschool children, plaque obtained from the gingival crevice resembled that of the adult. The exception was that spirochaetes and Bacteroides melaninogenicus were not present in all children (De Araujo and Macdonald 1964). Above the age of 5 years, Bact. melaninogenicus was found in 18–40 per cent of children. However, between the ages of 13–16 years, essentially all children harbour this micro-organism (Bailit et al. 1964; Kelstrup 1966). Spirochaetes also show a similar increase with age.

Studies of experimental gingivitis in children aged 36–66 months showed that, after prophylaxis, the first morphological group of bacteria to re-establish themselves were the cocci. During the second week without oral hygiene, the main cultivatable micro-organisms were the filamentous and fusospirochaetal forms. Spirochaetes were observed in a few children, but after 16 days they were found in all children. Similarly, Bact. melaninogenicus was cultivated from all children (Mackler and Crawford 1973). Quantitative relationships between the appearance of the different bacterial types and the clinical changes were not found.

A comparative microbiological study of experimental gingivitis in children (aged 4–6 years) and young adults has shown significant differences in their periodontal flora (Moore et al. 1982, 1984). The results are summarized in Table 5.2. This study also showed that the following bacteria—Fusobacterium nucleatum, Actinomyces WVa 963, Selenomonas DO4, and Treponema socranksii—were the predominant species that correlated with the increase in gingival inflammation observed in both children and adults during the period of investigation.

Although differences were found in the microbiology of plaque between children and adults subjected to experimental gingivitis, the correlation between certain predominant micro-organisms and the development of gingivitis suggests that differences in the host response may be a more important factor in the 'resistance' that children show to plaque and gingival inflammation.

Table 5.2 Synopsis of the bacteriological features of plaque obtained during an experimental gingivitis study in children and adults (after Moore *et al.* 1982, 1984)

Species in significantly greater numbers in children's plaque	Species in significantly greater numbers in adults' plaque
Leptotrichia spp.	*Fusobacterium*
Capnocytophaga	*Eubacterium*
Selenomonas spp.	
Bacterial species which require formate and fumarate	
Bacteroides spp.	

5.3 PREPUBERTAL PERIODONTITIS

5.3.1 INTRODUCTION

Periodontitis affecting the primary dentition is rare and has invariably been associated with other definable syndromes (e.g. Papillon–Lefèvre syndrome, hypophosphatasia) or an underlying medical disorder (e.g. diabetes mellitus, white blood-cell disorder, or histiocytosis X). These conditions in relation to periodontal disease are discussed in Chapter 3. Prepubertal periodontitis was described as a distinct clinical entity by Page and co-workers in 1983 (Page *et al.* 1983). It can be defined as periodontitis affecting the primary dentition where there is no other definable syndrome or underlying medical condition. This type of periodontitis can occur in a localised or generalized form.

5.3.2 LOCALIZED PREPUBERTAL PERIODONTITIS

The age of onset of the localized form is very young (approximately 4 years). In this condition, the gingival tissues show few inflammatory changes and plaque levels are usually low. Alveolar bone loss is rapid when compared to that in adults and teenagers. The pathogenesis of localized prepubertal periodontitis is uncertain (see later) but a defect in neutrophil or monocyte function (but not both) has been reported (Page *et al.* 1983).

5.3.3 GENERALIZED PREPUBERTAL PERIODONTITIS

The generalized form is characterized by a fiery-red, acute inflammatory change affecting the entire width of attached gingiva; other features include gingival hyperplasia, cleft formation, and recession. Onset is earlier than in the localized form and occurs on tooth eruption. There is rapid destruction of the alveolar bone and sometimes root resorption. Children with generalized prepubertal periodontitis are very susceptible to recurrent infections, especially otitis media and chest infections. This would suggest that there is a defect in their host response. Case reports depicting this condition have shown that affected children have an underlying defect in PMN and monocyte chemotaxis and adherence.

5.3.4 EPIDEMIOLOGY

Advanced alveolar bone loss affecting otherwise healthy children is most unusual. Several case reports have described periodontitis in the primary dentition (Goepferd 1981; Bystrom *et al.* 1983; Cogen *et al.* 1984; Ngan *et al.* 1985; Mandell *et al.* 1986; Mishkin *et al.* 1986). Page and co-workers, in their original paper, described five cases of periodontitis affecting the deciduous dentition (Page *et al.* 1983).

In an analysis of the radiographs of 2264 children, 19 were identified as having lost alveolar crestal bone (Sweeney *et al.* 1987). The age range of these 19 children was 5 years, 10 months—10 years, 9 months. This finding suggests that the incidence of prepubertal periodontitis is less than 1 per cent.

5.3.5 MICROBIOLOGY

The predominant micro-organisms obtained from pockets associated with the localized form of prepubertal periodontitis are *Actinobacillus actinomycetemcomitans*, *Bact. intermedius*, *Capnocytophaga* spp. *Bact. gingivalis*, *F. nucleatum* and *Eikenella corrodens* (Delaney and Kornman 1987). All these types are known for their periodontopathogenicity, and their common occurrence in the pockets of localized prepubertal periodontitis suggests an infective component to the disease (Sweeney *et al.* 1987).

5.3.6 PATHOGENESIS

Uncertainty surrounds the pathogenesis of prepubertal periodontitis, in particular its existence as a separate disease entity. Generalized prepubertal periodontitis is associated with a profound defect in monocyte and PMN adherence and chemotaxis. As discussed in Chapter 3, disorders of white blood cells are invariably accompanied by severe periodontal destruction. It could perhaps be argued that generalized prepubertal periodontitis is the periodontal manifestation of an underlying white blood-cell dysfunction. Laboratory studies have shown that PMNs from two children with generalized prepubertal periodontitis appeared to have missing from their particulate fraction, a glycoprotein of 180 000 Da (GP-180) (Bowen *et al.* 1982). The mothers and siblings of the two children had similar defects in PMN GP-180; their levels were approximately half of normal. This suggests that the PMN defect in GP-180 has an X-linked pattern of inheritance.

The identity of the localized form of prepubertal periodontitis has been similarly questioned (Sweeney *et al.* 1987). In many instances, the localized form resembles juvenile periodontitis. Both conditions have a localized nature, a similar microflora, and an underlying defect in PMN function. Case reports suggest that localized prepubertal periodontitis is an early manifestation of the juvenile form (Rosenthal 1951; Hawes 1960; Fourel 1974; Pleasants and Nelson 1975; Sonis 1980; Goepfred 1981).

A retrospective radiographic study on 17 patients with localized juvenile periodontitis and 17 matched controls showed that nearly all the patients and none of the controls had evidence of localized marginal bone loss in the primary dentition (Sjodin *et al.* 1989). Although there are shortcomings in the interpretation of retrospective radiographs, in particular standardization of views, the results suggest that localized juvenile periodontitis (see next section) may start in the primary dentition. Furthermore, the pathogenesis of juvenile periodontitis is thought to involve several components, i.e., specific bacteria, immunodeficiencies, PMN dysfunction, and a genetic predisposition. It is difficult to conceive that a series of components like these manifest themselves only in the permanent dentition, with little or no effect on the deciduous dentition.

If localized prepubertal periodontitis represents the early part of the spectrum of juvenile periodontitis, then the incidence of this problem may be greater than initially thought. However, diagnosis of juvenile periodontitis in the deciduous dentition may be difficult, as loosening and loss of the primary dentition (even prematurely) are considered normal occurrences.

5.3.7 TREATMENT

Generalized prepubertal periodontitis responds poorly to conventional periodontal treatment and antimicrobial therapy. In the cases reported by Page *et al.* (1983), a brief improvement in the periodontal status was achieved after a granulocyte transfusion. In a further case report (Shurin *et al.* 1979), an improvement in the patients general condition and PMN chemotaxis occurred after extraction of the periodontally involved teeth. They suggest that the pocket microflora (in particular *Capnocytophaga*) was responsible for producing the localized defect in PMN chemotaxis.

Localized prepubertal periodontitis responds to an improvement in oral hygiene, curettage, and antibiotic therapy. There have been few long-term studies of the effect of prepubertal periodontitis on the permanent dentition. Some studies suggest that the disease process continues and affects the permanent dentition (Rosenthal 1951; Hawes 1960; Jorgenson *et al.* 1975;), whilst another case report has shown that if all the deciduous teeth are extracted, the permanent dentition remains unaffected (Pleasants and Nelson 1975).

5.4 JUVENILE PERIODONTITIS

5.4.1 INTRODUCTION

Severe periodontal destruction affecting juveniles and young adults has been known for many years. The condition was first described in 1923 (Gottlieb 1923) as a chronic, degenerative, non-inflammatory disease of the periodontal tissues. Radiographs of affected teeth show a diffuse atrophy of the alveolar bone and an associated 'cementopathia'. For many years it was considered that systemic disease was important in the pathogenesis of this condition. Furthermore, the destruction of the periodontal tissues was thought to be due to degeneration (hence the name periodontosis), rather than of an inflammatory nature (Gottlieb

Table 5.3 Terminology used to describe rapid periodontal destruction in juveniles and young adults

Description	Reference
Diffuse atrophy of alveolar bone	Gottlieb (1923)
Deep cementopathia (cementopathia profunda)	Gottlieb (1928)
Paradontitis marginalis progressiva	Wannemacher (1938)
Paradontitis	Thoma and Goldman (1940)
Precocious advanced alveolar bone destruction	Miller *et al.* (1941)
Periodontosis	Orban and Weinmann (1942)
Periodontosis with periodontitis	Kaslick and Chasens (1968)
Juvenile periodontitis	Butler (1969)
Precocious periodontitis	Sugarman and Sugarman (1977)

1928; Orban and Weinmann 1942). These views are no longer held.

Since Gottlieb's original description, several other terms have been used to describe rapid periodontal destruction in juveniles and young adults (see Table 5.3). The terms periodontosis and juvenile periodontitis have been synonomous for many years, but in this chapter, the condition will be referred to as juvenile periodontitis.

A definition of juvenile periodontitis was given by Baer (1971), who described it as a disease of the periodontium occurring in otherwise healthy adolescents, which is characterized by a rapid loss of alveolar bone around more than one tooth of the permanent dentition. The condition exists in two forms—localized form where alveolar bone loss is mainly confined to the first molars and/or incisors, and a generalized form affecting many teeth (Hormand and Frandsen 1979). A more recent definition describes localized juvenile periodontitis (LJP) as a disease occurring in otherwise healthy individuals under the age of 30 with destructive periodontitis localized to the first permanent molars and incisors and not involving more than two other teeth. Generalized juvenile periodontitis (GJP) is defined as destructive periodontitis in individuals under the age of 30 years affecting more than 14 teeth, i.e., it is generalized to an arch or an entire dentition (Genco *et al.* 1986).

There is uncertainty as to whether LJP and GJP are distinct disease entities or different manifestations of the same disease process. There is some evidence that juvenile periodontitis commences as the localized form, and if untreated progresses to the generalized form (Baer and Socransky 1979; Hormand and Frandsen 1979; Saxen and Murtomaa 1985). However, this view was not supported by findings of Burmeister *et al.* (1984), who showed that 39 per cent of patients between the ages of 21 and 30 with evidence of juvenile periodontitis had lesions restricted to their incisors and molars.

The identity of generalized juvenile periodontitis is further confounded by the terms used by other workers. Page *et al.* (1983) described severe periodontal destruction in young adults (20–30 years) as rapidly progressive periodontitis, whereas Burmeister *et al.* (1984) used the term early-onset severe periodontitis. Similarly, severe periodontal destruction is a feature of recurrent attacks of acute necrotizing ulcerative gingivitis (ANUG) (Page and Schroeder 1982).

Whatever terminology is used, the condition is concerned with rapid periodontal destruction in adolescents and young adults. It may well transpire that GJP is an homogeneous group of diseases that encompasses rapidly progressive periodontitis, early onset of severe periodontitis, and periodontitis associated with recurrent attacks of ANUG. In some young patients the destruction may be preceded by localized lesions confined to the first molars and incisors.

5.4.2 Epidemiology

The epidemiology of juvenile periodontitis has been widely investigated in various populations from different ethnic backgrounds. Early studies suggested that the disease had an incidence from 0.1 to 17.6 per cent (Dawson 1948; Day and Shourie 1949; Day *et al.* 1955; Ramfjord 1961). More recent studies have reported the incidence to be 0.1–0.4 per cent (Saxen 1980*a*; Saxby, 1984*a*; Kronauer *et al.* 1986; Bial and Mellonig 1987). In these latter studies, more precise diagnostic criteria were applied to the populations screened, and this may account for the lower incidence than reported previously. The diagnostic criteria used were as follows:

1. The subject must be in good health.
2. More than one tooth in the dentition must be involved.
3. Alveolar bone loss of 2 mm or more should be found at more than one surface of the affected teeth.
4. The probing depth at the diseased site should exceed 5 mm.
5. Local irritants (calculus and overhanging margins of restorations) are not commensurate with the amount of bone loss.

Data from various epidemiological studies suggest that the incidence of juvenile periodontitis varies among different ethnic groups. In Saxby's study, subjects were obtained from different ethnic backgrounds and the incidence was 0.02 per cent for Caucasians, 0.8 per cent for Negroes, and 0.2 per cent for Asians (Saxby 1984*a*).

Early studies showed that juvenile periodontitis was more common in females (Rao and Tewani 1968; Manson and Lehner 1974; Hormand and Frandsen 1979), but these findings must be interpreted with caution. The clinical manifestations of juvenile periodontitis may well be related to the onset of puberty, which starts earlier in females. With an increase in age, the incidence of juvenile periodontitis shows no sex difference (Saxby 1984*b*).

5.4.3 Clinical features of LJP

The onset of LJP is between the ages of 11–15 years and characteristic clinical features include pocket formation, loss of attachment, and bone loss associated with the first permanent molars and incisors (Baer 1971). Around the molars, the bony defects are often angular on the mesial and distal aspects of the teeth and have a 'mirror image' distribution on both sides of the jaw (Fig. 5.1). The degree of gingival inflammation associated with the periodontal pockets shows marked variation. Clinically, the gingiva can appear healthy, but invariably bleed on probing. Supragingival plaque deposits and calculus formation are usually minimal.

As the disease progresses, there is increased mobility of affected teeth. Frequently, the first sign of LJP is spacing and mobility of the upper and lower incisors.

Histologically, the gingival tissues show ulceration of the pocket epithelium and inflammatory changes in the connective tissue associated with the base of the pocket. These inflammatory changes rarely extend to the marginal gingiva, which may account for the lack of overt clinical signs of inflammation. The cellular infiltrate in LJP is predominantly of plasma cells (60 per cent), with lymphocytes and a variable amount of neutrophils and polymorphs (Liljenberg and Lindhe 1980).

An electron microscopic investigation of the pocket epithelium in juvenile periodontitis showed gross distortion of the pocket walls, and separation of epithelial cells with a fine granular precipitate in the intercellular spaces (Shafik *et al.* 1988). It was suggested that these changes were more indicative of degeneration than the changes found in pocket epithelum from adult periodontitis.

The subgingival microflora in LJP is relatively sparse (20–200 μm thick), but covers the entire exposed root surface (Waerhaug 1976, 1977*a*; Westergaard *et al.* 1978). The specific microbiology of this flora is discussed later.

5.4.4 Clinical features of GJP

Although the natural history of GJP is uncertain, the disease has distinctive clinical features. The age of diagnosis is between 20 and 30 years, but the onset may be earlier. Severe, generalized bone loss is the characteristic feature; this may be restricted to the upper and/or lower arch. Patients with GJP often show good plaque control and the extent of bone loss is not commensurate with the level of oral hygiene (Davies *et al.* 1985). The extent of gingival inflammation varies from patient to patient and often from site to site. If the disease is active (i.e. there is a burst of activity), the gingival tissues will be hyperaemic and may show signs of cyanosis. There is increased vascularization of the gingival tissues, which accounts for the prominence of surface vessels passing below the attached gingiva.

In many patients the diagnosis of GJP often goes undetected. Invariably the first signs of disease are tooth mobility, migration, or periodontal abscess formation. The diagnosis may be reached from routine bitewing radiographs.

5.4.5 Pathogenesis of juvenile periodontitis

It would seem that the pathogenesis of juvenile periodontitis is related to the interplay of several factors. These include the specific microbiology of subgingival plaque, defects in

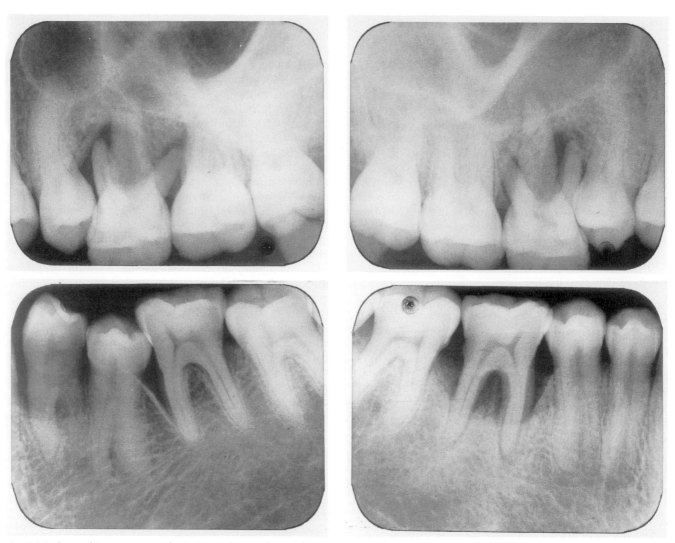

Fig. 5.1 Radiographic appearance of a patient with juvenile periodontitis showing bilaterally similar, localized infrabony defects associated with the first permanent molars.

cementum, hereditary factors, impaired PMN function, and disorders of the immune system.

Microbiology of LJP

There is now convincing evidence that LJP is associated with specific micro-organisms. Early studies identified capnophilic bacteria (i.e. *Capnocytophaga*) and Gram-negative rods from the subgingival flora of patients with LJP (Newman *et al.* 1976; Slots 1976). One of these Gram-negative organisms was subsequently identified as *A. actinomycetemcomitans* (Tanner *et al.* 1979). Subsequent studies have shown that *A. actinomycetemcomitans* is frequently associated with LJP and plays a significant role in its pathogenesis (Slots *et al.* 1980*b*; Zambon *et al.* 1983*a*; Haffajee *et al.* 1984; Zambon 1985).

A. actinomycetemcomitans is rarely found in subgingival plaque from juveniles or in patients with adult periodontitis, yet the organism is found in large numbers (up to 70 per cent of the total bacteria) in subgingival plaque from

patients with LJP. Of patients with LJP, 97 per cent will have this organism in their periodontal pockets (Zambon 1985). Furthermore, resolution of LJP coincides with a reduction and elimination of this bacterium in the subgingival plaque. Recurrence of the disease is associated with recolonization of the pocket by *A. actinomycetemcomitans* (Slots and Rosling 1983).

A. actinomycetemcomitans has long been recognized as a cause of severe, extraoral infections. These include endocarditis, osteomyelitis, meningitis, urinary tract infections, and abscesses involving the brain and thyroid gland (Genco *et al.* 1986). Thus, its pathogenicity is well established.

Role of A. actinomycetemcomitans

There are many lines of evidence that implicate *A. actinomycetemcomitans* as the causative agent in LJP. The high isolation rate of this bacteria from patients with LJP and the relationship between bacterial number and disease resolution and recurrence are important factors supporting this association.

Over 90 per cent of patients with LJP have elevated serum immunoglobulins to *A. actinomycetemcomitans* and high levels of antibodies to it in both crevicular fluid and gingival tissue (Haffajee *et al.* 1984; Genco *et al.* 1985). These antibodies may modulate the disease process by influencing the colonization and proliferation of the bacterium in the periodontal pocket. Levels of these antibodies also relate to disease activity, with a decline in antibody concentration after successful treatment (Ranney *et al.* 1982). There is also a significant inverse relationship between attachment levels and serum antibodies to *A. actinomycetemcomitans* and *Bact. gingivalis* in patients with juvenile periodontitis. This inverse relationship may suggest a failure by the host to mount a substantial antibody response, which in turn leads to more widespread periodontal destruction (Gunsolley *et al.* 1987). These various antibody studies all support the pathogenicity of *A. actinomycetemcomitans* in LJP.

A variety of virulent factors can be produced by *A. actinomycetemcomitans*. These have the potential to destroy, either directly or indirectly, the periodontium. Factors that can have a direct effect on the periodontal tissues include a bacterial collagenase that destroys gingival connective tissue (Robertson *et al.* 1982), an epitheliotoxin, which will facilitate bacterial penetration of junctional and pocket epithelium (Birkedal-Hansen *et al.* 1982), a fibroblast-inhibiting factor, which will impede repair (Stevens and Hammond 1982), and a lipopolysaccharide that causes bone resorption (Iino and Hopps 1984).

Virulent factors from this bacterium that can indirectly affect the periodontal tissues are those which essentially act on the host's immune response. These include a leukotoxin, which destroys PMNs (Taichman *et al.* 1980; Zambon *et al.* 1983*b*), and a chemotactic inhibitory factor, which impairs the chemotactic responses of PMNs (Van Dyke 1982). Both factors would deplete the protective role of PMNs in the periodontal tissues. The destruction of PMNs by leukotoxin will lead to the release of lysomal enzymes, which will potentiate further tissue destruction.

Other factors from *A. actinomycetemcomitans* will also activate T-suppressor cells, which in turn suppresses both the B-cell and T-cell responses (Shenker *et al.* 1982). An unusual feature of this micro-organism is its ability to resist destruction by serum bactericidal factors (Sundqvist and Johannson 1982; Evans and Genco 1983). Thus it will retain its viability in the periodontal pocket for longer than Gram-negative organisms. An *in vitro* study has shown that it can activate peripheral blood monocytes to produce significant amounts of the monokines interleukin-I and tissue necrosis factor (Lindemann and Economou 1988). Both monokines are able to induce osteoclastic bone resorption.

Apart from LJP, *A. actinomycetemcomitans* has also been isolated from cases of rapid periodontal destruction. These include juvenile patients with insulin-dependent diabetes (Mashimo *et al.* 1983) and young adults with advanced bone loss (Moore *et al.* 1982). Animal studies show that when this bacterium is inoculated into rats there is severe loss of periodontal attachment and bone (Irving *et al.* 1975).

From the various findings described above, it would seem that *A. actinomycetemcomitans* is intimately associated with

LJP and perhaps other forms of severe, destructive periodontal disease. The bacterium has the virulent factors to destroy directly the periodontal tissues by the production of enzymes and toxins, and suppresses the host defence mechanisms and immune response. A further feature of LJP is the ability of the bacteria to 'invade' the underlying connective tissue (Gillet and Johnson, 1982; Saglie *et al.* 1982; Christersson *et al.* 1987); this invasion may be significant in tissue breakdown. Tissue invasion by *A. actinomycetemcomitans* may, in part, explain the poor response of LJP to local treatment by scaling and root planing (Kornmann and Robertson 1985). Although this invasion may be a feature of LJP, its extent and the number of bacteria in the connective tissues have been questioned by Liakoni *et al.* (1987*a*,*b*), who examined gingival tissue from patients with LJP under the electron microscope and found that bacterial invasion was not as widespread as previously thought.

There is good evidence that genetic factors are important in the pathogenesis of LJP (see later). However, studies on families with LJP also suggest that the disease is transmissable via spread of *A. actinomycetemcomitans* (Zambon *et al.* 1983*a*). Adults who harbour this organism may pass it on to other members of the family. There is even a suggestion that it may be contracted from the family pet dog (Preus 1987).

The role of cementum

In Gottlieb's description of juvenile periodontitis, it was suggested that the underlying cause was a defect in cementum (Gottlieb 1928). This concept has been re-examined (Lindskog and Blomlof 1983; Blomlof *et al.* 1986) in a comparative histological study on teeth from patients with LJP, adult periodontitis, and healthy controls. Cementum from patients with LJP had extensive areas of hypoplasia on both the exposed and intra-alveolar root surfaces. This suggests that the defect is generalized and not related to the pathology of the pocket. Cemental hypoplasia may be due to impaired mineralization of the organic matrix or failure of the matrix to develop. It will result in poor attachment of the periodontal fibres and an increased susceptibility to breakdown. Defects in cementum may be hereditary and could be important in the initiation of LJP.

Genetic factors

A familial and racial tendency in the distribution of juvenile periodontitis has been recognized for some time, but the mode of inheritance is somewhat uncertain. The increased incidence of juvenile periodontitis in females would suggest an X-linked dominant inheritance with reduced penetrability (Melnick *et al.* 1976; Spektor *et al.* 1985). Other studies support the possibility of an autosomal-recessive mode of inheritance, as the segregation ratio did not exceed 25 per cent (Saxen 1980*b*; Long *et al.* 1987). It has also been suggested that juvenile periodontitis has an autosomal-dominant inheritance pattern (Boughman *et al.* 1986); in this case, one child presented with juvenile periodontitis and amelogenesis imperfecta. These two disorders show linkage to genetic markers on chromosome 4.

The conflicting results on the mode of inheritance of juvenile periodontitis highlight some of the problems associated with genetic analysis on this group of patients. The age bands of the disease are defined, which restricts information on phenotypic expression. The onset of the disease is variable, and in adults over the age of 35 years it is difficult to determine whether loss of attachment is attributable to previous episodes of juvenile periodontitis or current episodes of chronic adult periodontitis. Furthermore, elderly relatives may well be edentulous and, in some cases, the cause of tooth loss is difficult to determine.

These problems were considered in a further study on genetic-model testing involving 28 families with a history of juvenile periodontitis (Boughman *et al.* 1988). The analysis showed that the autosomal-recessive model of inheritance was most applicable in their data.

The various genetic studies show that if a patient has juvenile periodontitis, there is a 50 per cent chance that the disease will develop in a brother or sister (Saxen 1980*b*; Van Dyke *et al.* 1985). In the sibling of such a patient, the chance of the disease developing is in the range of 17–30 per cent (Saxen and Nevanlinna 1984; Boughman *et al.* 1988).

Other evidence in support of the genetic component of juvenile periodontitis comes from blood groups and HLA antigens. A large number of patients with juvenile periodontitis are of blood group B (Kaslick *et al.* 1971), but other findings have shown that patients with blood phenotype A_1 were more susceptible to periodontal disease than phenotype A_2. Although an association was shown between juvenile periodontitis and HLA antigens (Reinholdt *et al.* 1977), subsequent studies refuted this finding (Saxen 1980*b*; Saxen and Koskimies 1984).

Genetic factors are undoubtedly important in the pathogenesis of juvenile periodontitis. However, it is uncertain how these are expressed. As discussed above, the defect in cementum associated with LJP may be familial. Similarly, the transmission of *A. actinomycetemcomitans* from one member of a family to another may account for the familial tendency in LJP. Many patients with juvenile periodontitis and their families show an underlying defect in PMN chemotaxis (see below). This defect is not reversible with treatment and may therefore be under genetic control (Genco *et al.* 1980).

Impairment of PMN function

A large proportion of patients (70 per cent) with LJP have a defect in PMN chemotaxis, which is cell-associated, and depressed PMN phagocytosis, which is serum-mediated (Cianciola *et al.* 1977; Lavine *et al.* 1979; Van Dyke *et al.* 1980; Genco *et al.* 1980). Other functions of PMNs in juvenile periodontitis are normal. These include superoxide production, release of lysosomal enzymes, adherence, and random migration. The nature of the chemotactic defect has been extensively investigated. The PMNs show reduced cell-surface receptors to the synthetic polypeptide chemotactic factor *N*-formylmethionyl phenylalanine (FMLP) and the complement factor C5a (Van Dyke *et al.* 1983). PMNs from patients with LJP also have reduced amounts of the surface glycoprotein GP-110; this glycoprotein is likewise important in the chemotactic response.

This underlying defect in PMN chemotaxis response appears to be familial (Van Dyke *et al.* 1985). If patients with LJP have impaired PMN chemotaxis, then up to half of the siblings in the family will show a similar defect. Conversely, if a patient with LJP has normal PMN chemotactic function, then the rest of the family will be unaffected.

Impaired PMN chemotaxis associated with LJP will affect migration of these cells into the junctional epithleium and gingival crevices. Thus, the host's defences will be compromised which, may increase susceptibility to *A. actinomycetemcomitans*. Once this bacterium is established in the pocket, the production of bacterial leukotoxins will further inhibit the host response and facilitate colonization of the pocket.

PMNs from patients with juvenile periodontitis have been stimulated *in vitro* with opsonized bacteria (Asman 1988). This produced an increased release of free oxygen radicals and elastase. Free oxygen radicals have the potential to damage the surrounding tissues and degrade collagen. PMN elastase has been implicated in the pathogenesis of cystic fibrosis and Crohn's disease. The release of these substances from PMNs in juvenile periodontitis may contribute to the local tissue destruction.

Conclusions

This account on the pathogenesis of juvenile periodontitis has itemized several contributory factors. All the evidence would suggest an interplay between them. The racial difference in incidence, and the familial defect in PMN chemotaxis and mineralization in cementum increases susceptibility to periodontal breakdown. If *A. actinomycetemcomitans* is allowed to colonize the gingival margin, it produces enough toxins and enzymes to further compromise the host response and destroy periodontal tissues. Antibodies are produced to this bacterium and these may modulate the course of the disease. The localized form of juvenile periodontitis may be a reflection of an adequate host response that limits the bacterial colonization to the first molar and incisor teeth. The generalized form follows if the immune response has been inadequate (Zambon *et al.* 1983*a*). An alternative explanation of the localized and generalized forms of juvenile periodontitis may relate to bacterial antagonism in the pocket (Hillman and Socransky 1982).

5.4.6 TREATMENT OF JUVENILE PERIODONTITIS

A variety of treatment regimens have been suggested for the management of juvenile periodontitis; these have been the subject of an excellent review (Krill and Fry 1987). Antimicrobial agents have been shown to be of value. These drugs have been used as the sole treatment, but more often to supplement non-surgical or surgical management. Flap surgery, with or without bone grafts and tooth transplantation, are other treatments that have been used.

Antimicrobial therapy

The specific role of *A. actinomycetemcomitans* in the pathogenesis of LJP has been discussed in the preceding section. This bacterium is sensitive to tetracycline and minocycline (Slots *et al.* 1980*a*). A further advantage of tetracycline is its ability to undergo concentration in crevicular fluid (Gordon *et al.* 1981). Hence tetracycline has been extensively used in the management of juvenile periodontitis.

Tetracycline alone plus supragingival plaque control has been evaluated in four patients with LJP (Novak *et al.* 1988); dosage was 1 g/day for 3–6 weeks. At the 3-month assessment, 79 per cent of the periodontal sites showed a decrease in pocket depth >2 mm, and 69 per cent of these sites showed a gain of attachment. The improvement in clinical measures was supported by radiographic evidence of an increase in bone levels. Apart from the antimicrobial effect of tetracycline, the drug also inhibits collagenase activity and osteoclastic bone resorption (Golub *et al.* 1984; Gomes *et al.* 1984). These properties may account for the observed improvement in attachment levels and the bone repair.

Regular (bi-weekly) subgingival irrigation with a 3 per cent hydrogen peroxide solution has been shown to be effective in suppressing *A. actinomycetemcomitans* in periodontal pockets of LJP (Wikesjo *et al.* 1989). Although no clinical data were recorded in this study, it was reported that irrigation suppressed the levels of the bacterium for up to five months after cessation of treatment.

Antimicrobial therapy and non-surgical management

A combination of regular scaling and root planing with systemic tetracycline therapy has been shown to be an effective treatment for the control of LJP (Gold 1979; Genco *et al.* 1981). The clinical and microbiological effects of subgingival debridement, topical Betadine, and systemic tetracycline have been compared during the different stages in the management of LJP (Slots and Rosling 1983). Both subgingival debridement and tetracycline therapy significantly reduced *A. actinomycetemcomitans* and *Capnocytophaga*, but a more profound effect was observed after tetracycline. Topical Betadine solution had no effect on the plaque microflora. A clinical improvement followed subgingival debridement, but this treatment did not arrest attachment loss, whereas tetracycline therapy produced a slight gain in attachment. Non-surgical management on its own was not effective in controlling LJP. This finding was subsequently confirmed by Christersson *et al.* (1985), who showed that root instrumentation failed to reduce subgingival levels of *A. actinomycetemcomitans*. A combination of scaling, root planing, and systemic tetracycline appears to be an effective means of controlling LJP.

Metronidazole and penicillin have been shown to be of little value in the management of LJP (Mitchell 1984; Kunihira *et al.* 1985). However, the combination of metronidazole, 250 mg, plus amoxycillin, 375 mg, three times a day for seven days, together with subgingival debridement, has been shown to be an effective treatment of LJP (Winkelhoff *et al.* 1989). Clinical improvement (reduced probing depths and a reduction in bleeding on probing) was found in all patients treated with this combined therapy. At 9–11 months after treatment, *A. actinomycetemcomitans* was still undetectable in the subgingival plaque. All patients who participated in this study had received conventional periodontal treatment in the past, including systemic antibiotics.

Antimicrobial therapy and surgical management

The combination of flap surgery and systemic antimicrobial therapy (tetracycline) was first reported in 1979 (Baer and Socransky 1979). Since then, other studies have shown that this combined approach is a very effective means of treating LJP.

Lindhe and Liljenberg (1984) treated 16 LJP patients with tetracycline, 250 mg, four times day for 14 days, and modified Widman flaps. Initially, this combination of treatments halted the progression of the disease, but there was recurrence in four patients. These four were retreated in the same manner. The patients were monitored for five years and at the end of this period there was an improvement in all clinical measures, with radiographic evidence of bone fill.

Bacteriological sampling of sites with LJP can provide a useful indication to the appropriate treatment (Kornmann and Robertson 1985). In their study, three treatment regimens were evaluated: scaling and root planing; scaling and root planing with systemic tetracycline (1 g/day for 28 days); and flap surgery with the same regimen of tetracycline. Periodontal pockets with high levels of *A. actinomycetemcomitans* or black-pigmented *Bacteroides* showed a better response to the combination of flap surgery and tetracycline. As with previous studies, scaling and root planing alone was of little value in the management of LJP.

Similar promising results in the control of LJP have been shown when flap surgery is combined with doxycycline (Mandell *et al.* 1986; Mandell and Socransky 1988). This particular combination of treatments eliminated *A. actinomycetemcomitans* from pockets for up to 12 months and facilitated a gain in clinical attachment.

Surgical management

Few studies have been undertaken to evaluate the effectiveness of flap surgery alone in the management of juvenile periodontitis. This procedure is recommended to gain access to the subgingival microflora (Gjermo 1981) and to remove granulation tissue and infected connective tissue (Christersson *et al.* 1985). In a retrospective study, 21 patients with LJP were successfully treated with supra and subgingival plaque control and scaling. Flap surgery was undertaken on those sites with a probing depth >5 mm (Waerhaug 1977*b*). These patients were kept under review for a period of 8–34 years. A similar result was obtained with 20 LJP patients who were initially treated with oral hygiene, scaling, root planing, and surgery (Saxen *et al.* 1986). These patients were re-examined some 6–12 years after initial therapy and all showed a marked improvement in the various clinical measures. The investigators concluded that patients with LJP can be treated by conventional measures and periodontal health can be maintained with the use of antimicrobial agents.

Grafting procedures

The angular bony defects in LJP lend themselves to osseous grafting procedures. The following types of grafts have been used with varying success: autogenous bone chips (Oshrain and Kaslick 1981), osseous coagulum (Burnette and Stewart 1969), frozen autogenous hip marrow (De Marco and Scaletta 1970) and freeze-dried bone allografts plus tetracycline (Yukna and Sepe 1982). If grafting procedures are to be undertaken, then optimal results are obtained when the graft is combined with tetracycline. The drug should be given systemically and can be incorporated in the graft material. There is no information on the type of attachment gained after osseous grafting. The new regenerative periodontal techniques (guided tissue regeneration) may be useful in the treatment of local defects associated with LJP.

Tooth transplantation

In many instances, first permanent molars are so severely affected by LJP that the only treatment is extraction. The possibility of replacing such teeth with unerupted third molars was first advocated by Baer and Gamble (1966). In essence, the criteria for successful transplantation are as follows:

1. The third molar crown should be slightly smaller than the tooth it is replacing.

2. Root development of the third molar should be incomplete.

3. The transplanted tooth should be kept out of occlusion for 3–4 weeks post-transplantation.

Some success has been reported with tooth transplantation in the management of LJP. A 7-year follow-up study of 15 transplanted cases showed that all the teeth survived (Borring-Moller and Frandsen 1978). Clinically, none of the teeth had a pocket depth > 3 mm, there was no attachment loss, and radiographs showed evidence of repair of the osseous defects.

Transplanted teeth are subject to root resorption and pulpal death. However, they may have a value as space maintainers until the patient is old enough for a more permanent prosthesis.

Other dental considerations in LJP

If the first permanent molars are lost as a consequence of LJP, then it is possible to move the second and third molars forward to fill the space. One case report suggested waiting three months after extraction before attempting orthodontic movement, as a tooth moved into the socket may be similarly affected (Goldstein and Fritz 1976). Others suggest waiting up to 18 months before attempting orthodontic treatment so as to allow complete healing of the tooth sockets (Compton *et al.* 1983).

The extensive alveolar bone loss that is often a feature of LJP is likely to cause pulpal death, owing to exposure of a lateral root canal. In such instances, root canal therapy is essential if the tooth is to be saved. This treatment is also required if root amputation or hemi section is being considered.

Conclusions

Although several options are available for the treatment of LJP, the combination of systemic tetracycline (a 2–4 week course) with flap surgery or root surface debridement appears to be the most predictable. Perhaps surgery and tetracycline is the best option as the procedure involves the removal of granulation and connective tissue infected with *A. actinomycetemcomitans*. The cases that do not respond to this management may well benefit from the combination of metronidazole, amoxycillin, and root surface debridement (Winkelhoff *et al.* 1989).

Tetracycline and related drugs (i.e. minocycline and doxycycline) are not without unwanted effects, and in theory, resistance can develop to Gram-negative bacteria (Van Palenstein Helderman 1984). It has been advocated that microbiological testing should be carried when antimicrobials are being considered for the treatment of LJP (Gjermo 1986).

5.5 PERIODONTAL DISEASE IN THE ELDERLY

5.5.1 INTRODUCTION

The improvement in environmental conditions, public health measures, and medical care over the past 50 years has dramatically increased the number of people surviving into old age. In the Western world, the 65 and older age group is the fastest growing segment and is estimated to make up one-third of the population. In the United States it has been predicted that by the year 2000, persons 75 years and over will constitute 45 per cent of the overall aged population, with over 5 million of them 85 years of age or older (Federal Council on Aging 1986). This increase in the aged population and improvement in health care is reflected in more of the elderly retaining their teeth. Thus, the dental practitioners and periodontologists are going to treat proportionally more elderly patients than their predecessors.

In this section we will consider the effect of age changes on the periodontal tissues and their response to plaque, the epidemiology of periodontal disease in the elderly, and treatment problems in an elderly population.

5.5.2 EFFECTS OF AGE ON THE PERIODONTAL TISSUES

All the periodontal tissues are affected by age changes and each component tissue will be considered separately. In many instances, the clinical significance of these changes has yet to be determined.

Gingival epithelium

The gingival and oral epithelium becomes thinner with age, less keratinized, and shows an increase in cell density

(Shklar 1966; Ryan *et al.* 1974). The interface between the epithelium and connective tissue also changes with age from a ridge-type to a papilla-type interface (Loe and Karring 1972). There is uncertainty about the effect of age on the mitotic activity of gingival and oral epithelium, with some studies reporting an increase with age, others reporting a constant rate of mitosis, and still others showing a decrease in activity (for review, see Van der Velden 1984). These various differences may be related to the level of inflammation present in the tissues before biopsy.

Gingival connective tissue

It is well recognized that skin shows definite age changes, for example, the appearance of wrinkles and loss of elasticity. These features are mainly due to the loss of subcutaneous fat. Gingival connective tissue does not contain such fat and therefore such obvious changes do not occur. Age changes that do occur in the gingival connective tissue include one from a fine to a more dense and coarse texture, and a decrease in the cellular component (Wentz *et al.* 1952). Animal studies have shown that the rate of collagen synthesis and the proportion of labile or more immature collagen decrease with age. There appears to be no evidence to support this finding in human studies.

Periodontal ligament

The connective tissue component of the periodontal ligament undergoes age changes. The fibre and cellular components decrease and the structure of the ligament becomes more irregular (Severson *et al.* 1978). Other changes include a reduction in cell density and mitotic activity, a reduction in organic matrix production, and a loss of acid mucopolysaccharide.

There are further, conflicting findings concerning the effect of age on the width of the periodontal ligament. Some studies report an increase with age whilst others report a decrease (for review see Van der Velden 1984). However, it is now well established that the width of the ligament is related to the functional demands on the tooth, and differences in occlusal loading may account for these conflicting findings. Thus, fewer remaining teeth would take a greater proportion of the occlusal load. This may produce a widening of the periodontal ligament and an increase in tooth mobility. In such circumstances, mobile teeth do not necessarily have a poor prognosis. It has also been reported that masticatory forces decrease with age, which may contribute to a reduction in the width of the periodontal ligaments (Helkimo *et al.* 1977).

Cementum

The formation of cementum (mainly acellular) occurs continuously throughout life and the increase in width with age is most marked in the apical region of the tooth (Zander and Hurzeler 1958). It has been suggested that the apical increase may be a response to passive eruption (Severson *et al.* 1978). A slight increase in remodelling of cementum also

occurs with age and is characterized by areas of resorption and apposition (Henry and Weinmann 1951). This may account for the increased irregularity observed on the surfaces of older teeth (Grant and Bernick 1972).

Alveolar bone

This structure shows marked changes with age; these include an increase in the number of interstitial lamellae, which produces a denser interdental septum, and a decrease in the number of cells in the osteogenic layer of the cribriform plate. With increasing age, the periodontal surfaces of the alveolar bone become jagged and collagen fibres show a less regular insertion into bone (Severson *et al.* 1978). Animal studies suggest that the width of the cribriform plate may decrease with age, but this finding has not been confirmed in human studies.

Ageing and attachment loss

In health, the apical cell of the junctional epithelium is attached to the cementum-enamel junction. A feature of periodontal destruction is loss of connective tissue attachment to the root surface and apical migration of the junctional epithelium. There is controversy as to whether age also induces apical migration of the junctional epithelium because epidemiological evidence suggests that periodontal breakdown increases with age. The dilemma in an elderly patient with attachment loss is whether it is due to periodontal disease or part of the ageing process, or both.

Animal studies suggest that ageing is associated with a gradual, physiological recession of the gingival tissues, which is concomitant with an apical migration of the junctional epithelium. This idea would support the theory of continuous passive eruption, which proposes that gingival recession occurs as a result of occlusal migration of the teeth in the presence of a stable gingival margin. The migration compensates for occlusal wear. This is depicted diagrammatically in Fig. 5.2.

Subsequent studies have shown that the occlusal movement of teeth is not necessarily associated with apical migration of the junctional epithelium, provided that there is good gingival health (Manson 1963; Anneroth and Ericsson 1967). It has been shown that the location of the mucogingival junction does not change with age (Ainamo 1978), and, in the absence of gingival recession, the width of attached gingiva increases with age (Ainamo *et al.* 1961). These studies point to the conclusion that the junctional epithelium remains at the cementum-enamel junction and the width of attached gingiva increases with age, owing to the eruption of the teeth or the dento alveolar complex (Fig. 5.2). These events only occur if the periodontal tissues are healthy. There is little evidence to support the physiological apical migration of the junctional epithelium with age.

5.5.3 EFFECTS OF AGE ON PLAQUE

There are various biochemical and microbiological changes in dental plaque with increasing age. The calcium and

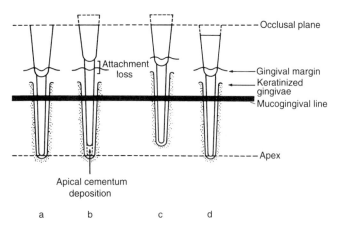

Fig. 5.2 Schematic diagram to show the relationship between attrition, attachment loss, and attached gingiva. (a) 'Normal': no attrition, no periodontal disease; (b) 'passive eruption': real attachment loss because of periodontal disease, attrition, and compensatory eruption; (c) dentoalveolar compensatory eruption: attrition, no periodontal disease, and increased width of attached gingiva; (d) no compensatory eruption: presence or absence of periodontal disease, attrition producing reduced occlusal face height.

phosphorus levels increase with the patient's age, and this may be related to similar increases in salivary calcium and phosphorus levels (Kleinberg *et al.* 1971).

The bacterial composition of plaque does show certain quantitative changes with age. Plaque from young patients contains more viable micro-organisms per mg than plaque from the elderly (Holm-Pederson *et al.* 1980). The number of spirochaetes is reported to increase in plaque with increasing age (Socransky *et al.* 1963). Conversely, there is a fall in the number of streptococci in plaque from elderly patients (Holm-Pedersen *et al.* 1980). It has also been shown that the rate of plaque accumulation increases with age (Holm-Pedersen *et al.* 1975). This may be due to physiological changes in saliva, or to an increase in gingival recession producing more plaque retentive areas and a greater exposed surface of roughened cementum.

The rate of plaque formation is also reported to be different between young and old patients (Brecx *et al.* 1985). In the early stages of plaque formation (4 h), there are significantly fewer bacteria in the elderly than the young patient. However, at 24 h, bacterial counts in both groups are similar. This may indicate a more rapid rate of plaque formation (i.e. from 4 h to 24 h) in the elderly.

Certain enzymic and immunological changes also occur in plaque from elderly patients. Levan hydrolase activity is markedly lower in plaque from elderly patients. This finding may be related to differences in the levels of streptococci between young and old (Holm-Pedersen *et al.* 1980).

The concentration of immune factors (IgA, IgM, C3, lactoferrin, lysozyme, and lactoperoxidase) is reported to be higher in plaque obtained from older people. The clinical significance of this finding and whether such changes alter the pathogenicity of plaque with regard to periodontal breakdown have yet to be determined.

5.5.4 EFFECTS OF AGE ON THE RESPONSE OF THE PERIODONTAL TISSUES TO PLAQUE

Various age-associated alterations occur in the body's immune and inflammatory responses that may affect the resistance of the periodontal tissues to bacterial plaque. A reduced immune response (as determined by the lymphocyte stimulation index) to plaque has been reported in the elderly (Church and Dolby 1978). Sensitization of peripheral blood leukocytes to lipopolysaccharides is a feature of experimental gingivitis in young adults. This sensitization does not appear to occur in the elderly (Holm-Pedersen *et al.* 1979). Also, an experimental model of gingivitis has shown that the rate of development of gingival inflammation (as assessed by crevicular fluid flow and bleeding on probing) increases with age (Holm-Pedersen *et al.* 1975). This could be associated with a diminished immune response; however, subsequent studies have shown that the susceptibility of an individual to periodontal disease is a more important determinant than age for the rate of development of periodontal inflammation (Van der Velden and Abbas, 1982).

5.5.5 EPIDEMIOLOGY

The increase in the elderly population has generated many investigations into the prevalence of dental disease in this group and their treatment needs.

One of the earliest epidemiological studies on the prevalence of periodontal disease and tooth loss in the adult population of the United States showed that periodontal disease was uncommon before the age of 18, and increased steadily with age (Marshall-Day *et al.* 1955). After the age of 40, there was a rapid rise in edentulousness, and by the age of 60, 60 per cent of the dentition had been lost and 20 per cent of the subjects were edentulous. This would suggest that periodontal destruction is age-associated. Further studies have shown that this is not the case and each succeeding generation is less affected by periodontal disease (Miller *et al.* 1987).

From the United Kingdom, there is little meaningful information on the incidence and severity of periodontal disease in elderly people. This may be due to the high incidence of edentulism (80 per cent) in the population aged 65 years and over, although there is regional variation in this figure. Findings from a survey carried out on 153 elderly subjects from the East Midlands showed an incidence of edentulism of 83 per cent. Of the remaining subjects, the investigators (Taylor *et al.* 1986) reported that their restorative, periodontal and surgical treatment needs were low. A further problem when investigating the periodontal status of elderly persons is differentiating between the effects of the 'normal' ageing process on the periodontal tissues and the effects of disease. This particular problem arises when attachment loss is considered.

There have been several reports from Scandinavian countries on the dental state of the elderly. In Finland, 40 per cent of elderly people aged 65 years and over had their natural teeth, but only 2 per cent of these had healthy periodontal tissues (Lappalainen *et al.* 1988). Of the dentate sample, 43 per cent of the men and 27 per cent of the women had severe periodontal disease with probing depths > 6 mm. Only half of the dentate men and three-quarters of the women brushed their teeth once a day. A similar figure for edentulism was found in a Norwegian study, with 46 per cent of subjects aged 67 years and older having their natural teeth (Rise and Heloe 1987).

Other studies from Scandinavian countries reported that periodontal treatment needs increase with age up to middle age. Thereafter, the periodontal health of most elderly people can be maintained by regular, non-surgical management (Plasschaert *et al.* 1978; Hugoson and Jordan 1982; Hugoson and Jordan 1982; Markkanen *et al.* 1983).

Studies from the United States have shown that approximately 60 per cent of the population aged 65 years and over are dentate (Hunt *et al.* 1985), with an average of 19 teeth remaining. Of the sample selected in at investigation, 90 per cent needed treatment of some type (oral hygiene instruction, scaling and root planing for pockets 3–6 mm in depth). Only 1 per cent of this cohort of patients had gingival bleeding and periodontal pockets greater than 6 mm. Another American study (Roper *et al.* 1972) showed that age did not significantly correlate with the following items: (a) presence of gingival inflammation; (b) the accumulation of plaque and calculus; (c) gingival recession; and (d) depth of periodontal pocket. On the other hand, in a group of 65-to74-year-olds, a correlation was demonstrated between the number of remaining teeth and the periodontal status (as measured by the periodontal index), and a high correlation with the standard of oral hygiene (Burt *et al.* 1985). The number of retained teeth in the same age group also showed a positive correlation with the remaining alveolar bone height supporting the teeth (Palmqvist and Sjodin 1987). This may indicate individual resistance to periodontal disease.

Other factors that may influence the retention of teeth in elderly people have been examined using multiple linear regression analysis (Levy *et al.* 1987). Physical and medical variables were relatively unimportant factors for determining the proportion of retained teeth in the population sample. The significant correlations were behavioural factors, especially tobacco consumption.

It may be inferred from the above studies that the periodontal needs of the elderly are relatively slight, and can be controlled by regular plaque control, dietary advice, and professional tooth cleaning. A further problem is that many elderly people are cared for in long-term stay hospital, or residential or nursing homes. One survey has shown that the dentate institutionalized elderly person has poor plaque control and severe gingival inflammation (Vigild 1988). Patients who received 'assistance' with oral hygiene measures had more plaque and gingival bleeding than those who managed to clean their own teeth. Vigild concluded that both the elderly and the staff who care for them are in need of regular instructions in plaque control and mouth care.

5.5.6 TREATMENT

Introduction

In the previous sections we have discussed the age changes that can affect the periodontal tissues and their response to plaque. All the statistics show that the elderly population is increasing and the rate of edentulism is falling. Thus, the management of periodontal problems in the elderly is going to take up an increasing amount of the dental surgeon's time. In this section we will consider the periodontal management problems that are particularly pertinent to elderly people.

Clinical aspects

Any periodontal treatment plan requires the appropriate diagnosis based on various indices and investigations. It is advisable to record and monitor simple plaque and bleeding indices, and pocket depths where possible. Such measures are essential for the assessment of cleaning efficiency, patient compliance, and disease progression. Furthermore, a visible record of performance can be just as powerful a motivational device for the elderly as for the young. The Community Periodontal Index of Treatment Needs (CPITN) is a valuable and viable means of monitoring in the elderly patient.

It has been reported that older patients develop plaque more quickly than the young (Holm-Pedersen *et al.* 1975, 1980). This phenomenon may be a feature of the greater area of exposed tooth surface, and/or of the grooved, tilted, single-standing, and less accessible teeth found in elderly people. Softer diets, reduced oral activity, and an increased incidence of xerostomia may similarly contribute to gross accumulation of plaque and calculus.

When plaque accumulates undisturbed, gingival inflammation appears to develop more rapidly in the older patients, but does not necessarily involve the deeper tissues. It is generally accepted that the dentate individual who has survived to their seventh or eighth decade is less susceptible to destructive periodontitis. Indeed, some individuals have considerable resistance to periodontal disease. Frequently, a severely worn dentition is supported by a periodontium showing few signs of destruction. It is therefore unusual to see generalized advanced periodontitis (i.e. with probing depths greater than 6 mm) in elderly patients. More commonly, a range of conditions is seen, from early to moderate chronic periodontitis, with varying degrees of gingival recession and localized advanced pocketing, especially where there are predisposing factors. In the older patient, these factors may include radicular grooves, exposed furcations, split roots, impinging restorations, or ill-fitting partial dentures.

Periodontal inflammation is a stimulus to overeruption and subsequent drifting and tilting of teeth. Furthermore, loss of alveolar support and inflammation within the periodontium can lead to increased tooth mobility, over and above that caused by excessive occlusal loading. Loose teeth may remain functional for many years and may be crucial to a complex treatment plan. Therefore, it remains essential in the first instance to establish periodontal health.

Atrophic or erosive lichen planus and benign mucous membrane pemphigoid are two conditions frequently seen in elderly individuals (see Chapter 3). Owing to the thinness and fragility of the overlying epithelium, both conditions can give the appearance of severe gingival inflammation, which may, in fact, only be superficial. In these patients, toothbrushing may produce discomfort and so discourage plaque control. Persistence with an atraumatic toothbrushing technique, supported by chlorhexidine mouthrinses and professional tooth cleaning, is usually sufficient to prevent further periodontal destruction. As discussed in Chapter 3, the more severe cases will require treatment with either topical or systemic corticosteroids.

Treatment options

Many factors will influence the periodontal treatment options for the elderly patient. These include their attitudes and expectations, previous dental treatment, existing oral and dental health, medical complications, their mobility, and their domestic or institutional support. The choice of treatment can usually be resolved into one of the following:

(1) minimum intervention for maintaining the *status quo*, for example, occasional hygiene therapy, fillings, and extractions as necessary;

(2) multiple extractions and the provision of dentures;

(3) more extensive periodontal and restorative treatment, including multiple root canal therapy and full coronal restorations.

In the United Kingdom, elderly patients have traditionally been offered the first two options, usually on the grounds of limited life expectancy, cost, and poor periodontal or dental prognosis. However, as far as prognosis is concerned, longitudinal studies have shown that in older patients suffering from advanced periodontitis, successful therapeutic results can be achieved and maintained for many years, provided there is optimal plaque control (Lindhe and Nyman 1975).

Plaque control

The demand for good instruction, demonstration, and motivation is just as important for the old as for the young. The following recommendations should improve communication with the elderly patient:

- Structure the plaque control message in a chronological, step-by-step manner; for example, the stages of a brushing routine.
- Avoid giving too much information at any one time—no patient, and certainly not an elderly person, can be expected to absorb instructions for disclosing, brushing, flossing, and so on, in a single session.
- Allow more time for explanation and clarification of terms. Use slower and clearer speech, but avoid shouting and over-exaggeration, both of which can cause offence. During instructions, the simple expedients of facing the patient, sitting closer, and

avoiding background noise are much appreciated by those with poor hearing.

- Listen for, and encourage feedback—if necessary by direct enquiry. Also, listen to the overtly, or covertly, expressed needs of the patient with regard to appearance, function, transport, and home support. A good rapport is more likely to result in compliance with instructions and return visits.
- Use several modes of communication to support the same message. Wherever possible, let the patients see and feel the presence of plaque, calculus, and inflammation for themselves. The 'tell, show, and feel' of correct toothbrushing can be supported by written advice. The written message should be simple, pithy, and printed in large, bold characters. Simple but realistic diagrams can be of value.
- Set realistic objectives. Crevicular and approximal brushing is desirable and achievable for patients of all ages if they have reasonable manual dexterity. For the less able, a simple scrub technique supplemented by once or twice daily rinsing with 0.2 per cent chlorhexidine would be appropriate. For the infirm patient, it is necessary to involve the family, or institutional staff, in a similar simple and regular regimen, augmented by hygienist treatment every 3–6 months.

Modified toothbrush handles for improved grip and access can be purchased or easily fabricated. A good range of handle-mounted interproximal brushes is now available. These are essential for cleaning of the wider interdental spaces and open furcations that are often present in the aged dentition. Contra-angled, single-tufted brushes are invaluable for reaching single-standing posterior teeth and those with long clinical crowns. A double-headed toothbrush designed for simultaneous cleaning of two tooth surfaces may find application in the physically handicapped elderly patient. Automatic toothbrushes, preferably of the rechargeable type and having an elliptical head movement, confer the real benefits of being less tiring and less painful for some elderly patients. In situations where finger and wrist or arm movements are restricted, a pulsed-jet water irrigator can be used once daily to deliver 400 ml of a 0.02 per cent solution of chlorhexidine gluconate. Floss holders also relieve less mobile fingers of what can be a difficult procedure. A plaque-control programme with reinforcement of oral hygiene and scaling is often all that is required in cases of early or moderate chronic adult periodontitis.

Surgical or non-surgical management

Age is not a contraindication to periodontal surgery. However, longitudinal studies have shown that in patients with moderately advanced periodontal disease, where adequate plaque control was achieved, there was no significant difference between sites treated surgically and those treated non-surgically (Pihlstrom *et al.* 1983). Although surgery produced a greater reduction in the depth of severe pockets, both types of treatment were capable of arresting periodontal destruction. Thus, for most elderly patients, especially those with medical complications or inadequate home care, a non-surgical approach is advisable. When root planing, it should be noted that repeated and excessive removal of cementum is unnecessary and may lead to dentinal sensitivity.

Gingivectomy, flap surgery, and root amputation are probably the most useful surgical techniques for the older patient. Although teeth with furcation involvements were once thought to have a poor prognosis, long-term surveys indicate a high survival rate into old age when managed surgically or non-surgically (Ross and Thompson 1978). Regeneration techniques using various forms of filters provide a new method of treating furcation lesions. Again, this technique would be applicable to the elderly.

Response to treatment

In both animal and human studies, wound healing is reported to be adversely affected by age. Factors include the rate of healing and the strength of the healed tissues. This may be a reflection of altered fibroblastic function and slower revascularization in elderly people. However, it appears that age is not a clinically significant factor in the healing of the periodontal tissues. It has been reported that healing after gingivectomy is not affected by age (Stahl *et al.* 1968). More evidence sugests that the amount of periodontal breakdown (and hence susceptibility to periodontal disease) is of greater importance in determining healing after periodontal surgery than is age (Abbas *et al.* 1984).

It is apparent that an older, dentate patient with an equivalent degree of periodontal breakdown may be regarded as being more resistant to the disease process than a younger person. Futhermore, such resistant individuals have been successfully treated surgically and non-surgically even with a less-than-ideal standard of plaque control (Van der Velden 1982). However, it should be emphasized that surgery performed on any patient with poor oral hygiene may constitute 'over-treatment', and result in greater damage to the periodontium (Nyman *et al.* 1977).

Splinting

Mobile teeth with no active periodontal disease may remain functional and in a stable position for many years. Splinting should not be undertaken lightly, as it frequently encourages plaque accumulation and inhibits its removal. Indications for splinting include increasing tooth mobility, the risk of exfoliation, or discomfort on eating or talking.

Psychosocial and medical aspects

The elderly may also suffer from psychosocial and/or medical problems that might encourage plaque accumulation, prevent or discourage its removal, or modify the body's response to its presence.

Psychosocial problems

It should not be assumed that older people are intellectually unable to cope with oral hygiene advice and instruction in plaque control. Longitudinal studies have shown that most of adult life is characterized by little change in intellectual capacity (Schaie 1974). However, biological decline and health problems may adversely influence some intellectual functions. For example, elderly people perform psychomotor tasks that require a high-speed response less efficiently than the young. Also, learning through information processing into memory is slower, especially when tasks are complex, or if the information is not meaningful or personally relevant (Fozard 1980; Hoyer and Plude 1980). It appears that in old age the memory is more susceptible to overload and 'interference' from stored, previous experiences. However, slower and repeated presentations produce a ready improvement in learning in older patients (Canestrari 1963).

Dramatic life-events and loss of personal roles (for example, loss of job, spouse, or independence) may be expected to occur more frequently in elderly persons. These events can have an adverse effect on self-concept and self-esteem. They can also induce breakdown and depression, especially when combined with declining general health (Gurland 1976).

Depression, like any other mental disorder, can impair the motivation to maintain oral hygiene, or to seek professional advice. The condition also reduces the capacity to comply with treatment. Such patients may be 'hard to reach', forget clear instructions, and find it difficult to make decisions about treatment. They may tire easily, and several short appointments are better than fewer long ones. In addition, antidepressant therapy often reduces salivary flow (especially tricyclic antidepressants), and the patients may resort to sucking sweets to moisten their mouths. Some patients have been prescribed ascorbic acid lozenges for the same reason. This can lead to a greater and more rapid plaque accumulation, to a deterioration in periodontal health, and to the development of root caries in susceptible individuals.

In dealing with elderly patients with depression and other mental disorders it is wise to have a concerned, thorough, low-key, and flexible attitude. Realistic objections need to be set for treatment, recall schedules, and domiciliary care. It is important to maintain contact with the patient or their family/friends. Such patients are easily 'lost' to the system and then reappear after a year or so with marked deterioration in their oral health.

The nervous system

Sensory loss—particularly visual and auditory—can seriously impair the patient's perception and participation during oral hygiene procedures. Visual accommodation deteriorates after the age of 45 years, and distance and depth perception decline rapidly after 75 years. Sight and adaptation in low light is poor. On the other hand, elderly patients may be particularly susceptible to the glare from dental lights. Thus, providing a hand mirror for oral hygiene instruction may be of limited value, and greater reliance must be placed on tactile detection of plaque with the tongue.

Loss of high-frequency tones (presbycusis) is a progressive condition experienced by 50–60 per cent of elderly people. Many depend on hearing aids and have to contend with the distraction of poorly discriminated background noise. The incidence of tinnitus also increases with age. In such cases it is necessary to deliver a slow, clearly enunciated message (without being too deliberate!) while sitting close to and facing the patient. Unnecessary, distracting background noise in the surgery should be eliminated.

Cerebrovascular problems are frequent in the aged. Facial palsy reduces the overall cleaning of gross debris by the oral musculature; and paresis of limbs may cause considerable physical handicap to satisfactory plaque control. In these circumstances it is essential to involve family, friends, or institutional staff in the oral hygiene motivation and instruction programme. Their commitment must be even greater if the patient has suffered a receptive dysphasia and is unable to be taught.

The incidence of Parkinson's disease and orofacial dyskinesias increases with age, and may be drug-induced. The unusual muscular activities of tremor, rigidity, tongue protusion, etc. may make access for cleaning difficult for both the patient and the operator.

The cardiovascular system

Increasing numbers of patients with rheumatic heart disease, degenerative valvular disease, and prosthetic heart valves are reaching old age. Appropriate antibiotic cover must be provided for blood-spilling procedures such as scaling, root planing, and periodontal surgery. Recall intervals should be at least one month. Clear case-note entries and prescriptions should be made, especially if a dental hygienist is to carry out treatment. Where possible, dental treatment should be avoided within six months of prosthetic heart-valve replacement.

In this age range, it is occasionally necessary to face the dilemma of whether to perform a dental clearance and risk intransigent denture problems and poorer quality of life, or retain a dentition showing varying degrees of periodontal and dental breakdown, with the attendant risk to general health. When all the medical and dental advice has been given, and if the patient opts to retain his/her dentition, there is a moral obligation for the profession to provide the necessary recall or domiciliary support.

The musculo skeletal system

Osteoarthritis, rheumatoid arthritis, and other connective tissue disorders, such as polymyalgia rheumatica, can severely limit attempts at plaque control. Automatic and modified, manual and interdental toothbrushes can improve grip and access. The use of a pulsed-jet irrigator to deliver a 0.02 per cent solution of chlorhexidine can also be recommended where wrist, arm, and shoulder movement is minimal. Again, the assistance of a third party for daily cleaning may be crucial.

Drugs

The well-documented effects of certain drugs on the periodontium may be seen with increasing frequency in the elderly population. Epanutin (anticonvulsant), cyclosporin (immunosuppressant) and nifedipine (calcium-channel blocker) can provoke gingival overgrowth in the susceptible individual (see Chapter 4). A more rigorous recall programme (3-monthly) should be considered because the rate of overgrowth may be related to the degree of gingival inflammation. Some antihypertensives, e.g. methyldopa, may produce lichenoid reactions in the gingival tissues.

Patients taking anticoagulants may require adjustment of dose before surgery, although scaling and root planing can usually be carried out within the therapeutic range (where the International Normalized Ratio, the INR, does not exceed 2.5).

5.5.7 Conclusions

The periodontium in dentate elderly patients invariably demonstrates the capacity to resist, overcome, and repair the ravages of periodontal disease, despite age changes that may suggest increased vulnerability. Dental surgeons often concern themselves with the amount of periodontal support that has been lost rather than the health of that which remains. In the elderly, as well as in all patients, periodontal health is still a prerequisite for successful restorative treatment. Effective and rewarding programmes of periodontal health are possible in general dental practice, institutional, and domiciliary settings. Perhaps the barriers to such care are not to be found principally with the patients, but in political and professional attitudes, and in understanding.

REFERENCES

PERIODONTAL DISEASE IN CHILDREN

Baer, P. N. (1957). Periodontal disease in children and adolescents: a clinical study. *Journal of the American Dental Association*, 55, 629–34.

Bailit, H. L., Baldwin, D. C., and Hunt, E. E. (1964). The increasing prevalence of gingival *Bacteroides melaninogenicus* with age in children. *Archives of Oral Biology*, 9, 435–8.

Biswas, S., Duperon, D. F., and Chebib, F. S. (1977). Study of periodontal disease in children and young adolescents. *Journal of Periodontal Research*, 12, 250–64.

Blankenstein, R., Murray, J. J., and Lind, O. P. (1978). Prevalence of chronic periodontitis in 13–15-year-old children. *Journal of Clinical Periodontology*, 5, 285–92.

Bowden, D. E., Davies, R. M., Holloway, P. J., Lennon, M. A., and Rugg-Gunn, A. J. (1973). A treatment need survey of a 15-year-old population. *British Dental Journal*, 134, 375–9.

Bowen, T. J. *et al.* (1982). Severe recurrent bacterial infections associated with defective adherence and chemotaxis in 2 patients with neutrophil deficiency in a cell-associated glyprotein. *Journal of Pediatrics*, 101, 932–40.

Bradley, R. E. (1961). Periodontal lesions in children: their recognition and treatment. *Dental Clinics of North America*, 5, 671–85.

Bystrom, A., Crossner, C-G., and Unell, L. (1983). 'Prepubertal' periodontitis: a case report. *Swedish Dental Journal*, 7, 254–6.

Clerehugh, V. and Lennon, M. A. (1986). The radiographic measurement of early periodontal bone loss and its relationship with clinical loss of attachment. *British Dental Journal*, 161, 141–4.

Cogen, R. B., Al-Joburi, W., Caufield, P. W., Stanley, H. P., and Donaldson, K. (1984). Periodontal disease in healthy children: two clinical reports. *Pediatric Dentistry*, **6**, 41–5.

Cohen, B. (1959). Morphological factors in the pathogenesis of periodontal disease. *British Dental Journal*, **107**, 31–9.

Cox, M. O., Crawford, J. J., Lundbald, R. L., and McFall, W. T. (1974). Oral leukocytes and gingivitis in the primary dentition. *Journal of Periodontal Research*, **9**, 23–8.

Davies, P. H. J., Downer, M. C., and Lennon, M. A. (1978). Periodontal bone loss in English secondary school children. *Journal of Clinical Periodontology*, **5**, 278–81.

Dé Araujo, W. C. and Macdonald, J. B. (1964). The gingival crevice microbiota in five preschool children. *Archives of Oral Biology*, **9**, 227–8.

Delaney, J. E. and Kornman, K. S. (1987). Microbiology of subgingival plaque from children with localised prepubertal periodontitis. *Oral Microbiology and Immunology*, **2**, 71–6.

Fish, W. (1961). Aetiology and prevention of periodontal breakdown. *Dental Progress*, **1**, 234–47.

Fourel, J. (1974). Periodontitis: juvenile periodontitis or Gottlieb's syndrome? Report of four cases. *Journal of Periodontology*, **45**, 240–4.

Fowler, C., Garret, S., Crigger, M., and Egelberg, J. (1982). Histological probe position in treated and untreated human periodontal tissues. *Journal of Clinical Periodontology*, **9**, 373–85.

Freed, H. K., Gapper, R. L., and Kalkwarf, K. L. (1983). Evaluation of periodontal probing forces. *Journal of Periodontology*, **54**, 488–92.

Gillett, R., Cruchley, A., and Johnson, N. W. (1986). The nature of the inflammatory infiltrates in childhood gingivitis, juvenile periodontitis and adult periodontitis: immunocytochemical studies using a monoclonal antibody to HLADR. *Journal of Clinical Periodontology*, **13**, 281–8.

Gjermo, P., Bellini, H. T., Santos, V. P., Martins, J. G., and Ferracyoli, J. R. (1984). Prevalence of bone loss in a group of Brazilian teenagers assessed on bite-wing radiographs. *Journal of Clinical Periodontology*, **11**, 104–13.

Goepfred, S. J. (1981). Advanced alveolar bone loss in the primary dentition. A case report. *Journal of Periodontology*, **52**, 753–7.

Hansen, B. F., Gjermo, P., and Bergwitz-Larsen, K. R. (1984). Periodontal bone loss in 15-year-old Norwegians. *Journal of Clinical Periodontology*, **11**, 125–31.

Hawes, R. (1960). Report of 3 patients experiencing juvenile periodontitis and early loss of teeth. *Journal of Dentistry for Children*, **27**, 169–77.

Hugosson, A., Koch, G., and Rylander, H. (1981). Prevalence and distribution of gingivitis—periodontitis in children and adolescents. Epidemiological data as a base for risk group selection. *Swedish Dental Journal*, **5**, 91–103.

Hull, P. S., Hillam, D. G., and Beal, J. F. (1975). A radiographic study of the prevalence of chronic periodontitis in 14-year-old English schoolchildren. *Journal of Clinical Periodontology*, **2**, 203–10.

Jorgenson, R. J., Leven, L. S., Hutcherson, S. T., and Salinas, C. F. (1975). Periodontitis in sibs. *Oral Surgery, Oral Medicine, Oral Pathology*, **39**, 396–402.

Kelstrup, J. (1966). The incidence of *Bacteroides melaninogenicus* in human gingival sulci and its prevalence in the oral cavity at different ages. *Periodontics*, **4**, 14–18.

Kleinberg, I., Chatterjee, R., Kaminsky, F. S., Cross, H. G., Goldenberg, D. J., and Kaufman, H. W. (1971). Plaque formation and the effect of age. *Journal of Periodontology*, **42**, 497–507.

Lennon, M. A. and Davies, R. M. (1974). Prevalence and distribution of alveolar bone loss in a population of 15-year-old school children. *Journal of Clinical Periodontology*, **1**, 175–82.

Listgarten, M. A. (1980). Periodontal probing, what does it mean? *Journal of Clinical Pharmacology*, **7**, 165–76.

Loe, H., Thelaide, E., and Jenkins, S. B. (1965). Experimental gingivitis in man. *Journal of Periodontology*, **36**, 177–87.

Loe, H., Anerud, A., Boysen, H., and Smith, M. (1978). The natural history of periodontal disease in man. The rate of periodontal destruction before 40 years of age. *Journal of Periodontology*, **49**, 607–20.

Longhurst, P., Johnson, N. W., and Hopps, R. M. (1977). Differences in lymphocyte and plasma cell densities in inflamed gingiva from adults and young children. *Journal of Periodontology*, **48**, 707–10.

Longhurst, P., Gillett, R., and Johnson, N. W. (1980). Electron microscopic quantitation of inflammatory infiltrates in childhood gingivitis. *Journal of Periodontal Research*, **15**, 255–66.

McCall, J. O. (1938). Gingival and periodontal disease in children. *Journal of Periodontology*, **9**, 7–15.

McHugh, W. D., McEwen, J. D., and Hitchin, A. D. (1964). Dental disease and related factors in 13-year-old children in Dundee. *British Dental Journal*, **117**, 246–53.

Mackler, S. B. and Crawford, J. J. (1973). Plaque development and gingivitis in the primary dentition. *Journal of Periodontology*, **44**, 18–24.

Majid, Z.B.A. (1983). Gingivitis in primary and preschool schoolchildren in Malaysia. *Dental Journal of Malaysia*, **6**, 77–84.

Mandell, R. L., Siegal, M. D., and Umland, E. (1986). Localised juvenile periodontitis of the primary dentition. *Journal of Dentistry for Children*, **53**, 193–6.

Massler, M. (1958). Periodontal disease in children. *International Dental Journal*, **8**, 323–6.

Massler, M., Schour, I., and Chopra, B. (1950). Occurrence of gingivitis in suburban Chicago school children. *Journal of Periodontology*, **21**, 146–64.

Matsson, L. (1978). Development of gingivitis in pre-school children and young adults. A comparative experimental study. *Journal of Clinical Periodontology*, **5**, 24–34.

Matsson, L. and Attstrom, R. (1979). Histologic characteristics of experimental gingivitis in the juvenile and adult beagle dog. *Journal of Clinical Periodontology*, **6**, 334–50.

Matsson, L. and Goldberg, P. (1985). Gingival inflammatory reaction in children at different ages. *Journal of Clinical Periodontology*, **12**, 98–103.

Matsson, L. and Goldberg, P. (1986). Gingival inflammation at deciduous and permanent teeth. *Journal of Clinical Periodontology*, **13**, 740–2.

Mieler, I. and Reimann, H. (1968). Die Haufigkeit der Parodontopathien bei Kindern und Jugendlichen im Alter von 3–18 Jahren. *Parodontologic Academy Review*, **2**, 101–9.

Mishkin, D. J., Grant, N. C., Bergeron, R. A., and Young, W. L. (1986). Prepubertal periodontitis: a recently defined clinical entity. *Pediatric Dentistry*, **8**, 235–8.

Moore, W. E. C., *et al.* (1982). Bacteriology of experimental gingivitis in young adult humans. *Infection and Immunity*, **38**, 651–67.

Moore, W. E. C. *et al.* (1984). Bacteriology of experimental gingivitis in children. *Infection and Immunity*, **46**, 1–6.

Muhlemann, H. R. (1958). Gingivitis in Zurich schoolchildren. *Acta Odontologica Helvetica*, **2**, 3–12.

Ngan, P. W. H., Tsai, C-C., and Sweeney, E. (1985). Advanced periodontitis in the primary dentition: case report. *Pediatric Dentistry*, **7**, 255–8.

Page, R. C. *et al.* (1983). Prepubertal periodontitis.1.Definition of a clinical disease entity. *Journal of Periodontology*, **54**, 257–71.

Parfitt, G. J., (1957). A five year longitudinal study of the gingival condition of a group of children in England. *Journal of Periodontology*, **28**, 26–32.

Parfitt, G. J. (1963). In *Clinical pedodontics* (ed. S.B. Finn), Saunders, Philadelphia.

Pedersen, P. O. (1944). Taendernes tilstand Nos. 2–6—aarige born. *Tandlaegebladet*, **48**, 485–565.

Pleasants, J. E. and Nelson, D. W. (1975). Pleasants disease. *Oral Surgery, Oral Medicine, Oral Pathology*, **39**, 686–694.

Rosenthal, S. L. (1951). Periodontitis in a child resulting in exfoliation of the teeth. *Journal of Periodontology*, **22**, 101–109.

Ruben, M. P., Frankl, S. N. M., and Wallace, S. (1971). The histopathology of periodontal disease in children. *Journal of Periodontology*, **42**, 473–84.

Schour, I. and Massler, M. (1947). Gingival disease in post-war Italy. *Journal of the American Dental Association*, **35**, 475–82.

Seymour, G. J., Crouch, M. S., and Powell, R. N. (1981). The phenotypic characterization of lymphoid cell sub populations in gingivitis in children. *Journal of Periodontal Research*, **16**, 582–92.

Seymour, G. J. *et al.* (1982). The identification of lymphoid cell subpopulations in sections of human lymphoid tissue and gingivitis in children using monoclonal antibodies. *Journal of Periodontal Research*, **17**, 247–56.

Shurin, S. B., Socransky, S. S, Sweenly, E., and Stossel, T. P. (1979). A neutrophil disorder induced by *Capnocytophaga*, a dental microorganism. *New England Journal of Medicine*, **301**, 849–54.

Sjodin, B., Crossner, C. G., Unell, L., and Ostlund, P. (1989). A retrospective radiographic study of alveolar bone loss in the primary dentition in patients with localised juvenile periodontitis. *Journal of Clinical Periodontology*, **16**, 124–7.

Socransky, S. S. and Manganiello, S. D. (1971). The oral microbiota of man from birth to senility. *Journal of Periodontology*, **42**, 485–96.

Sonis, A. L. (1980). Periodontosis of the primary dentition: a case report. *Pediatric Dentistry*, **2**, 53–5.

Stallard, R. E. (1967). Current concepts of periodontal disease. *Journal of Dentistry for Children*, **34**, 204–10.

Sutcliffe, P. (1968). Chronic anterior gingivitis. An epidemiological study in children. *British Dental Journal*, **125**, 17–25.

Sutcliffe, P. (1972). A longitudinal study of gingivitis in puberty. *Journal of Periodontal Research*, **7**, 52–8.

Sweeney, E. A., Alcoforado, G. A. P., Nyman, S., and Slots, J. (1987). Prevalence and microbiology of localised prepubertal periodontitis. *Oral Microbiology and Immunology*, **2**, 65–70.

Todd, J. E. and Dodd, D. (1983). *Children's dental health in the United Kingdom*, 1983. HMSO, London.

Waite, I. M. and Furniss, J. S. (1987). Periodontal disease in children, a review. *Journal of Paediatric Dentistry*, **3**, 59–67.

Zappler, S. E. (1948). Periodontal disease in children. *Journal of the American Dental Association*, **37**, 333–340.

JUVENILE PERIODONTITIS

Asman, B. (1988). Peripheral PMN cells in juvenile periodontitis. *Journal of Clinical Periodontology*, **15**, 360–4.

Baer, P. N. (1971). The case for periodontosis as a clinical entity. *Journal of Periodontology*, **42**, 516–19.

Baer, P. and Gamble, J. (1966). Autogenous dental transplants as a method of treating the osseous defect in periodontosis. *Oral Surgery, Oral Medicine, Oral Pathology*, **22**, 405–10.

Baer, P. N. and Socransky, S. S. (1979). Periodontosis: case report with long-term follow-up. *Periodontal Case Reports*, **1**, 1–6.

Bial, J. J. and Mellonig, J. T. (1987). Radiographic evaluation of juvenile periodontitis (periodontosis). *Journal of Periodontology*, **58**, 321–6.

Birkedal-Hansen, H., Caufield, P. W., Wannemeumler, Y., and Pierce, R. (1982). A sensitive screening assay for epitheliotoxins produced by oral micro-organisms. *Journal of Dental Research*, **61**, 192.

Blomlof, L., Hammarstrom, L., and Lindskog, S. (1986). Occurrence and appearance of cementum hypoplasias in localized and generalised juvenile periodontitis. *Acta Odontologica Scandinavica*, **44**, 313–20.

Borring-Moller, G. and Frandsen, A. (1978). Autologous tooth transplantation to replace molars lost in patients with juvenile periodontitis. *Journal of Clinical Periodontology*, **5**, 152–158.

Boughman, J. A., Halloran, S. L., and Roulston, D. (1986) An autosomal dominant form of juvenile periodontitis (JP): its localization to chromosome No. 4 and linkage to dentinogenesis imperfecta. *Journal of Craniofacial and Genetic Development Biology*, **6**, 341–50.

Boughman, J. A., Beaty, T. H., Yang, P., Goodman, S. V., Wooten, R. K., and Suzuki, J. B. (1988). Problems of genetic model testing in early onset periodontitis. *Journal of Periodontology*, **59**, 332–7.

Burmeister, J. A., Best, A. M., Palcanis, K. G., Caine, F. A., and Ranney, R. R. (1984). Localized juvenile periodontitis and generalised severe periodontitis: clinical findings. *Journal of Clinical Periodontology*, **11**, 181–92.

Burnette, E. and Stewart, K. (1969). Treatment of mandibular surgical defect complicated by periodontosis. *Texan Dental Journal*, **87**, 11–16.

Butler, J. H. (1969). A familiar pattern of juvenile periodontitis (periodontosis). *Journal of Periodontology*, **40**, 115–18.

Christersson, L., Slots, J., Rosling, B., and Genco, R. J. (1985). Microbiological and clinical effects of surgical treatment of localized juvenile periodontitis. *Journal of Clinical Periodontology*, **12**, 465–76.

Christersson, L. A., Wikesjo, U. M. E., Albini, B., Zambon, J. J., and Genco, R. J. (1987). Tissue localization of *Actinobacillus* actinomycetemcomitans in human periodontitis. II. Correlation between immunofluorescence and culture techniques. *Journal of Periodontology*, **58**, 540–5.

Cianciola, I. J., Genco, R. J., Patterson, M. R., McKenna, J., and Van Oss, C. J. (1977). Defective polymophonuclear leukocyte function in a human periodontal disease. *Nature*, **265**, 445–7.

Compton, D., Claiborne, W., and Hutchens, L. (1983). Combined periodontal, orthodontic and fixed prosthetic treatment of juvenile periodontitis: a case report. *International Journal of Periodontology and Restorative Dentistry*, **4**, 21–33.

Davies, R. M., Smith, R. G., and Porter, S. R. (1985). Destructive forms of periodontal disease in adolescents and young adults. *British Dental Journal*, **158**, 429–36.

Dawson, C. E. (1948). Dental defects and periodontal disease in Egypt, 1946–1047. *Journal of Dental Research*, **27**, 512–23.

Day, C. D. M. and Shourie, K. L. (1949). A roentgenographic survey of periodontal disease in India. *Journal of American Dental Association*, **39**, 572–88.

Day, C. D. M., Stephens, R. G., and Quigley, L. F. (1955). Periodontal disease: prevalence and incidence. *Journal of Periodontology*, **26**, 185–203.

De Marco, T. and Scaletta, L. (1970). The use of autogenous hip marrow in the treatment of juvenile periodontosis. *Journal of Periodontology*, **41**, 683–4.

Evans, R. T. and Genco, R. J. (1983). *Actinobacillus actinomycetemcomitans* resistant to serum bactericidal activity: a potential virulence mechanism. *Journal of Dental Research*, **62** (abstr. 70).

Genco, R. J., Van Dyke, T. E., Park, B., Ciminelli, M., and Horozewicz, H. (1980). Neutrophil chemotaxis impairment in juvenile periodontosis: evaluation of specificity, adherence, deformability and serum factors. *Journal of the Reticuloendothelial Society*, **28**, 81–91.

Genco, R., Cianciola, L., and Rosling, B. (1981). Treatment of localized juvenile periodontitis. *Journal of Dental Research*, **60**, 527.

Genco, R. J., Zambon, J. J., and Murray, P. A. (1985). Serum and gingival fluid antibodies as adjuncts in the diagnosis of *Actinobacillus actinomycetemcomitans*-associated periodontal disease. *Journal of Periodontology*, **56** (Spec. iss.), 41–50.

Genco, R. J., Christersson, L. A., and Zambon, J. J. (1986). Juvenile periodontitis. *International Dental Journal*, **36**, 168–76.

Gillet, R. and Johnson, N. W. (1982). Bacterial invasion of the periodontium in a case of juvenile periodontitis. *Journal of Clinical Periodontology*, **9**, 93–100.

Gjermo, P. (1981). The treatment of periodontal disease in the mixed dentition. *International Dental Journal*, **31**, 45–8.

Gjermo, P. (1986). Chemotherapy in juvenile periodontitis. *Journal of Clinical Periodontology*, **13**, 982–6.

Gold, S. (1979). Combined therapy in the treatment of periodontosis. Case report. *Periodontal Case Reports*, **1**, 12–15.

Goldstein, M. and Fritz, M. (1976). Treatment of periodontosis by combined orthodontic and periodontal approach: report of a case. *Journal of the American Dental Association*, **93**, 985–90.

Golub, L. M., Ramamurthy, N., and McNamara, T. F. (1984). Tetracyclines inhibit tissue collagenase activity: a new mechanism in the treatment of periodontal disease. *Journal of Periodontal Research*, **19**, 651–5.

Gomes, B. C., Golub, L. M., and Ramamurthy, N. S. (1984). Tetracyclines inhibit parathyroid hormone-induced bone resorption in organ culture. *Experientia*, **40**, 1273–5.

Gordon, J., Walker, C., and Murray, J. (1981). Tetracyline levels achievable in gingival crevice fluid and *in vitro* effect on subgingival organisms. Part II Susceptibilities of periodontal bacteria. *Journal of Periodontology*, **52**, 613–16.

Gottlieb, B. (1923). Die diffuse Atrophie des Alveolarknochens Weitere Beitrage zur Kenntnis des Alveolarschwandes und dessen Wiedergutmachung durch Zementwachstum. *Zeitschrift für Stomatologie*, **21**, 195–262.

Gottlieb, B. (1928). The formation of the pocket: diffuse atrophy of alveolar bone. *Journal of the American Dental Association*, **15**, 462–76.

Gunsolley, J. C., Burmeister, J. A., Tew, J. G., Best, A. M., and Ranney, R. R. (1987). Relationship of serum antibody to attachment level patterns in young adults with juvenile periodontitis or generalised severe periodontitis. *Journal of Periodontology*, **58**, 314–20.

Haffajee, A. D., Socransky, S. S, Ebersole, J. L., and Smith, D. J. (1984). Clinical, microbiological and immunological features associated with treatment of active periodontosis lesions. *Journal of Clinical Periodontology*, **11**, 600–18.

Hillman, J. D. and Socransky, S. S. (1982). Bacterial interference in the oral ecology of *Actinobacillus actinomycetemcomitans* and its relationship to human periodontosis. *Archives of Oral Biology*, **27**, 75–7.

Hormand, J. and Frandsen, A. (1979). Juvenile periodontitis. Localization of bone loss in relation to age, sex and teeth. *Journal of Clinical Periodontology*, **6**, 407–16.

Iino, Y. and Hopps, R. M. (1984). The bone resorbing activities in tissue culture of lipopolysaccharides from the bacteria *Actinobacillus actinomycetemcomitans*, *Bacteroides gingivalis* and *Capnocytophaga ochracea* isolated from human mouths. *Archives of Oral Biology*, **29**, 59–64.

Irving, J. T., Newan, M. G., and Socransky, S. S. (1975). Histological changes in experimental periodontal disease in rats, monoinfected with a Gram-negative microorganism. *Archives of Oral Biology*, **20**, 219–20.

Kaslick, R. S. and Chasens, A. I. (1968). Periodontosis with periodontitis: a study involving young adult males. *Oral Surgery, Oral Medicine, Oral Pathology*, **25**, 305–50.

Kaslick, R. S., Chasens, A. I., Tuckman, M. A., and Kaufman, B. (1971). Investigation of periodontosis with periodontitis: literature survey and findings based on ABO blood groups. *Journal of Periodontology*, **42**, 420–7.

Kornmann, K. S. and Robertson, P. B. (1985). Clinical and microbiological evaluation of therapy for juvenile periodontitis. *Journal of Periodontology*, **56**, 443–6.

Krill, D. B. and Fry, H. R. (1987). Treatment of localized juvenile periodontitis (periodontosis): a review. *Journal of Periodontology*, **58**, 1–8.

Kronauer, E., Borsa, G., and Lang, N.P. (1986). Prevalence of incipient juvenile periodontitis at age 16 years in Switzerland. *Journal of Clinical Periodontology*, **13**, 103–8.

Kunihira, D., Caine, F., and Palicanis, K. (1985). A clinical trial of phenoxymethyl penicillin for adjunctive treatment of juvenile periodontitis. *Journal of Periodontology*, **56**, 352–360.

Lavine, W. S. *et al.* (1979). Impaired neutrophil chemotaxis in patients with juvenile and rapidly progressive periodontitis. *Journal of Periodontal Research*, **14**, 10–19.

Liakoni, H., Barber, P. M., and Newman, H. N. (1987*a*). Bacterial penetration of the pocket tissues in juvenile/postjuvenile periodontitis after the presurgical oral hygiene phase. *Journal of Periodontology*, **58**, 847–55.

Liakoni, H., Barber, P., and Newman, H. N. (1987*b*). Bacterial penetration of pocket soft tissue in chronic adult and juvenile periodontitis cases. An ultrastructural study. *Journal of Clinical Periodontology*, **14**, 22–8.

Liljenberg, B. and Lindhe, J. (1980). Juvenile periodontitis: some microbial, histopathological and clinical characteristics. *Journal of Clinical Periodontology*, **7**, 48–61.

Lindemann, R. A. and Economou, J. S. (1988). *Actinobacillus actinomycetemcomitans* and *Bacteroides gingivalis* activate human peripheral monocytes to produce interleukin-1 and tumour necrosis factor. *Journal of Periodontology*, **59**, 728–30.

Lindhe, J. and Liljenberg, B. (1984). Treatment of localized juvenile periodontitis—results after 5 years. *Journal of Clinical Periodontology*, **11**, 399–410.

Lindskog, S. and Blomlof, L. (1983). Cementum hypoplasia in teeth affected by juvenile periodontitis. *Journal of Clinical Periodontology*, **10**, 443–51.

Long, J. C., Nance, W. E., and Waring, P. (1987). Early onset periodontitis: a comparison and evaluation of two proposed modes of inheritance. *Genetics and Epidemiology*, **4**, 13.

Mandell, R. L. and Socransky, S. S. (1988). Microbiological and clinical effects of surgery plus doxycycline on juvenile periodontitis. *Journal of Periodontology*, **59**, 373–9.

Mandell, R. L., Tripodi, L. S., and Savitt, E. D. (1986). The effect of treatment on *Actinobacillus actinomycetemcomitans* in localized juvenile periodontitis. *Journal of Periodontology*, **57**, 94–99.

Manson, J. D. and Lehner, T. (1974). Clinical features of juvenile periodontitis (periodontisis). *Journal of Periodontology*, **45**, 636–40.

Mashimo, P. A., Yamamoto, Y., and Slots, J. (1983). The periodontal microflora of juvenile diabetics culture, immunofluorescence and serum antibody studies. *Journal of Periodontology*, **54**, 420–30.

Melnick, M., Shields, E. D., and Bixler, D. (1976). Periodontosis: a phenotypic and genetic analysis. *Oral Surgery, Oral Medicine, Oral Pathology*, **42**, 32–41.

Miller, S. C., Wolf, W. and Seidler, B. B. (1941). Systemic aspects of precocious advanced alveolar bone destruction. *Journal of Dental Research*, **20**, 386.

Mitchell, D. (1984). Metronidazole: its use in clinical dentistry. *Journal of Clinical Periodontology*, **11**, 145–58.

Moore, W. E. C., Holdmena, L. V., Smibert, R. M., Hash, D. E., Burmeister, J. A., and Ranney, R. R. (1982). Bacteriology of severe periodontitis in young adult humans. *Infection and Immunity*, **38**, 1137–48.

Newman, M. G., Socransksy, S. S., Savitt, E. D., Propas, D. A., and Crawford, A. (1976). Studies of the microbiology of periodontosis. *Journal of Periodontology*, **47**, 373–9.

Novak, M. J., Polson, A. M., and Adair, S. M. (1988). Tetracycline therapy in patients with early juvenile periodontosis. *Journal of Periodontology*, **59**, 366–72.

Orban, B. and Weinmann, J. P. (1942). Diffuse atrophy of the alveolar bone (periodontosis). *Journal of Periodontology*, **13**, 31–45.

Oshrain, H. and Kaslick, R. (1981). Periodontosis—a sixteenth-year case report. *Periodontal Case Reports*, **3**, 18–21.

Page, R. C. and Schroeder, H. E. (1982). *Periodontitis in man and other animals. A comparative review*. Karger, Basle.

Page, R. C. *et al.* (1983). Rapidly progressive periodontitis, a distinct clinical condition. *Journal of Periodontology*, **54**, 197–209.

Preus, H. R. (1987). Possible exogenous source of *Aa* in rapid destructive periodontitis in man. *Journal of Dental Research*, **66**, 195.

Ramfjord, S. P. (1961). The periodontal status of boys 11–17 years old in Bombay, India. *Journal of Periodontology*, **32**, 237–48.

Rao, S. S. and Tewani, S. V. (1968). Prevalence of periodontosis among Indians. *Journal of Periodontology*, **39**, 27–34.

Ranney, R. R., Yanni, N. R., Burmeister, J. A., and Tew, J. G. (1982). Relationship between attachment loss and precipitating serum antibody to *Actinobacillus actinomycetemcomitans* in adolescents and young adults having severe periodontal destruction. *Journal of Periodontology*, **53**, 1–7.

Reinholdt, J., Bay, I., and Svejgaard, A. (1977). Association between HLA-antigens and periodontal disease. *Journal of Dental Research*, **56**, 1261–3.

Robertson, P. B., Lantz, M., Marucha, P. T., Kornman, T. S., Trummel, C. L., and Holt, S. C. (1982). Collagenolytic activity associated with *Bacteroides* species and *Actinobacillus actinomycetemcomitans*. *Journal of Periodontal Research*, **17**, 275–83.

Saglie, F. R., Carranza, F. A., Newman, M. G., Cheng, L., and Lewin, K. J. (1982). Identification of tissue invading bacteria in human periodontal disease. *Journal of Periodontal Research*, **17**, 452–5.

Saxby, M. (1984*a*). Prevalence of juvenile periodontitis in a British school population. *Community Dentistry and Oral Epidemiology*, **12**, 185–7.

Saxen, M. S. (1984*b*). Sex ratio in juvenile periodontitis: the value of epidemiological studies. *Community Dental Health*, **1**, 29–32.

Saxen, L. (1980*a*). Prevalence of juvenile periodontitis in Finland. *Journal of Clinical Periodontology*, **7**, 177–86.

Saxen, L. (1980*b*). Hereditary of juvenile periodontitis. *Journal of Clinical Periodontiology*, **7**, 276–88.

Saxen, L. and Koskimies, S. (1984). Juvenile periodontitis—no linkage with HLA-antigens. Journal of Periodontal Research, 19, 441–444.

Saxen, L. and Murtomaa, H. (1985). Age-related expression of juvenile periodontosis. *Journal of Clinical Periodontology*, **12**, 21–6.

Saxen, L. and Nevanlinna, H. R. (1984). Autosomal recessive inheritance of juvenile periodontitis: test of a hypothesis. *Clinical Genetics*, **25**, 332–5.

Saxen, L., Asikainen, S., Sandholm, L., and Kari, K. (1986). Treatment of juvenile periodontitis without antibiotics—a follow up study. *Journal of Clinical Periodontology*, **13**, 714–19.

Shafik, S. S., Zaki, A. E., Ashrafi, S. H., Nour, Z. M., and Elnesr, N. M. (1988). Comparison of scanning and transmission electron microscopy of the epithelial pocket wall in juvenile and adult periodontitis. *Journal of Periodontology*, **59**, 535–43.

Shenker, B. J., McArthur, W. P., and Tsai, C-C. (1982). Immune suppression induced by *Actinobacillus actinomycetemcomitans*. I.Effects on human peripheral blood lymphocyte responses to mitogens and antigens. *Journal of Immunology*, **128**, 148–54.

Slots, J. (1976). The predominant cultivable organisms in juvenile periodontitis. *Scandinavian Journal of Dental Research*, **84**, 1–10.

Slots, J. and Rosling, B. (1983). Suppression of the periodontopathic microflora in localized juvenile periodontitis by systemic tetracycline. *Journal of Clinical Periodontology*, **10**, 465–86.

Slots, J., Evans, R., Lobbins, P., and Genco, R. (1980*a*). *In vitro* antimicrobial susceptibility of *Actinobacillus actinomycetemcomitans*. *Antimicrobial Agents and Chemotherapy*, **18**, 9–12.

Slots, J., Reynolds, H. S., and Genco, R. J. (1980*b*). *Actinobacillus actinomycetemcomitans* in human periodontal disease: a cross-sectional microbiological investigation. *Infection and Immunity*, **29**, 1013–20.

Spektor, M. D., Vandesteen, G. E., and Page, R. L. (1985). Clinical studies of one family manifesting rapidly progressive juvenile and prepubertal periodontosis. *Journal of Periodontology*, **56**, 93–101.

Stevens, R. H. and Hammond, B. F. (1982). Inhibition of fibroblast proliferation by extracts of *Capnocytophaga* spp. and *Actinobacillus actinomycetemcomitans*. *Journal of Dental Research*, **61**, 347.

Sugarman, M. M. and Sugarman, E. F. (1977). Precocious periodontitis: clinical entity and a treatment responsibility. *Journal of Periodontology*, **48**, 397–409.

Sundqvist, G. and Johannson, E. (1982). Bactericidal effect of pooled human serum on *Bacteroides melaninogenicus*, *Bacteroides asaccharolyticus* and *Actinobacillus actinomycetemcomitans*. *Journal of Dental Research*, **90**, 29–36.

Taichman, N. S., Dean, R. T., and Sanderson, C. J. (1980). Biochemical and morphological characterization of the killing of human monocytes by a leukotoxin derived from *Actinobacillus actinomycetemcomitans*. *Infection and Immunity*, **28**, 258–68.

Tanner, A. C. R., Haffer, C., Bratthall, G., Visconti, R. A., and Socransky, S.S. (1979). A study of the bacteria associated with advancing periodontitis in man. *Journal of Clinical Periodontology*, **6**, 278–307.

Thoma, K. H. and Goldman, H. M. (1940). Wandering and elongation of the teeth, and pocket formation in parodontosis. *Journal of the American Dental Association*, **27**, 335–41.

Van Dyke, T. (1982). Inhibition of neutrophil chemotaxis by soluble bacterial products. *Journal of Periodontology*, **53**, 502–8.

Van Dyke, T. E., Horoszewicz, H. O., Cianciola, L. J., and Genco, R. J. (1980). Neutrophil chemotaxis dysfunction in human periodontitis. *Infection and Immunity*, **27**, 124–32.

Van Dyke, T. E., Levine, L. J., Tehak, L. A., and Genco, R. J. (1983). Juvenile periodontitis as a model for neutrophil function: reduced binding of the complement chemotactic factor C5a. *Journal of Dental Research*, **62**, 870–2.

Van Dyke, T. E., Schweinebraten, M., Cianciola, L. J., Offenbacher, S., and Genco, R. J. (1985). Neutrophil chemotaxis in families with juvenile periodontitis. *Journal of Periodontal Research*, **20**, 503–14.

Van Palenstein Helderman, W. H. (1984). Does modern microbiological knowledge imply antibiotic therapy in periodontal disease? *Deutsch Zahnaerztliche Zeitschrift*, **39**, 623–9.

Waerhaug, J. (1976). Subgingival plaque and loss of attachment in periodontosis as observed in autopsy material. *Journal of Periodontology*, **47**, 636–42.

Waerhaug, J. (1977*a*). Subgingival plaque and loss of attachment in periodontosis as evaluated on extracted teeth. *Journal of Periodontology*, **48**, 125–30.

Waerhaug, J. (1977*b*). Plaque control in the treatment of juvenile periodontitis. *Journal of Clinical Periodontology*, **4**, 29–40.

Wannenmacher, E. (1938). Umschau auf dem Gebiet der Paradentose. *Zentralblatt für die Gesamte Zahn-, Mund-, und Kieferheilkunde*, **3**, 81–96.

Westergaard, J., Frandsen, A., and Slots, J. (1978). Ultrastructure of the subgingival microflora in juvenile periodontitis. *Scandinavian Journal of Dental Research*, **86**, 421–9.

Wikesjo, U. M. E., Reynolds, H. S., Christersson, L. A., Zambon, J. J., and Genco, R. J. (1989). Effects of subgingival irrigation on *A. actinomycetemcomitans*. *Journal of Clinical Peiodontology*, **16**, 116–19.

Winkelhoff, Van A. J., Rodenburg, J. P., Goene, R. J. M., Abbas, F., Winkel, E. C., and Dé Graaff, J. (1989). Metronidazole plus amoxycillin in the treatment of *Actinobacillus actinomycetemcomitans*-associated periodontitis. *Journal of Clinical Periodontology*, **16**, 128–39.

Yukna, R. and Sepe, W. (1982). Clinical evaluation of localized periodontosis defects treated with freeze-dried bone allografts combined with local and systemic tetracyclines. *International Journal of Periodontology and Restorative Dentistry*, **5**, 9–21.

Zambon, J. J. (1985). *Actinobacillus actinomycetemcomitans* in human periodontal disease. *Journal of Clinical Periodontology*, **12**, 1–20.

Zambon, J. J., Christersson, L. A., Slots, J. (1983*a*). *Actinobacillus actinomycetemcomitans* in human periodontal disease: prevalence in patient groups and distribution of biotypes with families. *Journal of Periodontology*, **54**, 707–11.

Zambon, J. J., Deluca, C., Slots, J. and Genco, R. J. (1983*b*). Studies of leukotoxin from *Actinobacillus actinomycetemcomitans* using the pro-myelocytic HL-60 cell line. *Infection and Immunity*, 40, 205–12.

PERIODONTAL DISEASE IN THE ELDERLY

Abbas, F., Van Der Velden, U., and Hart, A. (1984). Relation between wound healing after surgery and susceptibility to periodontal disease. *Journal of Clinical Periodontology*, 11, 221–9.

Ainamo, A. (1978). Influence of age on the location of the maxillary mucogingival junction. *Journal of Periodontal Research*, 13, 189–93.

Ainamo, A., Ainamo, J. and Poikkens, R. (1961). Continuous widening of the band of attached gingiva from 23 to 65 years of age. *Journal of Periodontal Research*, 16, 595–9.

Anneroth, G. and Ericsson, S. G. (1967). An experimental histological study of monkey teeth without antagonist. *Odontological Reviews*, 18, 345–59.

Brecx, M., Holm-Pedersen, P., and Theilade, J. (1985). Early plaque formation in young and elderly individuals. *Gerodontics*, 1, 8–13.

Burt, B. A., Ismail, A. I., and Eklund, S. A. (1985). Periodontal disease, tooth loss and oral hygiene among older Americans. *Community Dentistry and Oral Epidemiology*, 13, 93–6.

Canestrari, R. E. (1963). Paced and self-paced learning in young and elderly adults. *Journal of Gerontology*, 18, 165–8.

Church, H. and Dolby, A. E. (1978). The effect of age on the cellular immune response to dento-gingival plaque extract. *Journal of Periodontal Research*, 13, 120–6.

Federal Council on Aging (1986). *Health Care Study for Older Americans*, DHHS Publication No. (OHDS) 86–20961. Washington DC.

Fozard, J. L. (1980). The time for remembering. In *Ageing in the 1980's: psychological issues* (ed. L.W.Poon). American Psychological Association, Washington DC.

Grant, D. and Bernick, S. (1972). The periodontium of aging humans. *Journal of Periodontology*, 43, 660–7.

Gurland, B. J. (1976). The comparative frequency of depression in various adult age groups. *Journal of Gerontology*, 31, 283–92.

Helkimo, E., Carlsson, G. E., and Helkimo, M. (1977). Bite force and state of dentition. *Acta Odontologica Scandinavica*, 35, 297–303.

Henry, J. L. and Weinmann, J. P. (1951). The pattern of resorption and repair of human cementum. *Journal of the American Dental Association*, 42, 270–90.

Holm-Pedersen, P., Agerbaek, N., and Theilade, E. (1975). Experimental gingivitis in young and elderly individuals. *Journal of Clinical Periodontology*, 2, 14–24.

Holm-Pedersen, P., Gaumer, M. R., and Folke, L. E. A. (1979). Aberrant blastogenic response to LPS in experimental gingivitis of elderly subjects. *Scandinavian Journal of Dental Research*, 87, 431–4.

Holm-Pedersen, P., Folke, L. E. A., and Gawronski, T. M. (1980). Composition and metabolic activity of dental plaque from healthy young and elderly individuals. *Journal of Dental Research*, 59, 771–6.

Hoyer, W. J. and Plude, D. J. (1980). Attentional and perceptual processes in the study of cognitive aging. In *Aging in the 1980's: psychological issues* (ed. L.W.Poon). American Psychological Association, Washington DC.

Hugoson, A. and Jordan, T. (1982). Frequency distribution of individuals aged 20–70 years according to severity of periodontal disease. *Community Dentistry and Oral Epidemiology*, 10, 187–92.

Hunt, R. J., Beck, J. D., Lemke, J. H., Kohout, J. F., and Wallace, R. B. (1985). Edentulism and oral health problems among elderly rural Iowans: the Iowa 65 + Rural Health Study. *American Journal of Public Health*, 75, 1177–81.

Kleinberg, I., Chatterjee, R., Kaminsky, F. S., Cross, H. G., Goldenberg, D. J., and Kaufmann, H. W. (1971). Plaque formation and the effect of age. *Journal of Periodontology*, 42, 497–507.

Lappalainen, R., Widstrom, E., and Markkanen, H. (1988). Periodontal condition, remaining teeth and dental health habits of the aged in Finland. *Gerodontics*, 4, 277–9.

Levy, S. M., Heckert, D. A., Beck, J. D., and Kohout, J. (1987). Multivariate correlates of periodontally healthy teeth in an elderly population. *Gerodontics*, 3, 85–8.

Lindhe, J. and Nyman, S. (1975). The effect of plaque control and surgical pocket elimination on the establishment and the maintenance of periodontal health. A longitudinal study of periodontal therapy in cases of advanced disease. *Journal of Clinical Periodontology*, 2, 67–79.

Loe, H. and Karring, T. (1972). The three-dimensional morphology of the epithelium–connective tissue interface of the gingiva as related to age and sex. *Scandinavian Journal of Dental Research*, 79, 315–26.

Manson, J. D. (1963). Passive eruption. *Dental Practice*, 14, 2–9.

Markkanen, H., Rajala, M. and Paunio, K. (1983). Periodontal treatment needs of the Finnish population aged 30 years and over. *Community Dentistry and Oral Epidemiology*, 11, 25–32.

Marshall-Day, C., Stephens, R., and Quickley, L. (1955). Periodontal disease: prevalence and incidence. *Journal of Periodontology*, 26, 185–203.

Miller, A., Brunelle, J. and Carlos, J. (1987). *Oral health of the United States*, NIH Publication No. 87–2868. National Institutes of Health, Bethesda MD.

Nyman, S., Lindhe, J., and Rosling, B. (1977). Periodontal surgery in plaque-infested dentitions. *Journal of Clinical Periodontology*, 4 240–9.

Palmqvist, S. and Sjodin, B. (1987). Alveolar bone levels in a geriatric Swedish population. *Journal of Clinical Periodontology*, 14, 100–4.

Pihlstrom, B. L., McHugh, R. B., Oliphant, T. H., and Otiz-Campos, C. (1983). Comparison of surgical and non-surgical treatment of periodontal disease. A review of current studies and additional results after $6\frac{1}{2}$ years. *Journal of Clinical Periodontology*, 10, 524–41.

Plasschaert, A. J. M., Folmer, T., Van den Heuvel, J. L. M., Jansen, J., Opijnen, L., and Wouters, S. L. J. (1978). An epidemiological survey of periodontal disease in Dutch adults. *Community Dentistry and Oral Epidemiology*, 6, 65–70.

Roper, R. E., Knerr, G. W., Gocka, E. F., and Stahl, S. S. (1972). Periodontal disease in aged individuals. *Journal of Periodontology*, 43, 304–10.

Rise, J. and Heloe, L. A. (1987). Oral conditions and need for dental treatment in an elderly population in Northern Norway. *Community Dentistry and Oral Epidemiology*, 15, 134–6.

Ross, I. and Thompson, R. (1978). A long-term study of root retention in the treatment of maxillary molars with furcation involvement. *Journal of Periodontology*, 49, 238–44.

Ryan, E. J., Toto, P. D., and Gargiulo, A. W. (1974). Aging in human attached gingival epithelium. *Journal of Dental Research*, 53, 74–6.

Schaie, K. W. (1974). Translations in gerontology—from lab to life-intellectual functioning. *American Psychology*, 29, 802–7.

Severson, J. A., Moffett, B. C., Kokich, V., and Selipsky, H. A. (1978). A histological study of age changes in the adult human periodontal joint (ligament). *Journal of Periodontology*, 49, 189–200.

Shklar, G. (1966). The effects of aging upon oral mucosa. *Journal of Investigative Dermatology*, 47, 115–20.

Socransky, S. S., Gibbons, R. J., Dale, A. C., Bortnick, L., Rosenthal, E., and MacDonald, J. B. (1963). The microbiota of the gingival crevice area of man. 1.Total microscopic and viable counts of specific organisms. *Archives of Oral Biology*, 8, 275–9.

Stahl, S. S., Witkin, G. J., Cantor, M., and Brown, R. (1968). Gingival healing. II. Clinical and histological repair sequences following gingivectomy. *Journal of Periodontology*, 39, 109–18.

Taylor, C. M., King, J. M., and Sheiham, A. A. (1986). A comparison of the dental needs of physically handicapped and non-handicapped elderly people living at home in Grimsby, England. *Gerodontics*, 2, 80–2.

Van der Velden, U. (1982). Regeneration of the interdental soft tissues following denudation procedures. *Journal of Clinical Periodontology*, **9**, 455–9.

Van der Velden, U. (1984). Effect of age on the periodontium. *Journal of Clinical Periodontology*, **11**, 281–94.

Van der Velden, U. and Abbas, F. (1982). Experimental gingivitis in relation to age. *Journal of Dental Research*, **62**, 488.

Vigild, M. (1988). Oral hygiene and periodontal conditions among 201 dentate institutionalised elderly. *Gerodontics*, **4**, 140–5.

Wentz, F., Maier, A., and Orban, B. (1952). Age changes and sex differences in the clinically normal gingiva. *Journal of Periodontology*, **23**, 13–24.

Zander, H. A. and Hurzeler, B. (1958). Continuous cementum apposition. *Journal of Dental Research*, **37**, 1035–44.

6. Smoking and periodontal disease

IAN D. M. MACGREGOR

6.1 INTRODUCTION

Tobacco smoking is an addictive habit first introduced into Europe in the sixteenth century. Cigarettes only became popular around the turn of the present century with the advent of machinery for their production and the use of milder, flue-cured tobaccos. Smoking is now recognized as the most important cause of preventable death and disease in the Western world. An enormous amount of data have now been accumulated that demonstrate unequivocally the relation between smoking and morbidity (for example, Royal College of Physicians 1971, 1977, 1983; World Health Organization 1975; American Medical Association 1978). Impressive evidence of the shortening of life in smokers has been provided by the classic studies of Doll and Peto (1976) in British doctors.

6.1.1 PREVALENCE

Currently, one-third of the adult population of the United Kingdom (33 per cent of men and 30 per cent of women over 16 years of age) smoke cigarettes, prevalence being higher in manual than in non-manual occupations (Office of Population Surveys and Censuses 1990). The number of cigarette smokers is slowly declining, but those who do smoke are smoking more. However, there is evidence that smokers are changing to lower-tar brands. Sales of pipe tobacco have remained at a constant level of about 5 per cent of total tobacco sales for many years.

Recent figures for the United States (Centers for Disease Control 1989) show that the proportion of adults who smoke cigarettes is lower than in the United Kingdom (31 per cent of men and 26 per cent of women) and that the habit continues to decline.

By contrast, consumption is rising in developing countries, particularly where tobacco production and taxation bring great economic benefits, and it will probably continue to rise for the foreseeable future (Royal College of Physicians 1983).

6.1.2 TOXICITY OF TOBACCO SMOKE

Hundreds of different compounds have been identified in tobacco smoke and some occur in concentrations judged to be harmful to health (US Department of Health, Education and Welfare 1976). Some of these substances are indisputably carcinogenic, and smoking has been implicated in the aetiology of oral neoplasia (for review, see Pingborg 1980). The important carcinogens are the polycyclic aromatic hydrocarbons and N-nitroso compounds found in the tar residue. 'Tar yield' is a common measure of the likely degree of toxicity of a particular tobacco; the higher the yield the greater the toxicity. Tobacco smoke also contains such noxious substances as benzanthracene and hydrogen cyanide, which undoubtedly have anti-bacterial properties (Wynder and Hoffmann 1967). Tobacco smoke appears to be selectively bactericidal, and as a result produces changes in the oral ecosystem, which, among other effects, may predispose smokers to increased risk of candidiasis (for review, see Macgregor 1989). The effects of smoking on oral bacteria and on the local immunological response will be considered later.

Prolonged irritation from tobacco smoke can lead to a variety of changes in the oral mucosa, from the benign smokers' keratosis to the white keratotic patches that characterize leukoplakia. Description of these changes is beyond the scope of this chapter and they have been extensively reviewed elsewhere (see Palmer 1987).

Nicotine

Among the substances found in tobacco smoke is the alkaloid nicotine, which appears to be responsible for the dependence that characterizes the smoking habit (Kumar and Lader 1981). In its pure form, nicotine is a strongly alkaline, volatile liquid and a powerful toxin. One drop placed on the skin is sufficient to kill a dog (or human) within minutes (Larson et al. 1961). During smoking, nicotine is rapidly absorbed into the bloodstream, where 30 per cent remains in its free form. It is highly lipid-soluble and readily penetrates cell membranes. Nicotine has actions on almost all the organs of the body (see Larson et al. 1961; Larson and Silvette 1975) but has a particular predilection for brain and other nervous tissues, which probably accounts for its marked psychological, as well as some of its important pharmacological, effects.

6.1.3 PHARMACOLOGY OF TOBACCO SMOKE PRODUCTS

The smoke from burning tobacco comprises two distinct phases, vapour and particulate. The vapour contains carbon dioxide and up to 5 per cent of carbon monoxide, which in heavy smokers may raise carboxyhaemoglobin levels up to 15 per cent of total haemoglobin (Royal College of Physicians 1977). Each puff of a cigarette draws in about 50 mg of material, of which 18 mg is solid, particulate matter (Wald et al. 1981). The particulate matter is in the form of an aerosol: liquid droplets and (in cigarette smoke) solid, submicroscopic particles with diameters in the range 18 mμ

– 1.6 μm (Kahler and Lloyd 1957; Harris 1960). The nicotine is contained in the particulate phase as droplets of the free substance suspended on these tar particles.

Nicotine is considered the most pharmacologically active compound in tobacco smoke. Most is absorbed through the lung alveoli, but nicotine can also be absorbed, though more slowly, through the oral mucosa in sufficient quantities to have a pharmacological effect (Armitage and Turner 1970). Nicotine mimics the actions of acetylcholine, to which it has a close structural resemblance, by a competitive type of blockade of acetylcholine at autonomic ganglia, initially stimulating and subsequently depressing synaptic transmission as a dose–response effect on the ganglion receptor. The effect of a lethal dose of nicotine is to block synaptic transmission altogether.

Nicotine has pronounced effects on the cardiovascular system. During smoking it increases the heart rate, cardiac output, and blood pressure by autonomic stimulation, which also effects peripheral vasoconstriction (Stimmel 1979). There is also evidence that nicotine acts directly on blood vessels and capillaries to produce vasoconstriction (Larson *et al.* 1961). The pharmacology and toxicology of nicotine have been extensively reviewed by Cohen and Roe (1981).

6.1.4 VARIABILITY OF SMOKING BEHAVIOUR

People smoke tobacco in many different ways. There are wide variations between smokers in the amount and proportions of constituents of tobacco smoke that enter the mouth. These differences depend on the frequency, size, and duration of the puffs and the depth of inhalation, as well as the rate of consumption and type of tobacco smoked. Such variability in the intake of toxic material needs to be borne in mind when considering the relation between tobacco smoking and disease.

6.1.5 PERSONALITY DIFFERENCES BETWEEN SMOKERS AND NON-SMOKERS

Smokers differ from non-smokers in their behaviour and lifestyle. Smokers are more impulsive, drink more alcohol, take more risks, and show less compliance with authority than non-smokers (see Royal College of Physicians 1977), traits that are consistently associated with extrovert behaviour. Smokers and non-smokers also differ to a small but statistically reliable extent in their personality characteristics. From a survey of 2400 people, in one of the first studies of its kind, Eysenck *et al.* (1960) reported that smokers showed more extroversion than non-smokers, and that cigarette consumption increased with the degree of extroversion in the subjects concerned. This has subsequently been confirmed by many other studies (for review, see Smith 1970). Cherry and Kiernan (1976) reported that smokers rated higher on the neuroticism scale, but this is at variance with earlier findings that suggest there is no difference in the degree of neuroticism in smokers and non-smokers (Smith 1970).

In comprehensive studies of family smoking patterns, and identical and non-identical twins, Eysenck and Eaves (1980) have shown that there is a genetic basis to smoking behaviour. They point out that people who are genetically predisposed to smoke may also be genetically predisposed to certain diseases, and that smokers may age faster than non-smokers, and so be more at risk. Part of this genetic variation affects other inherited differences, 'particularly individual differences in personality' (Eysenck and Eaves 1980). These personality differences may have an important bearing on dental health behaviour, and this will be discussed below.

6.2 EFFECTS ON DENTAL STRUCTURES

6.2.1 THE TEETH

Tobacco smoking produces black or brown stains on the tooth surface, which are caused by the tar products of tobacco consumption. Brown stains are also found on the teeth of non-smokers, but smokers have almost twice as much stain as non-smokers. However, the degree of staining in smokers does not correlate with the level of oral cleanliness (McKendrick *et al.* 1970) nor with the amount of tobacco consumed (Glickman 1964).

6.2.2 THE GINGIVA

Smoking does not normally lead to striking gingival changes. Heavy smokers may have greyish discoloration and hyperkeratosis of the gingiva; an increased number of keratinized cells has been reported in the gingiva of smokers (Calonius 1962). Regular application of tobacco smoke to the ears of mice resulted in epithelial hyperplasia, inflammation, and fibrosis in the area to which the smoke was applied (Kreschover 1952).

Histological changes in the gingiva associated with smoking in man do not appear to have been studied in any detail. Manhold *et al.* (1968) found no noteworthy differences in the microscopic appearance of gingival biopsies from 10 smoker and 12 non-smoker volunteer subjects, all of whom had 'clinically normal' gingiva. Changes in the epithelium were described as keratotic, hyperkeratotic, hyperplastic or dyskeratotic. More recently, studies of experimental gingivitis in man have suggested that smoking has deleterious effects on gingival blood vessels, and these are considered in more detail below.

6.3 ACUTE NECROTIZING ULCERATIVE GINGIVITIS

A possible connection between smoking and acute necrotizing ulcerative gingivitis (ANUG) was first suggested more than a century ago (Bergeron 1859). Stammers (1944) reported that smoking was an almost universal finding in 1017 recorded cases of ANUG. He found that healing was delayed in those patients who continued to smoke during the treatment period, compared with smokers who refrained from smoking. Pindborg (1947) found a positive association between tobacco smoking and ANUG in a survey of 1433 Danish marines: 10.7 per cent of subjects who smoked 10 g of tobacco (equals 10 cigarettes) per day had ANUG as compared with only 1.5 per cent of non-smokers. In a subsequent study of 5690 Danish marines, Pindborg (1949) found ANUG in 8.5 per cent of smokers (less than 10 g/day) as compared with 1.9 per cent of non-smokers. Smokers had more calculus than non-smokers, but the effect of smoking was independent of the amount of calculus present. The prevalence of ANUG in pipe smokers was similar to that in cigarette smokers (Frandsen and Pindborg 1949). In a later study, Pindborg (1951) found that 56 out of 57 individuals with ANUG were smokers. Ludwick and Massler (1952) found a low prevalence of ANUG in 3880 enlisted US Navy personnel, aged 17 to 21 years. Twenty subjects had ANUG, only one of whom did not smoke. Giddon *et al.* (1964) found ANUG in 2.5 per cent of 326 college students. Of 22 subjects with a history of presumed ANUG, 14 were smokers and 8 were non-smokers. Goldhaber and Giddon (1964) reported that all but 2 of 61 individuals with ANUG were smokers, of whom 41 per cent smoked 20 or more cigarettes per day. Three-quarters of 185 control subjects smoked, but only 5 per cent smoked more than 20 cigarettes per day. Shields (1977) reported that 88 per cent of 45 army personnel with ANUG smoked, compared with 68 per cent of smokers amongst the 50 age-matched controls.

In a more recent study in Edinburgh, Kowolik and Nisbet (1983) found that ANUG was almost invariably associated with tobacco smoking. Out of 100 consecutive patients presenting with ANUG, 98 were cigarette smokers. Only 14 of the patients with ANUG claimed to smoke 10 cigarettes per day or fewer; the remaining 84 smoked more than 10 cigarettes per day. These investigators also recorded the reported time the patients with ANUG had been smokers. The mean was 6–8 years before the onset of ANUG but the range was very wide and there was no relation between the severity of the condition and the length of time the patient had habitually smoked.

Why ANUG occurs more frequently in smokers is not clear. The aetiology of ANUG is complex; it includes poor plaque control and mental stress (Shannon *et al.* 1969) as well as smoking, and no doubt these factors are all closely related. Over the past few years there has been an appreciable decline in the incidence of ANUG possibly as a result of a general improvement in oral hygiene, although the reasons are not properly understood. Possible mechanisms for the increased susceptibility of ANUG in tobacco smokers include (a) vasoconstriction of gingival blood vessels, (b) reduced activity of oral leukocytes, and (c) proliferation of anaerobic, fuso-spirochaetal micro-organisms.

Kardachi and Clarke (1974) postulated that smoking potentiates the effects of mental stress in reducing blood flow in the gingiva, causing severe vasoconstriction of capillary loops in the marginal tissue and resulting in necrosis of the apex of the interdental papilla. This necrotic tissue, they suggest, would facilitate the rapid growth and invasion of anaerobic micro-organisms.

There is little experimental evidence to support this hypothesis. Nicotine infused into the bloodstream of experimental animals produced a sharp transient increase in gingival blood flow, followed by a fall below baseline levels (Clarke *et al.* 1981; Clarke and Shepherd 1984). In man, the results of experimental studies have been equivocal. While Baab and Oberg (1987) found that smoking a single cigarette produced a significant rise in gingival blood flow when compared with the effects of resting and sham-smoking (puffing on an unlit cigarette), Bergstrom *et al.* (1988) observed that vascular increase in smokers was only half that in non-smokers during a 28-day, experimental, plaque-induced gingivitis.

Although smoking is known to produce peripheral vasoconstriction, in some subjects this is preceded by vasodilation. In any particular instance, the effect produced is probably related to the degree of inhalation of the tobacco smoke and the rate of nicotine absorption (Mulinos and Shulman 1940). It must remain doubtful that gingival vasoconstriction is a prime mechanism for the onset of ANUG as the condition almost invariably arises in chronically inflamed gingiva, in which net blood flow is increased (Kaplan *et al.* 1982). Smoking has important effects on oral bacteria and oral polymorphonuclear leukocytes (PMNs) and these will be considered below.

6.4 CALCULUS FORMATION

6.4.1 EARLY EPIDEMIOLOGICAL STUDIES OF CALCULUS AND ORAL DEBRIS

There have been consistent reports of more calculus in smokers than in non-smokers from the earliest epidemiological studies made after World War II. Shay and Smart (1945), in a survey of Royal Air Force personnel, found less calculus in light smokers than in heavy smokers. Likewise, Pindborg (1947, 1949) found a positive correlation between smoking and calculus deposition: the more tobacco the subjects smoked, the greater were the quantities of supragingival and subgingival calculus. Calculus was simply scored as present or absent, which is a crude method of estimation by present-day standards. Nevertheless, Pindborg (1949) observed that 56 per cent of subjects who smoked more than 10 cigarettes per day had supragingival calculus compared with 41 per cent of non-smokers. Twice as many smokers (25 per cent) as non-smokers (13 per cent) had subgingival deposits. Kowalski (1971) re-examined Pindborg's data by statistical analysis of the contingency tables. Kowalski demonstrated that smokers were more likely to have calculus than non-smokers, but found no relation between the quantity of calculus present and the amount of tobacco consumed.

Frandsen and Pindborg (1949) reported that significantly more pipe smokers than cigarette smokers had supragingival calculus. This might be because the pH of pipe smoke is higher than that of cigarette smoke (Armitage and Turner 1970) and/or because pipe smokers circulate the smoke around the mouth, whereas cigarette smoke tends to be inhaled. Moreover, the smoking cycle is much longer in pipe smokers than in cigarette smokers, causing pipe smokers to salivate more (see below).

Brandtzaeg and Jamison (1964a, b), in their survey of periodontal disease in 200 Norwegian army recruits, found that amounts of calculus and oral debris increased significantly as tobacco consumption increased. They measured oral cleanliness using the Oral Hygiene Index (OHI) described by Greene and Vermillion (1960). This is a composite index in which both soft and hard deposits are scored for each segment. The index is the mean of the summed segmental scores; the higher the index, the worse the oral hygiene. Held (1967) reported higher OHI scores among smokers than non-smokers in 459 males from five urban populations in Iran, but the differences were not statistically significant. Similarly, McKendrick et al. (1970) reported a trend towards higher OHI scores in smokers than non-smokers. However, smokers had twice as much staining as non-smokers. Kristoffersen (1970), in a study of periodontal disease in Norwegian soldiers, found a positive association between OHI (both debris and calculus indices) and tobacco consumption. Similarly, Alexander (1970) found significantly more calculus in smokers and non-smokers, using the Calculus Surface Index derived from Ennever et al. (1961), in which calculus is scored as present or absent on the facial, lingual, and approximal surfaces of each tooth present. Ainamo (1971), using his Retentive Calculus Index (Ainamo 1970), found that the amount of calculus increased in a near-linear fashion with increasing tobacco consumption, except in six subjects who smoked more than 20 cigarettes per day.

In his comprehensive study of periodontal disease in England and Northern Ireland, Sheiham (1971) found significantly higher OHI scores in smokers than in non-smokers in both communities, the calculus component of OHI accounting for most of the difference. Preber and Kant (1973) also used the OHI in their examination of the periodontal status of Swedish teenagers. Smokers had poorer oral hygiene than non-smokers, but the difference was not statistically significant. Lavstedt (1975) reported a significant correlation between calculus, estimated from the calculus component of the OHI, and smoking in 1104 individuals in whom approximal bone resorption could be viewed on radiographs. More recently, Ismail et al. (1983) have reported results from the National Health and Nutrition Examination Survey in the United States undertaken between 1971 and 1974. Examination of 1328 smokers and 1104 non-smokers, using the simplified OHI (Green and Vermillion 1964), found that the smokers have significantly more calculus than non-smokers. Feldman et al. (1983) examined the periodontal status of 862 male volunteers in Boston, MA, 228 of whom were cigarette smokers and 153 pipe or cigar smokers. Calculus accumulation was one of six periodontal measures examined (Feldman et al. 1982), and was scored on a 0–3 basis: a score of 0 represented no calculus; score 1, flecks of supragingival or subgingival calculus on the tooth surface; score 2, a discontinuous band of calculus; score 3, a continuous circumferential band of calculus around the tooth. Calculus deposition was found to be significantly increased in smokers compared with non-smokers.

6.4.2 SALIVA AND SALIVATION

The calcium phosphates found in supragingival calculus are in the main derived from the saliva. The organic components may also arise from this source, the proteins and polypeptides constituting the major fraction. The increased amount of calculus found in smokers might therefore be due to an effect of tobacco smoke upon properties of saliva, and the evidence for this will now be considered.

Salivary flow rate

Smoking markedly increases the flow rate of saliva, an observation first made by Murray in 1776, and one well known to every novice smoker. Others have since described this effect in experimental studies. Winsor (1932) recorded the rate of parotid salivary flow in five smokers and five non-smokers, who each smoked a cigarette for 5 min. A marked increase in flow rate occurred in each subject during the smoking period, which continued to a lesser extent during the succeeding 5 min. During the next 25 min, increased secretion continued in the smokers, but there was a marked diminution below resting level in the non-smokers. Winsor and Richard (1935) recorded a marked increase in parotid secretion in three non-smokers when they smoked cigarettes. In both studies, subjects were requested to inhale. Barylko-Pikielna et al. (1968) found, in 50 smokers, that 'normal' cigarette smoking, which was not defined further, increased resting levels of parotid flow rate by between 1.5 and 2.8 times. Pangborn and Sharon (1971) reported a marked increase in parotid flow rate in eight smokers and eight non-smokers: they did not allow their subjects to inhale. Schnedorf and Ivy (1939) collected whole-mouth saliva from fifteen smokers and five non-smokers for 15 min periods before, during and after smoking two or three cigarettes, but they did not report whether their subjects inhaled. Salivary flow rate increased in all but two of their subjects, both smokers. Overall flow rate during smoking was double that before and after smoking.

Pangborn and Sharon also showed that when cigarettes are smoked through a filter assembly, which traps the particulate matter and allows only the gases to enter the mouth, the rate of salivary secretion is unaffected. This suggests that the salivation caused by smoking is a reflex phenomenon produced by irritant particulate matter in the smoke. From this account, pipe smokers might be expected to salivate more because they circulate smoke around the mouth, whereas cigarette smoke tends to be inhaled. Moreover, the smoking cycle is much longer in pipe smokers than in cigarette smokers. Pipe smokers might also salivate simply because they grip the pipe-stem between the teeth. These factors do not appear to have been investigated, but pipe smokers do accumulate more supragingival calculus than cigarette smokers (Frandsen and Pindborg 1949).

Regular smoking, however, is not associated with any significant alteration in salivary secretion (Chandler et al. 1974; Baum 1981; Heintze 1984; Parvinen 1984). Heintze (1984) also investigated the immediate effect of smoking on salivary flow in 20 smokers, measuring flow-rate upon cessation of smoking two cigarettes, and repeating measurements after 30 min and 1 h. Contrarily, smoking had no effect.

The common reflex effect of smoking on salivary flow-rate could explain the larger amounts of supragingival calculus found in smokers than in non-smokers. Calculus formation is normally preceded by plaque formation, the soft accumulations serving as a matrix for subsequent mineralization. However, the increase in mineralized deposits in smokers is unlikely to be due to alterations in the oral flora (see below); also calculus can form in the absence of micro-organisms (Baer and Newton 1959). The factors that initiate and regulate the nucleation of hydroxyapatite crystals appear to be entirely independent of the processes that govern the development of the microbial plaque.

Properties of saliva

Chemical composition

An increase in parotid salivary flow has been shown to raise the pH and the calcium concentration of parotid saliva (Jenkins 1978), and to produce changes that favour the precipitation of calcium phosphate (Gron 1973). A temporary increase in the calcium concentration of saliva, following smoking, was reported in 7 out of 10 cases studied by Strauss and Fockeler (1939). They also reported an increase in salivary potassium concentration in 5 out of 10 cases, and an increase in the salivary phosphate concentration in 10 out of 12 cases. However, the methods of estimating the concentrations of these components were not described, and by present-day standards, particularly in respect of calcium estimation, must be considered somewhat crude.

More recently, Macgregor and Edgar (1986) described a trend towards raised calcium concentration in fresh saliva in smokers immediately after smoking a cigarette. The difference between smokers and non-smokers was statistically significant in one of three studies of 12 smokers and 12 non-smokers. This study also found that salivary calcium concentration was significantly lowered after incubation of both smokers' and non-smokers' saliva for 24 h at 37°C. This reduction was greater in smokers than in non-smokers, although not to a significant extent. Phosphate concentrations did not show any variation with tobacco consumption and, unlike calcium concentration, did not show any significant fall after incubation.

Dogon *et al.* (1971) collected parotid secretion, by uniform stimulation, from 13 smokers and 12 non-smokers, every 4 h for 24 h. They found that the calcium concentration of the secretion was significantly lower, and the potassium concentration higher, in the smokers than in the non-smokers. Their finding of lower calcium concentrations in saliva at specific time-intervals does not necessarily conflict with reports of raised calcium concentration in smokers (Strauss and Fockeler 1939; Macgregor and Edgar 1986) because sampling was not carried out immediately after smoking.

Smoking may therefore increase the mineralizing potential of saliva. This is compatible with the finding that the calcium concentration in plaque is raised in heavy smokers (Macgregor *et al.* 1985, described below) although smoking appears to have no effect on the rate of salivary precipitation (Macgregor and Edgar 1986). Irrespective of any increase in calcium concentration in smokers' saliva, however, if smoking increases the salivary flow rate there will be an increase in the calcium dose during and immediately after smoking. This in itself could explain the increase in mineralized deposits in smokers.

Higher thiocyanate concentrations have consistently been reported in smokers' saliva (e.g. Dogon *et al.* 1971; Tenovuo and Makinen 1976). The reason for this increase is not known, but it is unlikely to have any influence on the formation or mineralization of plaque.

pH and oxidation–reduction potential

Kenney *et al.* (1975) reported a dramatic fall in the oxidation–reduction potential (Eh) of saliva in 19 smokers and 19 non-smokers immediately after smoking one cigarette. A small but significant rise in pH after smoking has also been recorded (Manhold *et al.* 1968; Kenney *et al.* 1975). Feyerabend *et al.* (1982) found salivary nicotine levels and pH to be negatively correlated. Parvinen (1984), in a study of 180 smokers, found the pH of stimulated whole saliva to be significantly lower than that in 462 non-smokers. Macgregor and Edgar (1986) found a barely discernible and statistically insignificant rise in pH immediately after smoking. A rise in pH would favour mineralization, while a fall in Eh provides evidence of the powerful reducing effect of cigarette smoke. As mentioned above, cigar smoke has a higher pH than cigarette smoke (Armitage and Turner 1970), which is consistent with the finding of more calculus in pipe smokers than in cigarette smokers (Frandsen and Pindborg 1949).

6.5 PLAQUE FORMATION

6.5.1 EPIDEMIOLOGICAL STUDIES

The early studies that examined the relation between smoking and oral cleanliness consistently found that smokers had poorer oral hygiene than non-smokers. Practically all of them used the OHI of Greene and Vermillion (1960), which is a combined measure of soft debris and calcified deposits. These have been described in the preceding section.

More recently, epidemiological and experimental studies have used specific measures of soft plaque accumulation in relation to other periodontal measures, including tobacco consumption. The bulk of the evidence indicates that people who smoke have more plaque than those who do not.

Ainamo (1971) in his periodontal survey of 167, randomly selected, Finnish male army recruits aged 18–26 years, 34 per cent of whom were cigarette smokers, used the Plaque Index (Pl I) of Silness and Loe (1964) to measure plaque. Mean Pl I scores were lowest in the group who did not smoke, and increased linearly with increasing consumption of cigarettes. The difference was statistically significant. Lavstedt (1975) reported a significant positive correlation between plaque, estimated according to the debris component of the OHI, and regular smoking in a study of 1104 individuals in whom approximal marginal bone loss could be measured on radiographs. Preber *et al.* (1980) investigated the periodontal condition of male army recruits in Sweden. The subjects, aged 19–27 years, numbered 134, of whom 81 per cent smoked cigarettes. Mean Pl I scores were significantly higher in the smokers than in the non-smokers. Modeer *et al.* (1980) reported significantly higher Pl I scores in boys aged 13–14 years who were heavy smokers (more than 10 cigarettes per day) than in their non-smoking counterparts.

Bergstrom and Floderus-Myrhed (1983) investigated the periodontal status of 163 identical twin-pairs, born in Sweden between 1886 and 1925, who had dissimilar smoking habits. In about 60 per cent of pairs, one twin was a smoker and the other was not. In the remaining pairs, one twin had a lifetime exposure to tobacco calculated, on the basis of daily cigarette consumption and the number of years the subject had been smoking, to differ from that of the co-twin. Plaque was assessed using the OHI. Out of 48 such pairs who showed differing plaque levels, in 30 cases the high-exposure twin had more plaque. Ismail *et al.* (1983) also found significantly more plaque in 1328 smokers than in 1104 non-smokers; plaque was measured with the simplified OHI (Greene and Vermillion 1964).

Macgregor (1984) measured the area of stained plaque, and the proportion of gingival margin in contact with plaque, on the buccal surfaces of six teeth in 128 dental patients, 64 of whom were cigarette smokers and 64 non-smokers matched for age and sex. In both sexes, smokers had significantly more plaque than non-smokers, and there was a trend towards increased plaque deposits with increasing cigarette consumption. Preber and Bergstrom (1985*a*), in a study of the effect of smoking on gingival bleeding in 20 periodontal patients, found a significantly higher mean Pl I in 10 of the subjects who consumed 20 or more cigarettes per day than in the remaining 10, who were non-smokers.

However, others have reported contrary findings. Alexander (1970) examined a group of 200 dental students and staff, and a group of 200 dental patients, and reported no difference in plaque levels between smokers and non-smokers in either group. The plaque scoring method he used was very gross, however. It relied on an estimate of whether stained plaque, where present, covered less or more than half of the buccal and lingual surface of the tooth scored. Thus the embrasure areas were ignored. This scoring system may not have been sufficiently sensitive to detect real though modest differences in plaque accumulations, particularly in dental personnel, who tend to have low plaque levels. Feldman *et al.* (1983), in the Boston study of periodontal measures in 862 males, also found significantly less plaque in smokers than in non-smokers. In this study, stained plaque (like calculus) was scored on a 0–3 scale. Where plaque was absent a score of 0 was assigned. Stained plaque scored 1 where only approximal surfaces were covered; a score of 2 was assigned where plaque was extended on to buccal or lingual surfaces, and a score of 3 was assigned where not less than two-thirds of the tooth surface was covered with plaque. The investigators concluded it was unlikely that the lower plaque levels in smokers were due to better oral hygiene practices, although these were unknown. More important, perhaps, was the fact

that the cigarette smokers were significantly younger than the non-smokers and pipe/cigar smokers, as oral hygiene is inclined to deteriorate with age.

Preber and Bergstrom (1986) measured plaque accumulations along with other periodontal items in 369 adult patients with moderate to severe periodontitis. Compared with a survey sample (2243) of the Stockholm population, there were proportionately twice as many smokers in the periodontitis group than in the survey sample. In the periodontitis group, mean Pl I values levels were similar in smokers and non-smokers, and no statistically significant difference was found.

Bergstrom and Eliasson (1987*a*) similarly found no difference in mean Pl I scores amongst 285 professional musicians aged 21–60 years, 31 per cent of whom were regular smokers and 69 per cent non-smokers, although alveolar bone height was decreased in smokers (see below). The level of oral hygiene was very high overall, with Pl I scores of less than 1 for smokers and non-smokers, at all ages.

6.5.2 EXPERIMENTAL PLAQUE-GROWTH STUDIES

The few studies of whether regular smoking alters the rate at which plaque develops have failed to find any effect. Bastiaan and Waite (1978) studied plaque growth in 10 smokers (10–20 cigarettes per day) and 10 non-smokers, over a 10-day, hygiene-free period. At baseline, all subjects were given professional prophylaxis to remove all tooth deposits. Pl I was recorded for each subject at 3, 7, and 10 days. Plaque was found to accumulate rapidly over the 10-day period in all subjects, but there was no significant variation in the rate of plaque growth with tobacco habit. Bergstrom (1981) measured the rate of plaque formation in seven subjects during a 5-day period of cigarette smoking and a 5-day non-smoking period; abstinence from all oral hygiene measures was maintained in each period. Stained plaque on the labial surface of a maxillary lateral incisor was photographed at baseline and at subsequent intervals of 24 h; the area of stained plaque was measured from the photographs. Bergstrom reported that the rate of plaque growth was slightly increased in the smokers, but the difference was not statistically significant.

Macgregor *et al.* (1985) described two separate studies in which plaque was harvested for gravimetric measurement, (i) from 15 cigarette smokers and 15 non-smokers after a 48-h period of abstinence from oral hygiene, and (ii) from 15 cigarette smokers and 12 non-smokers after a 48-h, hygiene-free period following complete plaque removal by toothbrushing. There was no significant association between wet weight of accumulated plaque and smoking in either study. In a further series of studies (Macgregor and Edgar 1986), whole saliva was collected from non-smokers, and from smokers immediately after smoking a single cigarette. Smokers' saliva did not differ from that of non-smokers in the turbidity developing after incubation (36°C for 24 h), which was considered to reflect mechanisms analogous to those involved in plaque formation.

Bergstrom and Preber (1986) studied the rate of plaque growth in 20 dental students, 10 of whom were smokers and 10 non-smokers, over a 28-day period of abstinence from all oral hygiene measures. Stained plaque area was measured from photographs of the anterior teeth at baseline, and thereafter at weekly intervals during the experimental period. Again, there was no quantitative difference between the growth rates of plaque in smokers and non-smokers.

In a recent study, following the experimental gingivitis model (see below) in healthy adult volunteers with good oral hygiene, Danielsen *et al.* (1990) found no significant differences in the rate of plaque accumulation between 12 smokers and 16 non-smokers after 21 days of abstention from all oral hygiene measures. At the commencement of the hygiene-free period, which followed thorough prophylaxis and instruction in oral hygiene once a week for four weeks, P1 I values were less than 0.2 in the 28 (out of 33) subjects who participated in the study. P1 I measurements were repeated after 5, 10, and 21 days; there were no significant differences in mean P1 I values between smokers and non-smokers at any examination.

These results indicate that the greater amounts of plaque found in smokers, as reported in most of the epidemiological surveys, are not due to any short-term effect on the rate of plaque development. That is not to say, there are no qualitative differences between plaques in smokers and non-smokers, but none has been described to date.

6.5.3 TOOTHBRUSHING BEHAVIOUR IN SMOKERS AND NON-SMOKERS

Why smokers have more plaque than non-smokers is not altogether clear, but recent studies suggest that oral hygiene behaviour in smokers may be less favourable than in non-smokers. Toothbrushing behaviour has a marked effect on oral cleanliness; people who brush their teeth frequently have less plaque than those who brush less frequently or only occasionally (e.g. Lang *et al.* 1973).

The first account of toothbrushing frequency in smokers and non-smokers by Ainamo (1971) in Finland, and subsequent studies by Modeer *et al.* (1980) and Preber *et al.* (1980) in Sweden, were inconclusive, although Ainamo considered that smokers did brush their teeth less frequently than non-smokers. Rajalo *et al.* (1980) obtained interview data from more than 3000 Finnish adolescents and found a weak association between smoking and sporadic toothbrushing.

In his study of 64 smoker and 64 non-smoker dental patients in north-east England, Macgregor (1984) found that male smokers spent significantly less time brushing their teeth, and had significantly more plaque remaining on their teeth after toothbrushing (estimated by area measurements from photographs) than age-matched, male, non-smokers. Similar trends were found in females, but not to a significant extent.

In an anonymous questionnaire survey in north-east England (Macgregor 1985), 646 adult males and 677 adult females, most of whom were dental patients, gave information about their toothbrushing habits and tobacco consumption. Male smokers reported brushing their teeth significantly less frequently than male non-smokers. In females,

there was a trend among heavy smokers (20 + per day) towards brushing less frequently, but light smokers showed an opposing trend.

Again in the north-east of England, Macgregor and Rugg-Gunn (1984, 1986) video-recorded 50 male agricultural students, 25 of whom were cigarette smokers and 25 non-smokers, brushing their teeth. The subjects, who had had no prior toothbrushing instruction, were filmed (with their knowledge) through a semisilvered mirror to avoid distraction by the filming. Comparisons between smokers and non-smokers of time spent brushing, and number of brushing strokes used overall and in each area of the mouth, showed no significant differences. However, smokers brushed fewer lingual areas than non-smokers, and were less inclined to brush buccal aspects of the teeth independently of the opposing arch. Moreover, the distribution of brushing strokes around the mouth was more uniform in the non-smokers than in the smokers.

Markkanen *et al.* (1985), in a study of periodontal status in 7190 Finnish adults, reported that smokers brushed their teeth less often than did non-smokers. They found that 26 per cent of smokers did not brush regularly, compared with only 15 per cent of non-smokers who did not brush regularly. Data from a survey of 3727 adolescent schoolchildren in England (Macgregor and Balding 1987*a*) also provided information about toothbrushing and smoking behaviour. Twenty per cent of the sample were smokers; they brushed their teeth significantly less often than did non-smokers.

These findings are compatible with the extrovert behaviour patterns observed in smokers; they tend to show less well-developed health-related behaviour than non-smokers, but more developed grooming behaviour, at least in adolescence (Balding and Macgregor 1987). Thus behavioural differences between smokers and non-smokers may largely account for the poorer oral cleanliness found in tobacco smokers.

6.6 CHRONIC PERIODONTAL DISEASE

Opinions have been divided about the effect of smoking on chronic inflammatory periodontal disease. Earlier reviews of the epidemiology of periodontal diseases concluded that smoking was a possible causative factor; by 1966, Waerhaug considered the accumulated evidence to be consistent and convincing. More recent work suggests that smoking may have a direct, though small, effect on the progression of periodontal destruction, independent of the level of oral hygiene.

6.6.1 TOOTH LOSS

It has been found consistently that smokers suffer more tooth loss than non-smokers. Daniell (1983), in a study of osteoporosis in 208 women, aged 60–9, attending his medical practice in California, found that 75 per cent of non-smokers and 67 per cent of smokers had natural teeth remaining at 50 years of age. Bergstrom and Floderus-Myrhed (1983) in their co-twin study, and Feldman *et al.* (1983) and Markkanen *et al.* (1985) in their surveys of periodontal disease, found that cigatette smokers had significantly fewer teeth than non-smokers. Osterberg and Mellstrom (1986) examined a random sample of 1377 Swedish 70-year-olds; toothlessness in men was more common in smokers (48 per cent) and ex-smokers (32 per cent) than in non-smokers.

6.6.2 EARLY EPIDEMIOLOGICAL STUDIES

Some of the earliest surveys reported a direct effect of smoking on periodontal status, but these early measurements of periodontal factors were relatively crude. Herulf (1950) found a higher prevalence of gingivitis in smokers than in non-smokers in a study of 535 Swedish dental students; heavy smokers had significantly more bone loss than non-smokers. Arno *et al.* (1958) reported a significant association between tobacco consumption and gingivitis in a survey of 1346 predominantly male employees in a manufacturing company in Norway, most of whom were aged 25–55 years. Gingivitis was measured by scoring presence or absence of inflammation at facial, lingual, and approximal tooth surfaces. Severity of gingivitis increased with increasing tobacco consumption, independent of age and oral hygiene status. Oral hygiene was estimated simply as 'good', 'fairly good' or 'not good'. These investigators did not discuss their findings in respect of the relation between smoking and oral hygiene in their report, but interestingly, χ^2 analysis of their raw data, subjective though they are, indicates that smokers have poorer oral cleanliness than non-smokers in individuals aged less than 45 years. This study was followed by a radiographic investigation of 728 male factory employees, aged 21–45 years (Arno *et al.* 1959). Ten periapical films were exposed for each subject and evaluated by means of a plastic ruler devised by Schei *et al.* (1959). A significant positive correlation was reported between the degree of bone resorption and the amount of tobacco smoked, but oral hygiene was a more important causative factor. Forsberg (1964) investigated the prevalence of gingivitis in 299 Swedish naval recruits aged about 20 years. Smokers had significantly deeper pockets than non-smokers, but there was no significant difference in the severity of gingivitis between smokers and non-smokers.

Brandtzaeg and Jamison (1964a) used the Periodontal Index (PI; Russell 1956) to measure the severity of periodontal disease in 200 Norwegian male army recruits aged 19–25 years. The PI assigns a score of 0–8 according to the periodontal status of each tooth; the higher the score the more severe the periodontal condition. However, the score for periodontal destruction (6 or 8) is so heavily weighted that it is not possible to identify early periodontitis. PI is a crude measure of periodontal disease, but was widely used in the earlier surveys. In the survey under consideration, higher PI scores were found in smokers than non-smokers. There was a strong and consistent relationship between PI and OHI; the higher PI scores found in smokers were explained by similar increases in OHI. Solomon *et al.* (1968) also reported higher PI scores in smokers than non-smokers in 7191 ambulatory medical patients, aged 20–79 years. However, this survey was conducted over a 9-year period by

an unspecified number of examiners, which rather detracts from its usefulness.

Summers and Oberman (1968) used the Periodontal Disease Index (PDI), described by Ramfjord (1959), to examine the relation between smoking and periodontal disease in 324 subjects, aged 20–50+ years. The PDI measures loss of tooth attachment, in contrast to the PI, which measures pocket probing depth. The advantage of the PDI is that it is a measure of accumulated periodontal destruction and is therefore unaffected by any periodontal treatment the individual may receive. In this study, smokers had higher mean PDI scores than non-smokers, but the difference was only significant in males over 40 years of age. Summers and Oberman considered that smoking was associated with increased severity of periodontal disease, independent of age. Herulf (1968) found a significant correlation between alveolar bone loss, estimated from radiographs, and tobacco consumption in 700 subjects aged 20–85 years: the more the subjects smoked the greater the bone loss, the difference being more marked in the younger age group. Severe bone loss was found in the heavy smokers without concomitant gingival inflammation; Herulf concluded that smoking had a direct adverse effect on the tooth-supporting tissues.

Alexander (1970), in his study of 200 dental students and staff and 200 dental patients, found that non-smokers had less severe gingivitis than smokers in the patient group, but no significant difference between student smokers and non-smokers. Sheiham (1971) found that smokers had significantly higher PI scores than non-smokers in his study of factory employees, 2119 of whom were dentate and gave information about their tobacco consumption. Sheiham noticed that more manual workers, who had worse periodontal disease than non-manual workers, were smokers, but the results indicated that the observed differences were associated with smoking behaviour rather than socio-economic status. When smokers and non-smokers were grouped by their OHI scores, PI scores in the smokers were only slightly higher than in non-smokers and the differences were not statistically significant. Sheiham was thus unable to demonstrate a direct effect of smoking on the periodontal tissues, but provided substantial evidence that smokers have worse oral hygiene than non-smokers, and as a consequence have more periodontal disease. Lavstedt (1975) reported a weak positive correlation between smoking and alveolar bone loss in a radiographic study of 1104 Swedish men and women, aged 18–65 years.

Other early studies, however, failed to find an association between smoking and periodontal disease status. Pindborg (1947, 1949) found that the prevalence of chronic gingivitis (unlike ANUG already mentioned) was not affected by smoking, although by present-day standards Pindborg's scoring system was very rudimentary. Subjects were simply scored as having 'normal' gingiva or 'chronic gingivitis', which was not defined further. Ludwick and Massler (1952) used the PMA index (Schour and Massler 1948) in their investigation of gingival disease in 2577 American naval recruits aged 17–21 years. They found no significant relation between smoking and chronic gingivitis. Lilienthal *et al.* (1965), in Australia, examined the periodontal status of

676 subjects aged 15 years and older, and reported that smoking had no effect on PI, although no details of smoking habits are described.

Waerhaug (1967) studied the effect of smoking on periodontal status (PI) in 8217 subjects in Sri Lanka (then Ceylon) and found that the periodontal condition of people who smoked cigarettes was better than those who did not smoke. Most of the non-smokers were betel chewers, who had worse periodontal disease than non-chewers. The smokers tended not to be betel chewers, so that any effects due to smoking were probably masked by the effects of betel chewing, which were far worse. Held (1967) used PI to measure the extent of periodontal involvement in his survey of urban populations in Iran. Amongst the 459 males aged 20–39 whom he examined, smokers had higher PI scores than non-smokers, but not to a significant extent. McKendrick *et al.* (1970) found no difference between mean PI of smokers and non-smokers among 103, dentally aware, university students in Scotland. Kristoffersen (1970) found the mean PI score to be higher in those subjects who smoked 10 cigarettes or more per day (heavy) than those who smoked fewer than 10 cigarettes per day (light) or none at all, in his study of 321 Norwegian soldiers, aged 19–23 years. Although Kristoffersen found that the difference in mean PI between light and heavy smokers was statistically significant, non-smokers had a higher mean PI than light smokers. Analysis of variance showed there was no relation between PI and smoking.

Ainamo (1971), in his study of 167, randomly selected, Finnish army recruits, used the Gingival Index (GI) (Loe and Silness 1963), which is a sensitive measure of gingival inflammation scored on a scale of 0–3 (where zero indicates health), to examine the relation between smoking and gingival disease. He found no difference in GI scores between smokers and non-smokers. Although, on the average, smokers had twice the amount of bone resorption of non-smokers, the range was wide and the differences not statistically significant. Preber and Kant (1973) recorded the GI in their study of 193 Swedish 15-year-olds, 51 of whom smoked one or more cigarettes per day. Radiographs were taken of the lower incisors; a trend towards more bone loss in smokers proved to be non-significant, but bone loss is likely to be minimal at this age. Modeer *et al.* (1980) made a similar study of gingivitis in 119 boys and 113 girls, aged 13–14 years, in Stockholm. In the boys, there was a significant difference in the GI between non-smokers and heavy smokers (more than 10 cigarettes per day), but when oral hygiene was taken into account there was no difference in severity of gingivitis. In their study of 134 Swedish army recruits, Preber *et al.* (1980) recorded GI and measured periodontal pocket depths in mm, as well as scoring Pl I. The lower incisors were radiographed. Mean GI scores for smokers were significantly higher than for non-smokers, but when smokers were compared with non-smokers with similar Pl I values, no difference in GI values was detected. There was no significant variation in severity of periodontal pocketing, nor in alveolar bone levels viewed on the radiographs, with tobacco consumption.

6.6.3 RECENT STUDIES

Clinical surveys

Ismail *et al.* (1983), reporting the results from the National Health and Nutrition Examination Survey, classified their subjects into current smokers, past smokers, and non-smokers who had never smoked. PI (measured in 2948 subjects) was significantly higher in current smokers than non-smokers, but there was no difference between past smokers and non-smokers. Among 2621 subjects in whom OHI-S (simplified) was measured, smokers had poorer oral hygiene than non-smokers. After grading subjects into four categories of oral hygiene: poor, fair, good, and excellent, only in the 'good' oral hygiene group were PI scores higher in smokers than in past smokers and non-smokers. There was no variation in PI with the amount of tobacco smoked, or between the use of cigarettes, cigars, or pipe tobacco, although the number of pipe and cigar smokers was low relative to cigarette smokers. Preber and Bergstrom (1986) examined periodontal measures in relation to smoking habits in 369 adult patients with moderate to severe periodontitis. Compared with a survey sample (2243) of the Stockholm population, there were proportionately twice as many smokers in the periodontitis group than in the survey sample. In the periodontitis group, PI levels were similar in smokers and non-smokers. However, experience of gingival bleeding and GI was less prounounced in smokers. Only 25 per cent of smokers reported gingival bleeding, compared with 51 per cent of non-smokers. Probing depths were similar in the different areas of the mouth, except for the palatal, which were significantly deeper in smokers. This finding is of interest as it might reflect greater exposure of the palatal than other gingiva to tobacco smoke. Bergstrom and Eliasson (1987b) made periodontal examinations in 242 subjects, aged 21–60 years, 31 per cent of whom were smokers. Plaque levels (Pl I) in smokers and non-smokers were similar. Probing depths were measured at six sites around each tooth. Both the number and the probing depths of pockets were greater in smokers than in non-smokers. On average, smokers had 36.0 sites with a probing depth of 4 mm or more, compared with 21.8 sites in non-smokers. The relatively greater occurrence of pockets in smokers remained after allowing for age and oral hygiene.

Radiographic surveys

Under this heading are included recent, comprehensive, clinical surveys that additionally used radiographs to measure bone loss. In an extensive study, Feldman *et al.* (1983) recorded six periodontal measures in their survey of 862 males (228 cigarette smokers, 153 pipe/cigar smokers, and 481 non-smokers) from the Veterans' Administration Dental Longitudinal Study. In addition to measurements of plaque and calculus, which have been described above, they recorded gingival inflammation and pocket depth (on scales of 0–3), and tooth mobility (scale 1–4). Alveolar bone loss was measured from full-mouth, long-cone periapical radiographs using a Schei *et al.* (1959) ruler. While this study found, contrarily, that plaque accumulations were significantly less in cigarette smokers than in non-smokers, mean periodontal pocket-depth and alveolar bone-loss scores were significantly higher in cigarette smokers than in non-smokers. Scores for gingival inflammation and tooth mobility did not differ significantly between cigarette smokers and non-smokers.

Bergstrom and Floderus-Myrhed (1983), in their study of 164 twin-pairs born 1886–1925 of whom one was a smoker and one a non-smoker, undertook a standardized full-mouth radiographic examination in each of their subjects; radiographs were read for 78 pairs. The heights of the interdental septa from first molar on the right side to first molar on the left side were measured, in each jaw, in relation to root length on a 4-point scale, using a Schei ruler. A mean score from all measured bone heights was obtained for each subject. Subjects with a high life-time exposure to smoking had significantly fewer teeth and significantly more bone loss than their non-smoking twins. Bolin *et al.* (1986) undertook clinical and full-mouth, long-cone radiographic examinations in 349 individuals in Stockholm born 1904–1952, 52 per cent of whom were smokers. Examinations were made in 1970 and 1980; and differences in measurements of alveolar bone height (Lavstedt *et al.* 1986) obtained at the two examinations were used in the analyses. The results suggested that smokers suffered more bone loss than non-smokers. Using multiple regression analyses, the investigators found that, as PI increased, the 10-year difference in alveolar bone height between smokers and non-smokers also increased.

In their study of 235 professional musicians, aged 21–60 years, in Stockholm, 31 per cent of whom were smokers, Bergstrom and Eliasson (1987*a*) examined each subject with full-mouth periapical radiographs, using the long-cone, paralleling technique. Alveolar bone height was measured mesially and distally on each tooth, excluding third molars, and expressed as a percentage of root length. At all ages there was a significant reduction in bone height in smokers, compared with non-smokers. This was true for all parts of the mouth. Regression analyses showed a gradual reduction in bone height with age in both smokers and non-smokers, but the reduction was significantly greater in smokers, irrespective of plaque levels. The subjects under study were a homogeneous occupational group with a high standard of oral hygiene and dental-care habits; even so, the investigators took care to eliminate the confounding effect of plaque from that of smoking. They concluded that smoking *per se* may have a detrimental effect on the tooth-supporting tissues.

Interestingly, Sparrow *et al.* (1982), reporting on a longitudinal study of bone density in the hand in 341 males, aged 40–80 years, who had two successive radiographs taken three to five years apart, observed that, under 55 years of age, smokers consistently showed greater bone loss than non-smokers. Probably all parts of the skeleton suffer loss of bone density with advancing age, but why it should be accelerated in smokers is not known. Daniell (1976) suggested that increased bone resorption might be due to smoking-related changes in blood pH, reduced oxygen tension, or lowered tissue levels of vitamin C. Whether Sparrow's observations are in any way related to reduced alveolar bone height in smokers, compared with non-smokers, is a matter of speculation.

Treatment need surveys

Markkanen *et al.* (1985), in their survey of 7190 subjects aged 30 years and older in Finland, found that non-smokers had less severe periodontal disease than smokers, although the differences were small. These workers used the Periodontal Treatment Need System (PTNS), described by Johansen *et al.* (1973), for scoring periodontal status. Each quadrant was scored on a scale of 0–4 according to the complexity of treatment required for that quadrant as a whole. Plaque levels were not recorded. The PTNS represented a new approach to quantifying periodontal treatment need, and was quick and simple to use. However, it provided only a crude measure of periodontal disease in a population and gained little acceptance. It was soon superseded by the Community Periodontal Index of Treatment Needs (CPITN), which follows the same basic principles but is altogether more refined. CPITN divides the mouth into six segments, rather than quadrants, for scoring purposes (Ainamo *et al.* 1982). The CPITN has gained universal acceptance and is widely used throughout the world.

In a recent study of 344 hospital personnel, aged 20–70 years, in Jerusalem, Goultschin *et al.* (1990) compared CPITN scores in cigarette smokers and non-smokers. Non-smokers had a significantly higher mean number of healthy sextants (Score 0: requiring no treatment) compared with smokers, and there was a significant decrease in the number of healthy sextants as the number of cigarettes smoked increased. However, sextants that at the most bled on probing with no calculus or pockets (Score one) decreased with smoking, with the largest reduction in bleeding among heavy smokers (more than 20 cigarettes per day) rather than non-smokers. Smokers had an average of 2.5 sextants with shallow pockets (Score 3), which was significantly higher than the 1.7 sextants in this category recorded for non-smokers, but there was no significant association between smoking and calculus (Score 2) or deep pockets (Score 4). The finding of decreased gingival bleeding in smokers is consistent with the observations of Bergstrom and Floderus-Myrhed (1983) and with results of other studies, described below, that have demonstrated reduced gingival blood flow in smokers.

Experimental gingivitis

Bastiaan and Waite (1978) recorded Pl I and GI in 10 smokers and 10 non-smokers over a 10-day, hygiene-free period. Plaque accumulated rapidly on the teeth of all subjects over the 10-day period. There was a trend towards more plaque accumulation in the smokers, but this was not statistically significant. GI scores did not increase as rapidly as Pl I scores, and there was no consistent trend or significant relation between GI and tobacco consumption.

Bergstrom and Preber (1986) followed the experimental gingivitis model in 20 dental students, 10 of whom were smokers and 10 non-smokers, over a 28-day period of abstension from oral hygiene. Disclosed plaque was scored from photographs of the labial surfaces of the anterior teeth, and visible inflammation of the gingiva was expressed as the number of labial gingival sites showing distinct redness, in each subject. These observations were supplemented by recording bleeding after probing with a constant-pressure probe, and by measurement of gingival fluid flow using filter strips. Registrations were made at baseline and 7, 14, 21, and 28 days during the experimental period. The rate of plaque formation was similar in both groups, but smokers showed less gingival inflammatory change than non-smokers. Gingival bleeding and gingival redness were significantly reduced in smokers from day 14, and gingival fluid flow, similarly, from day 21. These differences increased with time.

Danielsen *et al.* (1990) also used the experimental gingivitis model in their study of 33 healthy adult volunteers, aged 20–30 years, in Denmark; none was a member of dental personnel. After baseline recording of P1 I and GI, followed by thorough prophylaxis and instruction in oral hygiene once a week for four weeks, 28 subjects were found to have a PI of less than 0.2. These 28 subjects with good oral hygiene were allowed to continue in the study: they were required to abstain from all oral hygiene measures for 21 days. After 5, 10, and 21 days, P1 I and GI were again recorded. Oral hygiene measures were then reinstituted, and P1 I and GI finally recorded 35 days after the experimental period began. Unusually, smoking habits were not known until the completion of the study, when 12 of the 28 participants reported they smoked 5–15 (mean 8.5) cigarettes per day. There were no significant differences in mean P1 I values between smokers and non-smokers at any examination. Mean GI values were similar in smokers and non-smokers at the start of the experiment, but increased to a significantly greater extent in non-smokers during the 21-day, hygiene-free period. At day 35, after oral hygiene had been reinstituted for 14 days, GI values were again quite similar. Thus the inflammatory response, measured clinically, appears to have been reduced or delayed in smokers, and their gingival recovery rate appeared to be enhanced.

These studies add to the accumulating evidence that the gingival inflammatory response may be suppressed or masked as a result of smoking. This has important consequences for the detection of periodontal disease, for it may lead to underdetection, and suggests that the defence mechanisms against bacterial attack may be impaired.

6.7 ORAL MICRO-ORGANISMS

Although smokers have more plaque than non-smokers, there is no evidence to suggest that smoking increases the rate at which plaque develops. Indeed, it would seem more likely that the toxic substances in the smoke, such as benzanthracene and hydrogen cyanide, would act to slow the rate of bacterial growth (Wynder and Hoffman 1967).

6.7.1. *In vitro* STUDIES

In an engaging laboratory experiment in 1890, Miller passed tobacco smoke through a solution containing a bacterial culture. Smoke from a quarter of a cigar was sufficient to sterilize the solution. While Miller's observations must be interpreted with care, they are consistent with the findings of more recent controlled experiments in which marked reductions in counts of viable bacteria followed exposure to tobacco smoke. Eight puffs of smoke from four cigarettes were passed over a suspension of bacteria in a culture medium at 37°C during a 3-hour period in a first experiment (Bardell and Smith 1979), and eight puffs from one cigarette in a subsequent, similar experiment (Bardell 1981). Compared with controls, the experimental cultures showed marked reductions in the numbers of normal oropharyngeal bacteria from a healthy subject, streptococci and staphylococci being equally susceptible to tobacco smoke components (Bardell and Smith 1979). Neisseriae succumbed more than streptococci, and all species of bacteria were more vulnerable to smoke from non-filtered cigarettes than smoke from filter-tipped cigarettes (Bardell 1981).

6.7.2. *In vivo* STUDIES

Tobacco smoke has a strong reducing effect in the mouth. Kenney *et al.* (1975) reported a dramatic fall in the oxidation-reduction potential (Eh), both in the gingival region of the upper first molar and in the floor of the mouth, in 19 smokers and 19 non-smokers immediately after smoking one cigarette. Such a reducing effect might promote the growth of anaerobic micro-organisms.

The Eh of developing plaque falls as the bacterial population is supplemented by facultative and strict anaerobes (Kenney and Ash 1969). This might help to explain the higher incidence of ANUG found in smokers than non-smokers (see above), associated as it is with proliferation of anaerobic micro-organisms.

Laboratory cultures have failed to show any variation in the proportion of aerobic to anaerobic bacteria as a consequence of smoking. Colman *et al.* (1976) cultured bacteria taken from three sites, on four separate occasions, in each of five heavy smokers (20 or more cigarettes per day) and four non-smokers. No statistically significant differences emerged between the numbers of the different types of bacteria from smokers and non-smokers. However, in cultures of bacterial swabs taken from the tongue and the palate, neisseriae were less numerous in the samples from the smokers than from the non-smokers. The investigators concluded that neisseriae, which do not grow well in the laboratory under anaerobic conditions, may diminish in smokers, owing to more anaerobic conditions that prevail on mucosal surfaces. Additionally, they considered the fact that smoking may have a selectively toxic effect on neisseriae, and Bardell's findings (Bardell and Smith 1979; Bardell 1981) serve to confirm this.

Bastiaan and Waite (1979) counted Gram-stained bacteria in developing plaques from 10 smokers and 10 non-smokers. There was a statistically significant increase in the proportion of Gram-positive to Gram-negative bacteria in 3-day-old plaque from the smokers, when compared with the non-smokers, but no such variation with tobacco habit was observed in mature plaques. They concluded that the difference in staining characteristics between early plaques in

smokers and non-smokers may have been due to an alteration in the Eh. Again, this is consistent with the *in vitro*
studies described above (Bardell and Smith 1979; Bardell
1981).

6.7.3 ORAL *Candida*

The fungus *Candida albicans* occurs as an oral commensal in
about 44 per cent of healthy, dentate persons. There is
evidence that smoking predisposes to candidal infection, but
this is by no means conclusive. In healthy individuals, the
primary oral reservoir is the tongue, and in denture wearers,
additionally, the prosthesis, from which the rest of the oral
mucosa, plaque-coated surfaces of the teeth, and the saliva
may become secondarily colonized.

While Arendorf and Walker (1979) found that smoking
significantly increased the carrier rate of *C. albicans* in
healthy subjects, other reports have given conflicting results, possibly on account of differences in methodology
(Macgregor 1989). However, two recent retrospective studies, one of 53 consecutive cases in the United Kingdom
(Arendorf *et al.* 1983), and the other of 32 consecutive cases
in Denmark (Holmstrup and Besserman 1983), suggest that
smoking probably does play a role in the pathogenesis of
oral candidiasis, and that smoking and denture wearing
would seem to be potent, additive, local factors in the
aetiology of this condition.

6.8 HOST RESPONSE IN PERIODONTAL
DISEASE

6.8.1 VASCULAR CHANGES

Numerous studies have demonstrated that smoking causes
peripheral vasoconstriction. Wright (1933), who was the
first to use capillary microscopy to investigate the effects of
smoking on the microcirculation, and Wright and Moffat
(1934) observed marked slowing and stasis in capillaries in
the nail-fold in some individuals during the smoking of a
cigarette. This was appreciable only when the smoker inhaled. In some cases, normal circulatory activity returned
during smoking, in others microcirculatory changes showed
a temporal relationship to inhalation of smoke. Others have
reported similar findings. Mulinos and Shulman (1939,
1940), among others, have presented evidence that the
vasoconstriction associated with smoking is due to deep
inhalation during smoking rather than to pharmacological
properties of tobacco smoke products.

As early as 1890, Langley and Dickinson pointed out that
nicotine caused initial dilitation of blood vessels, followed by
constriction, probably of the whole area supplied by the Vth
cranial nerve. More recent research has confirmed this.
Smoking has been shown to cause a decrease in blood flow
in the nasal mucosa (Drettner 1965) and in the oral mucosa
(Shuler 1968).

The effect of smoking on blood flow in the gingiva has
only recently been investigated. Bergstrom and Floderus-
Myrhed (1983), in their study of 164 twin-pairs, one of
whom was a smoker and the other a non-smoker, were

intrigued to find that subjects who smoked regularly
reported less gingival bleeding, in spite of having higher
plaque scores, than did non-smokers. This observation is
supported by subsequent clinical studies. Preber and Bergstrom (1985*a*) recorded bleeding from the gingival crevice
on probing with a constant-pressure probe in 10 non-
smoker and 10 smoker (20 cigarettes per day or more)
patients with periodontal disease. Gingival bleeding was
significantly less in smokers than non-smokers, and the
differences were accentuated in the presence of plaque or
diseased tissue. Bergstrom *et al.* (1988) studied the vascular
reaction in plaque-induced experimental gingivitis in 16
dental students, eight of whom were smokers and eight non-
smokers, over 28 days. Changes in the number of gingival
vessels were measured using stereophotographs. The
number of vessels increased over time in both groups, but
after 28 days this increase in smokers was only half of the
increase in non-smokers.

Baab and Oberg (1987) measured the acute effect of
smoking a cigarette in 12 young adult smokers by means of
a laser fibre-optic probe inserted into the buccal gingival
sulcus of an upper first molar. This instrument measured the
flux of blood cells within a 1 mm radius of the tip of the
probe, using the principle of the Doppler shift. Sham smoking (puffing on an unlit cigarette) produced a slight mean
rise in gingival blood-flow rate, while smoking a lit cigarette
produced a sharp, significant rise in mean gingival blood-
flow rate when compared with resting and sham-smoking
values, which continued for 5 min after cessation of smoking. Blood-flow rate then slowly declined to resting levels
during the 25-min recovery period. However, relative blood
flow to the forearm skin decreased slightly during sham
smoking and continued to decline during the smoking
period. The finding of a prolonged, increased, blood-flow
rate in the gingiva appears to be at variance with the known
vasoconstrictive effect of smoking, but might have been a
result of the steep rise in heart rate and blood pressure
observed during the experimental period. Clearly, further
studies of the effect of tobacco smoke on the vascular
response of the gingiva are required.

Bleeding from the gum margin is an important early
symptom of gingivitis, and gingival bleeding on probing is
now widely used in clinical examination as a means of
identifying active lesions in periodontal disease. If gingival
bleeding is reduced as a result of smoking, this must be
considered detrimental because it may lead to an inaccurate
assessment of periodontal status, and fail to alert the patient
to the presence of disease. It may also indicate a diminution
of the defence capabilities of the gingival tissues.

6.8.2 EFFECTS ON ORAL POLYMORPHONUCLEAR
LEUKOCYTES

There is good evidence that smoking has an adverse effect
on the mechanisms responsible for the production of immunity (Royal College of Physicians 1977). Holt *et al.* (1974)
found that cells of the immune system were highly susceptible to exposure to tobacco smoke *in vitro* when compared
with epithelioid and fibroblastic cells from a number of

sources. This suggests that the immune response in smokers may be impaired as a result of smoke-induced damage.

The polymorphonuclear leukocyte (PMN) is the most abundant phagocyte found at the site of acute inflammation, and probably has an important role in the defence of the marginal periodontal tissues against bacterial invasion. The results of experiments in animals and man indicate that tobacco smoke may depress the activity of PMNs. Noble and Penny (1975) observed that circulating PMNs from habitual smokers showed a lower rate of chemotactic migration than those from non-smokers. Corberand *et al.* (1980) found PMN mobility to be severely depressed by a solution of tobacco-smoke concentrate, although phagocytosis and bactericidal activity were not affected. However, they point out that high concentrations of tobacco-smoke components may be attained in the mouth and more deleterious effects may be observed.

There is a normal flow of PMNs from the gingival crevice into the mouth, which is increased in gingival inflammation (Attstrom 1971). The rate at which PMNs migrate from the gingival crevice in dogs can be reduced by the application of a solution of tobacco-smoke condensate (Kraal *et al.* 1977). Moreover, oral PMNs from smokers have less phagocytic ability, measured by their capacity to engulf latex spheres, than those from non-smokers (Kenney *et al.* 1977), and smoking cigarettes reduces their mobility by 50–100 per cent (Eichel and Shahrik 1969). Kraal and Kenney (1979) found no significant difference in the migration rate of circulating PMNs from smokers and non-smokers, but any effect due to smoking may be obscured by natural variation in this migration rate in healthy individuals. Bridges *et al.* (1977) found that PMNs also lost their ability to react to chemotactic stimuli when exposed to small quantities of tobacco-smoke products *in vitro*.

6.8.3 GINGIVAL FLUID FLOW

The passage of fluid through the junctional epithelium into the gingival crevice is markedly increased in gingival inflammation and resembles an inflammatory exudate (see Chapter 1). It contains leukocytes and plasma proteins, and probably plays an important role in the defence of the marginal tissues against bacterial attack (Cimasoni 1983).

Measurement of gingival fluid exudate, using filter-paper strips, appears to be a satisfactory method of estimating the degree of gingival inflammation, and within certain limitations allows for sensitive measurement of changes in inflammatory response—in effect changes in vascular permeability—in the same gingival tissue in the same individual.

Smoking appears to reduce the flow of this gingival fluid exudate. Hedin *et al.* (1981) collected gingival fluid, using paper strips placed at the gingival margin for 3 min., from 30 habitual cigarette smokers (16 of whom smoked more than 15 cigarettes per day) and 26 non-smokers. Mean fluid-flow measurements were significantly lower in the smokers than non-smokers. Bergstrom and Preber (1986) studied 10 smokers and 10 non-smokers over a 4-week period during which the subjects abstained from all oral

hygiene measures. They found that the degree of gingival redness, the occurrence of bleeding from the gingival margin, and the gingival fluid exudate (measured using paper strips) all increased during the experimental period. However, for each measure, the observed increase was significantly lower in the smokers than in the non-smokers.

In a more recent study, McGuire *et al.* (1989) measured levels of continine, a metabolite of nicotine, in the saliva and gingival fluid of cigarette smokers. Using high-performance liquid chromatography, cotinine was detected in a wide range of concentrations in all 16 smokers, while no evidence of cotinine was found in any of the 13 non-smokers. Cotinine levels in gingival fluid of smokers were, on average, five or six times greater than corresponding salivary concentrations. This study demonstrates the extent of the systemic distribution of nicotine in smokers, and suggests that it may play a role in tissue destruction in inflammatory periodontal disease.

6.9 PERIODONTAL WOUND HEALING

Cessation of smoking is reported to favour wound healing after surgical treatment to the hand (Mosley and Finseth 1977) and in cardiovascular disease (US Department of Health and Human Services 1983). Smokers evidently suffer more than non-smokers from painful socket after the removal of impacted third molars (Sweet and Butler 1979) and other teeth (Meechan *et al.* 1988).

The effects of smoking on periodontal wound healing have only recently received attention, but there is now good evidence that smoking does have a detrimental effect on the outcome of periodontal treatment. Preber and Bergstrom (1985b) demonstrated that, after non-surgical periodontal therapy for moderate to severe periodontitis, there was less reduction in periodontal pocket probing depths in 40 heavy smokers (20 or more cigarettes per day) than in 35 non-smokers. Mean differences in probing-depth reduction were significant in the maxillary arch and anterior regions, and were most marked in the anterior maxillary region. In a subsequent investigation (Preber and Bergstrom 1990) on the outcome of surgical treatment in 24 smokers and 30 non-smokers, probing-depth reductions 12 months after modified Widman flap surgery were significantly less in the smokers than in the non-smokers. Miller (1987) found a strong correlation between cigarette smoking (10 or more cigarettes per day) and failure to obtain optimum root coverage after free soft-tissue autografts in 100 graft sites. However, he found that grafts in light smokers (no more than 5 cigarettes per day) responded as favourably as in non-smokers. Habitual smokers who refrained from smoking for two weeks after surgery gained similar root coverage to that obtained in non-smokers.

These clinical findings are supported by the results of laboratory studies of tooth root surfaces exposed to nicotine. Raulin *et al.* (1988) studied the effect of exposing human foreskin fibroblasts *in vitro* to varying concentrations of nicotine on their attachment to glass and to non-diseased root surfaces of extracted human teeth. Nicotine-treated fibroblasts attached to glass at all concentrations of nicotine, but the normal orientation of the cells was disrupted compared with nicotine-free controls. The degree and mode of attachment of fibroblasts to root surfaces in nicotine-contaminated culture varied with the concentration of nicotine. The number and length of cytoplasmic processes increased as the nicotine dose increased. Compared with control cultures, attachment of fibroblasts to root surfaces appeared to become more tenuous with increasing doses of nicotine. Raulin *et al.* concluded that, while nicotine does not actually prevent the attachment of fibroblasts to root surfaces, it may make them more susceptible to periodontal breakdown and less amenable to new attachment procedures. Cuff *et al.* (1989) examined the nicotine content of 29 periodontally diseased teeth extracted from 11 smokers; buried third molars removed from subjects who claimed to be non-smokers served as controls. The smoking habits of the smokers were not described, but the nicotine content of the roots of smokers' teeth varied widely both between and within subjects. Each tooth was bisected and root planing of one half resulted in a significant drop in recorded nicotine levels when compared with the unplaned control half. However, the results were not altogether consistent as in two cases the nicotine content was greater in the control than in the experimental half. Curiously, traces of nicotine were found in two of the buried third molars in the non-smokers, which raises the interesting possibility of contamination by passive smoking.

6.10 CONCLUSIONS

Epidemiological studies of dental disease have consistently found poorer oral hygiene in tobacco smokers than in non-smokers. All of the surveys conducted since the early postwar period have reported increased quantities of calculus in smokers. It has long been known that smoking causes a marked increase in salivary flow rate as a simple reflex effect and this could explain the tendency of smokers to accumulate increased amounts of calculus. There is some evidence that smoking also increases the mineralizing potential of saliva. Many of the water-soluble substances in the gas phase of the tobacco smoke become dissolved in the saliva and the particulate phase is probably dispersed in a similar way. These particles are extremely small and might conceivably act as nuclei for aggregation of protein complexes, or as seeding agents in crystal formation.

Virtually all of the studies that have measured plaque in smokers and non-smokers have found more in smokers. There is no evidence that smoking increases the rate at which plaque develops, or that it has any material effect on salivary precipitation. It seems likely that the major factor leading to greater plaque accumulation in smokers is inadequate oral hygiene. Toothbrushing habits in smokers tend to be less favourable than in non-smokers; less so in men that in women, between whom statistically significant differences in brushing frequency have been found. Male smokers

are less efficient toothbrushers, brush their teeth less frequently, and spend less time toothbrushing than male non-smokers.

Smoking does not ordinarily give rise to striking gingival changes. At a clinical level, smoking appears to suppress visible gingival inflammation in response to plaque accumulation and there is mounting evidence that gingival bleeding is reduced in smokers. Gingival bleeding is an important early sign of chronic gingivitis and the masking of this feature may result in failure to recognize the presence of disease.

Smokers have fewer teeth than non-smokers and more severe destructive periodontal disease; they have deeper periodontal pockets and more alveolar bone loss. The poorer periodontal status of smokers is thought to be largely due to their increased plaque levels, although some studies indicate that habitual smoking has a small but significant detrimental effect on periodontal health. If smoking tobacco does have any adverse effect on the periodontal tissues, it is much less important than accumulation of plaque.

Yet smoking does have small but noticeable effects on the oral ecology, although it does not alter to any extent the species of micro-organisms that constitute the oral flora. Tobacco smoke has a strong reducing capacity in the mouth and appears to contribute to anaerobiosis, possibly by altering the oxidation–reduction potential in favour of anaerobic micro-organisms, and possibly by a selective toxic effect on particular species. Certainly this predisposes smokers to oral infection by anaerobes, such that ANUG, which is associated with proliferation of anaerobic bacteria, is rarely seen in non-smokers, and it could contribute to the progress of destructive periodontal disease.

Tobacco may have a more pernicious effect in predisposing to periodontal disease by diminishing oral cellular immunity, and possibly suppressing other immune mechanisms that help to maintain the ecological balance. There is good evidence that smoking depresses the activity of oral PMNs, reducing their chemotactic response, mobility, and phagocytic ability. Blood flow in the gingiva and the output of crevicular fluid are also reduced, further decreasing cellular and humoral immune components in the region of the gingival crevice. It is not altogether surprising that smoking has recently been shown to impair periodontal wound healing, and this includes non-surgical as well as surgical therapy. These reports alone provide grounds for advising periodontal patients to reduce or stop their smoking.

Christen (1970) has called attention to the dentists' responsibility to advise their patients against smoking. He and others (Cohen *et al.* 1989) have shown that a few minutes spent counselling dental patients who smoke cigarettes can have a small but important effect in reducing overall cigarette consumption. Smoking does not ordinarily lead to tooth loss, but the prospect of losing teeth from periodontal disease can be a persuasive argument against smoking, particularly in young people. It is hoped that the evidence of the harmful effects of smoking presented in this chapter might serve to stimulate dentists to give informed advice to help their patients who smoke to stop.

REFERENCES

Ainamo, J. (1970). Concomitant periodontal disease and dental caries in young adult males. *Suomen Hammaslaaskariseuran Toimituksia*, **66**, 303–66.

Ainamo, J. (1971). The seeming effect of tobacco consumption on the occurrence of periodontal disease and dental caries. *Suomen Hammaslaakariseuran Toimituksia*, **67**, 87–94.

Ainamo, J., Barmes, D., Beagrie, G., Cutress, T., Martin, J., and Sardo Infirri, J. (1982). Development of World Health Organisation (WHO) Community Periodontal Index of Treatment Needs (CPITN). *International Dental Journal*, **32**, 281–91.

Alexander, A. G. (1970). The relationship between tobacco smoking calculus and plaque accumulation and gingivitis. *Dental Health*, **9**, 6–9.

American Medical Association Committee for Research on Tobacco and Health (1978). *Tobacco and health*. AMA Education and Research Foundation, Chicago.

Arendorf, T. M. and Walker, D. M. (1979). Oral candidal populations in health and disease. *British Dental Journal*, **147**, 267–72.

Arendorf, T., Walker, D. M., Kingdom, R. J., Roll, J. R. S., and Newcombe, R. G. (1983) Tobacco smoking and denture wearing in oral candidal leukoplakia. *British Dental Journal*, **155**, 340–3.

Armitage, A. K. and Turner, D. M. (1970). Absorption of nicotine in cigarette smoke through the oral mucosa. *Nature*, **266**, 1231–2.

Arno, A., Waerhaug, J., Lovdal, A., and Schei, O. (1958). Incidence of gingivitis as related to sex, occupation, tobacco consumption, toothbrushing and age. *Oral Surgery, Oral Medicine, Oral Pathology*, **11**, 587–95.

Arno, A., Schei, O., Lovdal, A., and Waerhaug, J. (1959). Alveolar bone loss as a function of tobacco consumption. *Acta Odontologica Scandinavica*, **17**, 3–9.

Attstrom, R. (1971). Studies on neutrophil polymorphonuclear leukocytes at the dento-gingival junction in gingival health and disease. *Journal of Periodontal Research*, suppl. 8.

Baab, D. A. and Oberg, P. A. (1987). The effect of cigarette smoking on gingival blood flow in humans. *Journal of Clinical Periodontology*, **14**, 418–24.

Baer, P. N. and Newton, W. L. (1959). The occurrence of periodontal disease in germ-free mice. *Journal of Dental Research*, **38**, 1238.

Balding, J. W. and Macgregor, I. D. M. (1987). Health-related behaviour and smoking in young adolescents. *Public Health*, **101**, 277–82.

Bardell, D. (1981). Viability of six species of normal oropharyngeal bacteria after exposure to cigarette smoke *in vitro*. *Microbios*, **32**, 7–13.

Bardell, D. and Smith, J. E. (1979). An *in vitro* study of mixed populations of normal oropharyngeal bacteria to cigarette smoke. *Microbios*, **26**, 159–64.

Barylko-Pikielna, N., Pangborn, R. M., and Sharon, I. L. (1968). Effect of cigarette smoking on parotid secretion. *Archives of Environmental Health*, **17**, 731–8.

Bastiaan, R. J. and Waite, I. M. (1978). Effects of tobacco smoking on plaque development and gingivitis. *Journal of Periodontology*, **49**, 480–2.

Baum, B. J. (1981). Evaluation of stimulated parotid saliva flow rate in different age groups. *Journal of Dental Research*, **60**, 1292–6.

Bergeron, E. J. (1859). *De la stomatite ulcereuse des soldats*, p. 70. Labe, Paris.

Bergstrom, J. (1981). Short-term investigation on the influence of cigarette smoking upon plaque formation. *Scandinavian Journal of Dental Research*, **89**, 235–8.

Bergstrom, J. and Eliasson, S. (1987a). Cigarette smoking and alveolar bone height in subjects with a high standard of oral hygiene. *Journal of Clinical Periodontology*, **14**, 466–9.

Bergstrom, J. and Eliasson, S. (1987b). Noxious effect of cigarette smoking on periodontal health. *Journal of Periodontal Research*, **22**, 513–17.

Bergstrom, J. and Floderus-Myrhed, B. (1983). Co-twin control study of the relationship between smoking and some periodontal disease factors. *Community Dentistry and Oral Epidemiology*, **11**, 113–16.

Bergstrom, J. and Preber, H. (1986). The influence of cigarette smoking on the development of experimental gingivitis. *Journal of Periodontal Research*, **21**, 668–76.

Bergstrom, J., Persson, L., and Preber, H. (1988). Influence of cigarette smoking on vascular reaction during experimental gingivitis. *Scandinavian Journal of Dental Research*, **96**, 34–9.

Bolin, A., Lavstedt, S., Frithiof, L., and Henrikson, C. O. (1986). Proximal alveolar bone loss in a longitudinal radiographic investigation. IV. Smoking and some other factors influencing the progress in a material of individuals with at least 20 remaining teeth. *Acta Odontologica Scandinavica*, **44**, 263–9.

Brandtzaeg, P. and Jamison, H. C. (1964a). A study of periodontal health and oral hygiene in Norwegian Army recruits. *Journal of Periodontology*, **35**, 302–7.

Brandtzaeg, P. and Jamison, H. C. (1964b). The effect of cleansing of the teeth on periodontal health and oral hygiene in Norwegian army recruits. *Journal of Periodontology*, **35**, 308–12.

Bridges, R. B., Kraal, J. H., Huang, L. J. T., and Chancellor, M. (1977). The effects of tobacco smoke on chemotaxis and glucose metabolism of polymorphonuclear leucocytes. *Infection and Immunity*, **15**, 115–23.

Calonius, P. E. B. (1962). A cytological study on the variation of keratinization in the normal oral mucosa of young males. *Journal of the Western Society of Periodontology*, **10**, 69.

Centers for Disease Control (1989). Tobacco use by adults—United States. *Journal of the American Medical Association*, **262**, 2364–9.

Chandler, D. C., Silverman, M. S., Lundblad, R. L., and McFall, W. T. (1974). Human parotid IgA and periodontal disease. *Archives of Oral Biology*, **19**, 733–5.

Cherry, N. and Kiernan, K. (1976). Personality scores and smoking behaviour—a longitudinal study. *British Journal of Preventive and Social Medicine*, **30**, 123–31.

Christen, A. G. (1970). The dentists role in helping a patient to stop smoking. *Journal of the American Dental Association*, **81**, 1146–52.

Cimasoni, G. (1983). *Crevicular fluid updated*. Karger, Basel.

Clark, N. G. and Shepherd, B. C. (1984). The effects of epinephine and nicotine on gingival blood flow in the rabbit. *Archives of Oral Biology*, **29**, 789–93.

Clarke, N. G. Shepherd, B. C., and Hirsch, R. S. (1981). The effects of intra-arterial epinephrine and nicotine on gingival circulation. *Oral Surgery, Oral Medicine, Oral Pathology*, **52**, 577–82.

Cohen, A. J. and Roe, F. J. C. (1981). *Monograph on the pharmacology and toxicology of nicotine*, Occasional Paper 4. Tobacco Advisory Council, London.

Cohen, S. J., Stookey, G. K., Katz, B. P., Drook, C. A., and Christen, A. G. (1989). Helping smokers quit: a randomised controlled trial with private practice patients. *Journal of the American Dental Association*, **118**, 41–5.

Colman, G., Beighton, D., Chalk, A. J., and Wake, S. (1976). Cigarette smoking and the microbial flora of the mouth. *Australian Dental Journal*, **21**, 111–18.

Corberand, J. *et al.* (1980). *In vitro* effect of tobacco smoke components on the function of normal human polymorphonuclear leukocytes. *Infection and Immunity*, **30**, 649–55.

Cuff, M. J. A., McQuade, M. J., Scheidt, M. J., Sutherland, D. E., and Van Dyke, T. E. (1989). The presence of nicotine on root surfaces of periodontally diseased teeth in smokers. *Journal of Periodontology*, **60**, 564–9.

Daniell, H. W. (1976). Osteoporosis of the slender smokers. *Archives of Internal Medicine*, **136**, 298–304.

Daniell, H. W. (1983). Postmenopausal tooth loss. *Archives of Internal Medicine*, **143**, 1678–82.

Danielsen, B., Manji, F., Nagelkerke, N., Fejerskov, O., and Baelum, V. (1990). Effect of cigarette smoking on the transition of dynamics in experimental gingivitis. *Journal of Clinical Periodontology*, **17**, 159–64.

Dogon, I. L., Amdur, B. H., and Bell, K. (1971). Observations on the diurnal variation of some inorganic constituents of human saliva in smokers and non-smokers. *Archives of Oral Biology*, **16**, 95–105.

Doll, R. and Peto, R. (1976). Mortality in relation to smoking: 20 years observations on male British doctors. *British Medical Journal*, **4**, 1525–36.

Drettner, B. (1965). The effect of cigarette smoking on blood flow of the skin, muscle and nasal mucosa. *Acta Societatis Medicorum Upsaliensis*, **70**, 49–58.

Eichel, B. and Shahrik, H. A. (1969). Tobacco smoke toxicity: loss of human oral leukocytic function and fluid-cell metabolism. *Science*, **166**, 1424–7.

Ennever, J., Sturzenberger, O. P., and Radike, A. W. (1961). Calculus surface index method for scoring clinical calculus studies. *Journal of Periodontology*, **32**, 54–7.

Eysenck, H. J. and Eaves, L. J. (1980). *The causes and effects of smoking*. Maurice Temple-Smith, London.

Eysenck, H. J., Tarrat, M., Woolf, M., and England, L. (1960). Smoking and personality. *British Medical Journal*, **1**, 1456–60.

Feldman, R. S., Douglass, C. W., Loftus, E. R., Kafur, K. K., and Chauncey, H. H. (1982). Interexaminer agreement in the measurement of periodontal disease. *Journal of Periodontal Research*, **17**, 80–9.

Feldman, R. S., Bravacos, J. S., and Rose, C. L. (1983). Association between smoking different tobacco products and periodontal disease indices. *Journal of Periodontology*, **54**, 481–7.

Feyerabend, C., Higenbottam, T., and Russell, M. A. (1982). Nicotine concentrations in urine and saliva of smokers. *British Medical Journal*, **284**, 1002–4.

Forsberg, A. (1964). En klinisk undersokning av tandkott och tander pa man i 20—arsaldern. *Svensk Tandlakare-Tidskrift*, **47**, 175–96.

Frandsen, A. and Pindborg, J. J. (1949). Tobacco and gingivitis III. Difference in the action of cigarette and pipe smoking. *Journal of Dental Research*, **28**, 464–5.

Giddon, D. B., Zackin, J. S., and Goldhaber, P. (1964). Acute necrotizing ulcerative gingivitis in college students. *Journal of American Dental Association*, **68**, 381–6.

Glickman, I. (1964). *Clinical periodontology*, (5th edn), p. 425. Saunders, Philadelphia.

Goldhaber, P. and Giddon, D. B. (1964). Present concepts concerning the etiology and treatment of acute necrotizing ulcerative gingivitis. *International Dental Journal*, **14**, 468–96.

Goultschin, J., Cohen, H. D. S., Donchin, M., Brayer, L., and Soskolne, W. A. (1990). Association of smoking with periodontal treatment needs. *Journal of Periodontology*, **61**, 364–7.

Greene, J. C. and Vermillion, J. R. (1960). Oral hygiene index; a method for classifying oral hygiene status. *Journal of the American Dental Association*, **61**, 172–9.

Greene, J. C. and Vermillion, J. R. (1964). The simplified oral hygiene index. *Journal of the American Dental Association*, **68**, 7–13.

Gron, P. (1973). The state of calcium and inorganic orthophosphate in human saliva. *Archives of Oral Biology*, **18**, 1365–78.

Harris, W. J. (1960). Size distribution of tobacco smoke droplets by a replica method. *Nature*, **186**, 537–8.

Hedin, C. A., Ronquist, G., and Forsberg, O. (1981). Cyclic nucleotide content in gingival tissue of smokers and non-smokers. *Journal of Periodontal Research*, **16**, 337–43.

Heintze, U. (1984). Secretion rate, buffer effect and number of lactobacilli and *Streptococcus mutans* of whole saliva of cigarette smokers and non-smokers. *Scandinavian Journal of Dental Research*, **92**, 294–301.

Held, A. J. (1967). A clinical survey about dental caries, periodontal diseases and oral hygiene in urban populations in Iran. *Paradontologie and Academy Review*, **1**, 159–92.

Herulf, G. (1950). Om det marginala alveolarbenet hos ungdom i studiealdern-en rontgenstudie. *Svensk Tandlakare-Tidskrift*, **43**, 42–82.

Herulf, G. (1968). On the marginal alveolar ridge in adults. *Svensk Tandlakare-Tidskrift*, **61**, 675–703.

Holmstrup, P. and Besserman, M. (1983). Clinical, therapeutic and pathogenic aspects of chronic multifocal candidiasis. *Oral Surgery, Oral Medicine, Oral Pathology*, **56**, 388–95.

Holt, P. G., Bartholomaeus, W. N., and Keast, D. (1974). Differential toxicity of tobacco smoke to various cell types including those of the immune system. *Australian Journal of Experimental Biological and Medical Science*, **52**, 211–14.

Ismail, A. I., Burt, B. A., and Eklund, S. A. (1983). Epidemiologic patterns of smoking and periodontal disease in the United States. *Journal of the American Dental Association*, **106**, 617–21.

Jenkins, G. N. (1978). *The physiology and biochemistry of the mouth*, (4th edn), p.298. Blackwell, Oxford.

Johansen, J. R., Gjermo, P., and Bellini, H. T. (1973). A system to classify the need for periodontal treatment. *Acta Odontologica Scandinavica*, **31**, 297–305.

Kahler, H. and Lloyd, B. J. (1957). The electron microscopy of tobacco smoke. *Journal of the National Cancer Institute*, **18**, 217–19.

Kaplan, M. L., Jeffcoat, M. K., and Goldhaber, P. (1982). Blood flow in gingiva and alveolar bone in beagles with periodontal disease. *Journal of Periodontal Research*, **17**, 384–9.

Kardachi, B. J. R. and Clarke, N. G. (1974). Aetiology of acute necrotising ulcerative gingivitis: a hypothetical explanation. *Journal of Periodontology*, **45**, 830–2.

Kenney, E. B. and Ash, M. M. (1969). Oxidation–reduction potential of developing plaque, periodontal pockets and gingival sulci. *Journal of Periodontology*, **40**, 630–3.

Kenney, E. B., Saxe, S. R., and Bowles, R. D. (1975). The effect of cigarette smoking on anaerobiosis in the oral cavity. *Journal of Periodontology*, **46**, 82–5.

Kenney, E. B., Kraal, J. H., Saxe, S. R., and Jones, J. (1977). The effect of cigarette smoke on human oral polymorphonuclear leukocytes. *Journal of Periodontal Research*, **12**, 227–34.

Kowalski, C. J. (1971). Relationship between smoking and calculus deposition. *Journal of Dental Research*, **50**, 101–4.

Kowolik, M. J. and Nisbet, T. (1983). Smoking and acute ulcerative gingivitis. *British Dental Journal*, **154**, 241–2.

Kraal, J. H. and Kenney, E. B. (1979). The response of polymorphonuclear leukocytes to chemotactic stimulation for smokers and non-smokers. *Journal of Periodontal Research*, **14**, 383–9.

Kraal, J. H., Chancellor, M. B., Bridges, R. B., Bemis, K. G., and Hawke, J. E. (1977). Variations in the gingival polymorphonuclear leukocyte migration rate in dogs induced by chemotactic autologous serum and migration inhibitor from tobacco smoke. *Journal of Periodontal Research*, **12**, 242–9.

Kreschover, S. J. (1952). The effect of tobacco on the epithelial tissues of mice. *Journal of the American Dental Association*, **45**, 528–40.

Kristoffersen, T. (1970). Periodontal conditions in Norwegian soldiers-an epidemiological and experimental study. *Scandinavian Journal of Dental Research*, **78**, 34–53.

Kumar, R. and Lader, M. (1981). Nicotine and smoking. *Current Developments in Psychopharmacology*, **6**, 127–64.

Lang, N. P., Cumming, B. R., and Loe, H. (1973). Toothbrushing frequency as it relates to plaque development and gingival health. *Journal of Periodontology*, **44**, 396–405.

Langley, J. N. and Dickinson, W. L. (1890). Pituri and nicotine. *Journal of Physiology (London)*, **11**, 265–306.

Larson, P. S. and Silvette, H. (1975). *Tobacco. Experimental and clinical studies*, suppl. 3. Williams & Wilkins, Baltimore.

Larson, P. S., Haag, H. B., and Silvette, H. (1961). *Tobacco. Experimental and clinical studies.* Williams & Wilkins, Baltimore.

Lavstedt, S. (1975). A methodological – roentgenological investigation on marginal alveolar bone loss. *Acta Odontologica Scandinavica*, 33/(Suppl. 67).

Lavstedt, S., Bolin, A., Henrikson, C. O, and Cartensen, J. (1986). Proximal alveolar bone loss in a longitudinal radiographic examination. I. Methods of measurement and partial recording. *Acta Odontologica Scandinavica*, 44, 149–57.

Lilienthal, B., Amerena, V., and Gregory, G. (1965). An epidemiological study of chronic periodontal disease. *Archives of Oral Biology*, 10, 553–66.

Loe, H. and Silness, J. (1963). Periodontal disease in pregnancy I. Prevalence and severity. *Acta Odontologica Scandinavica*, 21, 533–51.

Ludwick, W. and Massler, M. (1952). Relation of dental caries experience and gingivitis to cigarette smoking in males 17 to 21 years old. *Journal of Dental Research*, 31, 319–22.

Macgregor, I. D. M. (1984). Toothbrushing efficiency in smokers and non-smokers. *Journal of Clinical Periodontology*, 11, 313–20.

Macgregor, I. D. M. (1985). Survey of toothbrushing habits in smokers and non-smokers. *Clinical Preventive Dentistry*, 7, 27–30.

Macgregor, I. D. M. (1989). Effects of smoking on oral ecology. *Clinical Preventive Dentistry*, 11, 3–7.

Macgregor, I. D. M. and Balding, J. W. (1987a). Toothbrushing and smoking behaviour in 14-year-old English schoolchildren. *Community Dental Health*, 4, 27–34.

Macgregor, I. D. M. and Balding, J. W. (1987b). Toothbrushing frequency and personal hygiene in 14-year-old schoolchildren. *British Dental Journal*, 162, 141–4.

Macgregor, I. D. M. and Edgar, W. M. (1986). Calcium and phosphate concentrations and precipitate formation in whole saliva from smokers and non-smokers. *Journal of Periodontal Research*, 21, 429–33.

Macgregor, I. D. M. and Rugg-Gunn, A. J. (1984). Uninstructed toothbrushing behaviour in young adults in relation to cigarette smoking in Newcastle. *Community Dentistry and Oral Epidemiology*, 12, 358–60.

Macgregor, I. D. M. and Rugg-Gunn, A. J. (1986). Toothbrushing sequence in smokers and nonsmokers. *Clinical Preventive Dentistry*, 8, 17–20.

Macgregor, I. D. M., Edgar, W. M., and Greenwood, A. R. (1985). Effects of cigarette smoking on the rate of plaque formation. *Journal of Clinical Periodontology*, 12, 35–41.

McGuire, J. R. *et al.* (1989). Cotinine in saliva and gingival crevicular fluid of smokers with periodontal disease. *Journal of Periodontology*, 60, 176–81.

McKendrick, A. J. W., Barbenal, L. M. H., and McHugh, W. D. (1970). The influence of time of examination eating, smoking, and frequency of brushing on the oral debris index. *Journal of Periodontal Research*, 5, 205–7.

Manhold, J. H., Rustogi, K. N., Doyle, J. L., and Manhold, B. S. (1968). Microscopic and microrespirometer (Q_{O_2}) study of the effect of cigarette smoking on human oral soft tissues. *Oral Surgery, Oral Medicine, Oral Pathology*, 26, 567–72.

Markkanen, H., Paunio, I., Tuominen, R., and Rajala, M. (1985). Smoking and periodontal disease in the Finnish population aged 30 years and over. *Journal of Dental Research*, 64, 932–5.

Meechan, J. G., Macgregor, I. D. M., Rogers, S. N., Hobson, R. S., Bate, J. P. C., and Dennison, M. (1988). The effect of smoking on immediate post-extraction socket filling with blood and on the incidence of painful socket. *British Journal of Oral and Maxillofacial Surgery*, 26, 402–9.

Miller, P. D. (1987). Root coverage with free gingival graft. Factors associated with incomplete coverage. *Journal of Periodontology*, 58, 674–81.

Miller, W. D. (1890). *The micro-organisms of the human mouth*, pp. 246–7. S. S. White Dental Manufacturing Co., Philadelphia.

Modeer, T., Lavstedt, S., and Ahlund, C. (1980). Relation between tobacco consumption and oral health in Swedish school children. *Acta Odontologica Scandinavica*, 38, 223–7.

Mosely, L. H. and Finseth, F. (1977). Cigarette smoking: impairment of digital blood flow and wound healing in the hand. *The Hand*, 9, 97–101.

Mulinos, M. G. and Shulman, I. (1939). Vasoconstriction in the hand from a deep inspiration. *American Journal of Physiology*, 125, 310–22.

Mulinos, M. G. and Shulman, I. (1940). The effects of cigarette smoking and deep breathing on the peripheral vascular system. *American Journal of Medical Science*, 199, 708–20.

Murray, J. A. (1776–1792). *Apparatus medicaminum. Nicotina tabacum.* J. C. Dieterich, Göttingen.

Noble, R. C. and Penny, B. B. (1975). Comparison of leukocyte count and function in smoking and nonsmoking young men. *Infection and Immunity*, 12, 550–5.

Office of Population Censuses and Surveys (1990). *OPCS monitor. Cigarette smoking 1972–1988.* HMSO, London.

Osterberg, T. and Mellstrom, D. (1986). Tobacco smoking: a major risk factor for the loss of teeth in three 70-year-old cohorts. *Community Dentistry and Oral Epidemiology*, 14, 367–70.

Palmer, R. M. (1987). *Tobacco smoking and oral health*, Health Education Authority Occasional Paper, No. 6. HEA, London.

Pangborn, R. M. and Sharon, I. M. (1971). Visual deprivation and parotid response to cigarette smoking. *Physiology and Behaviour*, 6, 559–61.

Parvinen, T. (1984). Stimulated salivary flow rate, pH and lactobacillus and yeast concentrations in non-smokers and smokers. *Scandinavian Journal of Dental Research*, 92, 315–18.

Pindborg, J. J. (1947). Tobacco and gingivitis. *Journal of Dental Research*, 26, 261–4.

Pindborg, J. J. (1949). Tobacco and gingivitis. II. Correlation between consumption of tobacco, ulceromembranous gingivitis and calculus. *Journal of Dental Research*, 28, 460–3.

Pindborg, J. J. (1951). Influence of service in armed forces on incidence of gingivitis. *Journal of the American Dental Association*, 42, 517–22.

Pindborg, J. J. (1980). *Oral cancer and precancer.* Wright, Bristol.

Preber, H. and Bergstrom, J. (1985a). Occurrence of gingival bleeding in smoker and non-smoker patients. *Acta Odontologica Scandinavica*, 43, 315–20.

Preber, H. and Bergstrom, J. (1985b). The effect of non-surgical treatment on periodontal pockets in smokers and non-smokers. *Journal of Clinical Periodontology*, 13, 319–23.

Preber, H. and Bergstrom, J. (1986). Cigarette smoking in patients referred for periodontal treatment. *Scandinavian Journal of Dental Research*, 94, 102–8.

Preber, H. and Bergstrom, J. (1990). Effect of cigarette smoking on periodontal healing following surgical therapy. *Journal of Clinical Periodontology*, 17, 324–8.

Preber, H. and Kant, T. (1973). Effect of tobacco smoking on periodontal tissue of 15-year-old schoolchildren. *Journal of Periodontal Research*, 8, 278–83.

Preber, H., Kant, T., and Bergstrom, J. (1980). Cigarette smoking, oral hygiene and periodontal health in Swedish army conscripts. *Journal of Clinical Periodontology*, 7, 106–13.

Rajala, M., Honkala, E., Rimpela, M., and Lammi, S. (1980). Toothbrushing in relation to other habits in Finland. *Community Dentistry and Oral Epidemiology*, 8, 391–5.

Ramfjord, S. P. (1959). Indices for prevalence and incidence of periodontal disease. *Journal of Periodontology*, 30, 51–9.

Raulin, L. A., McPherson, J. C., III., McQuade, M. J., and Hanson, B. S. (1988). The effect of nicotine on the attachment of human fibroblasts to glass and human root surfaces *in vitro*. *Journal of Periodontology*, **59**, 318–25.

Royal College of Physicians (1971). *Smoking and health now*, Pitman Medical, Tunbridge Wells.

Royal College of Physicians (1977). *Smoking or health*, p. 100. Pitman Medical, Tunbridge Wells.

Royal College of Physicians (1983), *Health or smoking*, Pitman, London.

Russell, A. L. (1956). A system of classification and scoring for prevalence surveys of periodontal disease. *Journal of Dental Research*, **35**, 350–9.

Schei, O., Waerhaug, J., Lovdal, A., and Arno, A. (1959). Alveolar bone loss as related to oral hygiene and age. *Journal of Periodontology*, **30**, 7–16.

Schnedorf, J. G. and Ivy, A. C. (1939). The effect of tobacco smoking on the alimentary tract. An experimental study of man and animals. *Journal of the American Medical Association*, **112**, 898–904.

Schour, I. and Massler, M. (1948). Prevalence of gingivitis in young adults. *Journal of Dental Research*, **27**, 733–4.

Shannon, I. L., Kilgore, W. G., and O'Leary, T. J. (1969). Stress as a predisposing factor in necrotizing ulcerative gingivitis. *Journal of Periodontology*, **40**, 240–2.

Shay, H. B. and Smart, G. A. (1945). The association of local factors with gingivitis. *British Dental Journal*, **78**, 135–7.

Sheiham, A. (1971). Periodontal disease and oral cleanliness in tobacco smokers. *Journal of Periodontology*, **42**, 259–63.

Shields, W. D. (1977). Acute necrotizing ulcerative gingivitis. A study of some of the contributing factors and their validity in an Army population. *Journal of Periodontology*, **48**, 346–9.

Shuler, R. L. (1968). Effect of cigarette smoking on the circulation of the oral mucosa. *Journal of Dental Research*, **47**, 910–15.

Silness, J. and Loe, H. (1964). Periodontal disease in pregnancy. II. Correlation between oral hygiene and periodontal condition. *Acta Odontologica Scandinavica*, **22**, 131–5.

Smith, G. M. (1970). Personality and smoking: a review of the literature. In *Learning mechanisms in smoking* (ed. W. A Hunt), pp. 42–61. Aldine, Chicago.

Solomon, H. A., Priore, R. L., and Bross, I. D. J. (1968). Cigarette smoking and periodontal disease. *Journal of the American Dental Association*, **77**, 1081–4.

Sparrow, D., Beausoleil, N. I., Garvey, A. J., Posner, B., and Gilbert, J. E. (1982). The influence of cigarette smoking and age on bone loss in men. *Archives of Environmental Health*, **37**, 246–9.

Stammers, A. (1944). Vincent's infection: observations and conclusions regarding the aetiology and treatment of 1,017 civilian cases. *British Dental Journal*, **76**, 147–55.

Stimmel, B. (1979). *Cardiovascular effects of mood-altering drugs*. Raven Press, New York.

Strauss, L. H. and Fockeler, J. (1939). Über die Einwirkungen von Tabak auf die Zahne, *Zeitschrift für Klinische Medizin*, **136**, 468–73.

Summers, C. J. and Oberman, A. (1968). Association of oral disease with 12 selected variables. 1. Periodontal disease. *Journal of Dental Research*, **47**, 457–62.

Sweet, J. B. and Butler, D. P. (1979). The relationship of smoking to localised osteitis. *Journal of Oral Surgery*, **37**, 732–5.

Tenovuo, J. and Makinen, K. K. (1976). Concentration of thiocyanate and ionizable iodine in saliva of smokers and non-smokers. *Journal of Dental Research*, **55**, 661–3.

US Department of Health and Human Services (1983). *The health consequences of smoking and cardiovascular disease*, p. 190. DHHS, Washington DC.

US Department of Health, Education and Welfare. (1976). *Health consequences of smoking*. DHEW, Rockville, MD.

Waerhaug, J. (1966). Epidemiology of periodontal disease. In *World workshop in periodontics* (ed. S. P. Ramfjord, D. A. Kerr, and M. M. Ash), pp. 181–211. University of Michigan, Ann Arbor.

Waerhaug, J. (1967). Prevalence of periodontal disease in Ceylon. Association with age, sex, oral hygiene, socioeconomic factors, vitamin deficiencies, malnutrition, betal and tobacco consumption and ethnic group. Final report. *Acta Odontologica Scandinavica*, **25**, 205–31.

Wald, N., Doll, R., and Copeland, D. (1981). Trends in tar, nicotine and carbon monoxide yields of UK cigarettes manufactured since 1934. *British Medical Journal*, **282**, 763–6.

Winsor, A. L. (1932). The effect of cigarette smoking on secretion. *Journal of General Psychology*, **6**, 190–5.

Winsor, A. L. and Richard, S. J. (1935). The development of tolerance for cigarettes. *Journal of Experimental Psychology*, **18**, 113–20.

World Health Organization (1975). *Smoking and its effects on health*, Technical Report Series, No. 568. WHO, Geneva.

Wright, I. S. (1933). The clinical value of human capillary studies. *Journal of the American Medical Association*, **101**, 439–42.

Wright, I. S. and Moffat, D. (1934). The effects of tobacco on the peripheral vascular system: further studies. *Journal of the American Medical Association*, **103**, 318–23.

Wynder, E. L. and Hoffmann, D. (1967). *Tobacco and tobacco smoke*, pp. 85–133. Academic Press, New York.

7. The sex hormones

7.1 INTRODUCTION

Oestrogens and progesterone are hormones whose cyclic production is uniquely controlled by the female ovary. Oestrogens are responsible for the physiological changes that take place at puberty in women and, together with progesterone, play a vital role in the preparation of the female reproductive tract for the reception of sperm and the implantation of a fertilized ovum. Current understanding of the synthesis and actions of these hormones has led to a rationale for therapeutic intervention in certain diseases. Extensive clinical use has also been made of synthetic compounds that can mimic the effects of endogenous hormones and are frequently prescribed as oral contraceptives. Endogenous androgens such as testosterone are important in controlling the emotional constitution and sexual characteristics of the male. The hormone also has general metabolic actions in promoting protein synthesis and retaining salts such as calcium, sodium, and chloride in the body. Clinically, testosterone is used in the management of male sexual disorders such as hypogonadism, impaired spermatogenesis, and impotence.

7.2 THE EFFECTS OF SEX HORMONES ON PERIODONTAL TISSUES

The effects that exogenous and endogenous sex hormones have upon the oral mucosa and periodontal tissues have been studied extensively both in animal experiments and from clinical observation.

The results of early animal experiments suggested that oestrogens increased the keratinization of already keratinized oral tissues (Ziskin *et al.* 1936; Ziskin and Nesse 1946) although the opposite effect has been observed in postmenopausal women (Trott 1957). The mucosal tissues and skin of elderly human subjects are thickened considerably under the influence of oestrogen (Goldzeiher *et al.* 1952) and epithelial hyperplasia has been demonstrated following subcutaneous application of oestradiol benzoate in mice (Nutlay *et al.* 1954). Similar effects have also been observed in ovariectomized squirrel monkeys, where a tendency towards hypertrophy and increased activity of epithelial cells followed intramuscular injections of radio labelled oestradiol (Litwack *et al.* 1970).

The effects of oestrogen and progesterone upon non-epithelial tissues have also been studied. Oestrogen causes an increase in the acid mucopolysaccharide content of connective tissues in human oral mucosa (Schiff and Burn 1961). Progesterone increases the permeability of the gingival vasculature of rabbits by causing endothelial cell dysfunction and reversible gap formation (Mohammed *et al.* 1974).

An increased cellularity of the periodontal membranes of mice five weeks after subcutaneous injection of oestrogen has been reported, although after 10 weeks the cellularity and collagen content of the periodontium were reduced when compared to non-injected controls (Glickman and Shklar 1954). It was suggested that after 10 weeks, oestrogen inhibited the formation of new connective tissue. At five weeks, the animals attempted to accommodate to the artificially induced hormone pattern. Also, there appeared to be an inhibition of alveolar periosteal bone formation in the 10-week, post-injection animals. A further animal experiment that was conducted over a similar time period, however, failed to demonstrate any effects of oestrogen or progesterone on alveolar bone loss in hamsters (Lundgren and Lindhe 1971).

Testosterone has been shown to exert anabolic effects to stimulate osteoblastic activity in hypophysectomized rats (Shklar *et al.* 1967). The effects, however, are minimal in tissues of healthy animals, which suggests that, at least in these experiments, injections of the exogenous hormone served only to restore the depleted anabolic activity.

7.2.1 SEX HORMONES AND PROSTAGLANDIN PRODUCTION

The effects of various concentrations of oestradiol 17-β and progesterone, both alone and in combination, on the levels of a series of prostaglandins in gingival tissue samples has been studied by El Attar *et al.* (1982). Relatively low concentrations of both hormones, which represented physiological levels in pregnancy, were found to be stimulatory to prostaglandin synthesis. When the concentrations of both hormones were increased above those expected to be found *in vivo* there was an inhibitory effect upon prostaglandin production. Furthermore, when the hormones were used in combination, their effect upon prostaglandin output was purely inhibitory. These findings may help to explain the relatively high prevalence of gingivitis during pregnancy (see p.137) and the observations that gingivitis scores and crevicular fluid flow can remain unaffected by oral contraceptives (Jensen *et al.* 1981).

7.2.2 LOCAL METABOLISM IN THE GINGIVA

The implication that sex hormones are causal in producing or modifying the gingival response to dental plaque is dependent upon the demonstration of these hormones and their metabolic products within the tissues. There is now substantial evidence to suggest that receptors do exist in gingival tissues for oestrogen, progesterone, and metabolites of testosterone (Formicola *et al.* 1970; Bashirelahi *et al.* 1977; Southren *et al.* 1978; Hernandez *et al.* 1981; Wenk *et *al.* 1981). Furthermore, the gingiva are able to metabolize the sex hormones (El Attar 1974; El Attar and Hugoson 1974; Ojanotko and Harri 1978; Vittek *et al.* 1979).

Oesterone is converted in vitro to its main metabolite oestradiol 17-β by an oxidoreductase enzyme. The parent molecule is also metabolized through a minor pathway to oestriol by 16α-hydroxylase (Holmes and El Attar 1977). The conversion rates are two to three times faster in inflamed gingiva than in healthy tissue (El Attar and Hugoson 1974; Holmes and El Attar 1977).

Chronically inflamed gingiva is twice as active as healthy tissue in metabolizing progesterone, and the chemical nature of progesterone metabolites also differs between healthy and diseased tissues (El Attar 1971; El Attar *et al.* 1973; Harri and Ojanotko 1978). The metabolite 5-pregnanedione is a product of the conversion of progesterone in normal gingiva, whereas its isomer, 6-pregnanedione, is a metabolite in chronically inflamed tissue. In both instances, however, the major active metabolite of progesterone is 20-hydroxyprogesterone, which is increased fourfold in inflamed tissues (El Attar *et al.* 1973). This evidence suggests that the accumulation of metabolic products of the naturally occurring sex hormones is an important factor in the pathogenesis of chronic gingivitis.

A positive correlation has been found between plasma levels of progesterone and its metabolites with the degree of gingival inflammation (Vittek *et al.* 1978). The gingival concentration of progesterone and its metabolites may also increase during pregnancy. The accumulation of the metabolites aggravates the inflammatory response of pre-existing gingivitis (Ojanotko and Harri 1982). Although these biochemical analyses have been undertaken on naturally occurring hormones that are circulating at elevated levels in the pregnant state, there is no evidence available to suggest that different circumstances prevail in patients taking oral contraceptive drugs.

The major pathway for the metabolism of testosterone in gingiva is by enzymatic conversion to 17β-hydroxy- A-ring reduced androgens (Rappaport *et al.* 1976; Vittek *et al.* 1979, 1982). With healthy gingiva the conversion appears to be minimal in women, although inflamed tissues of both sexes are able to metabolize testosterone by about the same magnitude (Ojanotko *et al.* 1980).

7.2.3 EFFECTS ON WOUND HEALING

The influence of oestrogen and progesterone upon wound healing and granulation tissue formation has also been studied extensively in animal experiments (Nyman 1971). Progesterone aggravates an inflammatory reaction during the lag phase of wound healing in rabbits. There is also a delay in the onset of collagen formation, although collagen formation does proceed at an increased rate when vascularization and the subsequent increased supply of arterial oxygen are established. Similar findings have been demonstrated when both oestrogen and progesterone are administered together, although oestrogen, if given alone, has no influence upon periods of acute inflammation, wound strength, or collagen formation during wound healing (Nyman 1971).

7.2.4 SEX HORMONES AND PRE-EXISTING GINGIVITIS

Sex hormones appear to have a more marked effect upon levels of gingival exudate in the presence of a chronic gingivitis (Lindhe *et al.* 1968a; Hugoson 1970). This may result from an increased vascularization of the chronically inflamed tissues (Lindhe and Branemark 1968; Lindhe *et al.* 1968b) and an increase in the permeability of the gingival vessels (Lindhe *et al.* 1968b). Vascular permeability has also been shown to increase after local application of sex hormones to the hamster cheek pouch (Lindhe and Branemark 1967a,b; Lindhe *et al.* 1967). These findings indicate that oestrogen and progesterone affect primarily the vascular response of irritated tissues without necessarily aggravating the other components of the classical inflammatory reaction. Such changes, however, may be species dependent as there is no response of rabbits gingiva to either castration or subsequent oestrogen replacement therapy (Rubright *et al.* 1971).

7.2.5 SALIVARY SEX HORMONES AND PERIODONTAL DISEASE

The concentrations of testosterone, oestradiol, and progesterone have been analysed by radioimmunoassay in the saliva of groups of subjects with and without periodontal disease (Vittek *et al.* 1984). Oestradiol levels were reduced significantly and progesterone concentrations increased in subjects suffering from periodontitis. There was no difference in testosterone levels between the men with and without periodontitis, but the concentrations were raised in menstruating women with periodontitis.

Vittek speculated that because of the high correlation between 'free' circulating hormones and their concentration in saliva, it was unlikely that increased levels of the hormones reflected their leakage from protein carriers at periodontally inflamed sites. It was suggested that the increased (or decreased) levels of the hormones were more likely due to altered production and or metabolism of hormones at peripheral tissue sites.

Finally, it was suggested that the increased testosterone–oestrogen ratio in periodontitis could reflect on the hyperandrogenic state. The relatively predominent androgens could then enhance the activity of enzymes such as salivary proteases, which have been implicated in the pathogenesis of periodontal disease (Vittek *et al.* 1984).

7.2.6 MODIFYING ACTION OF CORTISOL

The modifying effects of other hormones, notably cortisol, should be considered whenever states of elevated sex hormone levels exist. Increased levels of plasma cortisol have been associated with increased oestrogen levels in pregnancy (Gemzell 1953). After administration of exogenous sex hormones (Plager *et al.* 1964), progesterone is able to displace cortisol from its plasma binding protein and therefore increase the physiological active levels of free cortisol (Rosenthal *et al.* 1969). Raised levels of plasma cortisol have anti-inflammatory effects leading to further modifications of the gingival response to increased levels of sex hormones. This may help to explain the findings of less inflamed connective tissues in some sex hormone-treated animals (Nyman 1971; Deasy *et al.* 1970).

7.2.7 PREGNANCY, PUBERTY, AND MENSTRUATION

The effects of physiological changes in sex hormone balance upon the response of the gingival tissues to dental plaque may be observed from repeated clinical observations in suitable patients. These effects can be compared and related to the oral manifestations consequential to oral sex-hormone therapy. The incidence of gingivitis (including pregnancy epulis) in pregnant women has been reported as being between 30 and 100 per cent (Ziskin *et al.* 1936; Maier and Orban 1949; Ringsdorf *et al.* 1962; Loe and Silness 1963; Loe 1965; Adams *et al.* 1973). The severity of inflammation increases gradually during pregnancy, with partial or complete resolution after parturition (Loe and Silness 1963; Silness and Loe 1964; Hugoson 1970; Samant *et al.* 1976). Gingivitis has also been reported to peak at six months' gestation and then resolve slightly in the final trimester (Cohen *et al.* 1971). It has been suggested that the elevated levels of oestrogen and progesterone found during pregnancy increase the sensitivity of the gingiva to irritants rather than initiate the inflammation (Jenkins 1978). Studies on plaque growth and composition, however, provide more detailed information.

Essentially, research has shown that plaque levels remain constant during pregnancy (Loe and Silness 1963; Cohen *et al.* 1971; Kornman and Loesche 1980). However, dark-field microscopic studies indicate that the subgingival microflora becomes progressively anaerobic as pregnancy progresses (Kornman and Loesche 1980). The prevalence of *Bacteroides melaninogenicus* ss. *intermedius* increases significantly and appears to be associated with the raised levels of oestradiol and progesterone. Plaque samples demonstrate an increase steroid uptake in pregnancy and this most likely relates to the oestradiol becoming a substitute for menadione, which is a growth requirement for *B. melaninogenicus* (Kornman and Loesche 1982).

Elevated levels of circulating sex hormones have also been linked to the increased severity and prevalence of gingivitis in puberty (Parfitt 1957; Sutcliffe 1972). This relationship is strengthened by the observation that, during adolescence, gingivitis peaks earlier in girls (11–13 years) than in boys (13–14 years).

Conversely, a 6-year longitudinal study of 18 hormonally stable girls failed to show any significant increase in gingivitis at pubertal maturation. There was no association between the onset of puberty and changes in levels of black pigmented *Bacteroides* (BPB) organisms in the subgingival plaque. However, in a concurrent cross-sectional study of girls suffering from precocious puberty, the detection of BPB correlated with serum levels of oestradiol and it was suggested that the hormone provides suitable growth conditions for these bacteria. Furthermore, the gingival indices of BPB-positive subjects were higher (but not significantly

so) than those of BPB-negative subjects (Yanover and Ellen 1986). The positive correlation between puberty and BPB levels, which was reported by Delaney (1986), was not confirmed in this study.

The gingival crevicular exudate increases at the time of ovulation in the menstrual cycle owing to the increased production of oestrogens and progesterone (Lindhe and Attstrom 1967). However, no such variation in exudate levels was seen in healthy tissues (Holm-Pedersen and Loe 1967). A deterioration of a pre-existing gingivitis was observed during the days of menstruation.

7.2.8 THE PREGNANCY EPULIS (GRANULOMA)

The pregnancy epulis is a soft, pendunculated swelling that may appear at any time during pregnancy, although is most commonly seen from about the third month onwards. The lesion, which is most prevalent on the labial aspect in the anterior part of the mouth, increases in size slowly throughout pregnancy and can regress partially or completely after parturition. A residual swelling should be removed surgically if necessary. The lesion can bleed profusely when excised and electrocautery may be indicated. An epulis should be removed during pregnancy if it is being traumatized by opposing teeth or restorations. There is, however, a high recurrence rate and unless otherwise indicated, epulides should be excised after parturition.

Histologically, the appearance is one of a mass of vascular spaces within a delicate, connective tissue stroma, which can intensify with age. The covering epithelium is thin and in areas of ulceration a fibrin exudate covers the surface. A moderate inflammatory infiltrate is usually present and suggests that the pregnancy epulis is a reactive proliferation of granulomatous tissue to a mild, traumatic stimulus.

7.2.9 ORAL CONTRACEPTIVES

The oral contraceptives are amongst the most widely used medical agents in the Western world. The most common type is a combined preparation of an oestrogen and a progesterone, whose actions are to prevent ovulation, predominantly by inhibiting the secretion follicle-stimulating hormone by the anterior pituitary gland. Additional therapeutic indications for oestrogen and progesterone include replacement therapy at the menopause, senile or atrophic vaginitis, dysfunctional uterine bleeding, failure of ovarian development, acne, hirsutism, and osteoporosis. In osteoporosis, several months of oestrogen therapy are required before calcium balance becomes positive and bone resorption returns to normal (Thalassinos *et al.* 1982). These effects are reversed rapidly when the treatment is discontinued (Aloia *et al.* 1985).

The effects of oral contraceptives upon gingival and periodontal tissues are well documented. Several case reports have described a hyperplastic, oedematous gingivitis following the use of oral contraceptives, which resolves when the drugs are withdrawn (Lynn 1967; Kaufman 1969; Sperber 1969; Chevallier 1970). This response appears to be a secondary reaction to the presence of local irritants, especially dental plaque. The exogenous hormones can also enhance the development of an anaerobic plaque in which *Bacteroides* species are prevalent, and this may occur in the absence of clinical changes in gingivitis scores and crevicular fluid flow (Jensen *et al.* 1981). However, levels of gingival exudate can be raised in females taking oral contraceptives (Lindhe and Bjorn 1967) and the influence of the contraceptives is most marked during the menstrual phase when the production of ovarian oestrogen and progesterone is minimal (Lindhe *et al.* 1969).

The maintenance of adequate plaque control is conducive to gingival health, despite continued administration of oral contraceptives (Pearlman 1974). These reports have been confirmed by the results of studies which have shown clearly that hormonal contraceptives are associated with an increase in severity of gingival inflammation (El Ashiry *et al.* 1970; Das *et al.* 1971). However, Knight and Wade (1974) failed to demonstrate significant differences in levels of either plaque or gingivitis between a group of women taking oral contraceptives over a period of one and a half years and age-matched controls. Subjects receiving the hormones for more than one and a half years, however, had greater periodontal destruction than either of the two previous groups and it was suggested that this was due to an altered host resistance seen in the long-term group.

7.3 CONCLUSION

Whenever there is an increase in circulating levels of sex hormones, the patients gingival tissues become susceptible to plaque-induced inflammatory changes. It is essential, therefore, that such patients maintain optimal plaque control to reduce the risk of further periodontal damage.

REFERENCES

Adams, D., Carney, J. S., and Dicks, D. A. (1973). Pregnancy gingivitis: a survey of 100 antenatal patients. *Journal of Dentistry*, **2**, 106–10.

Aloia, J. F., Cohn, S. G., Vaswani, A., Yeh, J. K., Yuen, J., and Ellis, K. (1985). Risk factors for postmenopausal osteoporosis. *American Journal of Medicine*, **78**, 95–100.

Bashirelahi, N., Organ, R. J., and Bergquist, J. J. (1977). Steroid binding protein in human gingiva. *Journal of Dental Research*, **56**, 125.

Chevallier, M. E. (1970). Mouth manifestations and oral contraceptives. *Revue Odonto-Stomatologie du Midi de la France*, **28**, 96–103.

Cohen, D., Shapiro, J., Friedman, L., Kyle, G., and Franklin, S. (1971). A longitudinal investigation of the periodontal changes during pregnancy and fifteen months post partum. Part II. *Journal of Periodontology*, **42**, 653–7.

Das, A. K., Bhowmick, S., and Dutta, A. (1971). Oral contraceptives and periodontal disease. *Journal of the Indian Dental Association*, **43**, 155–8.

Deasy, M., Grota, L., and Kennedy, J. E. (1970). Peripheral plasma progesterone levels in squirrel monkeys. *Journal of Dental Research*, **49**,

Delaney, J. E. (1986). Subgingival microbiota associated with puberty: studies of pre-, circum-, and postpubertal human females. *Paediatric Dentistry*, **8**, 268–75.

El-Ashiry, G. M., El-Kafrawy, A. H., Nasr, M. F., and Younis, N. (1970). Comparative study of the influence of pregnancy and oral contraceptives on the gingivae. *Oral Surgery, Oral Medicine, Oral Pathology*, **30**, 472–5.

El Attar, T. M. A. (1971). Metabolism of progesterone $7a^3H$ *in vitro* in human gingiva with periodontitis. *Journal of Periodontology*, **42**, 721–5.

El Attar, T. M. A. (1974). The *in vitro* conversion of male sex steroid, $1,2-^3H$-androstenedione in normal and inflamed human gingiva. *Archives of Oral Biology*, **19**, 1185–90.

El Attar, T. M. A. and Hugoson, A. (1974). Comparative metabolism of female sex steroids in normal and chronically inflamed gingiva of the dog. *Journal of Periodontal Research*, **9**, 284–9.

El Attar, T. M. A., Roth, G. D., and Hugoson, A. (1973). Comparative metabolism of $4-^{14}C$-progesterone in normal and chronically inflamed human gingival tissue. *Journal of Periodontal Research*, **8**, 79–85.

El Attar, T. M. A., Lin, S., and Tira, D. E. (1982). The relationship between the concentration of female sex steroids and prostaglandin production by human gingiva in vitro. *Prostaglandins, Leukotrienes and Medicine*, **8**, 447–58.

Formicola, A. J., Weatherford, T., and Grupe, H. Jr. (1970). Uptake of ^3H-estradiol by the oral tissues of rats. *Journal of Periodontal Research*, **5**, 269–75.

Gemzell, C. A. (1953). Blood levels of 17-hydroxycorticosteroids in normal pregnancy. *Journal of Clinical Endocrinology*, **13**, 898–902.

Glickman, I. and Shklar, G. (1954). Modification of the effect of cortisone upon alveolar bone by the systemic administration of oestrogen. *Journal of Periodontology*, **25**, 231–9.

Goldziether, J. W., Roberts, I. S., Rawls, W. B., and Goldziether, M. A. (1952). Local action of steroids on senile human skin. *Archives of Dermatology*, **66**, 304–15.

Harri, M.-P. and Ojanotko, A. O. (1978). Progesterone metabolism in healthy and inflamed female gingiva. *Journal of Steroid Biochemistry*, **9**, 826.

Hernandez, M. R., Wenk, E. J., Southern, A. L., Rappaport, S. C., and Vittek, J. (1981). Localisation of ^3H-androgens in human gingiva by radioautography. *Journal of Dental Research*, **60** 607 (abstr. 1193).

Holmes, L. G. and El Attar, T. M. A. (1977). Gingival inflammation assessed by histology, ^3H-estrone metabolism and prostaglandin E_2 levels. *Journal of Periodontal Research*, **12**, 500–9.

Holm-Pedersen, P. and Loe, H. (1967). Flow of gingival exudate as related to menstruation and pregnancy. *Journal of Periodontal Research*, **2**, 13–20.

Hugoson, A. (1970). Gingival inflammation and female sex hormones. *Journal of Periodontal Research* (Suppl. 5), 1–18.

Jenkins, G. N. (1978). The effects of hormones on the oral structures. In *The physiology and biochemistry of the mouth*, (4th edn), pp. 215–37. Blackwell Scientific, London.

Jensen, J., Liljemark, W., and Bloomquist, C. (1981). The effect of female sex hormones on subgingival plaque. *Journal of Periodontology*, **52**, 588–602.

Kaufman, A. Y. (1969). An oral contraceptive as an aetiologic factor in producing hyperplastic gingivitis and a neoplasm of the pregnancy tumour type. *Oral Surgery, Oral Medicine, Oral Pathology*, **28**, 666–70.

Knight, G. M. and Wade, A. B. (1974). The effects of hormonal contraceptives on the human periodontium. *Journal of Periodontal Research*, **9**, 18–22.

Kornman, K. S. and Loesche, W. J. (1980). The subgingival microbial flora during pregnancy. *Journal of Periodontal Research*, **15**, 111–22.

Kornman, K. S. and Loesche, W. J. (1982). Effects of oestradiol and progesterone on *Bacteroides melaninogenicus* and *Bacteroides gingivalis*. *Infection and Immunity*, **35**, 256–63.

Lindhe, J. and Attstrom, R. (1967). Gingival exudation during the menstrual cycle. *Journal of Periodontal Research*, **2**, 194–8.

Lindhe, J. and Bjorn, A.-L. (1967). Influence of hormonal contraceptives on the gingiva of women. *Journal of Periodontal Research*, **2**, 1–6.

Lindhe, J. and Branemark, P.-I. (1967a). Changes in microcirculation after local application of sex hormones. *Journal of Periodontal Research*, **2**, 185–93.

Lindhe, J. and Branemark, P.-I. (1967b). Changes in vascular permeability after local application of sex hormones. *Journal of Periodontal Research*, **2**, 259–65.

Lindhe, J. and Branemark, P.-I. (1968). The effect of sex hormones on vascularisation of granulation tissue. *Journal of Periodontal Research*, **3**, 6–11.

Lindhe, J., Branemark, P.-I., and Lundskug, J. (1967). Changes in vascular proliferation after local application of sex hormones. *Journal of Periodontal Research*, **2**, 266–72.

Lindhe, J., Attstrom, R., and Bjorn, A.-L. (1968a). Influence of sex hormones on gingival exudation in dogs with chronic gingivitis. *Journal of Periodontal Research*, **3**, 279–83.

Lindhe, J., Birch, J., and Branemark, P.-I. (1968b). Vascular proliferation in pseudo-pregnant rabbits. *Journal of Periodontal Research*, **3**, 13–20.

Lindhe, J., Attstrom, R., and Bjorn, A.-L. (1969). The influence of progestogen and gingival exudation during menstrual cycles. *Journal of Periodontal Research*, **4**, 97–102.

Litwack, D., Kennedy, J. E., and Zander, H. A. (1970). Response of oral epithelia to ovariectomy and oestrogen replacement. *Journal of Periodontal Research*, **5**, 263–8.

Loe, H. (1965). Periodontal changes in pregnancy. *Journal of Periodontology*, **36**, 209–16.

Loe, H. and Silness, J. (1963). Periodontal disease in pregnancy. I. Prevalence and severity. *Acta Odontologica Scandinavica*, **21**, 533–51.

Lundgren, D. and Lindhe, J. (1971). Lack of influence of female sex hormones on alveolar bone loss in hamsters. *Scandinavian Journal of Dental Research*, **79**, 113–18.

Lynn, B. D. (1967). 'The Pill' as an etiologic agent in hypertrophic gingivitis. *Oral Surgery, Oral Medicine, Oral Pathology*, **24**, 333–4.

Maier, A. W. and Orban, B. (1949). Gingivitis in pregnancy. *Oral Surgery*, **2**, 334–73.

Mohamed, A. H., Waterhouse, J. P., and Friederici, H. H. R. (1974). The microvasculature of the rabbit gingiva as affected by progesterone: an ultrastrucural study. *Journal of Periodontology*, **45**, 50–60.

Nutlay, A. G., Bhaskar, S. M., Weinmann, J. P., and Budy, A. M. (1954). Effects of estrogen on the gingiva and alveolar bone of molars in rats and mice. *Journal of Dental Research*, **33**, 115–27.

Nyman, S. (1971). Studies on the influence of estradiol and progesterone on granulation tissue. *Journal of Periodontal Research*, Suppl. 7, 1–24.

Ojanotko, A. O. and Harri, M.-P. (1978). Testosterone metabolism in chronically inflamed male gingival tissue. *Journal of Steroid Biochemistry*, **9**, 825.

Ojanotko, A. O. and Harri, M.-P. (1982). Progesterone metabolism by rat oral mucosa. II. The effect of pregnancy. *Journal of Periodontal Research*, **17**, 196–201.

Ojanotko, A., Neinstedt, W., and Harri, P. (1980). Metabolism of testosterone by human healthy and inflamed gingiva (*in vitro*). *Archives of Oral Biology*, **25**, 481–4.

Parfitt, G. J. (1957). A five year longitudinal study of the gingival condition of a group of children in England. *Journal of Periodontology*, **28**, 26–32.

Pearlman, B. A. (1974). An oral contraceptive drug and gingival enlargement; the relationship between local and systemic factors. *Journal of Clinical Periodontology*, **1**, 47–51.

Plager, J. E., Schmidt, K. G., and Staubitz, W. J. (1964). Increased unbound cortisol in the plasma of estrogen-treated subjects. *Journal of Clinical Investigations*, **43**, 1066–72.

Rappaport, S. C., Vittek, J., Altman, K., Gordon, G. G., and Southren, A. L. (1976). Sex differences in the metabolism of androgens by human gingiva. *Journal of Dental Research*, **55**, B71 (abstr. 37).

Ringsdorf, W. M., Ringsdorf, W.M., Jnr., Powell, B. J., Knight, L. A., and Cheraskin, E. (1962). Periodontal status and pregnancy. *American Journal of Obstetrics and Gynecology*, **83**, 258–63.

Rosenthal, H. E., Slaunwhite, W. R., and Sandberg, A. A. (1969). Transcortin: a corticosteroid-binding protein of plasma. X. Cortisol and progesterone interplay and unbound levels of these steroids in pregnancy. *Journal of Clinical Endocrinology*, **13**, 352–67.

Rubright, W. C., Higa, L. H., and Yanone, M. E. (1971). Histological quantification of the biological effects of estradiol benzoate on the gingiva and genital mucosa of castrated rabbits. *Journal of Periodontal Research*, **6**, 55–64.

Samant, A., Malik, C. P., Chabra, S. K., and Devi, P. K. (1976). Gingivitis and periodontal disease in pregnancy. *Journal of Periodontology*, **47**, 415–18.

Schiff, M. and Burn, H. F. (1961). The effect of intravenous estrogens on ground substance. *Archives of Otolaryngology*, **71**, 765–80.

Shklar, G., Chauncey, H. H., and Shapiro, S. (1967). The effect of testosterone on the periodontium of normal and hypophysectomised rats. *Journal of Periodontology*, **38**, 203–10.

Silness, J. and Loe, H. (1964). Periodontal disease in pregnancy. II. Correlation with oral hygiene and periodontal condition. *Acta Odontologica Scandinavica*, **22**, 121–35.

Southren, A. L., Rappaport, S. C., Gordon, G. G., and Vittek, J. (1978). Specific 5a-dihydrotestosterone receptors in human gingiva. *Journal of Clinical Endocrinology and Metabolism*, **47**, 1378–82.

Sperber, G. H. (1969). Oral contraceptive hypertrophic gingivitis. *Journal of the Dental Association of South Africa*, **24**, 37–40.

Sutcliffe, P. (1972). A longitudinal study of gingivitis and puberty. *Journal of Periodontal Research*, **7**, 52–8.

Thalassinos, N. C., Gutteridge, D. H., Joplin, D. F., and Fraser, T. R. (1982). Calcium balance in osteoporotic patients on long-term oral calcium therapy with and without sex hormones. *Clinical Science*, **62**, 221–6.

Trott, J. R. (1957). An histological investigation into keratinisation found in human gingivae. *British Dental Journal*, **103**, 421–7.

Vittek, J., Gordon, G. G., Rappaport, S. C., and Southern, A. L. (1978). Effect of plasma progesterone on ⁴-3-ketosteroid-5a-reductase activity in human gingiva and its biological significance. *Journal of Dental Research*, **57**, 311 (abstr. 948).

Vittek, J., Rappaport, S. C., Gordon, G. G., Munnanci, P. R., and Southren, A. L. (1979). Concentration of circulating hormones and metabolism of androgens by human gingiva. *Journal of Periodontology*, **50**, 254–64.

Vittek, J., Rappaport, S. C., Gordon, G. G., Hagendoorn, J. and Southren, A. L. (1982). Metabolism of androgens by human periodontal ligament. *Journal of Dental Research*, **61**, 1153–7.

Vittek, J., Kirsch, S., Rappaport, S. C., Bergman, M., and Southren, A. L. (1984). Salivary concentrations of steroid hormones in male and in cycling and postmenopausal females with and without periodontitis. *Journal of Periodontal Research*, **19**, 545–55.

Wenk, E. J., Hernandez, M. R., Vittek, J., Rappaport, S. C., and Southren, A. L. (1981). Localisation of ³H-estrogens in human gingiva by radioautography. *Journal of Dental Research*, **60**, 607–19.

Yanover, L. and Ellen, R. P. (1986). A clinical and microbiologic examination of gingival disease in parapubescent females. *Journal of Periodontology*, **57**, 562–7.

Ziskin, D. E. and Nesse, G. J. (1946). Pregnancy gingivitis. *American Journal of Orthodontics and Oral Surgery*, **32**, 390–432.

Ziskin, D. E., Blackberg, S. N., and Slanetz, C. A. (1936). Effects of subcutaneous injections of estrogenic and gonadrotopic hormones on gums and oral mucous membranes of normal and castrated rhesus monkeys. *Journal of Dental Research*, **15**, 407–28.

8. Dietary and nutritional aspects of periodontal disease

8.1 INTRODUCTION

The vitality of the periodontal tissues, in both health and disease, depends strongly upon an adequate source of essential nutrients being available to the host. The epithelium of the dentogingival junction and the underlying connective tissues are amongst the most dynamic tissues in the body. The maintenance of these tissues and, therefore, the integrity of the periodontium is dependent upon an adequate supply of proteins, carbohydrates, fats, vitamins, and mineral salts. A chronic deficiency in the availability of one or more of these nutrients may be expected to produce pathological alterations in the periodontal tissues.

The loss of connective tissue attachment evident during active periodontal disease is the result of a basic interaction between the virulence of the infecting organisms and the resistance of the host. This destruction is a consequence of infection and a nutritional deficiency alone is no longer believed to initiate periodontal disease. It is more likely, however, that a state of malnutrition will predispose a subject to the onset of a periodontal infection or, alternatively, will modify the rate of progression of established disease (Glickman 1964; Ferguson 1969).

The exact mechanisms by which nutritional deficiencies modify periodontal destruction have not been precisely defined. Alfano (1976) has suggested that any of the basic periodontal defence factors could be affected. These include the protein and urea content of both saliva and crevicular fluid, the integrity of the dentogingival barrier and the turnover of its constituent cells, the mobilization and activation of polymorphonuclear leukocytes in the early inflammatory response, and the activation of lymphocytes and the production of immunoglobulins in the immune response. In the following sections of this chapter, specific mention will be made of evidence about how the deficiency of a nutrient may influence one or more of these defences.

8.2 NUTRITION RESEARCH AND PERIODONTAL DISEASE

Initially, mention must be made of the extreme controversy that has emanated from much of the research into the role of nutrition in the aetiology of periodontal diseases. Alfano (1976) believes that this is primarily due to six basic problems that have not always been addressed when researchers have studied the interaction of the complex processes of disease and nutritional biochemistry.

First, the multifactorial aetiology of periodontal disease makes the study of a specific predisposing factor very difficult, if not impossible. The number of variables, such as rate of plaque formation, age of subjects, and local irritating factors, should be minimized as far as possible. Further, it is possible that the influence of extensive amounts of plaque could mask any effect of nutritional upset on periodontal status, at least in short-term studies and in epidemiological research on underprivileged populations.

Second, nutritional experiments on animals must be designed with both *ad libitum* and pair-fed control groups. When a component is restricted in an animal's diet, the daily food consumption tends to go down. Control animals on 'normal diets' may therefore be consuming more food (and nutrients) than the experimental group. Pair-fed animals given the same bulk of food as the experimental groups but with no deficient nutrient should also be used.

Third, the importance of using standardized periodontal indices and radiographic techniques must be recognized (Stepnick 1975). Many early studies used individually developed or very subjective indices. In addition, an accurate assessment of nutritional status must be made and it is important to realize that the status is not always indicated by the blood levels of a nutrient. Tissue levels of vitamin C, for example, can be reduced before there is any depletion of the vitamin in serum (Alfano *et al.* 1975).

Fourth, the animal model in experimental work should be chosen carefully, and the animal should be susceptible to a deficiency of the nutrient under study. The metabolism and potential interactions of any nutrient in the animal should be known.

Fifth, the observations from nutritional studies must be assessed in relation to the length of the trial. The acute changes that occur in animal experiments when a nutrient is totally withdrawn from the diet for a short period of time may not accurately reflect the changes that will occur in man. This is particularly so when the human changes are monitored in epidemiological studies which reflect chronic nutritional deficiencies that have developed over many years.

Sixth, and finally, the statistical analysis of data from nutrition–periodontitis studies is often complicated by a number of factors. These include the number of control groups in animal experiments, the death of animals as a direct result of nutritional upset (which leads to selection of animals by survival), interactions between nutrients, and the dominant and overriding effect of plaque on the recorded observations.

When these six points are considered it becomes clear that the study of diet, nutrition, and periodontal diseases can pose particular problems to the investigator in both human and animal experiments. Undoubtedly, a number of workers have taken great care in designing their studies to maintain scientific integrity. Unfortunately, substantial data have emanated from poorly controlled studies and such information has not been analysed vigorously by the appropriate statistical tests. Consequently, it is hardly surprising that many studies have produced equivocal results which have not been substantiated by later work.

8.3 NUTRITIONAL DEFICIENCIES IN HUMANS

Although many diets of populations in the so-called Westernized countries are far from ideal, it is reassuring to find that clinical states of nutritional deficiency such as scurvy and pellagra are very rare. Consequently, when nutritional problems are detected in humans they are often associated with predisposing conditions such as alcoholism, mental retardation, medical problems, or inadequately functioning dentures (Shaw 1970).

Most of the epidemiological studies directed towards the oral changes in deficiency states have been undertaken in Third World countries. When the findings of these studies are considered, two important points must be remembered. First, that the plaque control in such populations is very basic and the extensive microbial irritation makes the effects of nutrition on periodontal defence mechanisms difficult to determine (Alfano 1976). Secondly, in these populations it is very unlikely that subjects are deficient in just one or two nutrients. States of malnutrition reflect a deficiency of many factors. It is clearly impossible, therefore, to determine whether a change in the oral tissues is due to a lack of one, two, or a combination of factors.

8.4 HISTORICAL PERSPECTIVES OF DIET AND PERIODONTAL DISEASE

The study of the teeth and supporting structures of ancient populations provides some useful information about the effect of diet, and in particular its consistency, on rates of dental attrition and the progression of periodontal disease.

In populations such as the Egyptians, who had severe attrition from a very coarse diet, there was a greater prevalence of periodontal disease than caries (Deeley 1976). This was probably due to the very low incidence of caries rather than to a high incidence of periodontal disease. The bone loss that did occur may have been caused by multiple abscess formation, which was a consequence of pulpal exposure caused by attrition.

A study of dental disease in the Natufians at Kebara in Israel found a low rate of attrition with little calculus and periodontal disease (Smith 1972). This pattern of dental disease is more typical of hunting-based populations eating non-abrasive but self-cleansing diets based predominantly on meat rather than on cereals and vegetables alone.

Finally, an extensive study by Clark *et al.* (1986) showed that in many pre-modern populations, the evidence of periodontal disease was scarce. Over 90 per cent of teeth examined showed no discernible bone loss despite the presence of large deposits of calculus. It must also be remembered that, at such times in history, the seasonal availability of food could have predisposed to periodic nutritional deficiencies (Gilbert and Mielke 1985) although the effect on loss of bone appeared to be minimal (Clark *et al.* 1986).

8.5 THE CONSISTENCY OF DIET

From the viewpoint of promoting and maintaining gingival and periodontal health it is often stated that a firm and fibrous diet is more beneficial than an intake of softer, more loosely textured foods (Bastien 1960). Softer diets tend to produce greater deposits of plaque (Krasse and Brill 1964; Egelberg 1965) and this trend is even greater when the soft diets contain high proportions of sucrose (Carlsson 1965a,b). Indeed, experiments with hamsters have shown that it is the proportion of sucrose in the diet rather than the consistency of the diet itself that is more relevant to the quantity of plaque produced (Mikx *et al.* 1984). These findings are not surprising when it is remembered that sucrose is the main substrate for the plaque-forming streptococci. It can be concluded that although soft diets will cause minimal trauma to the periodontal tissues, produce less attrition to the teeth, and predispose to less food impaction, the consistency of the intake can produce greater quantities of more tenacious, adherent plaque, particularly when sucrose is a major constituent (Shaw 1965; Bowen and Cornick 1967; Folke *et al.* 1972).

Diets that are predominantly fibrous have been considered advantageous in their ability to impart a natural cleansing action to the teeth and periodontium. This was demonstrated by the periodontal destruction around the anterior teeth of a captive population of baboons which had been fed cubed food rations for between three and five years. When a fibrous supplement was introduced to the diet, gingival inflammation regressed and calculus deposits were dislodged by maize (Isserow 1978). These observations have not been repeated in humans, however, in whom fibrous dietary components were found not to have an effect on plaque formation, gingival fluid production, or the severity of gingival inflammation (Sreebny 1972, 1975; Birkeland and Jorkejend 1974).

With coarse diets, vigorous mastication is needed and the plaque that does form approximally tends to be toward the cleansible buccal and lingual surfaces of the teeth. Significant deposits do not accumulate beneath the contact points in sites that are associated with the onset of periodontal disease (Newman 1974). However, coarse and granular diets can predispose to direct traumatic injury to the supporting tissues (Mitchell and Johnson 1956; Klinsberg and Butcher 1959; Person 1961; Shaw and Griffiths 1961). This damage is most likely to be seen in the approximal regions where food impaction occurs (Cohen 1960). Histological observations on rats demonstrated that animals fed pellet diets had pronounced food impaction, gingival inflammation, and recession. Less food impaction was seen when the diet was given in powdered form, and minimal inflammation and impaction occurred in animals fed a liquid diet

(Stahl and Dreizen 1964). From similar experiments it was concluded that the consistency of the diet may be more important than its nutritional content in contributing to gingival irritation and subsequent inflammation (Riar *et al.* 1964).

Another long-considered advantage of coarse and fibrous diets is their ability to stimulate the oral lining tissues and enhance keratinization (Weinmann 1940; O'Rourke 1947). Alfano (1976) correctly points out, however, that the crevicular epithelium, which is under constant insult from bacterial plaque, is non-keratinized and no amount of dietary stimulation is likely to induce the epithelial cells to secrete keratin. This supposed advantage of a fibrous diet, therefore, cannot be substantiated.

8.6 MALNUTRITION AND GENERALIZED DIETARY INADEQUACY

Several studies have reported a high prevalence of periodontal disease in rural populations in countries where nutritionally inadequate diets are commonplace (Marshall-Day and Shourie 1944; Marshall-Day *et al.* 1955; Sanjana *et al.* 1958; Mehta *et al.* 1959; Green 1960; Ramfjord 1961). In this early epidemiological research the potential role of diet was not addressed. Further, the gross deposits of plaque and calculus that were reported would have made the interpretation of any nutritional effects difficult. However, a comparison of the periodontal status in young adult males in an Indian rural district with an aged and oral hygiene-matched group in Atlanta (USA) showed disease scores to be significantly more severe in the Asian population (Green 1960). Factors such as diet and nutrition were not reported but could have contributed to these observations.

Russell *et al.* (1961) investigated the periodontal conditions of Alaskan Eskimos and further assessed plasma levels of protein, ascorbic acid, vitamin A, and carotene. No association was detected between periodontal disease and the levels of any of these nutrients. A later study also failed to detect any strong relationship between plasma levels of the same nutrients and periodontal disease in South Vietnamese (Russell *et al.* 1965). However, there was a tendency for measures of disease to be higher in people from villages where the diet was deficient in protein, carbohydrate, riboflavin, and iron. Similar to many studies of this era, the overwhelming and controlling influence of plaque on periodontal disease in the underprivileged groups would have reduced greatly any chance of finding an association between nutrition and disease status.

One definite association between general malnourishment and an infectious periodontal disease has been reported in children who live in rural areas of Africa. In two separate and controlled studies the incidence of acute necrotizing ulcerative gingivitis was found to be as high as 25 per cent in undernourished children under 10 years of age (Enwonwu 1972, 1973; Sawyer and Nwoka 1985). Further, the prevalence and severity of gingivitis (which increased with the severity of malnourishment) improved considerably when 'proper' diets were provided to the undernourished children (Sawyer and Nwoka 1985). Paradoxically, the diets of these rural children were very high in fibrous foods (supposedly self-cleansing) and low in carbohydrates. The prevalence of caries was very low.

Another group of subjects who may suffer from a generalized nutritional inadequacy are the elderly. The Agriculture Human Nutrition Research Center at Tufts University (Massachusetts, USA) collected nutritional data from elderly people (at least 60 years of age) living independently in the community. When compared to standard values for adults, the study subjects had lower levels of vitamins K and B_{12}, riboflavine, thiamine, folate, and tocopherol. There was also a high degree of periodontal destruction and recession and a marked correlation between plaque index and gingival index (Papas *et al.* 1984). However, it would be wrong to attribute the periodontal destruction to the nutritional status, as a very high proportion of the attachment loss would have occurred over 30 to 40 years and before any nutritional problems. Only precise longitudinal data collected over a lifetime and relating rates of attachment loss to nutritional status would provide useful information.

8.7 PROTEIN DEFICIENCY AND PERIODONTAL DISEASE

Proteins are constituents of the organic matrices of all the dental tissues including the alveolar bone. The integrity of the periodontal ligament, the fibres of which are being remodelled constantly, is dependent upon a protein (amino acid) supply. A considerable amount of research in the 1950s and 1960s, therefore, investigated the effects of both protein deprivation and supplements upon the periodontal tissues.

The early research was carried out almost entirely on animals including rats, monkeys, dogs, and hamsters. Protein deprivation or restriction produced dystrophic changes in the periodontal ligament, a decrease in cementum formation, osteoporosis, and resorption of the alveolar bone (Stein and Ziskin 1949; Chawla and Glickman 1951; Frandsen *et al.* 1953; Goldman 1954; Person *et al.* 1958; Stahl *et al.* 1958; Baer and White 1961; Riar *et al.* 1964). The epithelial attachments remained largely unaffected. Further, when protein deprivation was combined with a diet of soft consistency, the pathological changes occurred extremely rapidly with marked degeneration of periodontal support (Ruben *et al.* 1962). These observations showed clearly that all of the periodontal structures (bone, ligament fibres, and cementum) are affected by protein depletion.

A series of studies of the effects of protein supplements on the periodontal structures in humans was conducted by Ringsdorf and Cheraskin in the early 1960s. Their initial reports indicated that a high-protein and low-carbohydrate diet had a significant effect in reducing sulcus depth and clinical tooth mobility, and in improving gingival health. These studies, which were conducted on dental students over only four days, had no control groups and the dietary changes were made only by recommendation of the investigators and without supervision. Two variables were involved, the high-protein and the low-carbohydrate factors

(Ringsdorf and Cheraskin, 1962*a,b*; Cheraskin and Ringsdorf 1963). Their later studies were more carefully designed. Different protein supplements were given and control groups included. The results were very similar to those of the earlier studies, as the protein supplements reduced mobilities and sulcus depths and resolved gingival inflammation (Ringsdorf and Cheraskin 1963, 1964; Cheraskin and Ringsdorf, 1964*a,b*; 1965).

8.7.1 DIETARY PROTEIN AND PERIODONTAL DISEASE IN DIABETES

Type I diabetes is often complicated by chronic renal failure, which reduces the synthesis of vitamin D. As a result, serum calcium levels are lowered and secondary hyperparathyroidism can contribute to alveolar bone loss. Under these circumstances a diet low in protein can slow the progression of renal failure by lowering serum phosphate and inhibiting glomerular hyperfiltration (Bergstrom 1984). Working on this hypothesis, Johnson and Thliveris (1989) produced histological evidence to show that a low-protein diet has a favourable effect in reducing alveolar bone resorption in streptozotocin-induced, diabetic rats. However, these are only preliminary observations and further work is needed to establish whether the regulation of protein in the diet can contribute to the management of periodontal disease in poorly controlled human diabetics.

8.8 VITAMINS AND PERIODONTAL DISEASE

Vitamins are essential and biologically active constituents of a diet, which cannot be replaced by other dietary components. The absence or scarcity of certain vitamins has been implicated as being a primary aetiological factor in the pathogenesis of periodontal diseases. Those that have been most extensively studied are vitamins C, A, E, and D.

8.8.1 VITAMIN C

Vitamin C (L-ascorbic acid) is the anti-scorbutic vitamin, which is present in a range of fresh fruits and vegetables and human milk. Man, non-human primates, and guinea-pigs are unable to synthesize vitamin C endogenously and are dependent totally upon dietary sources. A dietary deficiency of vitamin C that leads to scurvy is rare in contemporary society. However, scurvy is occasionally diagnosed amongst the elderly living alone at home, alcoholics, dietary faddists, and infants who are fed exclusively on sterilized milk and food.

A minimum daily intake of 10 mg ascorbic acid is protective against scurvy (Bartley *et al.* 1953). The precise daily requirement of ascorbic acid has not been defined but it is generally considered that an intake of about 30 mg will satisfy all metabolic requirements and allow for an individual's daily variations and for degradation of the vitamin during food preparation. A daily intake of more than 100 mg would saturate the plasma and much of the dose would be excreted in the urine (El Ashiry *et al.* 1969).

Ascorbic acid and connective tissue metbolism

The precise role of ascorbic acid in metabolism is not clear but it has been established that the vitamin contributes to the formation of collagen, bone matrix (glycosaminoglycans), and the intercellular cement substance of the endothelial compartment in the vascular tree (Follis 1948). One major function of the vitamin is its involvement in the hydroxylation of lysine and proline, which occurs in the formation of the collagen molecule. The vitamin may also be associated with the enzyme alkaline phosphatase, which is present in high concentrations in the vicinity of collagen formation (Jenkins 1978). Experiments have shown that the alkaline phosphatase activity is reduced significantly in ascorbic acid-deficient guinea-pigs (Kanouse 1966; Cabrini and Carranza 1963).

Formed collagen, however, is unaffected by a depletion of ascorbic acid and so alteration in the structure of the fibres of the periodontal ligament will result from the inability of the host to synthesize and repair rather than an inability to maintain mature fibres (Waerhaug 1958). Ascorbic acid deficiency does not appear to reduce the number of fibroblasts present in connective tissues (Gersh and Catchpole 1949; Chen and Postlethwait 1961).

Ascorbic acid and polymorphonuclear leukocytes

The concentration of ascorbic acid in white blood cells is about 16 mg/100 ml, which is both higher and more constant than the level in plasma (0.5–1.0 mg/100 ml). The plasma level is particularly sensitive to variations in diet, stress, nicotine intake, and the use of oral contraceptives (Rivers 1975; Pelletier 1977). On a vitamin C-free diet the plasma levels will fall to zero after about six weeks whereas the whole blood content will not be depleted until about three months.

These findings suggest that the vitamin is important in maintaining the function of the white cells, although the evidence for this is somewhat equivocal. In an *in vitro* study, Nungester and Ames (1948) found that a deficiency of ascorbic acid impaired the phagocytic capacity of leukocytes. Later, *in vivo* work, however, indicated that the bactericidal activity of leukocytes was impaired when the daily intake of ascorbate was increased to 2 g (Shilotri and Bhat 1977). A number of *in vitro* studies have shown that ascorbic acid supplements are able to stimulate the hexose monophosphate shunt of polymorphs and so increase their chemotactic ability (De Chatelet *et al.* 1972; Goetzl *et al.* 1974). The mobility of these cells is also increased. If polymorphs are dependent upon ascorbic acid to maintain their migratory (and possibly phagocytotic) abilities, then a deficiency of the vitamin would increase the susceptibility of the dentogingival area to bacterial attack. The first line of host defence would be impaired.

Clinical features of scurvy

The presenting signs and symptoms of scurvy are associated with the impaired production of collagen and intercellular ground substance and with the resulting weakness of capillary walls. Common signs include petechiae, ecchymoses, and spontaneous bruising of the extremities. Haematuria, epistaxis, and bleeding into tissues, joints, and muscles occur (Touyz 1984). Vascular congestion in the hair follicles leads to enlargement, keratosis, and a localized reddening of the skin. If the haemorrhages are in the subperiosteal region of the long bones, then severe pain and tenderness can occur.

Anaemia may result from the loss of blood. A generalized lethargy and increased susceptibility to infections have been reported (Ralli and Sherry 1941; Exton-Smith 1979). Wound healing is impaired, particularly in the deeper aspects of wounds that rely upon capillary growth and the production of collagen fibres for successful organization.

Periodontal features of scurvy

The oral symptoms that are associated with scurvy can be very similar to those of a chronic, oedematous gingivitis but occasionally their severity is conclusive in securing a diagnosis of the generalized condition (Falconer 1979; Touyz 1984).

The oral inflammation, which is exacerbated by poor oral hygiene, can involve the free gingiva, attached gingiva, and the alveolar mucosa. In severe cases the gingiva become brilliant red, tender, and grossly swollen. The spongy tissues are extremely hyperaemic and bleed spontaneously or on gentle stimulation such as occurs on chewing (Stolman 1961). In long-standing cases the tissues attain a darkish blue or purple hue, which can complicate the diagnosis and suggest more life-threatening conditions such as leukaemia. Ulceration may develop and lead to secondary infections.

Alveolar bone resorption with increased tooth mobility has been described (Shaw 1978), although true loss of attachment and pocket formation do not occur as a result of ascorbic acid deficiency alone (Boyle 1937; Waerhaug 1958).

Histopathology of oral scurvy

Pathological changes can be identified in both the epithelial and connective tissues. Gingival epithelium undergoes thinning and may show spongiosis. When severe atrophy occurs, blood will exude through breaks in the epithelial layer. The lamina propria of the gingiva shows structural disorganization with poorly formed collagen fibres and many thin-walled and leaking blood vessels (Touyz 1984).

Evidence for the role of ascorbic acid in periodontal disease

The most widely researched field within the subject of nutrition and periodontal disease is that of the role of ascorbic acid in the aetiology, prevention, and treatment of the disease. The details of many of the earlier studies in this field will not be reviewed here and the reader is referred to the appropriate review articles (El Ashiry *et al.* 1969; Woolfe *et al.* 1980). However, a summary of the findings will be useful before consideration is given to how ascorbic acid and periodontal disease are associated.

Animal studies

The early experimental animal studies of the effects of ascorbic acid deficiency on the periodontal tissues demonstrated that, in both monkeys and guinea-pigs, periodontal pathology could be induced by omitting the vitamin from the diet. Boyle believed that the deficiency produced atrophic changes in the gingiva and underlying bone in guinea-pigs (Boyle 1937, 1938). Others have described changes similar, but not identical, to those of a plaque-induced periodontitis in humans. They include bleeding and flabby gingiva, osteoporosis and resorption of alveolar bone, rupture of periodontal ligament fibres, widening of the periodontal membrane space, and increased tooth mobility (Tomlinson 1939; Topping and Fraser 1939; Glickman 1948; Turseky and Glickman 1954; Dunphy *et al.* 1956; Waerhaug 1958; Hunt and Paynter 1959). Dreizen and Stone (1961), however, were careful to point out that plaque and calculus need to be present before pocket formation can occur. This finding, when considered with the results of later research, is particularly significant. Indeed, Alvares *et al.* (1981) failed to induce spontaneous gingivitis or periodontitis after 23 weeks feeding with an ascorbate-deficient diet. However, when plaque-associated lesions were induced the pocket depths were significantly greater in animals with a subclinical ascorbate deficiency than in pair-fed controls. This would indicate that ascorbic acid deficiency is unlikely to be an initiating factor in inflammatory periodontal disease, although it may enhance a plaque-induced lesion that is already present (Woolfe *et al.* 1980).

Human studies

The findings of the numerous studies of vitamin C status and human periodontal disease have failed to produce clear scientific evidence of a relationship between these variables.

One group of proponents concluded that when the plasma levels of vitamin C are lowered then some degree of gingivitis or periodontal disease will ensue (Barahal and Priestman 1942; Blockley and Baenziger 1942; Stuhl 1943; Kyhos *et al.* 1944). The classical and perhaps most widely quoted study was that undertaken by Crandon *et al.* (1940). Crandon consumed a vitamin C-deficient diet for six months and only after the fifth month was a slightly boggy gingival appearance found. Irregularities of the lamina dura appeared at this time, although the oral changes occurred almost two months after skin lesions were detected. These observations have been contradicted by the findings of both extensive epidemiological and longitudinal clinical trials, which did not find a significant correlation between ascorbic acid status and either gingival health or periodontal destruction (Burrill 1942; Restarski and Pijoan 1944; Perlitsh *et al.* 1961; Russell 1962, 1963; Barros and Witkop 1963; Russell *et al.* 1965; Shannon 1965; Enwonwu and Edozien 1970; Buzina *et al.* 1973). Nevertheless, although low plasma levels of ascorbic acid may not alone initiate periodontal lesions and patients with severe scurvy can have healthy gingiva, it is possible that a deficiency of vitamin C will exacerbate an existing gingivitis (Hodges *et al.* 1971).

There are also conflicting results from studies in which supplementation with ascorbic acid has been used, either alone or when combined with local measures, in the treatment of periodontal diseases. Cohen (1955) showed that, in the absence of local periodontal treatment, a 500 mg oral dose of ascorbic acid improved markedly the gingival condition in teenagers after 90 days. Over a similar trial period, larger daily doses of ascorbic acid (1–3 g) have reduced irregularities in the lamina dura of young adults and it has been suggested that this is due to a consolidation of the collagen at the alveolar bone/cementum interface (Cowan 1976). Furthermore, daily supplements of only 25–75 mg have been reported to improve periodontal health (Kyhos *et al.* 1944). Ultrastructural observations tend to support these clinical findings. Aurer-Kozelj *et al.* (1982) found that daily supplements of 70 mg ascorbic acid given for six weeks produced marked changes in the structure of the epithelium and connective tissue of the gingival lamina propria. Desmosomal junctions between epithelial cells became longer and the contact surface between cells increased. They suggested that the number of collagen-producing fibroblasts increases with ascorbic acid intake, as excreted collagen was indentified in large numbers of bundles in the vicinity of the cells.

In addition to the administration of ascorbic acid in tablet form, a number of workers have reported that gingivitis can be resolved by supplementing a diet with pure fruit juices such as orange, lemon, and grapefruit (Hanke *et al.* 1933a,b; Mead 1944; Thomas 1954, Thomas *et al.* 1962). However, it is now known that the frequent and long-term imbibition of large quantities of citrus drinks can cause extensive dental erosion. The recommendation of such regimens to prevent or treat a localized disease such as gingivitis must be considered unwarranted.

In contrast to the studies that have shown that ascorbic acid supplements are beneficial in maintaining a healthy periodontium, a number of reports have failed to provide such evidence (Ungley and Horton 1943; Parfitt and Hand 1963; Dachi *et al.* 1966). In controlled trials, neither large-dose/short-term nor small-dose/long-term regimens have proved to be effective (Kutscher 1953; Pierce *et al.* 1960). Further, the topical application of ascorbic acid by rinsing has no significant action on plaque formation or gingivitis (Flotra *et al.* 1969).

Ascorbic acid has been found to be beneficial in the treatment of gingivitis when administration was combined with local measures. Linghorne *et al.* (1946) showed that high doses (375 mg/day) of the vitamin, when given alone, had no effect on established inflammation. When smaller doses (75 mg/day) were used as an adjunct to scaling and prophylaxis, then the incidence of the recurrence of inflammation was reduced. Combination therapy has also been shown to be more effective than prophylaxis or ascorbic acid alone in reducing gingivitis (El Ashiry *et al.* 1964a,b).

The use of vitamin C in the treatment of ascorbutic patients with periodontal disease must be considered outdated. Local treatments such as scaling and root planing are more effective and more predictable than dietary supplementation with ascorbic acid. Dietary supplementation is no longer considered to be associated with improved periodontal health (Ismail *et al.* 1983) and is certainly not fulfilling

an important principle of basic medicine—removal of the cause. Further, the excessive intake of ascorbic acid may precipitate problems such as renal calculi and diarrhoea (Briggs *et al.* 1973) and can also interfere with the action of certain drugs including warfarin and aspirin (Rosenthal 1971; Loh and Wilson 1975).

8.8.2 VITAMIN D, CALCIUM AND PHOSPHATE

The cardinal sign of periodontal disease is loss of connective tissue attachment including the resorption of alveolar bone. Consequently, a certain amount of research interest, principally during the 1960s, was directed towards the possible periodontal manifestations of a dietary (or metabolic) imbalance of vitamin D, calcium, and phosphate.

Vitamin D

Vitamin D (cholecalciferol) itself is inactive but is converted to the active form (1,25-dihydroxycholecalciferol) by two hydroxylation reactions. These occur primarily in the liver and kidney. The active form of vitamin D acts to promote the retention of calcium and phosphate in the body. The principal actions are to increase the absorption of calcium in the small intestine and to mobilize calcium from formed bone (in an attempt to maintain plasma levels). There is some evidence that the hormonal metabolite of vitamin D can be reduced in some individuals with advancing age. This may lead to reduced absorption of calcium, resulting in secondary hyperparathyroidism and bone resorption (Bland 1984).

Much of the scientific evidence for the periodontal changes that result from a vitamin D deficiency has been gained from animal experiments. Oliver (1969) and his co-workers (1972) studied the periodontal tissues of the rat because of similarities to the human tooth-supporting tissues. There were no significant changes in the periodontal tissues of rats deficient in vitamin D alone. However, in calcium-deficient rats and animals suffering from a deficiency of both calcium and vitamin D there was a reduction of alveolar bone mass and greater areas of unmineralized osteoid. In the periodontal ligament, the number and diameter of the dentoalveolar fibres were reduced and this may have resulted from an alteration in the masticatory activity due to the loss of the mineralized tissue. Later evidence showed, however, that the synthesis of insoluble collagen was reduced significantly in rats deficient in both factors, although not in rats deficient in calcium alone (Oliver *et al.* 1972).

The periodontal effects of overdosing with vitamin D in dogs have also been described (Becks 1942). Such changes, which appeared to be related to increased osteoblastic activity, included pathological calcification of the periodontal membrane and gingiva, osteosclerosis of the alveolar bone, and marked hypercementosis.

Calcium and phosphate

A great deal of controversy has surrounded the potential dietary role of calcium and phosphate in the initiation and spread of periodontal diseases. In theory, the hypocalcaemia and hyperphoshataemia that result from dietary imbalance of these ions will produce a nutritional, secondary hyperparathyroidism, which initiates alveolar bone resorption. The basis of this theory emanated from experiments on dogs by Henrikson (1968), who believed that these dietary factors are of greater importance than plaque in the pathogenesis of periodontal disease. Later experiments on rats and dogs failed to substantiate the theory. Findings suggest that, whereas a hypocalcaemic diet can produce inter-radicular alveolar osteoporosis and thinning of individual trabeculae, it will not initiate inflammation, migration of the epithelial attachment, loss of periodontal fibres or resorption of the alveolar margin (Svanberg *et al.* 1973; Bissada and DeMarco 1974).

The evidence implicating the importance of calcium in human periodontal disease is even more equivocal. Lutwak *et al.* (1971) found that daily supplements with calcium (100 mg/day) decreased gingivitis, pocket depths, and tooth mobility in an uncontrolled study of 10 patients. Further, in a controlled and cross-over radiographic study they also reported an increase in density of alveolar bone in patients receiving 1000 mg daily supplements for six months (Lutwak *et al.* 1971). Baer (1977), however, proposes that calcium does not play a significant role in the initiation or progression of periodontal disease and that the most important factor is the interaction between plaque and the host's immune response.

8.8.3 Vitamin E

Vitamin E (α-tocopherol) occurs in wheatgerm oil, animal fats, and grain, and was first isolated in 1936. Its physiological functions in man are not established, although animal experiments have shown that the deficiency state causes spontaneous abortion and impaired spermatogenesis. The precise role of the vitamin in the human reproductive system is uncertain. Evidence suggests that vitamin E may act as a lipid antioxidant and it has an important role in maintaining the stability of cell membranes and protecting red blood cells against haemolysis. The vitamin is widely consumed as part of multiple vitamin therapy.

Vitamin E and periodontal disease

The possible role of vitamin E in the management of periodontal disease is based upon its ability to interfere with the production of prostaglandins, which themselves are important in the development of inflammation (see chapter 11). On the basis of this assumption, Goodson and Bowles (1973) used vitamin E to treat 14 patients with periodontal disease and found a reduction in inflammation after 21 days, as determined by crevicular fluid flow. Cerna *et al.* (1984*a*) presented preliminary results which showed that long-term (12 weeks) administration of 300 mg vitamin E daily had a significant effect in reducing inflammatory changes in the periodontium when measured using the Periodontal Index of Russell. In contrast, a cross-sectional study failed to show a significant difference in serum level of

vitamin E in patients with periodontal disease when compared to healthy controls (Slade *et al.* 1976). Bland (1984) suggested, however, that more information might have been obtained from Slade's study if intracellular rather than serum levels of the vitamin had been determined. Serum vitamin E correlates with serum lipid, which was not standardized in that investigation.

Nevertheless, a specific correlation between vitamin E deficiency and periodontal disease will be difficult if not impossible to determine. This is due primarily to the wide distribution of the vitamin in oils, fats and grains (coupled with a recommended intake of only 30 IU) and the relatively high prevalence of periodontal disease (Slade *et al.* 1976).

8.8.4 Vitamin A

Vitamin A is essential for normal function of the retina; for the growth, differentiation, and maintenance of epithelial tissues; and for bone growth and embryonic development. These different physiological functions are mediated through distinct parts of the vitamin molecule, which are collectively known as retinoids. Animal experiments have shown that a deficiency of vitamin A can result in marked epithelial hyperplasia and reduced cellular differentiation (King, 1940), These changes are reversed when vitamin A is restored to the diet. However, in man, severe toxicity is associated with excessive use of the vitamin.

Vitamin A is present in a wide variety of food substances including dairy products, fish-liver oils, and meats. The storage of the vitamin in the body is enhanced by vitamin E.

Vitamin A and periodontal disease

The effects of a vitamin A deficiency on periodontal structures have been established for over 50 years as a result of animal experiments. In the soft tissues, avitaminosis A has been shown to produce localized gingival recession, epithelial hypertrophy, and hyperplasia in monkeys, guinea-pigs, and dogs (Mellanby and King 1934; King 1935, 1937; Topping and Fraser 1939; Mellanby 1941; Glickman and Stoller 1948; Miglani 1959). Hyperkeratinization was described in most but not all animals (Frandsen 1963*a,b*). Frandsen (1963*a*) expressed the view that, in species with markedly keratinized oral tissues in health, it would be difficult to assess accurately an increase in the thickness of keratin.

It is unlikely that a deficiency of the vitamin alone will cause gingivitis. Transient inflammation, gingivitis, and pocket formation have been reported in monkeys (Topping and Fraser 1939) and dogs (Mellanby and King 1934). However, later studies indicated that, in the deficiency state, infection and gingivitis are absent and that local irritation is necessary before an inflammatory response is observed (Boyle 1941; Glickman and Stoller 1948; Frandsen 1963*a,b*).

Changes in the alveolar bone are also evident in vitamin A deficiency. The reported observations have been contradictory and include the replacement of bone trabeculae with fibrous connective tissue (Marshall 1927; King 1935), reduced bone formation (Boyle 1941; Miglani 1959), and increased thickness of bone and greater deposition on the labial aspect of the cortical plates (Irving 1949, 1956; Schour *et al.* 1941). A theory was advanced by Frandsen (1963*b*) to explain, at least in part, these contradictory findings. He suggested that the main effect of vitamin A deficiency on bone is to suppress resorption by inhibiting osteoclast function. Osteoblast function may also be reduced (Frandsen and Becks 1962), although if the magnitude of suppression is greater in favour of the resorbing cells, then bone deposition will continue, albeit at a slower rate. The most significant factor for consideration in animal studies is, therefore, the time interval over which the bone changes occur.

Studies in humans have been unable to determine any significant correlation between the vitamin A deficiency state and periodontal changes (Russell *et al.* 1961; Waerhaug 1962; Cutress *et al.* 1976). Nevertheless, Cerna *et al.* (1984*b*) suggested that an increase in serum vitamin A may be responsible for improved periodontal health seen in studies on vitamin E, as that vitamin is known to inhibit the oxidation of vitamin A.

8.9 TRACE ELEMENTS

Alterations in serum levels of trace elements are more likely to be a result of the periodontal disease process rather than a consequence of variations in dietary intake. A positive and significant correlation has been demonstrated between serum copper and the severity of periodontal disease (Freeland *et al.* 1976). The inflammatory process itself is known to elevate serum copper (Gubler *et al.* 1958) and this may be related to a leukocyte factor that mobilises ceruloplasmin from the liver (Pekarek *et al.* 1972). Copper is also essential for the development and maturation of connective tissues (O'Dell *et al.* 1961). A copper metalloenzyme contributes to the stabilization of collagen (Burch *et al.* 1975), and Freeland *et al.* (1976) suggested that if this enzyme accumulates in blood or if copper is not transferred to the periodontal tissues, then an elevation in serum levels of copper will result.

Zinc levels in serum have also been studied and found to decrease with an increase in alveolar bone resorption (Frithiof *et al.* 1980). Zinc can inhibit several functions of polymorphonuclear leukocytes (Chapvil *et al.* 1977) and the ions also stabilize the cell membranes and inhibit the release of lysosome enzymes (Chapvil 1973). The reduction in serum zinc in periodontal disease, therefore, may stimulate both leukocyte function and the release of potent enzymes that will enhance the inflammatory process and lead to loss of periodontal collagen.

Not all workers have detected variations in levels of trace elements in periodontal disease. Kilgore *et al.* (1969) failed to find a relationship between serum levels of sodium, potassium, or chloride and periodontal status. Similarly, Miglani *et al.* (1969) could not relate serum copper to periodontal disease, although they did report a hypoferraemia with the advancement of disease. No obvious reason for this observation was given.

8.10 COENZYME Q AND CITRATES

Coenzyme Q is a crystalline quinone that was isolated from the lipids of beef heart mitochondria by Crane *et al.* in 1957. It is an important mediator in citric acid metabolism and has an essential role in the process of electron transfer during oxidative phosphorylation. The coenzyme also reduces the concentration of citrate in the tissues, possibly by stimulating the enzyme aconitate hydratase. The coenzyme is derived from dietary tyrosine and requires many vitamins and minerals to fulfil the enzymatic transfomations in its synthesis. A deficiency of any of these dietary factors could result in depletion of the coenzyme (Littarru *et al.* 1971). Coenzyme Q is now used as a collective term for five closely related compounds (Q_{10}, Q_9, Q_8, Q_7, and Q_6), which are designated according to the number of isoprenoid units at position 6 of the carbon ring.

Hypercitricaemia and abnormal citric acid metabolism have been suggested as aetiological factors in periodontal disease. Raised levels of citrate have been detected in serum of people with periodontal diseases (Tsunemitsu 1963; Tsunemitsu *et al.* 1964; Tanner 1967; Tsunemitsu and Matsumura 1967). Further, Simon *et al.* (1968) found a highly significant correlation between blood citrate and the severity of periodontal disease, which confirms that the increase in citrate is related to changes in bone metabolism (Suzuki *et al.* 1965). These findings were not confirmed in trisomy-21 subjects with periodontal disease (Cutress *et al.* 1969, 1971). Differences in metabolism and disease aetiology in Down's syndrome were forwarded as the reasons for the negative findings.

The increases in serum citrates mentioned above could be related to a deficiency of coenzyme Q that can occur in the gingiva of patients with periodontal disease (Littarru *et al.* 1971; Nakamura *et al.* 1973; Hansen *et al.* 1976). On the assumption that such a deficiency will impair oxidative phosphorylation, respiration, and citrate metabolism in the periodontal tissues, coenzyme Q supplements have been used to significantly reduce hypercitraemic conditions (Tsunemitsu and Matsumura 1967). Clinical improvement has also been reported (Littarru *et al.* 1971; Wilkinson *et al.* 1975) and Nakamuru and co-workers have stated that the therapeutic administration of coenzyme Q to patients with periodontal disease (and a nutritional inadequacy) should be combined with routine measures for maximum benefit.

8.11 GENERAL CONCLUSIONS

From the information presented in this chapter, it is apparent that the bulk of research into dietary and nutritional factors and periodontal disease was undertaken before the primary aetiological role of plaque (and its micro-organisms) became fully established. Dietary deficiencies, however, clearly have a mediating influence on the periodontal tissues and the nutritional status of periodontal patients should not be overlooked. Further, in special groups it is important to achieve a nutritional and a biochemical balance for maintenance of both the oral tissues and the host response to plaque. Such groups, which include the elderly (De Paola 1984) and those who may require dental implants (Greene 1977), may require nutritional screening and counselling, especially if elaborate and expensive treatment is to be considered. Whatever the case, dietary counselling and supplementation should only follow a complete nutritional assessment and, whenever possible, advice from a dietician (DePaola et al. 1984).

REFERENCES

Alfano, M. C. (1976). Controversies, perspectives and clinical implications of nutrition in periodontal disease. *Dental Clinics of North America*, **20**, 519–48.

Alfano, M. C., Miller, S. A., and Drummond, S. F. (1975). Effect of ascorbic acid deficiency on the permeability and collagen biosynthesis of oral mucosal epithelium. *Annals of New York Academy of Science*, **258**, 253–63.

Alvares, O., Altman, L. C., Springmeyer, S., Ensign, W., and Jacobson, K. (1981). The effect of subclinical ascorbate deficiency on periodontal health in non-human primates. *Journal of Periodontal Research*, **16**, 628–36.

Aurer-Kozelj, J., Kralj-Klobucar, N., Buzina, R., and Bacic, M. (1982). The effect of ascorbic acid supplementation on periodontal tissue ultrastructure in subjects with progressive periodontitis. *International Journal of Vitamin and Nutrition Research*, **52**, 333–41.

Baer, P. N. (1977). Calcium deficiency is responsible for the initiation of periodontal disease. (Letter.) *Journal of Periodontology*, **48**, 427.

Baer, P. N. and White, C. L. (1961). Studies on periodontal diseases in the mouse. IV. The effects of a high protein, low carbohydrate diet. *Journal of Periodontology*, **32**, 328–30.

Barahal, H. S. and Priestman, M. G. (1942). Relationship of vitamin C deficiency and dental condition in mental patients. *American Journal of Psychology*, **98**, 823–7.

Barros, L. and Witkop, C. J., Jr. (1963). Oral and genetic study of Chileans, 1960. III. Periodontal disease and nutritional factors. *Archives of Oral Biology*, **8**, 195–206.

Bartley, W., Krebs, H. A., and O'Brien, J. R. P. (1953). *Vitamin C requirements of human adults*, special Report Series, No.280, pp. 176–9. London, HMSO.

Bastien, V. G. J. (1960). Diet, its dynamics and dental disorders. *Journal of the Canadian Dental Association*, **26**, 332–40.

Becks, H. (1942). Dangerous effects of vitamin D overdosage on dental and paradental structures. *Journal of the American Dental Association*, **29**, 1947–68.

Bergstrom, J. (1984). Discovery and rediscovery of low protein diet. *Clinical Nephrology*, **21**, 29–35.

Birkeland, J. M. and Jorkejend, L. (1974). The effect of chewing apples on dental plaque and food debris. *Community Dentistry and Oral Epidemiology*, **2**, 161–2.

Bissada, N. F. and DeMarco, T. J. (1974). The effect of a hypocalcaemic diet on the periodontal structures of the adult rat. *Journal of Periodontology*, **45**, 739–45.

Bland, J. (1984). Childhood nutrition and oral diseases. *Journal of Paedodontics*, **8**, 319–36.

Blockley, C. H. and Baenziger, P. E. (1942). An investigation into the connection between the vitamin C content of the blood and periodontal disturbances. *British Dental Journal*, **73**, 57–62.

Bowen, W. H. and Cornick, D. (1967). Effect of carbohydrate restriction in monkeys with active caries. *Helvetica Odontologica Acta*, **11**, 27.

Boyle, P. E. (1937). Experimental alveolar bone atrophy produced by ascorbic acid deficiency. *Proceedings of the Society of Experimental Medicine*, **36**, 733–5.

Boyle, P. E. (1938). Deficiencies as a factor in diffuse alveolar atrophy. *Journal of the American Dental Association*, **25**, 1436–46.

Boyle, P. E. (1941). Effect of various dietary deficiencies on the periodontal tissues of the guinea-pig and of man. *Journal of the American Dental Association*, **28**, 1788–93.

Briggs, M. H., Garcia-Webb, P., and Davies, P. (1973). Urinary oxalate and vitamin C supplements. *Lancet*, **ii**, 201.

Burch, R. E., Hahn, K. J., and Sullivan, J. F. (1975). Newer aspects of the roles of zinc, manganese and copper in human nutrition. *Clinical Chemistry*, **21**, 501–20.

Burn, C. G., Orten, A. U., and Smith, A. H. (1941). Changes in the structure of the developing tooth in rats maintained on a diet deficient in vitamin A. *Yale Journal of Biological Medicine*, **13**, 817–30.

Burrill, D. Y. (1942). Relationship between blood plasma vitamin C level to gingival and periodontal health. *Journal of Dental Research*, **21**, 353–63.

Buzina, R., Bzodarec, M., Jusic, M., Milanovic, N., and Kolombo, V. (1973). Epidemiology of angular stomatitis and bleeding gums. *International Journal for Vitamin and Nutrition Research*, **43**, 401–5.

Cabrini, R. L. and Carranza, F.A., Jr. (1963). Alkaline and acid phosphatase in gingival and tongue wounds of normal and vitamin A deficient animals. *Journal of Periodontology*, **34**, 74–9.

Carlsson, J. (1965a). Effect of diet and early plaque formation in man. *Odontologisk Revy*, **16**, 112–25.

Carlsson, J. (1965b). Effect of diet on presence of *Streptococcus salivarius* in dental plaque and saliva. *Odontologisk Revy*, **16**, 336–47.

Cerna, H., Fiala, B., Fingerova, H., Pohanka, E., and Szwarcon, A. (1984a). Contribution to indication of total therapy with vitamin E in chronic periodontal disease (pilot study). *Acta Universitatis Palackianae Olomucensis Facultatis Medicae*, **107**, 167–70.

Cerna, H., Fiala, B., Fingerova, H., and Pohanka, J. (1984b). Vitamin A level in patients with chronic periodontal disease. Preliminary notice. *Acta Universitatis Palackianae Olomucensis Facultatis Medicae*, **107**, 163–5.

Chapvil, M. (1973). New aspects in the biological role of zinc: a stabiliser of macromolecules and biological membranes. *Life Science*, **13**, 1041–9.

Chapvil, M., Stankova, L., and Zukoski, C. (1977). Inhibition of some functions of polymorphonuclear leukocytes by *in vitro* zinc. *Journal of Laboratory and Clinical Medicine*, **89**, 135–46.

Chawla, T. N. and Glickman, I. (1951). Protein deprivation and periodontal structures of the albino rat. *Oral Surgery, Oral Medicine, Oral Pathology*, **4**, 578–602.

Chen, R. W. and Postlethwait, R. W. (1961). Ascorbic acid in the biosynthesis and maintenance of collagen. *Surgery, Gynecology and Obstetrics*, **112**, 667–74.

Cheraskin, E. and Ringsdorf, W. M., Jr. (1963). Periodontal pathosis in man. III. Effect of relatively high-protein-low refined carbohydrate diet upon clinical tooth mobility. *Annals of Dentistry*, **22**, 13–18.

Cheraskin, E. and Ringsdorf, W. M., Jr. (1964a). Periodontal pathosis in man. IX. Effect of combined versus animal protein supplementation upon gingival state. *Journal of Dental Medicine*, **19**, 82–4.

Cheraskin, E. and Ringsdorf, W. M., Jr. (1964b). Periodontal pathosis in man. VII. Effect of protein versus placebo supplementation upon clinical tooth mobility. *Periodontics*, **2**, 69–70.

Cheraskin, E. and Ringsdorf, W. M., Jr. (1965). Periodontal pathosis in man. X. Effect of combined versus animal protein supplementation upon sulcus depth. *Journal of Oral Therapeutics*, **1**, 497–500.

Clark, N. G., Carey, S. E., Srikandi, W., Hirsch, R. S., and Leppard, P. I. (1986). Periodontal disease in ancient populations. *American Journal of Physical Anthropology*, **71**, 173–83.

Cohen, B. (1960). Comparative studies in periodontal disease. *Proceedings of the Royal Society of Medicine*, **53**, 275–80.

Cohen, M. M. (1955). The effect of large doses of ascorbic acid on gingival tissues at puberty. *Journal of Dental Research*, **34**, 750–1.

Cowan, A. (1976). The influence of vitamin C on the periodontal membrane space—a radiographic study. *Irish Journal of Medical Science*, **145**, 273–84.

Crandon, J. H., Lund, C. C., and Dill, D. B. (1940). Experimental human scurvy. *New England Journal of Medicine*, **223**, 353–69.

Crane, F. L., Hatefi, Y., Lester, R. L., and Widmer, C. (1957). Isolation of a quinone from beef heart mitochondria. *Biochimica et Biophysica Acta*, **25**, 220–2.

Cutress, T. W., Suckling, G. W., and Brown, R. H. (1969). Periodontal disease and serum citric acid levels in trisomy-21 (mongolism). *Archives of Oral Biology*, **14**, 1129–31.

Cutress, T. W., Suckling, G. W., and Brown, R. H. (1971). Periodontal disease and serum citric acid levels in trisomy-21. A further study. *Archives of Oral Biology*, **16**, 1367–70.

Cutress, T. W., Mickleson, K. N. P., and Brown, R. H. (1976). Vitamin A absorption and periodontal disease in trisomy G. *Journal of Mental Deficiency Research*, **20**, 17–23.

Dachi, S. F., Saxe, S. R., and Bohannan, H. M. (1966). The failure of short-term vitamin supplementation to reduce sulcus depth. *Journal of Periodontology*, **37**, 221–3.

De Chatelet, L. R., Cooper, M. R., and McCall, C. E. (1972). Stimulation of the hexose monophosphate shunt in human neutrophils by ascorbic acid: mechanism of action. *Antimicrobial Agents and Chemotherapy*, **1**, 12–16.

Deeley, W. S. (1976). Diet caused early man's dental ills. *Dental Student*, **54**, 102–4.

DePaola, D. P. (1984). Diet, nutrition and oral health: a rational approach for the dental practice. *Journal of the American Dental Association*, **109**, 20–32.

DePaola, D. P., Alvares, O., and Etzel, K. R. (1984). Nutrition and periodontal disease. *Tic* (Albany NY), **43**, 5–7.

Dreizen, S. and Stone, R. E. (1961). *Nutritional deficiency stomatitis*, Practical Dental Monographs. Year Book Medical Publications, Chicago.

Dunphy, J. E., Udopa, K. N., and Edwards, L. C. (1956). Wound healing, a new prospective with particular reference to vitamin C deficiency. *Annals of Surgery*, **144**, 304–17.

Egelberg, J. (1965). Local effect of diet on plaque formation and development of gingivitis in dogs. I. Effect of hard and soft diets. *Odontologisk Revy*, **16**, 31–41.

El-Ashiry, G. M., Ringsdorf, W. M., Jr., and Cheraskin, E. (1964a). Local and systemic influences in periodontal disease. III. Effect of prophylaxis and natural versus synthetic vitamin C upon sulcus depth. *New York Journal of Dentistry*, **34**, 254–62.

El-Ashiry, G. M., Ringsdorf, W. R., Jr., and Cheraskin, E. A. (1964b). Local and systemic influences on periodontal disease. II. Effect of prophylaxis and natural versus synthetic vitamin C upon gingivitis. *Journal of Periodontology*, **35**, 520–9.

El-Ashiry, G. M., El-Kafrawy, A. H., Bissada, N. F., and El-Mostehy, M. R. (1969). Vitamin C and the periodontium. *Egyptian Dental Journal*, **15**, 15–32.

Enwonwu, C. (1972). Epidemiological and biochemical studies of necrotising ulcerative gingivitis and noma (cancrum oris) Nigerian children. *Archives of Oral Biology*, **17**, 1357–71.

Enwonwu, C. (1973). Influence of socio-economic conditions on dental development in Nigerian children. *Archives of Oral Biology*, **18**, 95–107.

Enwonwu, C. O. and Edozien, J. C. (1970). Epidemiology of periodontal disease in western Nigerians in relation to socio-economic status. *Archives of Oral Biology*, 1231–44.

Exton-Smith, A. N. (1979). The clinical diagnosis of vitamin deficiencies in everyday medical practice. In *The importance of vitamins to human health* (ed. T. C. Taylor). pp. 127–38. MTP Press, Lancaster.

Falconer, D. T. (1979). Scurvy presenting with oral symptoms. A case report. *British Dental Journal*, **146**, 313–14.

Ferguson, H. W. (1969). Effect of nutrition on the periodontium. In *Biology of the periodontium* (ed. A. H. Melcher and W. H. Bowen). Academic Press, New York.

Flotra, L., Johanssen, J. R., and Gjermo, P. (1969). The effect of Ascoxal–T on experimental gingivitis and plaque formation. *Journal of Periodontal Research*, **4**, 171–2.

Folke, L., Gawronski, T., Staat, R., and Harris, F. (1972). Effect of dietary sucrose on quantity of plaque. *Scandinavian Journal of Dental Research*, **80**, 529–33.

Follis, R. H. (1948). In *The pathology of nutritional disease* (ed. C. C. Thomas) Springfield Press, Illinois.

Frandsen, A. M. (1963a). Periodontal tissue changes in vitamin A deficient young rats. *Acta Odontologica Scandinavica*, **21**, 19–34.

Frandsen, A. M. (1963b). Experimental investigations of socket healing and periodontal disease in rats. Effects of local roentgen irradiation; effects of vitamin A deficiency. *Acta Odontologica Scandinavica*, **21**, 13–111.

Frandsen, A. M. and Becks, H. (1962). The effect of hypovitaminosis A on bone healing and endochondral ossification in rats. *Oral Surgery, Oral Medicine, Oral Pathology*, **15**, 474–87.

Frandsen, A. M., Becks, H., Nelson, M. M., and Evans, H. M. (1953). The effects of various levels of dietary protein on the periodontal tissues of young rats. *Journal of Periodontology*, **24**, 135–42.

Freeland, J. H., Cousins, R. J., and Schwartz, R. (1976). Relationship of mineral status and intake to periodontal disease. *American Journal of Clinical Nutrition*, **29**, 745–9.

Frithiof, L. *et al.* (1980). The relationship between marginal bone loss and serum zinc levels. *Acta Medica Scandinavica*, **207**, 67–70.

Gersh, I. and Catchpole, H. R. (1949). Organisation of ground substance and basement membrane and its significance in tissue injury, disease and growth. *American Journal of Anatomy*, **85**, 457–521.

Gilbert, R. I. and Mielke, J. H. (1985). *The analysis of prehistoric diets*, p. 164. Academic Press, Orlando, FA.

Glickman, I. (1948). Acute vitamin C deficiency and periodontal disease. II. The effect of acute vitamin C deficiency upon the response of the periodontal tissues of the guinea pig to artificially induced inflammation. *Journal of Dental Research*, **27**, 201–10.

Glickman, I. (1964). Nutrition in the prevention and treatment of gingival and periodontal disease. *Journal of Dental Medicine*, **19**, 179–83.

Glickman, I. and Stoller, M. (1948). The periodontal tissues of the albino rat in vitamin A deficiency. *Journal of Dental Research*, **27**, 758.

Goetzl, E. J., Wasserman, S. I., Gigli, I., and Austen, K. F. (1974). Enhancement of random migration and chemotactic response of human leukocytes by ascorbic acid. *Journal of Clinical Investigation*, **53**, 813–18.

Goldman, H. M. (1954). Effects of dietary protein deprivation and of age on the periodontal tissues of the rat and spider monkey. *Journal of Periodontology*, **25**, 87–96.

Goodson, J. M. and Bowles, D. (1973). The effect of α-tocopherol on sulcus fluid flow in periodontal disease. *Journal of Dental Research*, **52**, 217.

Green, J. C. (1960). Periodontal disease in India: report of an epidemiological study. *Journal of Dental Research*, **39**, 302–12.

Greene, A. H. (1977). Dental implants, periodontal disease and nutrition. *Oral Implantology*, **6**, 567–83.

Gubler, C. J., Lahey, M. E., Cartwright, G. E., and Winthrop, M. M. (1958). Studies on copper metabolism. X. Factors influencing the plasma copper level of the albino rat. *American Journal of Physiology*, **171**, 652–8.

Hanke, M. T. *et al.* (1933a). Nutritional studies on children. The effect upon gingivitis of adding orange and lemon juice to the diet. *Dental Cosmos*, **75**, 570–80.

Hanke, M. T., Ghent, C. L., Marberg, C. M., and Bartholomew, M. D. (1933*b*). Nutritional studies on children. Further observations on diet as a factor in growth and as an aid in the control of gingivitis and dental caries. *Dental Cosmos*, **75**, 933–46.

Hansen, I. L., Iwamoto, Y., and Folkers, K. (1976). Bioenergetics in clinical medicine. IX. Gingival and leukocyte deficiencies of coenzyme Q10 in patients with periodontal disease. *Research Communications in Chemical Pathology and Pharmacology*, **14**, 729–38.

Henrikson, P. A. (1968). Periodontal disease and calcium deficiency. *Acta Odontologica Scandinavica*, **26** (Suppl. 50).

Hodges, R. E., Hood, J., Canham, J. E., Sauberlich, H. E., and Baker, E. M. (1971). Clinical manifestations of ascorbic acid deficiency in man. *American Journal of Clinical Nutrition*, **24**, 432–43.

Hunt, A. M. and Paynter, K. Y. (1959). The effect of ascorbic acid deficiency on the teeth and periodontal tissues of guinea pigs. *Journal of Dental Research*, **38**, 232–43.

Irving, J. T. (1949). The effects of avitaminosis and hypervitaminosis A upon the incisor teeth and incisal alveolar bone of rats. *Journal of Physiology (London)*, **108**, 92–107.

Irving, J. T. (1956). Frühe histologische Veranderungen in der Knochenformation bei Vitamin-A-Mangel. *Medizinische Klinik (Munchen)*, **51**, 690–3.

Ismail, A. I., Burt, B. A., and Eklund, S. A. (1983). Relation between ascorbic acid intake and periodontal disease in the United States. *Journal of the American Dental Association*, **107**, 927–31.

Isserow, B. (1978). A preliminary study on the role of diet consistency as a cause of periodontal disease in laboratory primates. *Diastema*, **6**, 19–21.

Jenkins, G. N. (1978). Chemical composition of teeth. In *The physiology and biochemistry of the mouth*, (4th edn), pp. 97–8. Blackwell Scientific, London.

Johnson, R. B. and Thliveris, J. A. (1989). Effect of low-protein diet on alveolar bone loss in streptozotocin-induced diabetic rats. *Journal of Periodontology*, **60**, 264–70.

Kanouse, M. C. (1966). Oxytalan fibers in the periodontium of ascorbic acid deficient guinea pigs. *Journal of Dental Research*, **45**, 311–14.

Kilgore, W. G., Shannon, I. L., and Terry, J. M. (1969). Systemic factors and periodontal status: sodium, potassium and chloride. *Journal of the Indian Dental Association*, **41**, 13–15.

King, J. D. (1935). Nutrition on relation to structure, dental caries and pyorrhea. *Dental Record*, **55**, 522–30.

King, J. D. (1937). Dietary deficiency, nerve lesions and the dental tissues. *Journal of Physiology (London)*, **88**, 62–77.

King, J. D. (1940). Abnormalities in the gingival and subgingival tissues due to diets deficient in vitaming A and carotene. *British Dental Journal*, **68**, 349–60.

Klinsberg, J. and Butcher, E. O. (1959). Aging, diet and periodontal lesions in the hamster. *Journal of Dental Research*, **38**, 421.

Krasse, B. and Brill, N. (1964). Effect of consistency of diet on bacteria in gingival pockets in dogs. *Odontological Revy*, **15**, 152–65.

Kutscher, A. H. (1953). Massive vitamin C therapy of chronic marginal gingivitis. *New York Dental Journal*, **19**, 422–4.

Kyhos, E. D., Gordon, E. S., Kimble, M. S., and Servinghous, E. L. (1944). Minimum ascorbic acid need of adults. *Journal of Nutrition*, **27**, 271–85.

Littarru, P., Nakamuru, R., Ho, L., Folkers, K., and Kuzell, W. C. (1971). Deficiency of coenzyme Q in gingival tissue, from patients with periodontal disease. *Proceedings of the National Academy of Science (USA)*, **68**, 2332–5.

Linghorne, W. J. *et al.* (1946). The relationship of ascorbic acid intake to gingivitis. *Canadian Medical Association Journal*, **54**, 106–19.

Loh, H. S. and Wilson, C. M. (1975). The interactions of aspirin and ascorbic acid in normal man. *Journal of Clinical Pharmacology*, **15**, 16–25.

Lutwak, L. *et al.* (1971). Calcium deficiency and human periodontal disease. *Israel Journal of Medical Science*, **7**, 504–5.

Marshall, J. A. (1927). Dental caries and pulp sequelae resulting from experimental diets. *Journal of the American Dental Association*, **14**, 3–37.

Marshall-Day, C. D. and Shourie, K. L. (1944). Incidence of periodontal disease in Punjab. *Indian Journal of Medical Research*, **32**, 47.

Marshall-Day, C. D., Stephens, R. G., and Quigley, L. F., Jr. (1955). Periodontal disease prevalence and incidence. *Journal of Periodontology*, **26**, 185–203.

Mead, S. V. (1944). Studies of the effect of the ingestion of citrus fruit on gingival haemorrhage. *Journal of Dental Research*, **23**, 73–9.

Mehta, F. S., Sanhana, M. K., Shroff, B. C., and Doctor, R. H. (1959). Follow-up study of the gingival aspects of periodontal disease and the local factors involved in its etiology amongst a group of schoolchildren in India. *Journal of the All Indian Dental Association*, **31**, 55–62.

Mellanby, H. (1941). The effect of maternal dietary deficiency of vitamin A on dental tissues in rats. *Journal of Dental Research*, **20**, 489–509.

Mellanby, M. and King, J. D. (1934). Diet and the nerve supply to the dental tissues. *British Dental Journal*, **56**, 538–49.

Miglani, D. C. (1959). The effect of vitamin A deficiency on the periodontal structures of rat molars, with emphasis on cementum resorption. *Oral Surgery, Oral Medicine, Oral Pathology*, **12**, 1372–86.

Miglani, D. C., Rajasekher, A., Shyamala, S., and Krishna Prasad, P. S. (1969). Blood studies in periodontal disease. II. Serum iron and copper values. *Journal of the Indian Dental Association*, **41**, 189–93.

Mikx, F. H., Maltha, J. C., Wolters-Lutgerhorst, J. M. L., and Franken, H. C. M. (1984). Age and diet composition in relation to experimental periodontal destruction in hamsters. *Journal of Periodontal Research*, **19**, 51–60.

Mitchell, D. F. and Johnson, M. (1956). The nature of the gingival plaque in hamsters. Production, prevention and removal. *Journal of Dental Research*, **35**, 651–5.

Nakamura, R., Littarru, G. P., Folkers, K., and Wilkinson, E. G. (1973). Deficiency of coenzyme Q in gingiva of patients with periodontal disease. *International Journal of Vitamin and Nutrition Research*, **43**, 84–92.

Newman, H. N. (1974). Diet, attrition, plaque and dental disease. *British Dental Journal*, **136**, 491–7.

Nungester, W. J. and Ames, A. M. (1948). The relationship between ascorbic acid and phagocytic activity. *Journal of Infectious Diseases*, **83**, 50–4.

O'Dell, B. L., Hardwick, B. C., Reynolds, G., and Savage, J. E. (1961). Connective tissue defect in the chick resulting from copper deficiency. *Proceedings of the Society for Experimental Biology and Medicine*, **108**, 402–5.

Oliver, W. M. (1969). The effect of deficiencies of calcium, vitamin D or calcium and vitamin D and of variations in the source of dietary protein on the supporting tissues of the rat molar. *Journal of Periodontal Research*, **4**, 56–69.

Oliver, W. M., Leaver, A. G., and Scott, P. G. (1972). The effect of deficiencies of calcium or of calcium and vitamin D on the rate of oral collagen synthesis in the rat. *Journal of Periodontal Research*, **7**, 29–34.

O'Rourke, J. T. (1947). The relation of the physical character of the diet to the health of the periodontal tissues. *American Journal of Orthodontic and Oral Surgery*, **33**, 687–700.

Papas, A. *et al.* (1984). Oral health status of the elderly, with dietary and nutritional considerations. *Gerodontology*, **3**, 147–55.

Parfitt, G. J. and Hand, C. D. (1963). Reduced plasma ascorbic acid levels and gingival health. *Journal of Periodontology*, **34**, 347–51.

Pekarek, R. S., Wannemacher, R. W., and Beisel, W. R. (1972). The effect of leukocytic endogenous mediator (LEM) on the tissue distribution of zinc and iron. *Proceedings of the Society for Experimental Biology and Medicine*, **240**, 658–88.

Pelletier, O. (1977). Vitamin C and tobacco. *International Journal of Vitamin and Nutrition Research*, **16**, 147–69.

Perlitsh, M. J., Neilsen, A. G., and Stanmyer, W. R. (1961). Ascorbic acid plasma levels and gingival health in personnel wintering over in Antarctica. *Journal of Dental Research*, **40**, 789–99.

Person, P. (1961). Diet consistency and periodontal disease in old albino rats. *Journal of Periodontology*, **32**, 308–11.

Person, P., Wannamacher, R., and Fine, A. (1958). The response of adult rat oral tissues to protein depletion: histologic observations and mitogen analysis. *Journal of Dental Research*, **37**, 292–300.

Pierce, H. B., Newhall, C. A., Merrow, S. B., Lamden, M. P., Schweiker, C., and Laughlin, A. (1960). Ascorbic acid supplementation. I. Response of gum tissue. *American Journal of Clinical Nutrition*, **8**, 353–62.

Ralli, E. P. and Sherry, S. (1941). Adult scurvy and the metabolism of vitamin C. *Medicine*, **20**, 251–5.

Ramfjord, S. P. (1961). Periodontal status of boys 11 to 17 years old in Bombay, India. *Journal of Periodontology*, **32**, 237–48.

Restarski, J. S. and Pijoan, M. (1944). Gingivitis and vitamin C. *Journal of the American Dental Association*, **31**, 1323–7.

Riar, D. S., Stahl, S. S., and Blechman, H. (1964). Effect of major salivary glands extirpation on periodontal tissues of young rats on various nutritional intakes. *Periodontics*, **2**, 157–61.

Ringsdorf, W. M., Jr. and Cheraskin, E. (1962a). Periodontal pathosis in man. II. Effect of relatively high-protein low-refined-carbohydrate diet upon sulcus depth. *Journal of Periodontology*, **33**, 341–3.

Ringsdorf, W. M., Jr. and Cheraskin, E. (1962b). Periodontal pathosis in man. II. Effect of relatively high-protein low-refined-carbohydrate diet upon gingivitis. *New York State Dental Journal*, **28**, 244–7.

Ringsdorf, W. M., Jr. and Cheraskin, E. (1963). Periodontal pathosis in man. IV: Effect of protein versus placebo supplementation upon gingivitis. *Journal of Dental Medicine*, **18**, 92–4.

Ringsdorf, W. M., Jr, and Cheraskin, E. (1964). Periodontal pathosis in man. V. Effect of protein versus placebo supplementation upon sulcus depth. *Parodontologie*, **18**, 83–6.

Rivers, J. M. (1975). Oral contraceptives and ascorbic acid. *American Journal of Clinical Nutrition*, **28**, 550–4.

Rosenthal, G. (1971). Interaction of ascorbic acid and warfarin. *Journal of the American Medical Association*, **215**, 1671.

Ruben, M. P., McCoy, D. V. M., Person, N. J. P., and Cohen, D. W. (1962). Effect of soft dietary consistency and protein deprivation on the periodontium of the dog. A preliminary report. *Oral Surgery, Oral Medicine, Oral Pathology*, **15**, 1061–70.

Russell, A. L. (1962). Periodontal disease in well and malnourished populations. *Archives of Environmental Health*, **5**, 153–7.

Russell, A. L. (1963). International nutrition surveys: a summary of preliminary dental findings. *Journal of Dental Research*, **42**, 233–44.

Russell, A. L., Consalazio, F., and White, C. L. (1961). Periodontal disease and nutrition in Eskimo scouts of the Alaska National Guard. *Journal of Dental Research*, **40**, 604–13.

Russell, A. L., Leatherwood, E. C., Consolazio, C. F., and Van Reen, R. (1965). Periodontal disease and nutrition in South Vietnam. *Journal of Dental Research*, **44**, 775–82.

Sanjana, M. K., Mehta, F. S., Doctor, R. H., and Shroff, B. C. (1958). Study of the relative importance of the various local factors involved in the etiology of gingival aspect of periodontal disease. *Journal of the All India Dental Association*, **30**, 55–8.

Sawyer, D. R. and Nwoka, A. L. (1985). Malnutrition and the oral health of children in Ogbomosho, Nigeria. *Journal of Dentistry for Children*, **52**, 141–5.

Schour, I., Hoffman, M. M., and Smith, M. C. (1941). Changes in the incisor teeth of albino rats with vitamin A deficiency and the effect of replacement therapy. *American Journal of Pathology*, **17**, 529–61.

Shannon, I. L. (1965). I. V. ascorbic acid loading in subjects classified as to periodontal status. *Journal of Dental Research*, **44**, 355–61.

Shaw, J. H. (1965). Further studies on the use of nutritionally adequate diets for the production of the periodontal syndrome in the rice rat. *Journal of Dental Research*, **44**, 1278–84.

Shaw, J. H. (1970). New knowledge of nutrition and dental health. *Medical Clinics of North America*, **54**, 1555–65.

Shaw, J. H. (1978). Nutrition In *A texbook of oral biology* (ed. J. H. Shaw, S. A. Sweeney, C. C. Carleton, and M. M. Samuel), pp. 405–6. Saunders, Philadelphia.

Shaw, J. H. and Griffiths, D. (1961). Relation of protein, carbohydrate and fat intake to the periodontal syndrome. *Journal of Dental Research*, **40**, 614–21.

Shilotri, P. G. and Bhat, K. S. (1977). Effect of megadoses of vitamin C. on bactericidal activity of leukocytes. *American Journal of Clinical Nutrition*, **30**, 1077–81.

Simon, E., Gedalia, I., Shapiro, S., and Margolin, V. (1968). Citrate content of blood and saliva in relation to periodontal disease in man. *Archives of Oral Biology*, **13**, 1243–7.

Slade, E. W., Jr., Bartuska, D., Rose, L. F., and Cohen, D. W. (1976). Vitamin E and periodontal disease. *Journal of Periodontology*, **47**, 352–4.

Smith, P. (1972). Diet and attrition in the Natufians. *American Journal of Physical Anthropology*, **37**, 233–8.

Sreebny, L. M. (1972). Effect of physical consistency of food on the 'crevicular complex' and the salivary glands. *International Dental Journal*, **22**, 394–401.

Sreebny, L. M. (1975). Food consistency and periodontal disease. In *Diet, nutrition and periodontal disease* (ed. S. P. Hazen). American Society for Preventive Dentistry, Chicago.

Stahl, S. S. and Dreizen, S.(1964). Adaptation of the rat periodontium to prolonged feeding of pellet, powder and liquid diets. *Journal of Periodontology*, **35**, 312–19.

Stahl, S., Miller, S. C., and Goldsmith, E. D. (1958). Effects of various diets on the periodontal structures of hamsters. *Journal of Periodontology*, **29**, 7–14.

Stein, G. and Ziskin, D. E. (1949). The effect of protein free diet on the teeth and periodontium of the albino rats. *Journal of Dental Research*, **28**, 529.

Stepnick, R. J. (1975). Is nutrition relevant to periodontal disease? *Journal of the American Society for Preventive Dentistry*, **5**, 16–22.

Stolman, J. M. (1961). Ascorbic acid and blood vessels. *Archives of Pathology*, **72**, 535–45.

Stuhl, F. (1943). Vitamin C subnutrition in gingivostomatitis. *Lancet*, **i**, 640–2.

Suzuki, T., Tsunemitsu, A., and Fosdick, L. S. (1965). Periodontal lesions in hypercitricemia: effect of insulin and some aconitase-activating substances on the blood citrate citric-acid level and the periodontal tissues. *Journal of Dental Research*, **44**, 309–13.

Svanberg, G., Lindhe, J., Hugoson, A., and Grondahl, H–G. (1973). Effect of nutritional hyperparathyroidism on experimental periodontitis in the dog. *Scandinavian Journal of Dental Research*, **81**, 155–62.

Tanner, H. A. (1967). The relationship of citrates to periodontal disease. *Journal of Periodontology*, **38**, 242–50.

Thomas, A. E. (1954). Some observations on the influence of orange juice injection on the teeth and supporting structures. *Oral Surgery, Oral Medicine, Oral Pathology*, **7**, 471–9.

Thomas, A. E., Busby, M. C., Ringsdorf, W. M., Jr., and Cheraskin, E. A. (1962). Ascorbic acid and alveolar bone loss. *Oral Surgery, Oral Medicine, Oral Pathology*, **15**, 555–65.

Tomlinson, T. H., Jr. (1939). Oral pathology in monkeys in various experimental dietary deficiencies. *Public Health Report*, (Washington) **54**, 431–9.

Topping, N. H. and Fraser, H. F. (1939). Mouth lesions associated with dietary deficiencies in monkeys. *Public Health Report* (*Washington*), **54**, 416–31.

Touyz, L. Z. (1984). Vitamin C, oral scurvy and periodontal disease. *South African Medical Journal*, **65**, 838–42.

Tsunemitsu, A. (1963). Blood citrates in severe early destructive periodontal disease. *Journal of Dental Research*, **42**, 783–5.

Tsunemitsu, A. and Matsumura, T. (1967). Effect of coenzyme Q administration on hypercitricaemia of patients with periodontal disease. *Journal of Dental Research*, **46**, 1382–4.

Tsunemitsu, A., Honjo, K., Kani, M., and Matsumura, T. (1964). Citric acid metabolism in periodontosis. *Archives of Oral Biology*, **9**, 83–6.

Turseky, S. and Glickman, I. (1954). Histochemical evaluation of gingival healing in experimental animals on adequate and vitamin C deficient diet. *Journal of Dental Research*, **33**, 273–80.

Ungley, C. C. and Horton, J. S. F. (1943). Bleeding gums in naval personnel, vitamin C and nicotinic acid intake. *Lancet*, **i**, 397–99.

Waerhaug, J. (1958). Effect of C-avitaminosis on the supporting structures of the teeth. *Journal of Periodontology*, **29**, 87–97.

Waerhaug, J. (1962). Preliminary report on WHO periodontal survey in Ceylon. October – December, 1960. World Health Organisation Report. *World Health Organisation Chronicle*, **14**, 482–3.

Weinmann, J. (1940). Keratinisation of the human oral mucosa. *Journal of Dental Research*, **19**, 57–71.

Wilkinson, E. G., Arnold, R. M., and Folkers, K. (1975). Treatment of periodontal disease with coenzyme Q10. *Research Communications in Chemical Pathology and Pharmacology*, **12**, 111–23.

Woolfe, S. N., Hume, W. R., and Kenney, E. B. (1980). Ascorbic acid and periodontal disease: a review of the literature. *Periodontal Abstracts*, **28**, 44–56.

9. Anti-plaque and anti-calculus agents

9.1 INTRODUCTION

Absolute periodontal health can only be achieved by maintaining a very high standard of plaque control. Such standards are attainable in the most highly motivated patients who are able to demonstrate the manual dexterity and skills necessary to remove plaque from all areas of the mouth. Other patients require professional assistance to maintain periodontal health and this includes a regular scaling and oral prophylaxis. All methods of mechanical plaque removal, however, are time-consuming both for the patient and the dental staff and for this reason, many patients are unable to persevere with newly mastered techniques such as flossing.

It can be argued, of course, that a completely plaque-free dentition and absolute periodontal health are not just unattainable but are unnecessary for many of the population. However, in certain patients, such as those suffering from juvenile periodontitis or a particular medical condition (see Chapter 3), even very thin and often undetectable films of plaque may predispose to excessive periodontal destruction in a short period of time. In such cases, high standards of plaque control are essential if tooth loss in later life is to be avoided. Further, certain physically or mentally handicapped people are unable both to clean their teeth effectively and to regularly attend a dentist's surgery. These people may also suffer from extensive periodontal disease.

It is apparent, therefore, that a need exists for means of plaque control adjunctive or alternative to the time-honoured mechanical methods. Consequently, much research has been directed towards the use of chemical agents in the management of periodontal disease.

9.2 PROPERTIES AND AIMS OF ANTI-PLAQUE AGENTS

The principle of chemical control of dental plaque has been determined according to certain criteria (Gjermo 1974). Chemical agents should inhibit the microbial colonization of tooth surfaces and prevent the subsequent development of plaque. Plaques already present on the teeth should be eliminated by dissolution or altered into less or non-pathogenic deposits by the chemicals used. The calcification of plaque into dental calculus should also be inhibited.

A large number of chemicals, including enzyme preparations, antibiotics, antiseptics, and surface-active substances, have been investigated to determine their suitability as anti-plaque agents. Unfortunately, there is, as yet, no substance that satisfies all the criteria of the ideal antiplaque agent (Bral and Brownstein 1988) (Table 9.1).

9.3 FIRST- AND SECOND-GENERATION AGENTS

Anti-plaque compounds have been categorized into first- and second-generation agents depending primarily upon their antimicrobial efficacy and relative substantivity (Kornman 1986). First-generation compounds include antibiotics, phenols, quaternary ammonium compounds, and sanguinarine. These are capable of reducing plaque scores by about 20 to 50 per cent and their efficacy is limited by their poor retention within the mouth.

Second-generation agents, however, are more effectively retained by oral tissues and their slow-release properties provide overall reductions in plaque scores of between 70 and 90 per cent. The bisbiguanides are examples of second-generation compounds. A similar level of plaque inhibition is achieved when first-generation agents are used four to six times daily and the second-generation compounds once or twice a day (Kornman 1986).

A summary of the most commonly researched and commercially available anti-plaque and anti-calculus agents, which are discussed in the following sections, is presented as Table 9.2.

9.4 ENZYME PREPARATIONS

Research into the use of enzymes as the active agents of anti-plaque preparations has been largely discontinued. Their use was based upon the theory that they would be able to break down the matrix of already-formed plaque and calculus. Furthermore, it was supposed that certain proteolytic enzymes would be bactericidal to plaque organisms and so act as 'disinfectants' when applied topically in the mouth. However, the results of clinical trials on both animals and humans have been disappointing and inconclusive.

Table 9.1 Ideal properties of antiplaque agents (Bral and Brownstein 1988)

Eliminate pathogenic bacteria only
Prevent development of resistant bacteria
Exhibit substantivity
Safe to the oral tissues at the concentrations and dosages recommended
Significantly reduce plaque and gingivitis
Inhibit the calcification of plaque to calculus
Do not stain teeth or alter taste
No adverse effects on the teeth or dental materials
Easy to use
Inexpensive

Although many of the more recently investigated enzymes have been directed towards inhibiting plaque development, a number of earlier studies observed the effects of enzymes on calculus formation. The use of a mucinase-containing dentifrice resulted in a reduction of calculus formation in a small number of subjects. Further, the deposits that did mineralize were generally much softer in texture (Stewart 1952; Aleece and Forcher 1954).

Preparations of dehydrated pancreas (Viokase) have also attracted considerable attention as anti-plaque and -calculus agents. Raw pancreas was defatted and desiccated to produce a stable powder containing trypsin, chymotrypsin, carboxypeptidase, amylase, lipase, and nucleases (Shwachman *et al.* 1955). These proteolytic enzymes are able to digest the toxic protein material that constitutes a favourable substrate for bacterial growth. In a well-controlled, longitudinal study of 134 subjects, Jensen (1959) showed that daily brushing with the enzyme powder reduced calculus formation by about 60 per cent. Gingival inflammation was also reduced by between 70 and 90 per cent and it was concluded that Viokase may be a valuable adjunct in the maintenance of oral hygiene. The beneficial effect of dehydrated pancreas on the inhibition of calculus formation has been confirmed by the results of later studies (Ennerver and Sturzenberger 1961; Packman *et al.* 1963; Bauhammers *et al.* 1968). The enzyme was also found to be effective in retarding the deposition of soft deposits and stain on teeth

Table 9.2 Anti-plaque and anti-calculus agents

Enzymes	Mucinase
	Dehydrated pancreas
	Mutanase
	Dextranase
	Lactoperoxidase–hypothiocyanite (Zendium)
Antibiotics	Penicillin
	Vancomycin
	Erythromycin
	Niddamycin CC10232
	Kanamycin
Phenols	Thymol (Listerine)
Quaternary ammonium compounds	Benzethonium chloride
	Benzalkonium chloride
	Cetylpyridinium chloride
	Domiphen bromide
Bisbiguanides	Chlorhexidine (Corsodyl, Eludril, Elgydium, Peridex)
	Alexidine
Bispyridines	Octenidine
Metallics salts	Zinc (Mentadent P)
	Tin
	Copper
Herbal extracts	Sanguinarine (Viadent)
Aminoalcohols	Octapinol
	Decapinol
Other surfactants	Sodium lauryl sulphate (Plax)

(Packman *et al.* 1963). Viokase-containing chewing gum has a significant effect on reducing plaque formation, although in a study of 91 subjects more than half complained of soft tissue irritation and a burning sensation on the tongue whilst the gum was being chewed (Allen and Courtney 1972).

Another proteolytic enzyme, produced from a mutant strain of *Bacillus subtilis*, also had a favourable effect on reducing stainable, soft, tooth deposits. This preparation was a mixture of neutral protease, alkaline protease, and amylase and was used daily as a mouthwash (Shaver and Schiff 1970).

The importance of proteolysis in plaque inhibition has been confirmed by the use of enzymes of fungal origin (Packman *et al.* 1963; Harrison *et al.* 1963). When the enzymes were incorporated into toothpastes, evidence strongly suggested that those with high proteolytic activity were more beneficial in retarding plaque formation than those that were highly amylolytic or cellulase active (Harrison *et al.* 1963).

The topical use of urea as a bactericidal, debriding agent of infected wounds led to its investigation as an inhibitor, both of dental caries and calculus formation. A double-blind, cross-over trial showed that a significant degree of calculus formation could be inhibited by the twice-daily use of a toothpaste containing 30 per cent urea (Belting and Gordon 1966*a*). Further, it was demonstrated that urea had the capacity to reduce preformed, artificial calculus deposits either by dissolving the mucoproteinaceous calculus matrix and/or by increasing the solubility of calcium salts in saliva (Belting and Gordon 1966*b*).

One of the most widely researched aspects of anti-plaque, enzyme preparations has been based upon their potential ability to break down and disperse the extracellular polysaccharides of the plaque matrix (see Chapter 2). Glucan hydrolases have been extensively investigated in both animal models and human clinical trials to assess their effects on both the water-insoluble, α-1,3 glucans (mutans) and the α-1,6 glucans (dextrans), which are water soluble. In an experiment on two groups of rats, an α-1,3 glucan 3 glucanohydrolase (Guggenheim and Haller 1972) was found to have a significant plaque-reducing effect in those animals kept in relative gnotobiosis for *Streptococcus mutans*. However, the enzyme had no effect on plaque formation in rats with their normal indigenous oral flora (Guggenheim *et al.* 1972). These findings confirm that plaque matrix is made up of a number of polysaccharide components and suggest that a specific mutanase preparation is only effective against the α-1,3 glucan component.

In a human clinical trial, a mutanase synthesized by a strain of *Aspergillus nidulans* was added to a sucrose solution and its effects on plaque formation compared to those of a pure sucrose solution. There was no significant inhibition of plaque by the introduction of the mutanase into the sucrose. However, bacteriological examination revealed that plaque harvested from the subjects who used the enzyme preparation contained a lower proportion of *Strep. mutans*. This suggests that these bacteria may depend upon the α-1,3 component of matrix to achieve colonization of teeth in humans (Kelstrup *et al.* 1973).

In a later, double-blind cross-over, clinical trial, Kelstrup *et al.* (1978) showed that a mutanase-containing chewing gum had a significant effect in reducing both the formation of plaque and the severity of gingivitis. However, no significant differences were found in the bacteriological composition of interproximal plaque of subjects who used the enzyme gum and those who used a placebo preparation. These findings contradict those of the previous investigation (Kelstrup *et al.* 1973) and it was suggested that, in the earlier trial, only 'suboptimal' quantities of enzyme were incorporated in the sucrose solution and the conditions for the action of the enzyme were far from ideal.

The enzyme dextranase has been studied as a potential agent for breaking down the α-1,6-linked glucan (dextran) in plaque matrix. Experiments on hamsters and rats have shown conclusively that, if dextranase is added either to drinking water or as part of a high sucrose diet, then the formation of plaque and the prevalence of caries can be reduced significantly (Fitzgerald *et al.* 1968; Konig and Guggenheim 1968; Block *et al.* 1969). Further, Block *et al.* showed that dextranase could both eliminate plaque formation and break down plaque deposits that had already formed on teeth. However, dextranase-resistant plaque was found in older animals with increasing time, and it was suggested that this may be due to the increase in numbers of filamentous organisms relative to those of streptococci.

In human trials the effects of dextranase have been inconclusive. In two studies, one on young adults and one on children, dextranase mouthwash had no demonstrable effect on plaque scores or its dry weight (Caldwell *et al.* 1971). However, the results of other studies conducted at the same time indicated that a dextranase mouthwash can be beneficial in preventing plaque formation and hydrolysing the already-formed matrix (Keyes *et al.* 1971; Lobene 1971). These contradictory findings may be attributed to differences in experimental protocol, such as the concentrations of dextranase used, the duration of rinsing, the methods of plaque assessment, and the age groups of the subjects. Indeed, the findings of Lobene's study were that dextranase does have an effect in reducing dry weight of plaque but has no apparent effect in reducing the plaque-covered surface area of the tooth.

Dextranase has also been incorporated into chewing gum and was found to significantly reduce the thickness of developing plaque over a 10-day period when compared to a placebo gum (Jensen and Loe 1971). Interestingly, the area of tooth surface covered with plaque was again only slightly reduced. Further, although the enzyme gum had a significant effect on plaque thickness, the severity of the gingivitis that developed was independent of the use of the enzyme.

9.4.1 LACTOPEROXIDASE–HYPOTHIOCYANITE SYSTEM

A more recently researched enzymatic system for reducing plaque growth is based upon the production of an intrinsic salivary inhibitor by a series of humoral factors and biochemical pathways.

Certain oral bacteria are known to produce hydrogen peroxide (H_2O_2) by the oxidation of the glycolytic enzyme

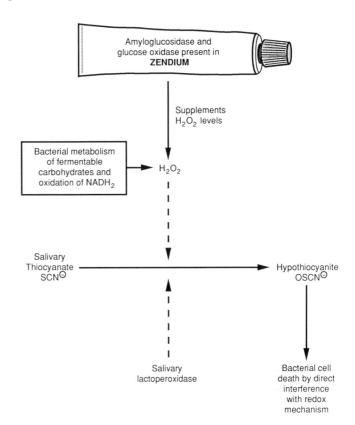

Fig. 9.1 The role of Zendium in the salivary thiocyanate–lactoperoxidase system of bacterial killing (see text).

$NADH_2$ by $NADH_2$ oxidase. Normally, this H_2O_2 is used to oxidize another $NADH_2$ molecule or is inactivated by the enzyme catalase. However, when the level of H_2O_2 in saliva is increased, it assists lactoperoxidase in the oxidation of thiocyanate (SCN^-) to produce the hypothiocyanite ion ($OSCN^-$), which is the hypohalite of thiocyanogen ($[SCN]_2$). The $OSCN^-$ interferes with the oxidation–reduction mechanisms of cells by upsetting the $NADH_2$–$NADPH_2$ balance. The lactoperoxidase and SCN^- essential to this reaction are both present in saliva.

The optimal H_2O_2 level required for $OSCN^-$ production is achieved by the introduction of a further enzyme system involving amyloglucosidase and glucose oxidase (Hoogendoorn and Moorer 1973). This system is the basis for the production of the commercially available dentifrice Zendium (Oral-B Laboratories). In addition to amyloglucosidase (1.2 per cent w/w) and glucose oxidase (0.3 per cent w/w), Zendium contains potassium thiocyanate (0.02 per cent w/w) and sodium fluoride BP (0.26 per cent). The role of Zendium in the lactoperoxidase–$OSCN^-$ system is summarized in Fig. 9.1.

In a series of laboratory experiments with rats the topical application of a paste containing amyloglucosidase and glucose oxidase was consistently found to be without inhibitory effects on plaque and the formation of early carious lesions when compared with a topical fluoride. However, significant beneficial effects of Zendium have been well reported in a number of controlled clinical studies using the dentifrice itself or a suspension of its contained enzymes as a mouth-rinse. The preparation has been successfully proven to be effective in the inhibition of plaque formation when compared either to placebo pastes containing no enzymes or to other commercially available pastes (Rotgans and Schmalz 1977; Rotgans et al. 1977; Koch and Strand 1979; Rotgans and Hoogendoorn 1979; Meskin et al. 1983; Schoenfeld et al. 1983; Midda and Cooksey 1986). Zendium has also been shown to have a significant effect on the reduction of gingivitis (Meskin et al. 1983; Midda and Cooksey 1986).

The results of studies in which the enzymes have been introduced into a solution have been contradictory. Koch et al. (1973) showed that a test rinse had a highly significant effect in reducing plaque formation when compared to a placebo rinse, whereas Afseth and Rolla (1983) failed to demonstrate any beneficial action of an enzyme rinse. A criticism of the latter study, however, is that the rinse was produced by making a suspension of the commercial tooth-paste. The vehicle of the preparation was, therefore, different to that intended by the manufacturers.

9.5 ANTIBIOTICS

The bacterial nature of dental plaque and its primary role in the aetiology of both caries and gingivitis has stimulated a considerable amount of research into the use of antibiotics in controlling these diseases.

The results of some early animal experiments indicated that the formation of plaque and the incidence of caries could be inhibited by adding antibiotic preparations to the diet (McClure and Hewitt 1946; Stephan et al. 1952; Fitzgerald and Jordan 1955). However, when penicillin was introduced into toothpastes and powders the effects upon caries incidence in children were inconclusive (Hill and Kniesner 1949; Zander 1950; Walsh and Smart 1951; Hill et al. 1953a). Furthermore, the constant use of such pastes did appear to enhance the development of penicillin-resistant streptococci in the mouth (Hill et al. 1953b). Consequently, the use of penicillin as a topical anti-plaque and anti-caries agent was abandoned.

Vancomycin is a bactericidal antibiotic that is poorly absorbed after oral dosing. The drug has been used topically both as an adhesive paste and a mouth-rinse in an attempt to control plaque formation. Mitchell and Holmes (1965) found that daily applications of a vancomycin-containing ointment markedly reduced the quantity of already-formed plaque in mentally retarded, institutionalized patients. When the applications were stopped the plaque scores returned to near baseline levels. As a mouth-rinse preparation, vancomycin has been shown to reduce the development of plaque, although the effect was not as dramatic as with tetracycline (Loe et al. 1967). The variation in the efficacy of the two drugs is because tetracycline is a broad-spectrum antibiotic whereas vancomycin is solely active against Gram-positive bacteria.

The administration of an erythromycin suspension, four times a day for seven days, reduced the quantity of plaque in adult volunteers by 35 per cent (Lobene et al. 1969).

Unfortunately, all the subjects suffered from diarrhoea during the study and a significant proportion of resistant streptococci were isolated for several weeks after drug administration.

Interest also developed in the macrolide antibiotic niddamycin (cc 10232), which was thought to be suitable for dental use because of its limited systemic applications in medicine. The drug was incorporated as a 0.01 per cent mouth-rinse in a double-blind clinical trial to assess anti-plaque and anti-calculus activity (Stallard et al. 1969). When the active mouth-rinse was used, reductions in plaque scores ranged between 11 and 23 per cent. Corresponding reductions also occurred in calculus formation (70–90 per cent) and gingivitis (55–72 per cent). Additional studies using varying concentrations of niddamycin rinses confirmed these findings and substantial plaque-inhibitory effects of up to 77 per cent were reported (Volpe et al. 1969). However, because of cross-sensitization between niddamycin and erythromycin, the clinical use of the drug was not developed (Mandel 1988).

Kanamycin is an aminoglycoside antibiotic that has a broad spectrum of activity. The drug was introduced as a 5 per cent, kanamycin–orabase, topical paste, which was studied extensively as an anti-plaque formulation (Loesche et al. 1971, 1977; Loesche and Nafe, 1973; Loesche 1976). When the paste was applied three times daily for five days, the development of plaque during the following three weeks was inhibited by 57 per cent (Loesche et al. 1971). Bacteriological studies showed that the reduction in plaque mass was primarily due to the inhibitory action upon streptococcal organisms (Loesche et al. 1977).

Kanamycin paste was also effective against established plaque and gingivitis when applied periodically for 40 weeks (Loesche and Nafe 1973). Plaque and gingival indices were stabilized at about 60 and 30 per cent of their baseline values, respectively, and no mechanical methods of plaque control were used during the study. Gingivitis was not eliminated and it was suggested that this was because the paste was not delivered into the gingival pockets (Loesche 1976). However, if the paste had been applied subgingivally, the additional effect upon gingivitis may have been only minimal as kanamycin is not effective against anaerobic bacteria.

Since the mid-1970s, interest in the use of antibiotic preparations to inhibit plaque growth and control gingivitis has waned considerably. The potential problems of bacterial resistance and hypersensitivity reactions are greater than the potential benefits of using antibiotics long term. Furthermore, there are now many alternative anti-plaque agents on the market and consequently a renewed interest in antibiotics for plaque control is unlikely.

9.6 PHENOLS

The phenols are a group of antiseptic compounds that have been used in medicine for over 100 years. Preparations of phenols and their derivatives have had widespread application as disinfectants, antiseptics, antipruritics, antifungals, and antimicrobials. The basic molecular structure of the

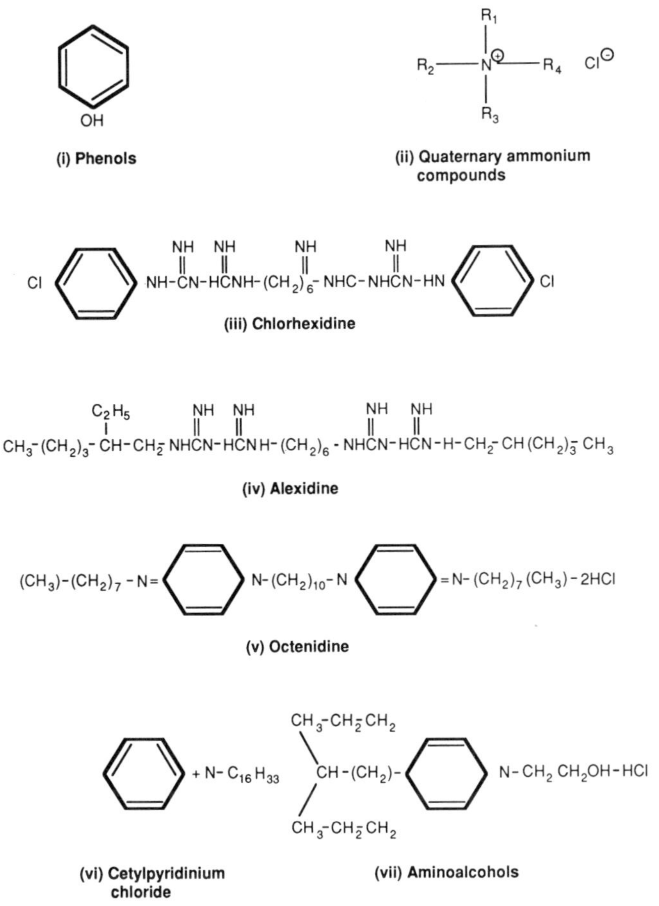

Fig. 9.2 Molecular structures of anti-plaque agents.

phenolic compounds is shown in Fig. 9.2. Most phenols exert a non-specific antibacterial action, which is dependent upon the ability of the drug, in its non-ionized form, to penetrate the lipid component of the cell walls of Gram-negative organisms. The resulting structural damage will affect the permeability control of micro-organisms in addition to several metabolic processes that are dependent upon enzymes contained within the cell membranes. Phenolic compounds have also been shown to exhibit anti-inflammatory properties, which may result from their ability to inhibit neutrophil chemotaxis, the generation of neutrophil superoxide ion, and the production of prostaglandin synthetase (Goodson 1985; Azuma *et al.* 1986).

Phenols have been incorporated into mouth-rinses for topical use as antimicrobial/antiseptic agents to inhibit plaque formation. Listerine (Warner-Lambert Pharmaceutical Co., USA) is an over-the-counter phenol preparation that contains thymol, eucalyptol, methyl salicylate, benzoic acid, and boric acid in a hydro-alcoholic vehicle.

The results of a number of short-term clinical trials demonstrated clearly that Listerine is an effective inhibitor of both plaque formation and the development of gingivitis (Kennedy and Kravets 1970; Gomer *et al.* 1972; Lusk *et al.* 1974; Fornell *et al.* 1975; Menaker *et al.* 1979; Mankodi *et al.* 1987). However, in two studies of 7 and 21 days, respectively, Listerine was used twice daily and no anti-plaque activity was demonstrated (Muhlemann *et al.* 1973;

Siegrist *et al.* 1986). Further, using the experimental gingivitis model, Siegrist *et al.* (1986) showed that when Listerine is used according to the manufacturer's instructions there is no effect on the occurrence and severity of gingivitis, or upon the prevalence of gingival bleeding on probing.

In a six-week study when Listerine was used as an adjunctive plaque-control method in patients with established gingivitis a significantly greater reduction in plaque and gingival index scores was seen in test patients than in controls (Axelsson and Lindhe 1987). However, it must be acknowledged that there are distinct differences in protocol between the Siegrist and the Axelsson studies. In the three-week Siegrist study the mouth-rinse was used in the absence of toothbrushing in an attempt to prevent gingivitis. In the six-week study by Axelsson and Lindhe, Listerine was used in addition to toothbrushing and in patients with established gingival inflammation. Consequently, it is difficult to confidently make direct comparisons between the studies.

In more recent, long-term trials, the efficacy of Listerine as an anti-plaque agent has been confirmed. Lamster *et al.* (1983), in a six-month, double-blind trial on 145 subjects, showed that Listerine reduced plaque scores by about 20 per cent when compared to the hydro-alcoholic vehicle and to water alone. The reduction of gingivitis scores was about 28 per cent. These results were affirmed in a similar, nine-month study by the same workers (Gordon *et al.* 1985), although the beneficial effects of Listerine in significantly reducing gingivitis were not apparent until after nine months. This was attributed to the better gingival health at baseline of subjects in the nine-month trial as a result of multiple prophylaxes undertaken at the start of the study.

As part of this latter clinical study, additional information was obtained about the effects of Listerine on plaque. When compared to hydro-alcoholic vehicle or to water alone, Listerine was found to reduce both the wet and dry weights of plaque by more than half after nine months' usage. The antiseptic also reduced both the protein content of plaque by about 60 per cent and the toxicity by 75 per cent, as determined by the limulus lysate assay (Fine *et al.* 1985). This suggests that the active agents in Listerine significantly affect the pathogenicity of plaque by reducing its overall endotoxin activity.

9.7 QUATERNARY AMMONIUM COMPOUNDS

Quaternary ammonium compounds (QACs) are cationic antiseptics and surface-active agents. The basic chemical structure is of a central nitrogen atom linked to four alkyl groups by covalent bonds. An electrovalent bond connects the anion to the nitrogen atom (see Fig. 9.2). The molecules have a net positive charge, which reacts with the negatively charged, cell membrane phosphates. The cell wall structure of the micro-organism is disrupted and increased permeability results. Quaternary amines tend to be more effective against Gram-positive than Gram-negative organisms. This may suggest that these antiseptics would be more beneficial as anti-plaque agents when used against early developing plaque, which contains predominantly Gram-positive bacteria. Benzethonium chloride, benzalkonium chloride, and cetylpyridinium chloride are the QACs that have received most attention as agents for plaque inhibition.

Early studies, which were conducted over just seven days, showed that cetylpyridinium and benzethonium chloride produced plaque inhibition of between 30 and 40 per cent (Sturzenburger and Leonard 1969; Volpe *et al.* 1969). However, Sturzenburger and Leonard found that cetylpyridinium chloride was only effective when used as a 0.05 per cent solution and combined with another QAC, domiphen bromide. A 0.025 per cent rinse of cetylpyridinium chloride alone had no anti-plaque activity, although it was not determined whether this was due to the weaker concentration or to the absence of domiphen bromide. In a later trial, cetylpyridinium chloride with added domiphen bromide was shown to have only slightly better anti-plaque activity than cetylpyridinium chloride alone (Barnes *et al.* 1976). No indication was given of the relative concentrations of the commercial cetylpyridinium mouth-rinses used. A good inhibiting effect of benzalkonium chloride was reported by Gjermo *et al.* (1970), but similar *in vitro* activity was not found with cetylpyridinium chloride. Both QACs did inhibit the growth of streptococci and staphylococci *in vitro*. It was concluded that the anti-plaque property of benzalkonium chloride was as a consequence of factors other than those associated with its antibacterial activity. A 0.075 per cent solution of benzethonium chloride was reported to inhibit plaque growth by 42 per cent in a study of 43 adults over 10 days (Compton and Beagrie 1975). This activity was significantly reduced when the benzethonium was combined with a 0.22 per cent solution of zinc chloride.

Other short-term studies confirm the anti-plaque nature of QACs (Carter and Barnes 1975; Ciancio *et al.* 1975; Lobene *et al.* 1979; Gargiulo *et al.* 1980; Llewelyn 1980), although the short-term effect on the development of gingivitis appears to be minimal (Ciancio *et al.* 1975; Compton and Beagrie 1975).

However, in trials of the effects of cetylpyridinium chloride on established gingivitis during periods of six to eight weeks, resolution of the inflammatory responses was observed. De la Rosa and Sturzenburger (1976) found significant reductions in gingivitis scores of between 25 and 58 per cent, but they recorded no observations of anti-plaque activity. In a placebo-controlled clinical trial in which patients with established gingivitis were instructed to supplement normal tooth-cleaning procedures with a twice daily rinse of 1 per cent cetylpyridinium chloride, a significant reduction in gingival inflammation was seen (Ashley *et al.* 1984*a*). When the plaques of the test and control patients were compared there were no significant differences in either the clinical scores or the microbial composition as determined by dark-field microscopy. The dry weight of plaque was 25 per cent less in the patients using the rinse. It is noteworthy that the mouth-rinse used in this study also contained 0.05 per cent zinc chloride but this may not have been of sufficient concentration to affect the germicidal properties of the cetylpyridinium (Compton and Beagrie 1975). Further, the absence of an effect of the cetylpyridinium on clinical plaque scores was a contradictory finding

to that reported by the same workers in a study on the effect of 0.1 per cent cetylpyridinium chloride on plaque growth over a 48-period (Ashley *et al.* 1984*b*).

The long-term effects of QACs on gingivitis and plaque have not been adequately investigated. In the only reported study over six months, Lobene *et al.* (1977) found that a twice-daily, 1-min rinse with cetylpyridinium chloride significantly reduced both gingivitis ($p < 0.001$) and plaque indices ($p < 0.001$).

The studies reviewed here indicate that QACs are effective inhibitors of plaque formation. However, if their efficacy is compared to that of chlorhexidine preparations (pp. 161–163), then their clinical usefulness would appear to be somewhat limited. The oral retention of QACs when assessed by their release into water rinses is about twice that of chlorhexidine. The desorption of QACs into saliva, however, is much more rapid (Bonesvoll and Gjermo 1978). Factors in saliva could influence the relative desorption of the drugs. It has been shown *in vitro* that calcium ions will displace cetylpyridinium chloride from carboxyl groups at lower calcium concentrations than those needed to displace chlorhexidine (Rolla and Melsen 1975). Further, the doubly charged chlorhexidine may bond more effectively to oral sites than the monovalent QACs molecules.

9.7.1 UNWANTED EFFECTS

Subjective side-effects of QAC mouth-rinses have been noticed primarily as burning sensations of the oral mucosa (Ciancio *et al.* 1975; Bonesvoll and Gjermo 1978). Objectively reported effects have included brownish discoloration of the teeth similar to that caused by chlorhexidine (Gjermo *et al.* 1970), a yellow-brown discoloration of the tongue (Gjermo *et al.* 1970; Compton and Beagrie 1975; Bonesvoll and Gjermo 1978), and a recurrent, aphthous-type of ulceration of the oral mucosa (Ashley *et al.* 1984*a*).

9.8 BISBIGUANIDES

The bisbiguanide compounds, which include chlorhexidine gluconate and alexidine, are the most effective anti-plaque agents currently in use. Bisbiguanides are the primary, second generation, anti-plaque agents as they exhibit considerable substantivity (Kornman 1986) and have very broad antibacterial properties.

9.8.1 CHLORHEXIDINE GLUCONATE

Chlorhexidine is a cationic chlorophenyl biguanide with outstanding bacteriostatic properties. The drug was synthesized and first reported by ICI in 1954, following extensive investigations of the biological properties of polydiguanide compounds (Davies *et al.* 1954). The molecular structure of chlorhexidine is shown above in Fig. 9.2.

Chlorhexidine is a well-tolerated and long-lasting antiseptic which is not neutralized by soaps, body fluids, or other organic compounds (Snyder and Finch 1982). Consequently, this compound was introduced for medical use in

1953 as an antiseptic cream for wounds. Its later applications included those of a presurgical skin cleanser, a surgical scrub, an obstetric cream, and an instrument sterilization fluid. The application of chlorhexidine as an anti-plaque and calculus agent was suggested by Schroeder in 1969.

Metabolism

When chlorhexidine is used as an anti-plaque mouth-rinse the mode of action is purely topical. The drug does not penetrate oral epithelium (Lindhe *et al.* 1970 *a,b*) and if some solution is inadvertently swallowed, initial binding of the drug will be to the mucosal surfaces of the alimentary tract. Chlorhexidine is poorly absorbed and almost all of the swallowed dose would then be excreted in the faeces. The small amount of chlorhexidine that may be absorbed is metabolized in the liver and kidney, but metabolic cleavage of the molecule is minimal (Winrow 1973).

Toxicity

Although the oral use of chlorhexidine can be accompanied by a number of characteristic unwanted effects (p.164), from a toxicity standpoint it is a relatively safe drug. This property is probably related to its poor systemic absorption. Topical use of chlorhexidine products in humans has established that concentrations of greater than 2 per cent may cause discomfort to the skin and that concentrations of up to 0.2 per cent are tolerated by the eye (Foulkes 1973).

Retention in the mouth

Chlorhexidine is the most effective anti-plaque agent. Its efficacy with respect to other compounds is related primarily not to its ability to kill oral micro-organisms (Gjermo *et al.* 1970) but rather to the specific pharmacodynamics that are associated with the retention of the drug in the mouth.

After a mouth-rinse of 10 ml, 0.2 per cent aqueous solution of chlorhexidine for 1 min. approximately 30 per cent of the drug is retained in the mouth (Bonesvoll *et al.* 1974*c*; Gjermo *et al.* 1975). The drug is believed to bond electrostatically to the acidic protein groups, such as phosphates, sulphates, and carboxyl ions, that are found extensively on the oral tissues (Gjermo 1975). Calcium ions in saliva are able to displace the chlorhexidine from the carboxyl binding sites and this mechanism may help to explain the prolonged bacteriostatic effect of the drug in the mouth (Gjermo 1975; Rolla and Melsen 1975). Further, chlorhexidine can displace calcium ions that are bound to the sulphated glycoproteins of dental plaque (Rolla and Melsen 1975). These findings suggest three possible mechanisms for the inhibition of plaque by chlorhexidine.

1. The effective blocking of acidic groups of salivary glycoproteins will reduce their adsorption to hydroxyapatite and the formation of acquired pellicle.

2. The ability of bacteria to bind to tooth surfaces may be reduced by the adsorption of chlorhexidine to the extracellular polysaccharides of their capsules or glycocalyces. This mechanism is of particular interest as further studies have demonstrated that when sucrose is added to bacterial suspensions *in vitro* the antibacterial effect of chlorhexidine is actually reduced (Davies 1973; Hennessey 1977). Production of extracellular polysaccharide increases dramatically in the presence of sucrose. A greater proportion of the drug will be absorbed by the cell coatings and less will be available to act upon the cell membrane to effect direct killing of the micro-organism (Hennessey 1977).

3. The chlorhexidine may compete with calcium ions for acidic agglutination factors in plaque (Rolla and Melsen 1975).

Laboratory studies have shown that chlorhexidine can bond to hydroxyapatite (Rolla *et al.* 1970, 1971; Bonesvoll *et al.* 1974a). The conditions under which this bonding occurs, however, are not usually comparable to those that may occur *in vivo*. For example, Rolla *et al.* (1970) demonstrated adsorption of chlorhexidine to teeth that had had their surface protein ground away before being immersed in 2 per cent solutions of the antiseptic for 5 min. From *in vivo* observations, Davies *et al.* (1970) suggested that the clinical benefits of chlorhexidine arise from its capacity to bind to both the inorganic and organic components of the tooth surface. However, it is now considered that it is the affinity of chlorhexidine for the acidic proteins in pellicle, plaque, and calculus and on the surfaces of bacteria and oral mucosa which is of greater clinical significance than its affinity for hydroxyapatite (Rolla *et al.* 1970; Waaler and Rolla 1985).

Factors that affect retention

A number of factors have been clearly shown to affect the binding capacity and plaque-inhibiting effect of chlorhexidine *in vivo*. After an oral rinse, the concentration of the drug in saliva falls rapidly and logarithmically during the first 4–8 h and shows marked variation between individuals. Over the following 12 h the rate of fall in concentration is reduced and the drug may still be detected after 24 h (Fig. 9.3) (Bonesvoll 1977). The proportion of chlorhexidine retained is directly dependent upon both the concentration and volume of the rinse solution. Approximately half of the quantity retained during a 60-s rinse will have bonded to receptor molecules in the first 15 s (Bonesvoll *et al.* 1974*b*).

The pH in the mouth significantly affects both the binding and release of chlorhexidine. Reducing the pH of the rinsing solution from 6.4 to 3.0 will reduce greatly the drug retention. The mechanism probably involves a reduction in the available, negatively charged receptor sites for chlorhexidine binding when the environment becomes more acidic. Increasing the pH, however, does not appear to affect retention (Fig. 9.4) (Bonesvoll *et al.* 1974*b*; Bonesvoll 1977). Reducing the oral pH by using acidic after-rinses also reduces retention of the drug and subsequent plaque inhibition (Gjermo *et al.* 1974). Free calcium ions have the capacity to reduce oral binding of chlorhexidine. The mechanism is likely to involve direct competition between the ions and the drug for available carboxyl groups on oral tissues (Rolla and Melsen 1975; Bonesvoll 1977). Bonesvoll further showed that the detergent sodium dodecyl sulphate strongly reduces chlorhexidine retention. As both calcium salts and detergents are invariably present in toothpastes, their use should be considered inadvisable either immediately before or after a chlorhexidine rinse or gel application.

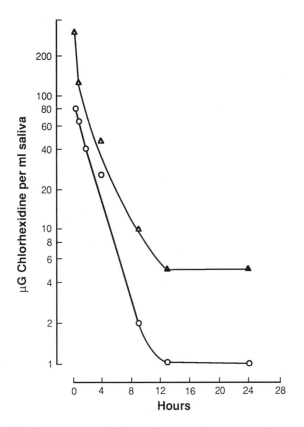

Fig. 9.3 Concentration of chlorhexidine in saliva, estimated from the [^{14}C]-activity of saliva samples, after rinsing for 1 minute with 10 ml of solution. $-\triangle-$ High retention subject. $-\bigcirc-$ Medium retention subject. Redrawn from Bonesvoll, P. (1977). *Journal of Clinical Periodontology*, **4**, 49–65. Permission from Munksgaard International Publishers Limited.

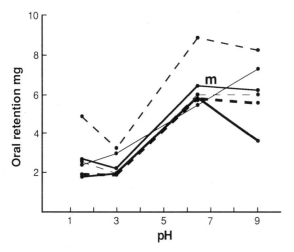

Fig. 9.4 Influence of pH of rinsing solution on the oral retention of [^{14}C]-chlorhexidine-digluconate. Mouth-rinses with 10 ml of a 0.2 per cent concentration for 1 min. 5 subjects. M = mean. Redrawn from Bonesvoll, P. *et al.* (1974c) *Archives of Oral Biology*, **19**, 1025–9. Permission from Pergamon Press.

Finally, there is evidence that teeth which are acid-etched, primed with sulphate solution, and then treated with chlorhexidine show more prolonged antibacterial activity than a series of control teeth in which any one of the above stages is omitted. This activity has been explained by the formation of crystals of calcium sulphate on the acid-treated enamel, which may then precipitate the drug as insoluble chlorhexidine sulphate (Turesky *et al.* 1977).

Bacterial killing

The mode of action of chlorhexidine in killing bacterial cells is dependent initially upon the drug having access to the cell walls. This is facilitated by the electrostatic forces between the negatively charged cells and the net positively charged chlorhexidine molecules. Having gained access to the cell membrane, chlorhexidine disorientates its lipoprotein structure, causing destruction of the osmotic barrier of the bacterium. Cell permeability increases and intracellular components such as potassium ions leak through the damaged membrane (Hugo and Longworth 1964).

A secondary action of chlorhexidine is to cause intracellular coagulation, which effectively slows down the rate of leakage of cell contents (Hennessey 1977). This cytoplasmic coagulation is responsible for the bactericidal effect of chlorhexidine and is directly dependent upon the concentration of the drug in solution.

Effect on oral bacteria

The short-term use of chlorhexidine causes a striking reduction in the number of oral micro-organisms. In the absence of other oral hygiene measures, chlorhexidine has been shown to reduce the number of bacteria in saliva by 85 per cent after only 24 h. A maximum reduction of 95 per cent occurred around five days, after which the numbers gradually increased to maintain an overall reduction of 70–80 per cent at 40 days (Schiott *et al.* 1970; Schiott 1973). With long-term daily rinses the reduction in numbers of salivary bacteria was between 30 and 50 per cent. This change was shown to be quantitative only, as the relative proportions of anaerobic, aerobic, and streptococcal organisms remained unaffected (Schiott *et al.* 1976b). In these studies, cessation of chlorhexidine therapy resulted in a return of bacterial counts to those that were found in matched control subjects.

The susceptibility of different strains of bacteria to chlorhexidine has been reported by Emilson (1977) in a study of a series of clinical specimens including dental plaque. A broad range of susceptibility was demonstrated amongst both Gram-positive and Gram-negative strains. Of the isolates tested, low minimal inhibitory concentrations (MIC) were found for staphylococci, *Strep. mutans*, *Strep. salivarius*, *Escherichia coli* and *Selenomonas*, whilst least susceptible strains were Gram-negative cocci resembling *Veillonella* (Emilson 1977). The effects of the structural modification of the chlorhexidine molecule on its activity against specific bacteria are discussed in detail on p.165.

The long-term use of any antibacterial agent can be associated with increased microbial resistance and reduced sensitivity. Bacterial resistance to chlorhexidine has been studied in depth by several workers, but the results have been inconsistent. In a two-year trial on the effects of a chlorhexidine dentifrice in humans, Gjermo and Eriksen (1974) showed that, on completion of the study, the oral flora of subjects was still sensitive to chorhexidine. However, in a controlled experiment on beagle dogs in which a 0.2 per cent chlorhexidine solution (or placebo) was applied topically each day for 12 months, Hamp *et al.* (1973) found that after 6 months the plaque, debris, calculus, and gingival indices appeared to escape the inhibitory effect of the drug.

Further, in another experiment on beagles, Briner and Wunder (1977) found that, although plaque organisms from dogs treated with chlorhexidine did show a slightly reduced sensitivity to the drug after 7 and 42 months, the reduction was not associated with a reduction in the efficacy of chlorhexidine against plaque or gingivitis. These findings have been confirmed in human clinical trials (Loe *et al.* 1976; Schiott *et al.* 1976*a*).

Although the findings are slightly inconsistent they have led Schiott and co-workers to suggest that the prolonged use of chlorhexidine tends to be selective towards strains of the more resistant bacteria in the oral flora. In effect, therefore, there is no actual change from susceptible organisms to resistant ones and so the effect on long-term plaque inhibition is negligible.

Clinical trials

The importance and efficiency of chlorhexidine as an antiplaque agent has emerged from the results of a large number of clinical trials. Investigations have been made on animals and human patients, and the vehicles of application for the drug have included mouth-rinse solutions, gels, and toothpastes.

Animal studies

In a study on beagle dogs the daily application of a 0.5 per cent chlorhexidine gel for 12 weeks significantly reduced the development of plaque, the quantity of established plaque, the formation of calculus, and the onset of gingivitis (Hull and Davies 1972*a*, *b*; Davis and Hull 1973). Similar effects on plaque and gingivitis were reported by Hamp *et al.* (1973), when a 0.2 per cent solution was used and the duration of the study increased to 12 months. However, after one year, the gingivitis and gingival exudate scores of the dogs that were given chlorhexidine had increased and were approximately half those of control animals. This suggests that the development or selection of chlorhexidine-resistant colonies in the oral flora had occurred.

The effects of chlorhexidine on the percentage of gingival connective tissue infiltrated with inflammatory cells are also significant. Histomorphometric analysis of gingival biopsy specimens showed that daily application of a 2 per cent chlorhexidine solution in rhesus monkeys for seven to eight weeks led to an infiltration of 0–6 per cent. Specimens that remained untreated had an infiltration of 16–40 per cent (Johnson and Kennedy 1972). The cells found in the infiltrate (plasma cells, polymorphs, lymphocytes) were those

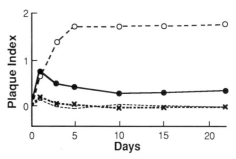

Fig. 9.5 Plaque index for the gingival areas of all teeth of the participants in the four experimental groups. ○−−−○ sucrose ●——● sucrose and chlorhexidine ×−·−× oral hygiene −−−− chlorhexidine. Redrawn from Loe, H. *et al.* (1972). *Scandinavian Journal of Dental Research*, **80**, 1–9.

normally associated with developing gingivitis in this species (Listgarten and Ellegaard 1973).

Human studies
Mouth-rinses.

The effects of chlorhexidine mouth-rinses on the development of plaque and gingivitis in humans have been well documented in clinical trials. In what is now considered to be a classical experiment, Loe and Schiott (1970) showed that twice-daily rinsing with a 0.2 per cent solution was effective in total plaque inhibition over 22 days. A once-daily rinse with the same concentration was not as effective and plaque deposits were evident between the posterior teeth. When the concentration of the solution was increased to 2 per cent and it was applied topically each day for 15 days, the inhibition of plaque development was again complete. The investigators concluded that a once-daily application of chlorhexidine is sufficient to inhibit plaque formation providing the active agent reaches all surfaces of the dentition. In a follow-up experiment, the twice-daily, 0.2 per cent rinse reduced plaque formation, even when it was supplemented by rinsing with a 50 per cent sucrose solution nine times each day. The inhibition of plaque, however, was not as effective as for subjects who rinsed with chlorhexidine only, or who practised mechanical oral hygiene procedures and had no sucrose supplements (Fig. 9.5) (Loe *et al.* 1972).

Chlorhexidine is able to reduce plaque formation and gingival inflammation even in the presence of existing tooth deposits and overhanging restorations. However, the effect is not as striking as when the rinse is used as a supplement to scaling and the reduction of overhangs (Flotra *et al.* 1972).

The anti-plaque effect of chlorhexidine can be affected by varying the concentration of the solution, the volume used, and the method of application (Cumming and Loe 1973). Generally, larger volumes of less concentrated rinses are as effective as smaller volumes of more concentrated solutions (Fig. 9.6). When the application of the solution is controlled by using an oral irrigating device, the resulting plaque inhibition, especially on posterior teeth, is improved (Cumming and Loe 1973). Under such conditions, 400 ml of a 0.2 per cent solution have been shown to be the lowest dose and concentration to inhibit plaque completely (Lang and Ramseier-Grossman 1981). Further, concentrations of

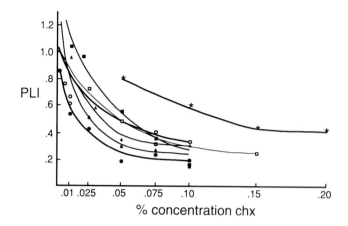

Fig. 9.6 Mean plaque index scores when irrigating or rinsing with various concentrations and volumes of chlorhexidine gluconate.
Oral irrigator
●——● 700ml
▲——▲ 400ml
■——■ 200ml
Rinsing
○——○ 200ml
△——△ 100ml
□——□ 50ml
—— 20ml
Redrawn from Cumming, B.R. and Loe, H. (1973). *Journal of Periodontal Research*, **8**, 57–62. Permission from Munksgaard International Publishers Limited

0.0033 per cent chlorhexidine or less do not differ significantly from placebo in their plaque-inhibitory capacity (Agerbaek *et al.* 1975). Longer clinical trials have confirmed that either brushing or rinsing with chlorhexidine solution have significant and beneficial effects upon the inhibition of plaque and the prevention of gingivitis. Loe *et al.* (1976) instructed 61 young adults in the daily use of 10 ml, 0.2 per cent chlorhexidine over two years as a supplement to routine oral hygiene measures. They compared these with a control group of 59 subjects who exercised routine plaque control only. The solution was applied with a toothbrush for the first eight months and thereafter given as a rinse. Chlorhexidine produced significantly lower plaque indices ($p < 0.05$) in the test subjects throughout the study; the corresponding gingival indices of the experimental group were significantly less than for the controls during the first 18 months ($p < 0.05$), although the difference became non-significant after 24 months. An additional observation was that the calculus indices were higher in the test group. It was suggested that a build-up and hardening of stain was responsible for this finding.

Very similar trends were reported when different concentrations of chlorhexidine were used as supervised rinses in children (aged 10–12 years) over a six-months period (Lang *et al.* 1982). Again, the rinses were an adjunct to routine oral hygiene methods. The effectiveness of different applications in reducing gingivitis scores was according to the ranking: 0.2 per cent, six times/week; 0.1 per cent, six times/week; 0.2 per cent, once/week. However, the plaque

reduction in the different groups did not differ significantly from one another.

One of the main problems with the long-term use of chlorhexidine is the severity of the unwanted effects that can develop (p. 164). Consequently, the more recent longitudinal studies have investigated extensively the potential use of 0.12 per cent mouth-rinses instead of the more concentrated 0.2 per cent solutions. In one of the largest clinical trials undertaken using chlorhexidine (on 600 adults), Segreto *et al.* (1986) concluded that a 0.12 per cent rinse, used twice daily over three months, offers the same clinical benefits as a 0.2 per cent solution. These benefits have also been reported when the period of observation was increased to six months (Grossman *et al.* 1986) and in the short-term, at least, a 0.12 per cent rinse has been proven to be superior to commercial products of both phenol and sanguinarine compounds (Fig. 9.7) (Siegrist *et al.* 1986). These findings tend to confirm the suggestions that the twice-daily use of a chlorhexidine solution of about 0.1 per cent concentration can adequately control plaque and gingivitis whilst minimizing the prevalence of side-effects (Bay 1978; Briner and Leonard 1980; de la Rosa *et al.* 1987).

The antimicrobial effects of the 0.12 per cent mouth-rinses are also similar to those of 0.2 per cent solutions. Trials conducted over six months have shown that a twice-daily 0.12 per cent rinse causes significant reductions in aerobes, anaerobes, streptococci, and particularly *Actinomyces* whilst producing no significant changes in bacterial resistance (Fig. 9.8) (Briner *et al.* 1986*a,b*).

Gels and toothpastes.

The results of investigations into the efficacy of chlorhexidine-containing gels and toothpastes have been largely inconclusive. In short-term, placebo-controlled studies conducted over four-week periods, the introduction of a 1 per cent chlorhexidine gel as an adjunct to mechanical plaque control had only a slight inhibitory effect on plaque growth and no effect on gingivitis (Hansen *et al.* 1975). However, subgingival deposits were not removed before or during the study, and consequently a significant reduction of gingival inflammation would not be expected.

The absence of an effect of gels on gingivitis was confirmed in another four-week study, although a significant effect on plaque inhibition was recorded (Bain and Strahan 1978). Similarly, in a series of three-day studies, Addy and Bates (1977) found that a 1 per cent chlorhexidine gel significantly inhibited plaque formation in denture wearers.

The observations made from a number of Scandinavian studies further complicate the situation. In a two-month, double-blind clinical trial on 53 students, two experimental toothpastes containing 0.6 and 0.8 per cent chlorhexidine both markedly reduced plaque formation (Gjermo and Eriksen 1972). When the period of observation was increased to two years, the effects of 0.4 and 1.0 per cent pastes on plaque and gingival indices were small and not significant (Johansen *et al.* 1975) but the lack of effect could be attributed to the development of chlorhexidine-resistant bacteria (Gjermo & Eriksen 1974). However, in previous trials the same pastes had shown anti-plaque properties

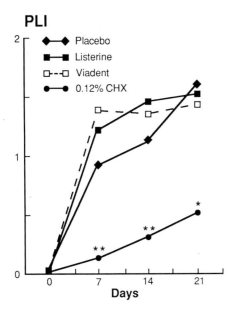

PLI

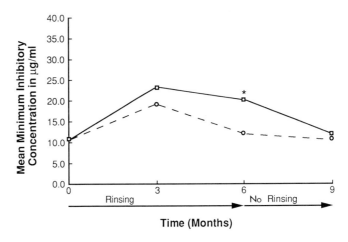

Fig. 9.7(a) Mean plaque index for all treatment groups rinsing with either placebo, Listerine, Viadent, or 0.12% chlorhexidine digluconate at all time intervals. *Significantly different [$p \leqslant 0.05$] from all other groups. **Significantly different [$p \leqslant 0.05$] from Listerine and Viadent.

Fig. 9.8(a) Mean MICS of chlorhexidine for streptococci isolates from individuals rinsing with 0.12% chlorhexidine gluconate mouth-rinse or a placebo mouth-rinse for 6 months. *Significantly different from placebo at $p = 0.05$ ☐ Isolates from chx-treated subjects. ○ Isolates from placebo-treated subjects.

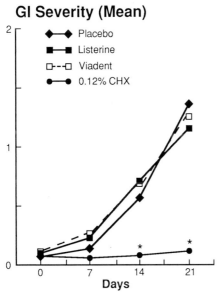

GI Severity (Mean)

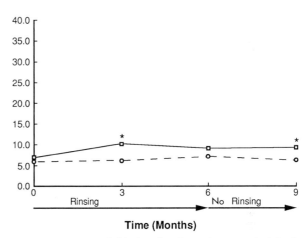

Fig. 9.7(b) Gingivitis severity [Mean GI] for all treatment groups rinsing with either placebo, Listerine, Viadent, or 0.12% chlorhexidine digluconate at all time intervals. *Significantly different [$p \leqslant 0.05$] from all other groups. Redrawn from Siegrist, B. E. *et al.* (1986). *Journal of Periodontal Research*, **21** [Supp. 16], 60–73. Permission from Munksgaard International Publishers Limited.

Fig. 9.8(b) Mean MICS of chlorhexidine for actinomyces isolates from individuals rinsing with a 0.12% chlorhexidine gluconate mouth-rinse or a placebo mouth-rinse for 6 months. Redrawn from Briner, W. W. *et al.* (1986). *Journal of Periodontal Research*, **21** [Supp. 16], 53–9. Permission from Munksgaard International Publishers Limited.

similar to those found when equivalent amounts of chlorhexidine in mouth-rinses were used (Gjermo and Rolla, 1970, 1971).

In summary, the results of trials using gels and toothpastes are equivocal. Short-term, anti-plaque effects appear

to be more favourable than those seen in longer-term trials but differences in trial designs make useful comparisons difficult. Such differences include the concentration of chlorhexidine, the base for the drug, the method and duration of application, and the indices used to assess the effects and changes. Further, the use of dental students in trials of the additional effects of chlorhexidine upon mechanical measures of plaque control can produce misleading information. Inherent motivation and dexterity usually leads to excellent mechanical tooth-cleaning in both test and control subjects. Consequently, the beneficial effects of chemical plaque-control agents are essentially masked (Flotra *et al.* 1972; Hansen *et al.* 1975; Johansen *et al.* 1975).

A summary of some of the more extensive, human clinical trials of chlorhexidine is presented in Table 9.3.

Unwanted effects

The main adverse effect of the oral use of chlorhexidine is extrinsic staining of teeth (Flotra *et al.* 1971*a*). A dark-yellow or brownish stain is often present on both natural and artificial teeth after only a few days use of any chlorhexidine preparation. The amount of staining shows great individual variation and it tends to be more severe with higher concentrations of chlorhexidine (Heyden 1973). The discoloration has been associated with locally high concentrations of the drug, which can occur on pellicle-covered tooth surfaces, carious lesions, mechanical defects, and unpolished amalgam restorations (Heyden 1973). The surface of the tongue can also be affected when chlorhexidine is used as a mouth-rinse (Loe and Schiott 1970).

The precise cause of the tooth discoloration is not clear but three possible mechanisms may be involved (for detailed review, see Eriksen *et al.* 1985):

1. Carbohydrates and amino acid-containing compounds present in acquired pellicle undergo a series of polymerization reactions to produce pigmented substances called melanoidins (Berk 1976). Such browning reactions are catalysed by chlorhexidine, which produces a thick pellicle containing more amino groups than ordinary pellicle (Nordbo 1979).

2. Chlorhexidine denatures the proteins in pellicle by splitting sulphide bridges to produce free sulphydryl groups. The latter then react with iron or tin ions to produce brown and yellow pigmented products (Ellingsen *et al.* 1982*a*, *b*).

3. Chlorhexidine reacts with ketones and aldehydes in dietary breakdown or intermediary products to form insoluble, coloured compounds (Nordbo 1971).

Although dietary factors may not be the only factors contributing to staining, there is strong evidence to suggest that certain drinks such as tea, coffee, red wine, and port cause more severe discoloration of teeth in the presence of chlorhexidine when compared with its effects when these beverages are not consumed (Addy *et al.* 1979; Prayitno *et al.* 1979). Such stain as does occur, however, can be removed by regular dental prophylaxis.

A further adverse effect of chlorhexidine mouth-rinses is the occurrence of painful, desquamative lesions on the oral mucosa, which may be associated with a burning sensation (Flotra *et al.* 1971*a*). Rushton (1977), however, considered that these lesions represent an occasional adverse response rather than an adverse effect, as histological examination of oral mucosa after prolonged exposure to chlorhexidine failed to demonstrate any changes in the normal structure (MacKenzie *et al.* 1976). Impairment of taste sensation has been reported by volunteers using 0.2 per cent chlorhexidine rinses (Flotra *et al.* 1971). Recent evidence suggests that this impairment is both short-lasting and specific for the discrimination of salty tastes (Lang *et al.* 1988).

No adverse systemic effects have been attributed to the prolonged oral use of chlorhexidine. During the two-year study undertaken by Schiott *et al.* (1976*c*) once-daily rinses with 0.2 per cent chlorhexidine had no effect on number of red cells and their haemoglobin content, erythrocyte sedimentation rate, differential white-cell counts, urine content, or liver and kidney function.

Parotid swelling is a rare, unwanted effect of chlorhexidine mouth-rinses. The condition appears to subside spontaneously within a few days after discontinuing use. The clinical features have the appearance of mechanical obstruction of the parotid duct. Overvigorous mouth-rinsing may predispose a patient to the condition. Such rinsing may create a negative pressure in the duct and the aspiration of chlorhexidine.

Dental applications

The clinical indications for the use of chlorhexidine are associated both with its anti-plaque properties and its capacity to act as a more general, bactericidal antiseptic.

Immediately after flap surgery or gingivectomy the periodontal environment is particularly susceptible to infection. Wounds are usually protected by a standard periodontal dressing and their rate of healing, when assessed by exudate and bleeding tendency, is quicker when chlorhexidine is included in the dressing (Asboe-Jorgensen *et al.* 1974). Gingivectomy wounds heal adequately when subjected to a twice-daily rinse with a 0.2 per cent solution (Hamp *et al.* 1975), although patients usually experience greater comfort when a dressing is applied (Addy and Dolby 1976). Chlorhexidine rinses have no effect on plaque formation beneath a periodontal dressing (Pluss *et al.* 1975; Langebeck and Bay 1976). However, if chlorhexidine powder is sprinkled into the dressing, a plaque-inhibitory effect is evident (Pluss *et al.* 1975).

The main advantage of a chlorhexidine mouth-rinse from a surgical standpoint is during the postoperative period immediately after pack removal. Complete plaque control can then be achieved without extensive use of proximal cleaning aids, which can be painful to use and may delay healing. In the longer term, however, the use of chlorhexidine mouth-rinses has no advantage over regular scaling and prophylaxis. Chlorhexidine treatment alone is more likely to result in a slightly deeper residual pocket, less gain of attachment in deeper sites, and greater attachment loss in shallow pockets (Westfelt *et al.* 1983).

In addition to the post-surgical management of periodontal wounds, chlorhexidine has also been advocated to improve healing after routine oral surgical procedures and in the postoperative management of immediate denture construction (Macalister 1961; Roed-Petersen and Hjorting-Hansen 1976).

The long-term use of chlorhexidine mouth-rinses may be indicated for patients whose mechnical plaque control is severely impaired. Patients wearing fixed orthodontic appliances or intermaxillary fixation devices will benefit from a daily rinse with a 0.2 per cent chlorhexidine solution (Krenkel and Rothler 1979). Furthermore, the inevitable tooth staining can be removed at the final appointment when active treatment has been completed.

Chlorhexidine is an extremely useful adjunct to routine oral hygiene measures for handicapped patients whose plaque control and gingival status are often very poor (Storhaug 1977). The cooperation of mentally handicapped patients is variable and in the most difficult cases the application of chlorhexidine gel in a soft splint can be beneficial (Usher 1975; Cutress *et al.* 1977). The home use of toothpastes and mouth-rinses will require cooperation from the patients and their parents or guardians but daily applications will help to control gingival inflammation (Flotra *et al.* 1971*b*; Bay and Russell 1975; Denver 1979). Further, the plaque-inhibitory effect of chlorhexidine can be beneficial in reducing caries activity (Loe *et al.* 1972; Zickert *et al.* 1982) but this action may be dependent upon the mode and concentration of the application (Emilson and Fornell 1976).

Chlorhexidine will help to control plaque accumulation in patients with drug-induced gingival overgrowth, although chlorhexidine has no apparent effect in minimizing the enlargement (Russell and Bay 1978).

The antiseptic properties of chlorhexidine have led to its suggested use in severely medically compromised patients who suffer from recurrent, generalized oral infections (Spiers *et al.* 1980; Ferreti *et al.* 1987). Local, oral infections such as denture-induced stomatitis, aphthous ulceration, dry socket, and acute ulcerative gingivitis also respond to chlorhexidine applications (Budtz-Jorgensen and Loe 1972; Olsen 1975; Addy 1977; Tjernberg 1979). However, it must be emphasized that in these instances chlorhexidine should be used only as an adjunct to the traditional modes of therapy.

In the management of periodontal disease, chlorhexidine could be used to reduce the numbers of pathogenic bacteria that populate periodontal pockets. Pockets may either be irrigated subgingivally with a chlorhexidine solution after scaling and root planing (Wennstrom *et al.* 1987) or applied as part of a home-care maintenance programme (Soh *et al.* 1982). Gingival inflammation can be controlled by daily applications by the patient but the long-term, antibacterial effect of infrequent professional irrigations in the dental surgery is likely to be minimal (Wennstrom *et al.* 1987). Further, in an attempt to prolong the time of contact between the drug and the bacteria, chlorhexidine has been incorporated into slow-release devices, such as acrylic strips, which are left *in situ* within the pockets (Addy *et al.* 1982). These methods have been shown to be effective *in vivo* (Addy and Langeroudi 1984; Addy *et al.* 1988), although their widespread clinical use has not yet been developed.

Finally, the general antiseptic properties of chlorhexidine have encouraged its use as a prophylactic rinse in the prevention of post-extraction bacteraemia (Jokinen 1978) and dry sockets (Field *et al.* 1988), and to reduce the bacterial content of the aerosol spray during ultrasonic scaling.

9.8.2 ALEXIDINE AND OTHER BISBIGUANIDES

Alexidine (2 ethyl hexyl bisbiguanidine dihydrochloride) is structurally related to chlorhexidine and has very similar properties (see Fig. 9.2, p.157). Alexidine is an antimicrobial agent active against yeasts. The drug is poorly absorbed from the gastrointestinal tract and the oral toxicity is low.

The anti-plaque activity of 0.035 and 0.05 per cent alexidine mouthwashes has been established from the results of clinical trials in which oral hygiene measures were

suspended for two to three weeks (Carlsson and Porter 1973; Lobene and Soparker 1973; Spolsky *et al.* 1975). A similar effect was seen when the rinses were used as an adjunct to routine plaque-control measures over two months (Formicola *et al.* 1978). The effects of short-term rinsing with alexidine on gingivitis, however, have generally been inconclusive.

In a longer study conducted over six months, twice-daily rinsing with 0.035 per cent alexidine significantly reduced plaque indices throughout the trial period. Gingivitis scores were also significantly lower after 90 days of rinsing, although the difference between test and control groups was not significant at the end of six months (Weatherford *et al.* 1977). When compared to 0.2 per cent chlorhexidine, Roberts and Addy (1981) showed that 0.035 per cent alexidine was significantly less effective in inhibiting plaque accumulation over 10-day, cross-over periods. It was suggested that the reduced anti-plaque activity was due to the lower concentration of the alexidine rinse, a factor determined by the low water solubility of the drug. The results of a number of clinical trials indicate that alexidine mouth-rinses also predispose to staining of the teeth and tongue (Carlsson and Porter 1973; Lobene and Soparker 1973; Spolsky *et al.* 1975; Addy and Roberts 1981). Consequently, there are few, if any, indications for using alexidine in preference to chlorhexidine as a plaque-control agent.

Alexidine is an alkyl bisbiguanide in which the *p*-chlorophenyl groups of chlorhexidine are replaced by alkyl terminal moieties. A number of other alkyl bisbiguanides including hexoctidine, heptihexidine, heptoctidine, hexidecidine, and hexhexidine also have activity against oral microorganisms similar to that of chlorhexidine. The activity appears to be related to the structure of the molecules. For example, agents with branched terminal alkyl groups are more active against *Actinomycetes* than those with unbranched groups. Similarly, increasing the length of the methylene bridge increases the activity against species of *Bacterioides* and *Fusobacterium* (Baker *et al.* 1987).

From a clinical viewpoint, the structural modification of anti-plaque agents to optimize their activity against specific bacterial species may prove a valuable field for future research.

9.9 BISPYRIDINES

Octenidine hydrochloride ((*N*,*N*'-(1, 10-decanediyldi-1(4H)-pyridynl-4-ylidene) bis-[1-octanamine] dyhydrochloride) is a bispyridine compound that has antimicrobial activity (see Fig. 9.2 on p. 157). *In vitro* observations (O'Connor *et al.* 1980; Slee and O'Connor 1983) and the results of very short-term animal experiments (Emilson *et al.* 1980) have suggested that this agent has significant anti-plaque activity. However, only a limited number of clinical trials have so far been undertaken in humans. In a seven-day study of experimental gingivitis, Patters *et al.* (1983) showed that twice-daily rinsing with 0.1 per cent octenidine in a mouthwash vehicle almost completely inhibited plaque formation. A 0.05 per cent rinse was not as effective and plaque was

Table 9.3 Synopsis of periodontal findings from controlled clinical studies on the use of chlorhexidine (CHX) as an anti-plaque agent

Study	Number of subjects	Type of subjects	Periodontal measures	CHX concentration, vehicle; frequency and duration of applications	Findings
Loe and Schiott (1970)	24	Dental students	Plaque index[b] Gingival index[a]	0.2% and 2.0% CHX rinses applied once and twice daily over 15–40 days	Twice-daily rinses with 0.2% CHX inhibit plaque and gingivitis Once daily rinse with 0.2% CHX does not inhibit plaque in all areas of mouth Once-daily application of 2.0% CHX totally inhibits plaque and gingivitis
Flotra et al. (1972)	50	Norwegian Air Force recruits	Plaque index Gingival index	0.1% and 0.2% CHX rinses applied twice daily over 17 weeks in the presence and absence of calculus and rough tooth surfaces	Comparable reductions in plaque indices for different concentration rinses CHX rinses reduce gingival index but not by the same magnitude as plaque index More effective reductions of both indices in the absence of calculus and rough tooth surfaces CHX is more effective adjacent to pockets of < 3 mm
Johansen et al. (1975)	73	Dental students	Plaque index Gingival index Caries index (Johansen et al. 1975)	0.4% and 1.0% CHX in toothpastes with and without abrasives; applications twice daily for 2 years	No significant differences in plaque inhibition between subjects using toothpastes and placebos Lowest plaque scores in subjects using abrasive pastes containing 0.4% and 1.0% CHX No significant differences in effects on gingival indices 1% CHX appeared to have an inhibitory effect on caries
Loe et al. (1976)	120	Dental and medical students	Plaque index Gingival index Calculus index (Volpe et al. 1965)	0.2% CHX applied daily by toothbrush (8 months) and then as a rinse (14 months); total observation, 2 years.	Significantly lower plaque index throughout in subjects using CHX Significantly lower gingival index values in CHX group for first 18 months only CHX group had higher calculus index scores than controls

Reference	N	Subjects	Indices / methods	Regimen	Findings
Lang et al. (1982)	158	Schoolchildren	Plaque index Gingival index PMGI (de la Rosa and Sturzenberger 1976)	0.1% and 0.2% CHX rinses daily for 6 days each week	Plaque reduced significantly in all CHX groups Gingival indices reduced significantly in all CHX groups
			CSI; CSSI (Ennerver et al. 1961)[c]	0.2% CHX twice a week only	Most effective reduction of gingival index in subjects using 0.2% CHX 6 times each week (as opposed to twice weekly) Calculus scores higher in all CHX subjects than controls
				All applications supervised	No differences in DMFS scores between groups
Segreto et al. (1986)	597	Adult volunteers	Plaque disclosing (Turesky et al. 1970) Gingival index PMGI[d]	0.12% and 0.2% CHX rinses over 3 months	Both CHX rinses significantly reduced plaque and gingivitis scores when compared to controls. There are no clinical advantages in using the 0.2% rinse over the 0.12% rinse
Grossman et al. (1986)	430	Adult volunteers	Plaque disclosing Gingival index	0.12% CHX rinse, twice daily over 6 months	Significantly less plaque in CHX group than controls Significantly less gingivitis and gingival bleeding in the CHX group Accumulation of calculus greater in CHX group
Siegrist et al. (1986)	31	Dental personnel	Plaque index Gingival index	0.12% CHX rinse, twice daily over 21 days	CHX rinse was superior to both phenol and plant alkaloid compounds in reducing plaque formation CHX had a greater capacity to maintain optimal gingival health than the phenols and plant alkaloids
Briner et al. (1986 a,b)	430	Adult volunteers	Microbiological assessment of plaque samples	0.12% CHX rinse, twice daily over 6 months	0.12% CHX significantly reduced the numbers of aerobes, anaerobes and streptococci in plaque samples 0.12% CHX had an especially pronounced inhibitory effect (up to 97%) on Actinomyces spp. There were no residual effects of CHX on plaque bacteria after cessation of rinsing

[a] Gingival index: Loe and Silness (1963) unless otherwise stated.
[b] Plaque index: (Silness and Loe (1964) unless otherwise stated.
[c] CSI: calculus surface index; CSSI; calculus surface severity index.
[d] PMGI; Papillary-marginal-gingivitis index.

detected on the gingival third of teeth. When the observation period was extended to 21 days, these findings were confirmed and a significant effect was also demonstrated on the inhibition of gingivitis (Patters *et al.* 1986).

The effects of daily octenidine rinses (0.5 and 1.0 per cent) on dental plaque in monkeys have been measured over a two-week period by Shern *et al.* (1988). Both concentrations reduced the plaque mass by about 60 per cent. The octenidine treatments also decreased the proportions of motile forms in subgingival plaque, which suggests that the pathogenic potential of plaque can be favourably reduced. Octenidine has been shown to be well tolerated by the oral mucosa when applied in a glycerol-based vehicle, although epithelial desquamation and burning occurred when a 0.1 per cent aqueous solution was used (Patters *et al.* 1986). As with chlorhexidine, however, a significant side-effect is the development of a yellow-brown stain on the teeth and occasionally the dorsum of the tongue.

The *in vitro* anti-plaque properties of a series of alkylamines that are related to octenidine have recently been evaluated (Wentland 1988). The di-*n*-octyl analogue (pirtenidine) is highly efficacious against several plaque-forming organisms of the streptococcal and *Actinomyces* species. This compound, which is up to 18 times as potent as chlorhexidine against some bacteria, is currently being prepared for use in clinical trials.

9.10 METALLIC SALTS

The salts of certain heavy metals can inhibit the growth of dental plaque and calculus. Salts of zinc, tin, and copper have received most attention in recent years and a number of commercial toothpastes now include these compounds in their formulations.

9.10.1 ZINC SALTS

The initial studies on zinc salts tested mixtures of zinc tribromsalan (0.125 per cent) with zinc phenolsulphonate (1.0 per cent) or zinc citrate (5 per cent) as potential anti-calculus and anti-plaque agents, respectively (Picozzi *et al.* 1972; Fischman *et al.* 1973). Significant reductions in both hard and soft deposits were reported, although the specific effects of the zinc ions would have been difficult to assess because tribromsalan is itself an antibacterial compound. Later *in vitro* studies attempted to define more precisely the anti-plaque activity of zinc ions but the results were contradictory. Evans *et al.* (1977) found that zinc phenolsulphonate and zinc chloride had no effect on plaque formation or growth. Bates and Navia (1979), however, showed that zinc sulphate did inhibit the initial formation of plaque (probably by a direct action on *Strep. mutans*) but had no effect on the growth of established plaque. Harrap *et al.* (1983) confirmed the *in vitro*, anti-plaque activity with a series of salts including zinc citrate, demonstrating a concentration-dependent inhibition of plaque growth.

Clinical tests with zinc mouth-rinses have produced further evidence to substantiate their effects on plaque development. Rinsing twice daily with zinc chloride solutions of about 0.2 per cent for periods up to seven days produced a 38–40 per cent reduction in plaque when measured by weight or index scores (Schmid *et al.* 1974; Skjorland *et al* 1978). However, when rinses were used only once daily, 0.22 per cent solutions of zinc chloride were found not to be effective (Compton and Beagrie 1975). When zinc citrate solutions (9.5 mM) were used as twice-daily rinses for only seven days, an 8 per cent reduction in plaque growth was obtained (Addy *et al.* 1980), although when the citrate concentration was doubled the inhibition increased to 30 per cent (Harrop *et al.* 1983). Additional evidence for concentration-dependent inhibition of plaque growth by zinc salts was produced by Disney *et al.* (1989), who evaluated six dentrifice formulations containing levels of zinc citrate of between 0 and 4 per cent. Greater anti-plaque and anti-calculus activity was seen with higher zinc concentrations, although this was only a demonstrable trend, which did not reach statistical significance.

These inconsistent observations again demonstrate the difficulty in drawing conclusions from a series of projects using different zinc salts, concentrations of solution, times of application, frequencies of rinsing, and methods of scoring plaque growth. Consequently, standardization of protocols with multicentre collaboration is essential if useful guidelines are to emerge from short-term clinical trials.

Zinc citrate has been combined with the non-ionic anti-microbial Triclosan (2,4,4'-trichloro-2'-hydroxydiphenyl ether) and investigated for anti-plaque activity as a toothpaste formulation. Such pastes are efficacious against plaque formation and the onset of gingivitis (Saxton 1986; Saxton and van der Ouderaa, 1989). Furthermore, observations from clinical trials undertaken over 6–12 months have suggested that zinc citrate/Triclosan pastes are more effective than placebo pastes in maintaining gingival health (Svatun *et al.* 1977, 1989).

The combination of zinc citrate and Triclosan has a greater plaque inhibitory action than either constituent used separately (Saxton *et al.* 1987), and its efficacy is related to the concentrations of the active agents rather than to the dose of the paste used (Saxton *et al.* 1986, 1987). However, in many clinical trials, the concentrations of zinc citrate and/or Triclosan were greater than those in the commercial toothpastes marketed today. It is of interest, therefore, that although twice-daily rinsing with slurries of 0.2 per cent Triclosan/0.5 per cent zinc citrate (commercial paste) does reduce plaque growth over four days (Addy *et al.* 1989), such effects are not significantly greater than those observed when rinsing with conventional toothpastes containing neither agent (Jenkins *et al.* 1989).

Finally, a toothpaste containing zinc chloride has been shown to have significant anti-calculus activity. At the end of a six-month period, subjects who used the test paste had 40 per cent less calculus than those who used a control paste (Lobene *et al.* 1987).

9.10.2 TIN SALTS

The ability of tin ions to inhibit plaque formation has been studied primarily with stannous fluoride (SnF_2) mouth-rinses. Early animal experiments showed that the daily topical application of a 0.1 per cent SnF$_2$ rinse significantly reduced bacterial accumulation on teeth (Konig 1959). Later, *in vivo*, human studies confirmed that the antibacterial effects were more likely due to the tin ions rather than the fluoride ions, although a synergistic effect of the two components cannot be overlooked (Andres *et al.* 1974; Tinanoff *et al.* 1976).

In a 12-day, comparative study on the effects of SnF$_2$ (0.2 per cent and 0. 3 per cent) and chlorhexidine mouth-rinses, Svatun *et al.* (1977) found that the tin solutions had definite anti-plaque properties, although chlorhexidine was more effective. They suggested that the mechanism of action of the tin ions is mediated through their ability to bind to the lipotechoic acid present on the surfaces of Gram-positive bacteria. The net surface charge of the organisms is therefore reversed and the adsorption of the cells to teeth is consequently reduced (Svatun *et al.* 1977). Furthermore, the effectiveness of SnF$_2$ solutions in reducing bacterial adhesion is related to the stability of the tin ions in aqueous solution and the rate at which they are taken up and retained by specific organisms (Tinanoff and Camosci 1980; Camosci and Tinanoff 1984). The accumulation of the tin in bacteria may alter their metabolism and other physicochemical chacteristics (Tinanoff and Camosci 1980).

Long-term trials have also demonstrated anti-plaque properties of SnF$_2$ rinses. Two groups of children rinsed daily for 28 months with 0.1 per cent SnF$_2$ or 0.05 per cent NaF solutions (Leverett *et al.* 1984). The children using SnF$_2$ had less plaque at four months than the NaF group but no differences were found at 16 and 28 months. In addition the SnF$_2$ group had consistently lower gingival indices than the NaF group, although the differences failed to reach statistical significance.

SnF$_2$ and NaF solutions have also been tested in preselected subjects with high levels of *Strep. mutans*. Subjects rinsed twice daily with either SnF$_2$ or NaF (200 p.p.m. F$^-$) for two years. After one year the SnF$_2$ group had significantly less gingivitis and fewer *Strep. mutans*/ml saliva than the subjects using NaF. The difference in *Strep. mutans* was maintained after two years but the reduction of gingivitis scores in the SnF$_2$ group was no longer significant (Klock *et al.* 1985).

9.10.3 COPPER SALTS

Limited research has been undertaken to assess the anti-plaque activity of copper ions. Using the 21-day, experimental gingivitis model, Waerhaug *et al.* (1984) found that subjects who used a copper sulphate mouth-rinse twice daily had a mean plaque index (PI) of 0.79 and a gingival index (GI) of 0.83 at the end of the test period. When a chlorhexidine rinse was used, the corresponding values were PI, 0.29, GI, 0.57 and when a water placebo was used the mean PI was 1.25 and mean GI, 1.02. Clearly the metallic solution did have anti-plaque activity but this was not as marked as when chlorhexidine was used.

More recently, in only a two-day study, a baseline application of a copper-containing prophylactic paste was found

to inhibit plaque growth after 24 h by 92 per cent. Only 33 per cent inhibition was reported after 48 h and it was concluded that to maintain efficacy, such pastes should be applied on a daily basis (Moore *et al.* 1989).

9.10.4 UNWANTED EFFECTS

The unwanted effects that have been reported with the use of mouth-rinses containing heavy metal salts are a metallic aftertaste, dryness of the mouth, and a yellow-brown discoloration of the teeth and tongue. However, the staining is mild and easily removed from the teeth using a pumice-based prophylaxis paste (Svatun *et al.* 1977; Waerhaug *et al.* 1984).

9.11 SANGUINARINE

Sanguinarine is a benzophenathridine alkaloid derived from the plant *Sanguinaria canadensis*. It is structurally related to alkaloids found in the plant *Fagara zanthoxyloides* which is chewed in Third world countries as a method for cleaning teeth (Odebiyi and Sofowara 1979; Elvin-Lewis *et al.* 1980). Sanguinarine, in its quaternary iminium form, has antimicrobial properties that have led to its relatively recent introduction as an anti-plaque agent. The *in vitro* analysis of MIC values of sanguinarine has determined that, within the range of 1–16 μg/ml, the drug can inhibit the growth of a wide range of oral bacteria. These include *Actinobacillu actinomycetemcomitans*, *Bacteroides gingivalis*, *Eikenella corrodens*, *Fusobacterium nucleatum* and *Strep. mutans* (Dzink and Socransky 1985).

In addition to its antimicrobial properties, a further important feature of sanguinarine is its retention in dental plaque when used as a mouth-rinse. The levels in plaque can exceed the MIC values for up to 2 h after rinsing, although the retention does show individual variability (Southard *et al.* 1984). Sanguinarine also has fluorescent properties, enabling it to be disclosed under long-wave, ultraviolet light (Southard *et al.* 1984).

9.11.1 CLINICAL TRIALS

The efficacy of sanguinarine has been tested in both short- and long-term trials. The extract has been introduced into mouth-rinses and toothpastes, and 0.03 per cent is the most frequently tested concentration.

Short-term studies, conducted over varying periods of up to 14 days and in the absence of other plaque-control measures, have demonstrated that sanguinarine preparations have significant anti-plaque properties when compared to placebo controls (Klewansky and Vernier 1984; Greenfield and Cuchel 1984; Lindhe 1984; Nygaard-Oestby and Persson 1984; Southard *et al.* 1984, 1985; Wennstrom and Lindhe 1985). Under such conditions, sanguinarine has also been shown to reduce the severity of the developing gingival inflammation (Lindhe 1984; Southard *et al.* 1985; Wennstrom and Lindhe 1985). Furthermore, sanguinarine is effective in controlling both the development of plaque and the continued growth of established deposits (Parsons *et al.* 1987; Southard *et al.* 1987). These effects can be achieved with oral rinses (0.03 per cent extract) and with supragingival irrigations made under pressure (0.00225 per cent extract). However, similar reductions in gingivitis scores of about 70 per cent were observed when irrigations were made with either weak sanguinarine solutions or with water, whereas rinsing with 0.03 per cent sanguinarine produced only a 30 per cent reduction in gingivitis (Parsons *et al.* 1987). This would suggest that the effects of weak solutions applied topically under pressure are greater than the effects of more concentrated solutions used as mouthrinses.

Not all short-term trials have shown that sanguinarine products have anti-plaque activity. Etemadzadeh and Ainamo (1987) found that twice-daily mouth-rinsing with 0.03 per cent solutions containing sanguinarine extract and 1000 p.p.m. zinc ions had no effect on plaque growth inibition. The anti-plaque activity was not affected by increasing the concentration of sanguinarine threefold. It was suggested that the anti-plaque properties of the particular sanguinarine product (Viadent) may be due to its zinc content rather than the herbal extract. A later study was designed to address specifically this problem (Southard *et al.* 1987a). A series of oral rinses containing varying concentrations of sanguinarine and zinc ions was evaluated over a two-week period. The inhibition of plaque growth and the development of gingivitis were influenced more by the concentrations of sanguinarine than zinc ions. However, the addition of zinc did enhance the effectiveness of the sanguinarine rinses. Further negative findings were reported by Schonfeld *et al.* (1986) when subjects brushed twice daily with a sanguinarine toothpaste (or placebo) for a month. Analysis of plaque samples by phase-contrast microscopy failed to show any beneficial effect of the test paste. However, plaque-control measures were maintained throughout the test period and the effects of sanguinarine may not have been apparent after only four weeks. Mallatt *et al.* (1989) also failed to demonstrate significant differences in plaque and gingivitis scores between two groups of young adults who used either a sanguinarine–zinc chloride toothpaste or a sodium fluoride paste for 21 days.

The few long-term studies so far undertaken have been concerned primarily with sanguinarine-containing toothpastes. Palcanis *et al.* (1986) studied only nine subjects who brushed twice daily with a sanguinarine paste and followed the brushing with sanguinarine rinse. The six month, plaque and gingivitis scores were lower than those of a control group of 10 subjects. In two other controlled, six-month studies, twice-daily brushing with a sanguinarine paste had no significant effect upon plaque scores (Lobene *et al.* 1986; Mauriello and Bader 1988). However, Lobene *et al.* found that gingivitis scores were lower in subjects who used the test paste and this may suggest that the drug affected the pathogenicity but not the quantity of the plaque.

Clearly sanguinarine products have definite anti-plaque properties. However, the efficacy of sanguinarine is low when compared to that of chlorhexidine (see Fig. 9.7) (Siegrist *et al.* 1986; Wennstrom and Lindhe 1986; Gazi 1988; Moran *et al.* 1988). For example, Wennstrom and

Lindhe found that over a four-week period, sanguinarine reduced the number of plaque scores of 2 and 3 by 38 per cent whereas the reduction with chlorhexidine was 82 per cent. Such low relative efficiency may preclude sanguinarine from being used as an anti-plaque agent in the short-term management of gingivitis (Gazi 1988).

9.11.2 UNWANTED EFFECTS

The main advantage of sanguinarine products over chlorhexidine is the relative absence of side-effects. A mild to moderate burning sensation in the mouth was reported in one study (Gazi 1988). However, the staining of the teeth and mucosal surfaces that accompanies the use of chlorhexidine does not appear to be a problem with sanguinarine.

In one *in vitro* study (Barczynski *et al.* 1988) the commercial product Viadent significantly reduced epithelial cell growth when cells were exposed for short periods of up to 24 h. The clinical relevance of these findings is doubtful as a 24-h exposure to Viadent would only occur after eight years' daily use.

9.12 SURFACTANTS

Surfactants or 'wetting agents' were introduced as an alternative method of plaque inhibition to the widely used antimicrobial compounds. Agents with low surface tension and lipophilic—hydrophilic properties can interfere with plaque growth without affecting the ecological balance of the oral flora (Willard *et al.* 1983). A number of the antimicrobial agents, including chlorhexidine, do possess surfactant properties. This section, however, is concerned primarily with products whose effects are mediated mainly through their 'wetting' abilities.

9.12.1 AMINOALCOHOLS

The substituted aminoalcohols (see Fig. 9.2 p.157) have comparatively low antibacterial properties. They also have a lower surface tension than that of the tooth surface and so the low antimicrobial effect may be compensated by a high local concentration on the enamel surface (Willard *et al.* 1983).

The initial *in vitro* experiments with the substituted aminoalcohol Octapinol demonstrated complete plaque inhibition during periods of between 3 and 12 days. Octapinol also prevented further plaque growth and was able to partly dissolve plaque that had already formed on teeth (Willard *et al.* 1983). The anti-plaque properties were confirmed both in short-term and long-term animal experiments when it was found that Octapinol counteracted the development of gingivitis in the absence of mechanical oral hygiene (Matsson *et al.* 1983; Willard *et al.* 1983). Similar observations were made in a three-week, experimental gingivitis study in humans. A 1 per cent Octapinol solution, applied twice daily with a brush, significantly reduced plaque formation and restricted the development of gingivitis when compared to a placebo (Matsson *et al.* 1983).

More recently, another substituted aminoalcohol, Decapinol, has shown promising anti-plaque properties in short-term clinical trials. Planimetric analysis demonstrated that plaque growth was restricted to 6.8 per cent of Decapinol-treated tooth surfaces during seven days abstinence from oral hygiene. Control surfaces had 40 per cent plaque coverage (Attstrom *et al.* 1989). Furthermore, 1 per cent Decapinol reduced the quantity of formed plaque by about 75 per cent (Attstrom *et al.* 1989). The effect of Decapinol on developing gingivitis is also impressive. Twice-daily rinsing with a 0.2 per cent solution has a similar effect upon gingival bleeding as a 0.2 per cent chlorhexidine solution applied with the same frequency (Klinge *et al.* 1989).

The unwanted effects of aminoalcohols include a slight local anaesthetic effect on soft tissues, a slightly bitter taste, and light-brown staining of the teeth (Attstrom *et al.* 1983). After three weeks' development, the staining is easily removed with a toothbrush and ordinary toothpaste.

9.12.2 PLAX

Plax is a commercial mouth-rinse with surfactant properties that has been marketed recently amid an extensive advertising campaign. The rinse is a combination of anionic and ionic surfactants including sodium lauryl sulphate and polysorbate 20. These ingredients act upon already-formed plaque to loosen and remove the deposits and use of the rinse is recommended before daily toothbrushing.

The clinical efficacy of Plax has been demonstrated in a series of trials undertaken in conjunction with Oral Research Laboratories Inc., USA. A single, 30-s oral rinse with Plax removed 16–22 per cent of already-formed plaque when compared to placebo. When the rinse was used in conjunction with toothbrushing, however, a 73 per cent reduction of plaque occurred in one study (7 days' duration) although other results (14 per cent plaque reduction over 14 days) were not as impressive.

Clearly, Plax does appear to be a useful adjunct to toothbrushing. However, the claim of a 300 per cent reduction of plaque when compared with control surfaces does not imply complete plaque inhibition and a number of long-term, controlled and independent trials are required before the effects of Plax can be compared accurately with other agents.

9.13 METHODS OF APPLICATION

The efficacy of any anti-plaque agent is dependent not only upon the relative activity of the drug but also upon the length of time for which the drug is in direct contact with tooth surfaces. Furthermore, it is essential that the agent gains access to the specific sites on the teeth where the maximum anti-plaque effects will be achieved. In health, these sites are, primarily, interproximally at the gingival margins, whereas in periodontally diseased mouths, subgingival applications are required.

The most frequently used modes of application for anti-plaque agents are mouth-rinses and toothpastes. The main problem with both these methods, however, is the relatively short contact time between the active agents and the teeth. Consequently, the well-proven success of chlorhexidine as a plaque inhibitor is related to its substantivity rather than to any unique action upon the oral flora.

Mouth-rinses are unable to penetrate subgingivally (Flotra *et al.* 1972) and so, where there are periodontal pockets, direct subgingival irrigation is required so that the agents can penetrate their depths (Pitcher *et al.* 1980; Hardy *et al.* 1982). Toothpastes to some extent may be applied directly into pockets using a crevicular brushing technique. However, it is doubtful whether such methods can introduce anti-plaque agents satisfactorily to the bases of deep periodontal lesions.

Interproximal applications of chlorhexidine can be made with gel preparations together with floss, wood-sticks, or interdental brushes. Chlorhexidine-impregnated floss has been shown to be more effective interproximally than conventional floss (Schuller and Yeung 1982). In an attempt to increase the contact times, drugs have been incorporated into chewing gums, lozenges, and periodontal dressings with varying degrees of success (Asboe-Jorgensen *et al.* 1974; Pluss *et al.* 1975; Kelstrup *et al.* 1978; Ainamo and Etemadzadeh 1987). Further, a number of so-called slow release devices have been used to increase the length of time the drugs are *in situ* in the gingival crevice (or periodontal pocket). Anti-plaque agents have been incorporated into pieces of dialysis tubing (Addy *et al.* 1982), hollow cellulose-acetate fibres (Coventry and Newman 1982), acrylic strips (Addy *et al.* 1982), and ethylcellulose films (Friedman and Golomb 1982) to prolong delivery times. Clinically and microbiologically, the effects of such systems have been promising.

A summary of the methods that have been used to apply anti-plaque agents is given in Table 9.4.

REFERENCES

Addy, M. (1977) Hibitane in the treatment of aphthous ulceration. *Journal of Clinical Periodontology*, **4**, 108–16.

Addy, M. M and Bates, N. J. F. (1977). The effect of partial dentures and chlorhexidine gluconate gel on plaque accumulation in the absence of oral hygiene. *Journal of Clinical Periodontology*, **4**, 41–7.

Addy, M. and Dolby, A. E. (1976). The use of chlorhexidine mouthwash compared with periodontal dressing following the gingivectomy procedure. *Journal of Clinical Periodontology*, **3**, 59–65.

Addy, M. and Langeroudie, M. (1984). Comparison of the immediate effects on the sub-gingival microflora of acrylic strips containing 40% chlorhexidine, metronidazole or tetracycline. *Journal of Clinical Periodontology*, **11**, 379–86.

Addy, M., and Roberts, W. R. (1981). Comparison of the bisbiguanide antiseptics alexidine and chlorhexidine. II. Clinical and *in vitro* staining properties. *Journal of Clinical Periodontology*, **8**, 220–30.

Addy, M., Prayitno, S., Taylor, L., and Caddgan, S. (1979). An *in vitro* study of the role of dietary factors in the aetiology of tooth staining associated with the use of chlorhexidine. *Journal of Periodontal Research*, **14**, 403–10.

Addy, M., Richards, J., and Williams, G. (1980). The effect of zinc citrate mouthwash on dental plaque and salivary bacteria. *Journal of Clinical Periodontology*, **7**, 309–15.

Addy, M., Rawle, L., Handley, R., Newman, H. N., and Coventry, J. R. (1982). The development and *in vitro* evaluation of acrylic strips and

Table 9.4 Methods of application of anti-plaque and calculus agents

Method of Delivery	Anti-plaque/Calculus Agent	Reference	Comments
Mouth-rinses	Enzymes Antibiotics Phenols Quarternary ammoniums Bisbiguanides Bispyridines Sanguinarine Heavy metals Aminoalcohols	References are given in the text to the use of these agents in mouth-rinse form	The most widely used method of application; most of the agents are now marketed as mouth-rinses, e.g. Corsodyl (chlorhexidine), Listerine (phenol), Veadent (sanguinarine)
Toothpastes and gels	Enzymes Phenols Bisbiguanides Sanguinarine Heavy metals	References are given in the text to the use of these agents in gel and toothpaste form	Another popular and commercial method of applying anti-plaque/calculus agents, e.g. Zendium (thiocyanate), Corsodyl, Veadent (sanguinarine)
Irrigation systems	Most studies of subgingival and pulsated jet systems have used 0.2% chlorhexidine as the active agent	Cumming and Loe (1973) Soh et al. (1982) Khoo and Newman (1983) Westling and Tynelius (1984) Watts and Newman (1986)	Can be applied by the dentist/hygienist or by the patient on a daily basis Control of subgingival plaque is most effective using subgingival pulsated jet systems
Slow-release devices (dialysis tubing, acrylic strips, ethylcellulose, films, varnishes)	Chlorhexidine, tetracycline and metronidazole are the most commonly researched drugs	Goodson et al. (1979 Addy et al. (1982) Coventry and Newman (1982) Friedman and Golomb (1982) Balanyk et al. (1983 Goodson et al. (1984) Newman et al. (1984) Friedman et al. (1985)	Increased contact time between drug and tooth surface; used primarily to affect the ecology of subgingival microflora rather than as anti-plaque agents
Periodontal dressings	Chlorhexidine	Asboe-Jorgensen et al. (1974) Pluss et al. (1975)	The rate of postoperative healing is increased and plaque-inhibition is evident when chlorhexidine is incorporated into dressings.
Chewing gums and lozenges	Enzyme (mutanase) Chlorhexidine	Kelstrup et al. (1978) Ainamo and Etemadzadeh (1987)	Attempts to increase contact times between agents and teeth; significant plaque-inhibitory effects reported in short-term trials
Dental restorative materials (composites and glass ionomers)	Chlorhexidine	Jedrychowski et al. (1983)	Addition of small quantities of chlorhexidine to composites and glass ionomers increases their anti-plaque effects without significantly altering the physical properties
Alginate powder	Chlorhexidine and fluoride	Hattab (1984)	Found to be effective as a cariostatic medium in animal experiments; no reference to plaque inhibition
Dental floss	Chlorhexidine	Schuller and Yeung (1982)	Significant reductions in plaque when compared to the use of conventional floss

dialysis tubing for local drug delivery. *Journal of Periodontology*, **53**, 693–9.

Addy, M., Hassan, H., Moran, J., Wade, W., and Newcombe, R. (1988). Use of antimicrobial containing acrylic strips in the treatment of chronic periodontal disease. A three month follow up study. *Journal of Periodontology*, **59**, 557–64.

Addy, M., Jenkins, S., and Newcombe, R. (1989). Studies on the effect of toothpaste rinses on plaque regrowth (I). Influence of surfactants on chlorhexidine efficacy. *Journal of Clinical Periodontology*, **16**, 380–4.

Afseth, J. and Rolla, G. (1983). Clinical experiments with a toothpaste containing amyloglucosidase and glucose oxidase. *Caries Research*, **17**, 472–5.

Agerbaek, N., Nelsen, B., and Rolla, G (1975). Application of chlorhexidine by oral irrigation systems. *Scandinavian Journal of Dental Research*, **83**, 284–7.

Ainamo, J. and Etemadzadeh, H. (1987). Prevention of plaque growth with chewing gum containing chlorhexidine acetate. *Journal of Clinical Periodontology*, **14**, 524–7.

Aleece, A. A. and Forcher, B. K. (1954). Calculus reduction with a mucinase dentifrice. *Journal of Periodontology*, **25**, 122–5.

Allen, D. L. and Courtney, R. M. (1972). A clinical study of plaque reduction by Viokase. *Journal of Periodontology*, **43**, 170–5.

Andres, C. J., Shaeffer, J. C., and Windeler, A. S. (1974). Comparison of antibacterial properties of stannous fluoride and sodium fluoride mouthwashes. *Journal of Dental Research*, **53**, 457–60.

Asboe-Jorgensen, V., Attstrom, R., Lang, N. P., and Loe, H. (1974). Effect of chlorhexidine dressing on healing after periodontal surgery. *Journal of Periodontology*, **45**, 13–17.

Ashley, F. P., Skinner, A., Jackson, P. Y, Woods, W., and Wilson, R. F. (1984a). The effect of a 0.1% cetylpyridinium chloride mouthrinse on plaque and gingivitis in adult subjects. *British Dental Journal*, **157**, 191–6.

Ashley, F. P., Skinner, A., Jackson, P. Y., and Wilson, R. F. (1984b). Effect of a 0.1% cetylpyridinium chloride mouthrinse on the accumulation and biochemical composition of dental plaque in young adults. *Caries Research*, **18**, 465–71.

Attstrom, R., Matsson, L., Edwardsson, S., Willard, L. O., and Klinge, B. (1983). The effect of Octapinol on dentogingival plaque and development of gingivitis. III. Short term studies in humans. *Journal of Periodontal Research*, **18**, 445–51.

Attstrom, R., Collaert, B., DeBruyn, H. and Movert, R. (1989). Effect of Decapinol on plaque development and gingivitis healing. *Journal of Dental Research*, **68**, 971 (abstr. 837).

Axelsson, P. and Lindhe, J. (1987). Efficacy of mouthrinses in inhibiting dental plaque and gingivitis in man. *Journal of Clinical Periodontology*, **14**, 205–12.

Azuma, Y., Ozaza, N., Ueda, Y., and Takgai, N. (1986). Pharmacological studies on the anti-inflammatory action of phenolic compounds. *Journal of Dental Research*, **65**, 53–6.

Bain, M. J. and Strahan, J. D. (1978). The effect of a 1% chlorhexidine gel in the initial therapy of chronic periodontal disease. *Journal of Periodontology*, **49**, 469–74.

Baker, P. J., Coburn, R. A., Genco, R. J., and Evans, R. T. (1987). Structural determinants of activity of chlorhexidine and alkyl bisbiguanides against the human oral flora. *Journal of Dental Research*, **66**, 1099–106.

Balanyk, T. E., Sandham, H. J., and Chan, D. (1983). Dental varnishes for slow intraoral release of antimicrobial agents. *Journal of Periodontal Research*, **62**, 672 (abstr. 205).

Barczynski, J. L., Fletcher, R. D., Segal, A. H., and Conway, J. C. (1988). Viadent, ethanol, and pH effects upon gingival epithelial-like cells, *in vitro*. *Journal of Periodontology*, **57**, 622–7.

Barnes, G. P., Roberts, D. W., Katz, R. V., and Woolridge, E. D. (1976). Effects of two cetylpyridinium chloride-containing mouthwashes on bacterial plaque. *Journal of Periodontology*, **47**, 419–22.

Bates, D. G. and Navia, J. M. (1979). Chemotherapeutic effects of zinc on *Streptococcus mutans* and rat dental caries. *Archives of Oral Biology*, **24**, 799–805.

Bauhammers, A., Landay, M. A., and Pinkos, D. T. (1968). Dental calculus inhibition in rats through pancreatin application. *Archives of Oral Biology*, **13**, 353–6.

Bay, L. (1978). The effect of toothbrushing with different concentrations of chlorhexidine on the development of dental plaque and gingivitis. *Journal of Dental Research*, **57**, 181–5.

Bay, L. M. and Russell, B. G. (1975). Effect of chlorhexidine on dental plaque and gingivitis in mentally retarded children. *Community Dentistry and Oral Epidemiology*, **3**, 267–70.

Belting, C. M. and Gordon, D. L. (1966a). *In vivo* effect of a urea-containing dentrifice on dental calculus formation. I. *Journal of Periodontology*, **37**, 20–5.

Belting, C. M. and Gordon, D. L. (1966b). *In vivo* effect of a urea-containing dentifrice on dental calculus formation. II. *Journal of Periodontology*, **37**, 26–33.

Berk, Z. (1976). Non-enzymatic browning. In *Braveman's introduction to biochemistry of foods*, pp. 149–67. Elsevier, Amsterdam.

Block, P. L., Dooley, C. L., and Howe, E. E. (1969). The retardation of spontaneous periodontal disease and the prevention of caries in hamsters with dextranase. *Journal of Periodontology*, **40**, 105–10.

Bonesvoll, P. (1977). Oral pharmacology of chlorhexidine. *Journal of Clinical Periodontology*, **4**, 49–65.

Bonesvoll, P. and Gjermo, P. (1978). A comparison between chlorhexidine and some quaternary ammonium compounds with regard to retention, salivary concentration and plaque inhibiting effect in the human mouth after mouthrinses. *Archives of Oral Biology*, **23**, 289–94.

Bonesvoll, P., Hjeljord, L. G., Gjermo, P., Rolla, G., and Olsen, I. (1974a). Binding of ^{14}C-chlorhexidine to plaque and teeth *in vitro* and *in vivo*. *Journal of Dental Research*, **53** (spec. iss.), Abstr. 360.

Bonesvoll, P., Lokken, P., and Rolla, G. (1974b). Influence of concentration, time, temperature and pH on the retention of chlorhexidine in the human oral cavity after mouthrinses. *Archives of Oral Biology*, **19**, 1025–9.

Bonesvoll, P., Lokken, P., Rolla, G., and Paus, P. N. (1974c). Retention of chlorhexidine in the oral cavity after mouthrinses. *Archives of Oral Biology*, **19**, 209–12.

Bral, M. and Brownstein, C. N. (1988). Antimicrobial agents in the prevention and treatment of periodontal diseases. *Dental Clinics of North America*, **32**, 217–41.

Briner, W. W. and Wunder, J. A. (1977). Sensitivity of dog plaque microorganisms to chlorhexidine during longitudinal studies. *Journal of Periodontal Research*, **12**, 135–9.

Briner, W. W. and Leonard, G. J. (1980). Antiplaque and antigingivitis effects as a function of chlorhexidine dose in beagles. *Journal of Dental Research*, **59** (spec. iss. A), 536.

Briner, W. W. *et al.* (1986a). Effect of chlorhexidine gluconate mouthrinse on plaque bacteria. *Journal of Periodontal Research*, **21** (Suppl. 16), 44–52.

Briner, W. W. *et al.* (1986b). Assessment of susceptibility of plaque bacteria to chlorhexidine after six months' oral use. *Journal of Periodontal Research*, **21** (Suppl. 16), 53–9.

Budtz-Jorgensen, E. and Loe, H. (1972). Chlorhexidine as a denture disinfectant in the treatment of denture stomatitis. *Scandinavian Journal of Dental Research*, **80**, 457–64.

Caldwell, R. C., Sandham, H. J., Mann, W. V., Finn, S. B., and Formicola, A. J. (1971). The effect of a dextranase mouthwash on dental plaque in young adults and children. *Journal of the American Dental Association*, **82**, 124–31.

Camosci, D. A. and Tinanoff, N. (1984). Antibacterial determinants of stannous fluoride. *Journal of Dental Research*, **63**, 1121–5.

Carlsson, H. C. and Porter, C. K. (1973). Inhibitory effect of a synthetic antibiotic mouthwash (QR-711) on dental plaque and gingivitis in young adults. *Journal of Periodontology*, 44, 225–7.

Carter, H. G. and Barnes, G. P. (1975). Effects of three mouthwashes on existing dental plaque accumulations. *Journal of Preventive Dentistry*, 2, 6–11.

Ciancio, S. G., Mather, M. L., and Bunnell, H. L. (1975). Clinical evaluation of a quaternary ammonium containing mouthrinse. *Journal of Periodontology*, 46, 397–401.

Compton, F. H. and Beagrie, G. S. (1975). Inhibitory effect of benzethonium and zinc chloride mouthrinses on human dental plaque and gingivitis. *Journal of Clinical Periodontology*, 2, 33–43.

Coventry, J. and Newman, H. N. (1982). Experimental use of a slow release device employing chlorhexidine gluconate in areas of acute periodontal inflammation. *Journal of Clinical Periodontology*, 9, 129–33.

Cumming, B. R. and Loe, H. (1973). Optimal dosage and method of delivering chlorhexidine solutions for the inhibition of dental plaque. *Journal of Periodontal Research*, 8, 57–62.

Cutress, T. W., Brown, R. H., and Barker, D. S. (1977). Effects on plaque and gingivitis of a chlorhexidine dental gel in the mentally retarded. *Community Dentistry and Oral Epidemiology*, 5, 78–83.

Davies, A. (1973). The mode of action of chlorhexidine. *Journal of Periodontal Research*, 8 (Suppl. 12), 68–75.

Davies, G. E., Francis, J., and Martin, A. R. (1954). 1:6-di-4′ chlorophenyl-diguanido-hexane ('Hibitane'): laboratory investigation of a new antibacterial agent of high potency. *British Journal of Pharmacology*, 9, 192–6.

Davies, R. M. and Hull, P. S. (1973). Plaque inhibition and distribution of chlorhexidine in beagle dogs. *Journal of Periodontal Research*, 8 (Suppl. 12), 22–7.

Davies, R. M., Jensen, S. B., Schiott, C. R., and Loe, H. (1970). The effect of topical application of chlorhexidine on the bacterial colonisation of teeth and gingiva. *Journal of Periodontal Research*, 5, 96–101.

De la Rosa, M. and Sturzenburger, O. P. (1976). Clinical reduction of gingivitis through the use of a mouthwash containing two quaternary ammonium compounds. *Journal of Periodontology*, 47, 535–7.

De la Rosa, M., Sturzenburger, O. P., and Moore, D. J. (1987). The use of chlorhexidine in the management of gingivitis in children. *Journal of Periodontology*, 59, 387–9.

Denver, J. G. (1979). Oral hygiene in mentally retarded children. A clinical trial using a chlorhexidine spray. *Australian Dental Journal*, 24, 301–5.

Disney, J. A., Gravers, R. C., Cancro, L., Payonk, G., and Stewart, P. (1989). An evaluation of 6 dentrifice formulations for supragingival anticalculus and anti-plaque activity. *Journal of Clinical Periodontology*, 16, 525–8.

Dzink, J. L. and Socransky, S. S. (1985). Comparative *in vitro* activity of sanguinarine against oral microbial isolates. *Antimicrobial Agents and Chemotherapy*, 27, 663–5.

Ellingsen, J. E., Eriksen, H. M., and Rolla, G. (1982a). Extrinsic dental stain caused by stannous fluoride. *Scandinavian Journal of Dental Research*, 90, 9–13.

Ellingsen, J. E., Rolla, G., and Eriksen, H. M. (1982b). Extrinsic dental stain caused by chlorhexidine and other denaturing agents. *Journal of Clinical Periodontology*, 9, 317–22.

Elvin-Lewis, M. (1980). The dental health of chewing stick users of Southern Ghana: preliminary findings. *Journal of Preventive Dentistry*, 6, 151–9.

Emilson, C. G. (1977). Susceptibility of various microorganisms to chlorhexidine. *Scandinavian Journal of Dental Research*, 85, 255–65.

Emilson, C. G. and Fornell, J. (1976). The effect of toothbrushing with chlorhexidine gel on salivary microflora, oral hygiene and caries. *Scandinavian Journal of Dental Research*, 84, 308–19.

Emilson, C. G., Bowen, W. H., Robrish, S. A., and Kemp, C. W. (1980). Effect of the antimicrobial agent octenidine on the plaque flora in primates. *Journal of Dental Research*, 59A, 489.

Ennever, J. and Sturzenberger, O. P. (1961). Inhibition of dental calculus formation by use of enzyme chewing gum. *Journal of Periodontology*, 32, 331–3.

Ennever, J., Sturzenberger, O. P., and Radike, A. W. (1961). The calculus surface index method for scoring clinical calculus studies. *Journal of Periodontology*, 32, 54–7.

Eriksen, H. M. Nordbo, H., Kantanen, H., and Ellingsen, J. E. (1985). Chemical plaque control and extrinsic tooth discolouration. *Journal of Clinical Periodontology*, 12, 345–50.

Etemadzadeh, H. and Ainamo, J. (1987). Lacking anti-plaque efficacy of 2 sanguinarine mouthrinses. *Journal of Clinical Periodontology*, 14, 176–80.

Evans, R. T., Baker, P. J., Coburn, R. A., Fischman, S. L., and Genco, R. J. (1977). *In vitro* antiplaque effects of antiseptic phenols. *Journal of Periodontology*, 48, 156–62.

Ferreti, G. A., Ash, R. C., Brown, A. T., Largent, B. M., Kaplan, A., and Lillich, T. T. (1987). Chlorhexidine for prophylaxis against oral infections and associated complications in patients receiving bone marrow transplants. *Journal of the American Dental Association*, 114, 461–7.

Field, E. A., Nind, D., Varga, E., and Martin, M. V. (1988). The effect of chlorhexidine irrigation on the incidence of dry socket. A pilot study. *British Journal of Oral and Maxillofacial Surgery*, 26, 395–401.

Fine, D. H., Letizia, J., and Mandel, I. D. (1985). The effect of rinsing with Listerine antiseptic on the properties of developing dental plaque. *Journal of Clinical Periodontology*, 12, 660–6.

Fischman, S. L., Picozzi, A., Cancro, L. P., and Pader, M. (1973). The inhibition of plaque by two experimental oral rinses. *Journal of Periodontology*, 44, 100–2.

Fitzgerald, R. J. and Jordan, H. V. (1955). Effects of antibiotics on experimentally-induced caries in rats. *Journal of Dental Research*, 34, 685–6.

Fitzgerald, R. J., Keyes, P. H., Stoudt, T. H., and Spinell, D. M. (1968). The effects of a dextranase preparation on plaque and caries in hamsters. A preliminary report. *Journal of the American Dental Association*, 76, 301–4.

Flotra, L., Gjermo, P., Rolla, G., and Waerhaug, J. (1971a). Side effects of chlorhexidine mouthwashes. *Scandinavian Journal of Dental Research*, 79, 119–25.

Flotra, L., Poppe, K. S. and Sangnes, G. (1971b). Plaque-kontroll hos handikappede pasienter. *Tandlakartidningen*, 63, 781–5.

Flotra, L., Gjermo, P., Rolla, G., and Waerhaug, J. (1972). A 4-month study on the effect of chlorhexidine mouthwashes on 50 soldiers. *Scandinavian Journal of Dental Research*, 80, 10–17.

Formicola, A. J., Deasy, M. J., Graessle, O. E., Johnson, D. H., and Howe, E. E. (1978). The effect of an alexidine mouthwash on plaque and gingivitis. *Journal of Periodontology*, 49, 145–7.

Fornell, J., Sundin, Y., and Lindhe, J. (1975). Effect of Listerine on dental plaque and gingivitis. *Scandinavian Journal of Dental Research*, 83, 18–25.

Foulkes, E. (1973). Some toxicological observations an chlorhexidine. *Journal of Periodontal Research*, 8 (Suppl. 12), 55–7.

Friedman, M. and Golomb, G. (1982). New sustained release dosage form of chlorhexidine for dental use. I. Development and kinetics of release. *Journal of Periodontal Research*, 17, 323–8.

Friedman, M., Harari, D., Raz, H., and Golomb, G. (1985). Plaque inhibition by sustained release of chlorhexidine from removable appliances. *Journal of Dental Research*, 64, 1319–21.

Gargiulo, V. *et al.* (1980). Protective effect against bacterial plaque accumulation of a mouthwash containing cetylpyridinium. *Minerva Stomatology*, 29, 39–44.

Gazi, M. I. (1988). Photographic assessment of the antiplaque properties of sanguinarine and chlorhexidine. *Journal of Clinical Periodontology*, **15**, 106–9.

Gjermo, P. (1974). Chemical cleaning of teeth, In *Oral hygiene* (ed. A. Frandsen). Munksgaard, Copenhagen,

Gjermo, P. (1975). Some aspects of drug dynamics as related to oral soft tissue. *Journal of Dental Research*, **54**, (spec. iss.), B44–56.

Gjermo, P. and Eriksen, H. (1972). Effects of chlorhexidine-containing dentrifices. *Caries Research*, **6**, 72–3.

Gjermo, P. and Eriksen, H. M. (1974). Unchanged plaque inhibiting effect of chlorhexidine in human subjects after 2 years of continuous use. *Archives of Oral Biology*, **19**, 317–19.

Gjermo, P. and Rolla, G. (1970). Plaque inhibition by antibacterial dentrifices. *Scandinavian Journal of Dental Research*, **78**, 464–70.

Gjermo, P. and Rolla, G. (1971). The plaque inhibiting effect of chlorhexidine-containing dentrifices. *Scandinavian Journal of Dental Research*, **79**, 126–32.

Gjermo, P., Baastad, K., and Rolla, G. (1970). The plaque-inhibiting capacity of 11 antibacterial compounds. *Journal of Periodontal Research*, **5**, 102–9.

Gjermo, P., Bonesvoll, P., and Rolla, G. (1974). Relationship between plaque inhibiting effect and retention of chlorhexidine in the human oral cavity. *Archives of Oral Biology*, **19**, 1031–4.

Gjermo, P., Bonesvoll, P., Hjeljord, L. G., and Rolla, G. (1975). Influence of variation of pH of chlorhexidine mouthrinses on oral retention and plaque inhibiting effect. *Caries Research*, **9**, 74–82.

Gomer, R. M., Holroyd, S. V., Fedi, P. F., and Ferrign, P. D. (1972). The effects of oral rinses on the accumulation of dental plaque. *Journal of the American Society of Preventive Dentistry*, **2**, 12–14.

Goodson, J. M. (1985). In *Dental plaque control measures and oral hygiene practices* (ed. H. Loe and D.V. Kleinman), pp. 143–6. IRL Press, Oxford.

Goodson, J. M., Haffajee, A., and Socransky, S. S. (1979). Periodontal therapy by local delivery of tetracycline. *Journal of Clinical Periodontology*, **6**, 83–92.

Goodson, J. M., Hogan, P., and Dunham, S. (1984). Clinical responses in a four quadrant study of periodontal therapy. *Journal of Dental Research*, **63**, 268 (abstr. 874).

Gordon, J. M., Lamster, I. B., and Sieger, M. C. (1985). Efficacy of Listerine antiseptic in inhibiting the development of plaque and gingivitis. *Journal of Clinical Periodontology*, **12**, 697–704.

Greenfield, W. and Cuchel, S. J. (1984). The use of an oral rinse and dentrifice as a system for reducing plaque. *Compendium of Continuing Education In Dentistry* (Supplement), **5**, 82–7.

Grossman, E. *et al.* (1986). Six month study of the effects of a chlorhexidine mouthrinse on gingivitis in adults. *Journal of Periodontal Research*, **21** (Suppl. 16), 33–43.

Guggenheim, B. and Haller, R. (1972). Purification and properties of an α-(1–3) glucanohydrolase from *Trichoderma harzianium*. *Journal of Dental Research*, **51**, 394–402.

Guggenheim, B., Regolati, B., and Muhlemann, H. R. (1972). Caries and plaque inhibition by mutanase in rats. *Caries Research*, **6**, 289–97.

Hamp, S. E., Lindhe, J., and Loe, H. (1973). Long-term effect of chlorhexidine on developing gingivitis in the beagle dog. *Journal of Periodontal Research*, **8**, 63–70.

Hamp, S. E., Rosling, B., and Lindhe, J. (1975). Effect of chlorhexidine on gingival wound healing in the dog. A histometric study. *Journal of Clinical Periodontology*, **2**, 143–52.

Hansen, F., Gjermo, P., and Erikssen, H. M. (1975). The effect of a chlorhexidine-containing gel on the oral cleanliness and gingival health in young adults. *Journal of Clinical Periodontology*, **2**, 153–9.

Hardy, J. H., Newman, H. N., and Strahan, J. D. (1982). Direct irrigation and subgingival plaque. *Journal of Clinical Periodontology*, **9**, 57–65.

Harrap, G. J., Saxton, C. A., and Best, J. S. (1983). Inhibition of plaque growth by zinc salts. *Journal of Periodontal Research*, **18**, 634–42.

Harrison, J. W. E., Salisbury, G. B., Abbott, D. D., and Packman, E. W. (1963). Effect of enzyme toothpastes upon oral hygiene. *Journal of Periodontology*, **34**, 334–7.

Hattab, F. (1984). Effect of topical application of alginate containing fluoride and chlorhexidine on dental caries in rats. *Caries Research*, **18**, 367–74.

Hennessey, T. D. (1977). Antibacterial properties of Hibitane. *Journal of Clinical Periodontology*, 4 (extra iss.), 36–48.

Heyden, G. (1973). Relation between locally high concentration of chlorhexidine and staining as seen in the clinic. *Journal of Periodontal Research*, **8** (Suppl. 12), 76–80.

Hill, T. J. and Kniesner, A. H. (1949). Penicillin dentrifice and dental caries experience in children. *Journal of Dental Research*, **28**, 263–6.

Hill, T. J., Sims, J., and Newman, M. (1953a). Effect of penicillin dentrifice on the control of dental caries. *Journal of Dental Research*, **32**, 448–52.

Hill, T. J., Rasch, C., and Wollpert, B. (1953b). The development of organisms with penicillin resistance associated with the use of a penicillin dentrifice. *Journal of Dental Research*, **32**, 453–7.

Hoogendoorn, H. and Moorer, W. R. (1973). Lactoperoxidase in the prevention of plaque accumulation, gingivitis and dental caries I. *Odontologisk Revy*, **24**, 355–66.

Hugo, W. B. and Longworth, A. R. (1964). Some aspects of the mode of action of chlorhexidine. *Journal of Pharmacy and Pharmacology*, **16**, 655–62.

Hull, P. S. and Davies, R. M. (1972a). The effect of a chlorhexidine gel on tooth deposits in beagle dogs. *Journal of Small Animal Practice*, **13**, 207–12.

Hull, P. S. and Davies, R. M. (1972b). Effect of chlorhexidine and a benzyl analogue of chlorhexidine on plaque, calculus and gingivitis in beagle dogs. *Journal of Dental Research*, **51**, 1243–4.

Jedrychowski, J. R., Caputo, A. A., and Kerper, S. (1983). Antibacterial and mechanical properties of restorative materials combined with chlorhexidines. *Journal of Oral Rehabilitation*, **10**, 373–81.

Jenkins, S., Addy, M., and Newcombe, R. (1989). Studies on the effect of toothpaste rinses on plaque regrowth (II). Triclosan with and without zinc citrate formulation. *Journal of Clinical Periodontology*, **16**, 385–7.

Jensen, A. L. (1959). Use of dehydrated pancreas in oral hygiene. *Journal of the American Dental Association*, **59**, 923–30.

Jensen, S. B. and Loe, H. (1971). The effect of dextranase on plaque and gingivitis in man. In *The prevention of periodontal disease* (ed. J.E. Eastoe, D.C.A. Picton, and A.G. Alexander), pp. 131–5, Kimpton, London.

Johansen, J. R., Gjermo, P., and Eriksen, H. M. (1975). Effect of 2 years' use of chlorhexidine-containing dentrifices on plaque, gingivitis and caries. *Scandinavian Dental Journal*, **83**, 288–92.

Johnson, N. W. and Kenney, E. B. (1972). Effect of topical application of chlorhexidine on plaque and gingivitis in monkeys. *Journal of Periodontal Research*, 7, 180–8.

Jokinen, M. A. (1978). Prevention of post extraction bacteraemia by local prophylaxis. *International Journal of Oral Surgery*, 7, 450–2.

Kelstrup, J., Funder-Nielsen, T. P., and Moller, E. N. (1973). Enzymatic reduction of the colonisation of *Streptococcus mutans* in human dental plaque. *Acta Odontologica Scandinavica*, **31**, 249–53.

Kelstrup, J., Holm-Pedersen, P., and Poulsen, S. (1978). Reduction of the formation of dental plaque and gingivitis in humans by crude mutanase. *Scandinavian Journal of Dental Research*, **86**, 93–102.

Kennedy, P. T. and Kravets, T. F. (1970). Plaque removal and the use of an antibacterial mouthwash. *United States Navy Medical Newsletter*, **55**, 39–40.

Keyes, P. H., Hicks, M. A., Goldman, B. M., McCabe, R. M., and Fitzgerald, R. J. (1971). Dispersion of dextranous bacterial plaque on human teeth with dextranase. *Journal of the American Dental Association*, **82**, 136–41.

Khoo, J. G. L. and Newman, H. N. (1983). Subgingival plaque control by a simplified oral hygiene regime plus local chlorhexidine or metronidazole. *Journal of Periodontal Research*, **18**, 607–19.

Klewansky, P. and Vernier, D. (1984). Sanguinarine and the control of plaque in dental practice. *Compendium of Continuing Education in Dentistry* (Supplement) **5**, 94–7.

Klinge, B., Matsson, L., Attstrom, R., Edwardsson, S., and Willard, L. O. (1989). Effect of local applications of Decapinol on developing and early established dental plaque in humans. *Journal of Dental Research*, **68**, 970 (Abstr. 829).

Klock, B., Serling, J., Kinders, S., Manwell, M. A., and Tinanoff, N. (1985). Comparison of effect of SnF$_2$ mouthrinses on caries incidence, salivary *S. mutans* and gingivitis in high caries prevalent adults. *Scandinavian Journal of Dental Research*, **93**, 213–17.

Koch, G., Edland, K., and Hoogendoorn, H. (1973). Lactoperoxidase in the prevention of plaque accumulation, gingivitis and dental caries. *Odontologisk Revy*, **24**, 367–72.

Koch, G. and Strand, G. (1979). Effect of an enzyme dentrifice on caries. *Swedish Dental Journal*, **3**, 9–13.

Konig, K. G. (1959). Dental caries and plaque accumulation in rats treated with stannous fluoride and penicillin. *Acta Odontologica Helvetica*, **6**, 39–44.

Konig, K. G. and Guggenheim, B. (1968). *In vivo* effects of dextranase on plaque and caries. *Acta Odontologica Helvetica*, **12**, 48–54.

Kornman, K. S. (1986). The role of supragingival plaque in the prevention and treatment of periodontal diseases. *Journal of Periodontal Research*, **21** (Suppl. 16), 5–22.

Krenkel, C. and Rothler, G. (1979). Erfahrungen mit 'chlorhexidin' bei intermaxillar verschnurten patienten. *Oesterreichische Zeitschrift für Stomatologie*, **76**, 408–13.

Lamster, I. B., Alfano, M. C., Seiger, M. C., and Gordon, J. M. (1983). The effect of Listerine antiseptic on existing plaque and gingivitis. *Journal of Clinical Preventive Dentistry*, **5**, 12–16.

Lang, N. P. and Ramseier-Grossmann, K. (1981). Optimal dosage of chlorhexidine digluconate in clinical plaque control when applied by the oral irrigator. *Journal of Clinical Periodontology*, **8**, 189–202.

Lang, N. P. *et al.* (1982). Effects of supervised chlorhexidine mouthrinses in children. A longitudinal trial. *Journal of Periodontal Research*, **17**, 101–11.

Lang, N. P., Catalanotto, F. A., Knopfli, R. U., and Antczak, A. A. A. (1988). Quality-specific taste impairment following the application of chlorhexidine mouthrinses. *Journal of Clinical Periodontology*, **15**, 43–8.

Langebeck, J. and Bay, L. (1976). The effect of chlorhexidine mouthrinses on healing after gingivectomy. *Scandinavian Journal of Dental Research*, **84**, 224–8.

Leverett, D. H., McHugh, W. D., and Jensen, O. E. (1984). Effect of daily rinsing with stannous fluoride on plaque and gingivitis. *Journal of Dental Research*, **63**, 1083–6.

Lindhe, J. (1984). Clinical assessment of antiplaque agents. *Compendium of Continuing Education in Dentistry* (Supplement) **5**, 594.

Lindhe, J., Hamp, S-E., Loe, H., and Schiott, C. R. (1970a). Influence of topical application of chlorhexidine on chronic gingivitis and gingival wound healing in the dog. *Scandinavian Journal of Dental Research*, **78**, 471–8.

Lindhe, J., Heyden, G., Svanberg, G., Loe, H., and Schiott, C. R. (1970b). Effect of local applications of chlorhexidine on the oral mucosa of the hamster. *Journal of Periodontal Research*, **5**, 177–82.

Listgarten, M. and Ellegaard, B. (1973). Experimental gingivitis in the monkey. *Journal of Periodontal Research*, **8**, 199–214.

Llewelyn, J. (1980). A double-blind cross-over trial on the effect of cetylpyridinium chloride 0.05 per cent (Merocet) on plaque accumulation. *British Dental Journal*, **148**, 103–4.

Lobene, R. R. (1971). A clinical study of the effect of dextranase on human dental plaque. *Journal of the American Dental Association*, **82**, 132–5.

Lobene, R. R., and Soparker, P. M., (1973). The effect of an alexidine mouthwash on human plaque and gingivitis. *Journal of the American Dental Association*, **87**, 848–51.

Lobene, R. R., Brian, M., and Socransky, S. S. (1969). Effect of erythromycin on dental plaque forming microorganisms. *Journal of Periodontology*, **40**, 287–91.

Lobene, R. R., Lobene, S. and Soparker, P. M. (1977). The effect of cetylpyridinium chloride mouthwash on plaque and gingivitis. *Journal of Dental Research*, **56**, B195 (abstr. 575).

Lobene, R. R., Kashket, S., Soparker, P. M., Schloss, J., and Sabine, Z. M. (1979). The effect of cetylpyridinium chloride on human plaque bacteria and gingivitis. *Pharmacology and Therapeutics in Dentistry*, **4**, 33–47.

Lobene, R. R. and Soparker, P. M., and Newman, M. B. (1986). The effects of a sanguinarine dentrifice on plaque and gingivitis. *Compendium of Continuing Education in Dentistry* (Supplement) **7**, 185–8.

Lobene, R. R., Soparkar, P. M., Newman, M. B., and Kohut, B. E. (1987). Reduced formation of supragingival calculus with use of fluoride-zinc chloride dentrifice. *Journal of the American Dental Association*, **114**, 350–2.

Loe, H. and Schiott, C. R. (1970). The effect of mouthrinses and topical application of chlorhexidine on the development of dental plaque and gingivitis in man. *Journal of Periodontal Research*, **5**, 79–83.

Loe, H. and Silness, J. (1966). Periodontal disease in pregnancy I. Prevalence and severity. *Acta Odontologica Scandinavica*, **21**, 533–51.

Loe, H., Theilade, E., Jensen, S. B., and Schiott, C. R. (1967). Experimental gingivitis in man. III. The influence of antibiotics on gingival plaque development. *Journal of Periodontal Research*, **2**, 282–9.

Loe, H., Von Der Fehr, F. R., and Schiott, C. R. (1972). Inhibition of experimental caries by plaque prevention. The effect of chlorhexidine mouthrinses. *Scandinavian Journal of Dental Research*, **80**, 1–9.

Loe, H., Schiott, C. R., Glavind, L., and Karring, T. (1976). Two years' oral use of chlorhexidine in man. I. General design and clinical effects. *Journal of Periodontal Research*, **11**, 135–44.

Loesche, W. J. (1976). Chemotherapy of dental plaque infections. *Oral Science Reviews*, **9**, 65–107.

Loesche, W. J., Green, E., Kenny, E. B., and Nafe, D. (1971). Effect of topical kanamycin sulphate on plaque accumulation. *Journal of the American Dental Association*, **83**, 1063–9.

Loesche, W. J. and Nafe, D. (1973). Reduction of supragingival plaque accumulations in institutionalised Down's syndrome patients by periodic treatment with topical kanamycin. *Archives of Oral Biology*, **18**, 1131–43.

Loesche, W. J., Hockett, R. N., and Syed, S. A. (1977). Reductions in the proportions of dental plaque Streptococci following a 5-day kanamycin treatment. *Journal of Periodontal Research*, **12**, 1–10.

Lusk, S. S, Bowers, G. M., Tow, H. D., Watson, W. J., and Moffitt, W. C. (1974). Effects of an oral rinse on experimental gingivitis, plaque formation and formed plaque. *Journal of the American Society of Preventive Dentistry*, **4**, 31–7.

Macalister, A. D. (1961). Post-operative dressings for immediate dentures. *New Zealand Dental Journal*, **57**, 82–4.

Mackenzie, I. C., Nuki, K., Loe, H., and Schiott, R. M. (1976). Two years' oral use of chlorhexidine in man. V. Effects on stratum corneum or oral mucosa. *Journal of Periodontal Research*, **11**, 165–71.

McClure, F. J. and Hewitt, W. L. (1946). The relationship of penicillin to induced rat dental caries and oral *L. acidophilis*. *Journal of Dental Research*, **25**, 441–3.

Mallatt, M. E., Beiswanger, B. B., Drook, C. A., Stookey, C. A., Stookey, G. K., Jackson, R. D., and Bricker, S. L. (1989). Clinical effect of a Sanguinaria dentrifice upon plaque and gingivitis in adults. *Journal of Periodontology*, **60**, 91–5.

Mankodi, S., Ross, N. M., and Mostler, K. (1987). Clinical efficacy of Listerine in inhibiting and reducing plaque and experimental gingivitis. *Journal of Clinical Periodontology*, **14**, 285–8.

Matsson, L., Klinge, B., Willard, L. O., Attstrom, R., and Edwardsson, S. (1983). The effect of Octapinol on dentogingival plaque and the development of gingivitis. II. Long term studies in beagle dogs. *Journal of Periodontal Research*, **18**, 438–44.

Mauriello, S. M. and Bader, J. D. (1988). Six-month effects of a sanguinarine dentifrice on plaque and gingivitis. *Journal of Periodontology*, **59**, 238–43.

Menaker, L., Weatherford, T. W., Pitts, G., Ross, N. M., and Lamm, R. (1979). The effects of Listerine antiseptic on dental plaque. *Alabama Journal of Medical Science*, **16**, 71–7.

Meskin, L. H., Silverstone, L. M., and Schoenfeld, S. (1983). Further studies on an enzyme-containing dentifrice. *Journal of Dental Research*, **62**, 693 (abstr. 389).

Midda, M. and Cooksey, M. W. (1986). Clinical uses of an enzyme-containing dentifrice. *Journal of Clinical Periodontology*, **13**, 950–6.

Mitchell, D. F. and Holmes, L. A. (1965). Topical antibiotic control of dentogingival plaque. *Journal of Periodontology*, **36**, 202–8.

Moore, R. L., Feldman, S. M., Abbott, L. J., Read, C. J., Williams, J. N., and Wittwer, J. W. (1989). Evaluating the antiplaque capabilities of a copper-containing prophylaxis paste. *Journal of Periodontology*, **60**, 78–80.

Moran, J., Addy, M., and Newcombe, R. (1988). A clinical trial to assess the efficacy of sanguinarine-zinc mouthrinse (Veadent) compared with chlorhexidine mouthrinse (Corsodyl). *Journal of Clinical Periodontology*, **15**, 612–16.

Muhlemanh, H. R., Schmid, R., and Firestone, A. R. (1981). Effect on rat caries of endogenous and exogenous hydrogen peroxide. *Caries Research*, **15**, 46–53.

Newman, H. N., Yeung, F. I. S, Wan Yusof, W. Z. A. B., and Addy, M. (1984). Slow release metronidazole and a simplified mechanical oral hygiene regime in the control of chronic periodontitis. *Journal of Clinical Periodontology*, **11**, 576–82.

Nordbo, H. (1971). Discolouration of human teeth by a combination of chlorhexidine and aldehydes and ketones *in vitro*. *Scandinavian Journal of Dental Research*, **79**, 356–61.

Nordbo, H. (1979). Ability of chlorhexidine and benzalkonium chloride to catalyse browning reactions *in vitro*. *Journal of Dental Research*, **58**, 1429.

Nygaard-Oestby, P. and Persson, I. (1984). Evaluation of sanguinarine chloride in control of plaque in the dental practice. *Compendium of Continuing Education in Dentistry* (Supplement) **5**, 90–3.

O'Connor, J. R., Paris, D. A., and Bailey, D. M. (1980). Octenidine hydrochloride, an effective dental plaque inhibitor. *Journal of Dental Research*, **59A**, 743.

Obeiyi, O. O. and Sofowara E. A. (1979). Antimicrobial alkaloids from Nigerian chewing stick (*Fagara zanghoxyloides*). *Plant Medica*, **36**, 204–7.

Olsen, I. (1975). Denture stomatitis: the clinical effects of chlorhexidine and amphotericin B. *Acta Odontologica Scandinavica*, **33**, 47–52.

Packman, E. W., Abbott, D. D., Salisbury, G. B., and Harrison, J. W. E. (1963). Effect of enzyme chewing gums upon oral hygiene. *Journal of Periodontology*, **34**, 255–8.

Palcanis, K. G., Formica, J. G., Miller, R. A., Brooks, C. N., and Gunsolley, J. C. (1986). Longitudinal evaluation of sanguinaria: clinical and microbiological studies. *Compendium of Continuing Education in Dentistry* (Supplement) **7**, 179–84.

Parsons, L. G., Thomas, L. G., Southard, G. L., Woodall, I. R. and Jones, B. J. B., (1987). Effect of sanguinaria extract on established plaque and gingivitis when supragingivally delivered as a manual rinse or under pressure in an oral irrigator. *Journal of Clinical Periodontology*, **14**, 381–5.

Patters, M. R., Anerud, K., Trummel, C. L., Kornman, K. S., Nalbandian, J., and Robertson, P. 8. (1983). Inhibition of plaque formation in humans by octenidine mouthrinse. *Journal of Periodontal Research*, **18**, 212–19.

Patters, M. R. *et al.* (1986). Effects of octenidine mouthrinse on plaque formation and gingivitis in humans. *Journal of Periodontal Research*, **21**, 154–62.

Picozzi, A., Fischman, S. L., Pader, M., and Cancro, L. P. (1972). Calculus inhibition in humans. *Journal of Periodontology*, **43**, 692–5.

Pitcher, G. R., Newman, H. N., and Strahan, J. D. (1980). Access to subgingival plaque by disclosing agents using mouthrinsing and direct irrigation. *Journal of Clinical Periodontology*, **7**, 300–8.

Pluss, E. M., Engelberger, P. R., and Rateitschak, K. H. (1975). Effect of chlorhexidine on dental plaque formation under periodontal pack. *Journal of Clinical Periodontology*, **2**, 136–42.

Prayitno, S., Taylor, L., Cadogan, S., and Addy, M. (1979). An *in vivo* study of dietary factors in the etiology of tooth staining associated with the use of chlorhexidine. *Journal of Periodontal Research*, **14**, 411–17.

Roberts, W. R. and Addy, M. (1981). Comparison of the bisbiguanide antiseptics alexidine and chlorhexidine. I. Effect on plaque accumulation and salivary bacteria. *Journal of Clinical Periodontology*, **8**, 213–19.

Roed-Petersen, B. and Hjorting-Hansen, E. (976). Avendelse of klorheksidin i traumatologien samt ved operativ behandling af granulomatose protesestomatitter. *Tandlaegebladet*, **80**, 367–9.

Rolla, G. and Melsen, B. (1975). On the mechanisms of the plaque inhibition by chlorhexidine. *Journal of Dental Research*, **54** (Spec. iss.), B57–62.

Rolla, G., Loe, H., and Schiott, C. R. (1970). The affinity of chlorhexidine for hydroxyapatite and salivary mucosa. *Journal of Periodontal Research*, **5**, 90–5.

Rolla, G. R., Loe, H., and Schiott, C. R. (1971). Retention of chlorhexidine in the human oral cavity. *Archives of Oral Biology*, **16**, 1109–16.

Rotgans, J. and Hoongedoorn, H. (1979). The effect of toothbrushing with a toothpaste containing amyloglucosidase and glucose oxidase on plaque accumulation and gingivitis. *Caries Research*, **13**, 144–9.

Rotgans, J. and Schmalz, G. (1977). Der effect einer amyloglucosidase und glucose oxidase enthaltenden Zahnpaste auf Plaquebildung und Gingivitis. *Deutsche Zahnaertzliche Zeitschrift*, **32**, 755–6.

Rotgans, J., Hoongedoorn, H., and Riethe, P. (1977). Effect of toothbrushing with toothpaste containing amyloglucosidase and glucose oxidase on plaque accumulation on teeth. *Caries Research*, **11**, 123–4.

Rushton, A. (1977). Safety of Hibitane. II. Human experience. *Journal of Clinical Periodontology*, **4** (Extra iss.), 73–9.

Russell, B. G. and Bay, L. M. (1978). Oral use of chlorhexidine gluconate toothpaste on epileptic children. *Scandinavian Journal of Dental Research*, **86**, 52–7.

Saxton, C. A. (1986). The effects of a dentrifice containing zinc citrate and 2,4,4 trichloro-2-hydroxydiphenyl ether. *Journal of Periodontology*, **57**, 555–61.

Saxton, C. A. and van der Ouderaa, F. J. G. (1989). The effect of a dentrifice containing zinc citrate and Triclosan on developing gingivitis. *Journal of Periodontal Research*, **24**, 75–80.

Saxton, C. A., Harrap, G. J., and Lloyd, A. M. (1986). The effect of dentrifices containing zinc citrate on plaque growth and oral zinc levels. *Journal of Clinical Periodontology*, **13**, 301–6.

Saxton, C. A., Lane, R. M., and van der Ouderaa, F. (1987). The effects of a dentrifice containing zinc salt and a non-cationic anti-microbial agent on plaque and gingivitis. *Journal of Clinical Periodontology*, **14**, 144–8.

Schiott, C. R. (1973). Effect of chlorhexidine on the microflora of the oral cavity. *Journal of Periodontal Research*, **8** (Suppl. 12), 7–10.

Schiott, C. R., Loe, H., Jensen, S. B., Kilian, M., Davies, R. M., and Glavind, K. (1970). The effect of chlorhexidine mouthrinses on the human oral flora. *Journal of Periodontal Research*, **5**, 84–9.

Schiott, C. R., Briner, W. W., Kirkland, J. J., and Loe, H. (1976a). Two-year use of chlorhexidine in man. III. Changes in sensitivity of the salivary flora. *Journal of Periodontal Research*, 11, 153–7.

Schiott, C. R., Briner, W. W., and Loe, H. (1976b). Two year use of chlorhexidine in man. II. The effect on the salivary bacterial flora. *Journal of Periodontal Research*, 11, 145–152.

Schiott, C. R., Loe, H., and Briner, W. W. (1976c). Two years oral use of chlorhexidine in man. IV. Effect on various medical parameters. *Journal of Periodontal Research*, 11, 158–64.

Schmid, M. O., Schait, A., and Muhlemann, H. R. (1974). Effect of a zinc chloride mouthrinse on calculus deposits formed on foils. *Helvetica Odontologica Acta*, 11, 22–4.

Schonfeld, S., Stamm, J. W., Meskin, L. H., and Silverstone, L. M. (1983). The effect of an enzyme-containing dentrifice on plaque and gingivitis. *Journal of Dental Research*, 62, 178.

Schonfeld, S., Farnoush, A., and Wilson, S. G. (1986). *In vivo* antiplaque activity of a sanguinarine-containing dentrifice: comparison with conventional toothpastes. *Journal of Periodontal Research*, 21, 298–303.

Schroeder, H. E. (1969). *Formation and inhibition of dental calculus*, p.129. Hans Huber, Stuttgart.

Schuller, P. and Yeung, P. (1982). Comparing plaque effectiveness between chlorhexidine impregnated floss and conventional floss. *Journal of Dental Research*, 61, 274 (abstr. 857).

Segreto, V. A., Collins, E. M., Beiswanger, B. B., de la Rosa, M., Isaacs, R. L., and Lang, N. P. (1986). A comparison of mouthrinses containing two concentrations of chlorhexidine. *Journal of Periodontal Research*, 21 (Suppl. 16), 23–32.

Shaver, K. J. and Schiff, P. (1970). Oral clinical functionality of enzyme Ap used as a mouthwash. *Journal of Periodontology*, 41, 333–6.

Shern, R. J., Little, W. A., Kennedy, J. B., and Mirth, D. B. (1988). Effects of octenidine on dental plaque and gingivitis in monkeys. *Journal of Periodontology*, 57, 628–33.

Shwachman, H., Leubner, H., and Catzel, P. (1955). Muscoviscidosis. In *Advances in pediatrics*, Vol. 7, pp. 249–323. Year Book Publishers, Chicago.

Siegrist, B. E., Gusberti, F. A., Brecx, M. C., Weber, H. P., and Lang, N. P. (1986). Efficacy of supervised rinsing with chlohexidine digluconate in comparison to phenolic and plant alkaloid compounds. *Journal of Periodontal Research*, 21 (Suppl.16), 60–73.

Silness, J. and Loe, H. (1964). Periodontal disease in pregnancy. II. Correlation between oral hygiene and periodontal condition. *Acta Odontologica Scandinavica*, 22, 121–35.

Skjorland, K., Gjermo, P., and Rolla, G. (1978). Effect of some polyvalent cations on plaque formation *in vivo*. *Scandinavian Journal of Dental Research*, 86, 103–7.

Slee, A. M. and O'Connor, J. R. (1983). *In vitro* antiplaque activity of octenidine hydrochloride (WIN41464–2) for preformed plaques of selected plaque forming micro-organisms. *Antimicrobial Agents and Chemotherapy*, 23, 379–84.

Snyder, I. S. and Finch, R. G. (1982). Antiseptics, disinfectants and sterilisation. In *Modern pharmacology* (ed. C. R. Craig and R. E. Stitzel), p.743. Little, Brown & Co., Boston.

Soh, L. L., Newman, H. N., and Strahan, J. D. (1982). Effects of subgingival chlorhexidine irrigation on periodontal inflammation. *Journal of Clinical Periodontology*, 9, 66–74.

Southard, G. L., Boulware, R. T., Walbourn, D. R., Croznik, W. J., Thorne, E. E., and Yankell, S. L. (1984). Sanguinarine, a new antiplaque agent: retention and plaque specificity. *Journal of the American Dental Association*, 108, 338–41.

Southard, G. L., Parsons, L. G., Thomas, L. G., Jnr. (1985). The antiplaque efficacy of a sanguinarine oral rinse. *Journal of Dental Research*, 64, 236 (abstr. 549).

Southard, G. L., Parsons, L. G., Thomas, L. G., Boulware, R. T., Woodall, I. R., and Jones, B. J. B. (1987a). The relationship of sanguinaria extract concentration and zinc ion to plaque and gingivitis. *Journal of Clinical Periodontology*, 14, 315–19.

Southard, G. L., Parsons, L. G., Thomas, L. G., Woodall, I. R., and Jones, B. J. B. (1987b). Effect of Sanguinaria extract on development of plaque and gingivitis when supragingivally delivered as a manual rinse or under pressure in an oral irrigator. *Journal of Clinical Periodontology*, 14, 377–80.

Spiers, A. S. D., Dias, S. F., and Lopez, J. A. (1980). Infection prevention in patients with cancer: microbiological evaluation of portable laminar air flow isolation, topical chlorhexidine and oral non-absorbable antibiotics. *Journal of Hygiene*, 84, 457–65.

Spolsky, V. W., Bhatia, H. L., Forsythe, A., and Levin, D. (1975). The effect of an antimicrobial mouthwash on dental plaque and gingivitis in young adults. *Journal of Periodontology*, 46, 685–90.

Stallard, R., Volpe, A. R., Orban, J. E., and King, W. J. (1969). The effect of an antimicrobial mouthwash on dental plaque, calculus and gingivitis. *Journal of Periodontology*, 40, 683–94.

Stephan, R. M., Fitzgerald, R. J., McClure, F. S., Harris, M. R. and Jordan, H. (1952). The comparative effects of penicillin, bacitracin, chlormycetin, aureomycin and streptomycin on experimental dental caries and on certain oral bacteria in the rat. *Journal of Dental Research*, 31, 421–7.

Stewart, G. G. (1952). Mucinase—a possible means of reducing calculus formation. *Journal of Periodontology*, 23, 85–90.

Storhaug, K. (1977). Hibitane in oral disease in handicapped patients. *Journal of Clinical Periodontology*, 4, (Extra Iss.), 102–7.

Sturzenburger, O. P. and Leonard, G. J. (1969). The effect of a mouthwash as an adjunct in tooth cleaning. *Journal of Periodontology*, 40, 299–304.

Svatun, B., Gjermo, P., Eriksen, H., and Rolla, G. (1977). A comparison of plaque inhibiting activity of stannous fluoride and chlorhexidine. *Acta Odontologica Scandinavica*, 35, 247–50.

Svatun, B., Saxton, C. A., van der Ouderaa, F., and Rolla, G. (1987). The influence of a dentrifice containing a zinc salt and a non ionic antimicrobial agent on the maintenance of gingival health. *Journal of Clinical Periodontology*, 14, 457–61.

Svatun, B., Saxton, C. A., Rolla, G., and van der Ouderaa, F. (1989). A 1-year study on the maintenance of gingival health by a dentrifice containing a zinc salt and non-anionic antimicrobial agent. *Journal of Clinical Periodontology*, 16, 75–80.

Tinanoff, N. and Camosci, D. A. (1980). Microbiological, ultrastructural and spectroscopic analyses of the anti-tooth-plaque properties of fluoride compounds *in vitro*. *Archives of Oral Biology*, 25, 531–43.

Tinanoff, N., Brady, J. M., and Gross, A. (1976). The effects of sodium fluoride and stannous fluoride mouthrinses on bacterial contamination of both enamel TEM and SEM studies. *Caries Research*, 10, 415–26.

Tjernberg, A. (1979). Influence of oral hygiene measures on the development of alveolitis sicca dolorosa after surgical removal of mandibular third molars. *International Journal of Oral Surgery*, 8, 430–4.

Turesky, S., Gilmore, N. D., and Glickman, I. (1970). Reduced plaque formation by the chloromethyl analogue of Vitamin C. *Journal of Periodontology*, 41, 41–3.

Turesky, S., Warner, V., and Slinsun, P. (1977). Prolongation of antibacterial activity of chlorhexidine adsorbed to teeth: effect of sulphates. *Journal of Periodontology*, 48, 646–9.

Usher, P. J. (1975). Oral hygiene in mentally handicapped children. A pilot study of the use of chlorhexidine gel. *British Dental Journal*, 138, 217–21.

Volpe, A. R., Manhold, J. H., and Hazen, S. P. (1965). *In vivo* calculus assessment. I. A method and its examiner reproducibility, *Journal of Periodontology*, 36, 292–4.

Volpe, A. R., Kuplzak, L. J., Brant, J. H., King, W. J., Kestenbaum, R. C., and Schussel, H. J. (1969). Antimicrobial control of bacterial plaque and calculus and the effects of these agents on oral flora. *Journal of Dental Research*, **48**, 832–41.

Waaler, S. M. and Rolla, G. (1985). Importance of teeth and tongue as possible receptor sites for chlorhexidine in relation to its clinical effect. *Scandinavian Journal of Dental Research*, **93**, 222–6.

Waerhaug, M., Gjermo, P., Rolla, G., and Johansen, J. R. (1984). Comparison of the effect of chlorhexidine and copper sulphate on plaque formation and development of gingivitis. *Journal of Clinical Periodontology*, **11**, 176–80.

Walsh, J. P. and Smart, R. S. (1951). Clinical trial of a penicillin tooth powder. *New Zealand Dental Journal*, **47**, 118–22.

Watts, E. A. and Newman, H. N. (1986). Clinical effects on chronic periodontitis of a simplified system of oral hygiene including subgingival pulsated jet irrigation with chlorhexidine. *Journal of Clinical Periodontology*, **13**, 666–70.

Weatherford, T. W., Finn, S. B., and Jamieson, H. C. (1977). Effects of an alexidine mouthwash on dental plaque and gingivitis in humans over a 6-month period. *Journal of American Dental Association*, **94**, 528–36.

Wennstrom, J. and Lindhe, J. (1985). Some effects of a sanguinarine-containing mouthrinse on developing plaque and gingivitis. *Journal of Clinical Periodontology*, **12**, 867–72.

Wennstrom, J. and Lindhe, J. (1986). The effects of mouthrinses on parameters characterising human periodontal disease. *Journal of Clinical Periodontology*, **13**, 86–93.

Wennstrom, J. L., Heye, L., Dahlen, G., and Grondahl, K. (1987). Periodic subgingival antimicrobial irrigation of periodontal pockets. I. Clinical observations. *Journal of Clinical Periodontology*, **14**, 541–50.

Wentland, M. P. (1988). The *in vitro* dental plaque inhibitory properties of a series of N-[¹-alkyl-4(IH)-pyridinylidene] alkylamines. *Journal of Medical Chemistry*, **31**, 2024–7.

Westfelt, E., Nyman, S., Lindhe, J., and Socransky, S. S. (1983). Use of chlorhexidine as a plaque control measure following gingival treatment of periodontal disease. *Journal of Clinical Periodontology*, **10**, 22–36.

Westling, M. and Tynelius-Bratthall, G. (1984). Microbiological and clinical short-term effects of repeated intracrevicular chlorhexidine rinsings. *Journal of Periodontal Research*, **9**, 202–9.

Willard, L. O., Edwardsson, S., Attstrom, R., and Matsson, L. (1983). The effect of Octapinol on dento-gingival plaque and development of gingivitis. I. *In vitro* experiments and short-term studies in beagle dogs. *Journal of Periodontal Research*, **18**, 429–37.

Winrow, M. J. (1973). Metabolic studies with radiolabelled chlorhexidine in animals and man. *Journal of Periodontal Research*, **8**, 45–8.

Zander, H. A. (1950). Effects of a penicillin dentrifice on caries incidence in school children. *Journal of the American Dental Association*, **40**, 569–74.

Zickert, I., Emilson, C. C., and Krasse, B. (1982). Effect of caries preventive measures in children highly infected with *Streptococcus mutans*. *Archives of Oral Biology*, **27**, 861–8.

10. Antibiotics in the management of periodontal disease

10.1 INTRODUCTION

Antibiotics are typically used in medicine to eliminate infections caused by the invasion of the host by a foreign, pathogenic micro-organism. The microbial aetiology of inflammatory periodontal diseases has provided the basis for the introduction of antibiotics in their overall management. The role of antibiotics as anti-plaque agents has been discusssed in Chapter 9 and will not be considered further here. This chapter will assess the ability of specific antibiotics to reduce the pathogenicity of the subgingival microflora and subsequently affect the clinical signs of disease. The pharmacokinetics and pharmacodynamics of the most frequently used agents will be discussed, and the clinical evidence of their efficacy presented. However, in the first instance, consideration must be given both to the rationale for the use of antibiotics in periodontal treatment and also to the possible routes of administration.

10.2 RATIONALE FOR THE USE OF ANTIBIOTICS

The academic argument over the importance of a specific or a non-specific bacterial aetiology for periodontal diseases may never be totally resolved (see Chapter 2). However, there is little doubt that certain specific organisms are closely associated with some forms of periodontal disease and perhaps 6–12 microbial species are responsible for the majority of cases of periodontitis (Table 10.1) (Theilade 1986). Unlike the majority of general infections, all the suspected periodontal pathogens are indigenous to the oral flora (Slots et al. 1980b; Zambon et al. 1983; Wolff et al. 1985). Consequently, the long-term and total elimination of

Table 10.1 Pathogens that have been associated with different forms of periodontal disease

Disease	Micro-organisms
Adult periodontitis	*Bacteroides gingivalis* *Bacteriodes melaninogenicus* *Fusobacterium nucleatum*
Localised juvenile periodontitis	*Actinobacillus* *actinomycetemcomitans* *Capnocytophaga*
Rapidly progressive periodontitis	*Bacteroides gingivalis* *Actinobacillus* *actinomycetemcomitans*

these organisms with antibiotics will be very difficult to achieve as immediate repopulation with the indigenous bacteria will occur when the therapy is concluded (Van Palenstein Heldermann 1986). Therefore, antibiotics as the only form of therapy are unlikely to be successful in the long term. Indeed, they are inferior to the time-honoured methods of treatment such as scaling and root planing alone (Listgarten et al. 1978; Lindhe et al. 1979). Nevertheless, in certain forms of periodontitis the loss of connective tissue attachment is rapid. Extremely virulent, Gram-negative organisms populate the deep pockets, and bacteria can actually invade the connective tissues (Gillett and Johnson 1982; Saglie et al. 1982). Under these circumstances, antibiotics provide a useful adjunct to root planing, which by itself may not remove all subgingival deposits and certainly would not affect any invading organisms that had already penetrated soft tissues. Furthermore, it is reassuring to know that all of the pathogens shown in Table 10.1 have been shown, *in vitro*, to be sensitive to a number of different antibiotics (Genco, 1981).

10.3 ROUTES OF ADMINISTRATION

The singular aim of using antibiotics as part of a treatment regimen is to achieve, within the periodontal environment, a concentration of the drug that is sufficient either to kill or arrest the growth of the pathogenic micro-organisms. The most effective and reliable method of achieving these concentrations is by systemic administration whereby the drug is able to bathe the subgingival flora by passing into the gingival crevicular fluid. Indeed, certain drugs such as tetracycline have been found to concentrate in crevicular fluid at higher levels than those found in serum after the same oral dose (Walker et al. 1981b; Baker et al. 1985). The drug can then bind to tooth sufaces, from which it is released in active form (Baker et al. 1983).

In an attempt to minimize the chances of adverse reactions, antibiotics have been applied topically to periodontal pockets by techniques such as subgingival irrigation (Pitcher et al. 1980), acrylic strips (Addy et al. 1982), and hollow, permeable, cellulose acetate fibres filled with the drug (Goodson et al. 1979; Lindhe et al. 1979). These methods allow lower doses of antibiotics to be administered than by oral dosing, although the extent to which the drugs penetrate the pockets will be less predictable. Further, the multiple insertion and removal of acrylic strips and fibres is time-consuming and this may preclude their widespread clinical use.

Table 10.2 Contraindications and unwanted effects of antibiotics that have been used in the management of periodontal diseases.

	Contraindications	Unwanted effects
Tetracyclines	Impaired renal function; pregnancy; children under 12 years	Abdominal discomfort, nausea, vomiting, diarrhoea, pseudomembranous colitis (rare), staining of teeth, candidal infections of mucous membranes, delayed closure of fontanelles Minocycline and doxycycline produce fewer renal side-effects and may be used in patients with renal failure Minocycline may also induce vertigo, dizziness, ataxia, and tinnitus
Metronidazole	Central nervous system disorders and severe hepatic disease. Avoid in the first trimester of pregnancy and with concurrent intake of alcohol	An unpleasant bitter or metallic taste, nausea, vomiting, indigestion, diarrhoea, constipation, and abdominal discomfort. Dizziness and headaches are less common
Penicillins	History of penicillin allergy	Hypersensitivity reactions ranging from mild rashes and urticaria to severe anaphylactic shock
Clindamycin Lincomycin	Impaired hepatic or renal function Diarrhoeal states	Abdominal discomfort, nausea, vomiting, diarrhoea, pseudomembranous colitis
Spiramycin Erythromycin	Hepatic impairment	Nausea, vomiting, diarrhoea

10.4 TETRACYCLINES

(e.g. tetracycline, chlortetracycline, clomocycline, demeclocycline, doxycycline, lymecycline, minocycline, and oxytetracycline)

The tetracyclines are a group of closely related, bacteriostatic antibiotics that provide a 'broad spectrum' of activity against both Gram-positive and Gram-negative micro-organisms. Gram-positive organisms are affected by lower concentrations of tetracyclines than are Gram-negative species, although more suitable antibiotics are usually preferred for Gram-positive infections. Tetracyclines are effective against many anaerobic and facultative bacteria, which is especially relevant from a periodontal standpoint. Tetracyclines are also active against most spirochaetes.

10.4.1 PHARMACODYNAMICS

Tetracyclines gain access to bacterial cells by the combined processes of passive diffusion through outer-membrane pores and active transfer utilizing an energy-dependent pump in the inner membrane. The drugs then act by inhibiting protein synthesis on the surfaces of the ribosomes. In brief, the synthesis of proteins starts when ribosomal subunits aggregate at the end of an mRNA molecule to produce a ribosome–mRNA complex. This complex can bind tRNA molecules that carry the appropriate amino acids for protein construction. Tetracyclines appear to bind to one of the subunits in the ribosomes and, by so doing, prevent the access of tRNA to the ribosomal–mRNA complex. Polypeptide synthesis is thus arrested.

10.4.2 PHARMACOKINETICS

Tetracyclines are usually given orally, although topical applications have been used in periodontal treatment regimens (Goodson *et al.* 1979, 1983; Lindhe *et al.* 1979). Tetracyclines are absorbed from the gastrointestinal tract and absorption is reduced when the drugs are taken with milk products or with substances containing calcium, magnesium, iron, or aluminium. However, even when the drugs are taken on an empty stomach, a certain amount remains in the bowel.

Tetracycline itself has been the most commonly researched member of this group in periodontal treatment, although minocycline and doxycycline have also been investigated. The oral dose for tetracycline is 1 g/day, which is administered as 250 mg tablets at six-hourly intervals. The peak plasma concentration occurs after 2–4 h and the half-life is between 6–10 h. The half-lives of minocycline and doxycycline are between 16 and 18 h, which allows a lower initial dose and less frequent administrations thereafter than for tetracycline.

All tetracyclines are distributed widely in the tissues and are localized in developing dental structures and bone. Tetracycline, minocycline, and doxycycline are detectable in crevicular fluid after oral dosing and their respective concentrations can reach levels of 10 times and 5 times those in serum (Bader and Goldhaber 1965; Ponitz *et al.* 1970; Ciancio *et al.* 1976; Gordon *et al.* 1980, 1981; Pascale *et al.* 1986). This is of particular importance when the drugs are used for the treatment of periodontal disease.

Tetracycline is excreted in the urine and should not be given to patients whose renal function is compromised. Doxycycline is excreted predominantly in the faeces and consequently does not accumulate in the blood of patients with renal disease. Excretion of minocycline is also unaffected by the state of renal function as the drug appears to be metabolized in the liver and then excreted in the faeces.

10.4.3 Tetracycline and periodontal diseases

Cases of moderately severe and advanced periodontal disease are traditionally treated with the time-honoured regimens of oral hygiene instruction, scaling, and root planing. These methods usually result in reducing scores for plaque and for gingival indices, decreasing pocket probing depths, and in the establishment of a periodontal microbial flora that is compatible with the maintenance of healthy tissues (Listgarten *et al.* 1978). In such cases, the adjunctive use of tetracycline therapy is not indicated because it is unlikely to achieve any short-term or long-lasting clinical effects not provided by mechanical debridement alone (Listgarten *et al.* 1978; Hellden *et al.* 1979; Slots *et al.* 1979). Occasionally, however, a case of chronic adult periodontitis will show no clinical improvement after routine therapy and the periodontal flora will continue to be a mixture of spirochaetes and Gram-negative, anaerobic rods. These so-called refractory cases of periodontitis can benefit from a two-week course of systemic tetracycline therapy of 1 g/day (Slots *et al.* 1979; Rams and Keyes 1983).

The effects of tetracycline therapy upon the subgingival flora associated with periodontitis have been well documented. The result of a two-week course of 1 g tetracycline/day is a shift from an essentially complex, Gram-negative flora to one that is predominantly Gram-positive and associated with healthy tissues (Williams *et al.* 1979). Bacterial resistance amongst the indigenous flora is not uncommon, both before and after tetracycline therapy (Hawley *et al.* 1980). Species of *Streptococcus* and *Actinomyces* have been shown to be resistant, although their association with gingival health and less progressive forms of periodontitis (Listgarten 1976; Williams *et al.* 1976) may negate the importance of this resistance. In the refractory cases of periodontitis, a short course of systemic tetracycline will cause a significant reduction in spirochaetes and Gram-negative rods to low or undetectable levels (Rams and Keyes 1983).

Tetracycline has been shown to be of considerable benefit in the treatment of localized juvenile periodontitis (LJP) in which the prime pathogen, *Actinobacillus actinomycetemcomitans*, is very susceptible to the antibiotic (Slots *et al.*

1980*a*). This capnophilic, Gram-negative rod is difficult to eliminate from LJP patients by mechanical debridement alone (Christersson *et al.* 1985), presumably because of its ability to invade the soft tissues. Systemic administration of 1 g/day tetracycline for three to six weeks in conjunction with supragingival plaque control can halt the progression of the LJP lesions (Novak *et al.* 1988), although it is more usual to give the tetracycline in a two-week course as an adjunct to non-surgical (Genco *et al.* 1981; Slots and Rosling 1983) or surgical management (Lindhe and Liljenberg 1984). However, Slots and Rosling recommend that tetracycline for treatment of LJP should be continued for one week after obtaining negative culture results for *A. actinomycetemcomitans* and that this would routinely involve a three-week course of the antibiotic. Such a regimen minimizes the chance of recolonization with the actinobacilli that might originate from a residual infection of the gingival tissues.

A number of clinical trials have been undertaken to determine the effects of using long-term and low-dose tetracycline therapy as an adjunct primarily to treatment of refractory periodontitis (Scopp *et al.* 1980; Kornman and Karl 1982; Lindhe *et al.* 1983*a*). Observations suggest that a daily dose of 250 mg tetracycline will control the progression of periodontal disease for periods of up to seven years and that this can be achieved even in the absence of mechanical debridement (Lindhe *et al.* 1983*a*). Despite the apparently healthy tissues, however, the subgingival flora in such patients can be complex and contain a number of potentially pathogenic, tetracycline-resistant organisms such as *Fusobacterium nucleatum*, *Eikenella corrodens* and *Selenomonas sputigena* (Williams *et al.* 1979; Kornman and Karl 1982). Furthermore, the clinical and bacterial status characteristic of the disease become reinstated from approximately six months after cessation of long-term, low-dose tetracycline therapy (Kornman and Karl 1982). When these points are considered with the fact that periodontal disease is a local infection, the use of long-term tetracycline as a treatment regimen is unwarranted.

In addition to the antimicrobial effects of tetracyclines, a further mechanism has been proposed to explain their efficacy in the treatment of periodontal disease. In a series of laboratory experiments and clinical trials on diabetic humans, Golub and co-workers have shown that tetracycline, doxycycline, and minocycline can all suppress the activity of the tissue enzyme collagenase as determined by its presence in crevicular fluid (Golub *et al.* 1983, 1984, 1985*a*, *b*, 1987). Mammalian collagenases are calcium-dependent enzymes and as tetracyclines are able to chelate multivalent metal cations, this may be the mechanism through which the inhibition occurs (Golub *et al.* 1983). The conversion of tetracycline to a non-antimicrobial analogue, de-dimethylaminotetracycline, does not reduce the anticollagenolytic action of the drug, indicating that these actions are independent of antimicrobial activity.

Bone regeneration in sites of periodontitis has been reported after tetracycline therapy (Fasciano and Fazio 1981; Hoerman *et al.* 1985; Moskow 1986) but the relative contributions of the antimicrobial and anticollagenase properties of the drug towards the regeneration is not known. Therefore, extensive longitudinal clinical trials are required to determine whether inhibiting collagenase alone will lead to a significant reduction in loss of attachment and bone resorption in the long term.

10.4.4 LOCAL DELIVERY OF TETRACYCLINE

A number of slow-release devices have been used to facilitate the local delivery of tetracycline (and other antimicrobials) in periodontal sites (see p. 180). Of such devices, monolithic ethylene vinyl acetate fibres have been found to be most efficacious in achieving prolonged delivery of the drug from the entire length of the fibres (Goodson *et al.* 1983). Furthermore, the concentrations of tetracycline in crevicular fluid achieved by controlled local delivery are up to 100 times those attained from systemic dosing (1500 μg/ml v. 15 μg/ml), and so the chances of complete suppression of bacterial growth (or collagenase activity) are increased.

10.4.5 OTHER TETRACYCLINES

Minocycline is a semi-synthetic derivative of tetracycline that is highly active against most periodontopathic organisms (Reynolds *et al.* 1981). The results of short-term studies in which minocycline was administered for seven to eight days to patients with periodontal disease indicate that the drug produces long-lasting shifts in the subgingival microflora, similar to those achieved by tetracycline (Ciancio *et al.* 1982). Minocycline also has the effect of resolving gingival inflammation, although its long-term effects on pocket depths and attachment levels are not known (Ciancio *et al.* 1980, 1982).

Another semi-synthetic tetracycline, doxycycline, has been used as an adjunct to periodontal surgery in the management of juvenile periodontitis. A two week course of doxycline with surgery produces a significant reduction in the prevalence of *A. actinomycetemcomitans* and this suppression can persist for up to 12 months (Mandell *et al.* 1986; Mandell and Socransky 1988). Long-term improvements in attachment levels were also reported, although the absence of a true control group (surgical therapy/no doxycycline) makes an accurate interpretation of the findings impossible.

10.5 METRONIDAZOLE

Metronidazole is a nitroimidazole compound with a broad spectrum of activity against protozoa and anaerobic bacteria. In medicine, it is used in the treatment of trichomonal genital infections, as a prophylactic agent before abdominal surgery, and in the management of severe anaerobic infections. The antibacterial activity against anaerobic cocci, anaerobic Gram-negative bacilli, and anaerobic Gram-positive bacilli has led to its use in the treatment of periodontal diseases.

10.5.1 PHARMACODYNAMICS

Metronidazole readily permeates bacterial cell membranes to achieve a steady-state, intracellular concentration. The antimicrobial effects of the drug depend upon its selective reactivity in the unstable and reduced form, which is achieved through the actions of electron-transport proteins of susceptible bacteria. Once in the cells, metronidazole binds to DNA and disrupts the helical structure of the molecules. Breakage of the DNA strands occurs, which ultimately leads to death of the cells. This process results in very rapid killing of anaerobic micro-organisms.

10.5.2 PHARMACOKINETICS

In periodontal treatment, metronidazole has been used both in tablet form and, less commonly, as a topical application. The drug is well-absorbed after oral administration and the peak plasma level is usually reached in about one hour. After a single dose of 200 mg the peak concentration in plasma is about 5 μg/ml. However, when repeated doses are given there is an accumulation of the drug for about two days, after which a steady state of about 6 μg/ml is reached (Rood 1980).

Metronidazole is widely distributed throughout the body and, after an oral dose, can be detected in saliva and crevicular fluid. The concentration in saliva can reach 200 μg/ml within about four hours of a single loading dose of 200 mg/ml (Altman 1980). When a single standard dose of 250 mg/ml is administered, levels of the drug in gingival crevicular fluid peak at between 3, and 4 μg/ml, again after three to four hours (Britt and Pohlod 1986). After five days, oral dosing with 250 mg/ml thrice daily, the levels of metronidazole in crevicular fluid show a much greater range and can be nearly 50 per cent higher than the concurrent serum concentrations (Giedrys-Leeper *et al.* 1985). This is presumably due to the accumulation of the drug in the crevicular fluid. Levels of between 10 and 20 μg/ml have also been reported in crevicualr fluid, albeit after a larger, single dose of 750 mg (Notten *et al.* 1982).

The half-life of metronidazole is about 8 h and the principal site of metabolism is the liver, where the drug is oxidized mainly into its glucuronide conjugates. These, together with the unchanged parent molecule, are excreted in the urine.

10.5.3 METRONIDAZOLE AND PERIODONTAL DISEASES

The rationale for the use of metronidazole in the treatment of periodontal diseases and other oral infections has revolved around the drug's specificity for anaerobes and the apparent inability of susceptible organisms to develop resistance (Mitchell 1984). However, the plasma (or crevicular fluid) levels of metronidazole required for the drug to be effective against the majority of anaerobes have not been clearly established. Rood (1980) stated that levels of about 6 μg/ml are adequate to deal with most anaerobic infections and that these levels would be achieved by a regimen of 200 mg thrice daily. However, Walker *et al.* (1983) showed that a concentration of 8 μg/ml was inhibitory to more than 90 per cent of bacteria in subgingival plaque in less than half the samples tested, and they suggested that gingival fluid levels of 15 µg/ml would be necessary for maximal inhibition. These levels may be achieved after multiple oral doses of metronidazole (Walker *et al.* 1983).

In one of the first studies on metronidazole and periodontal disease, Loesche *et al.* (1981) administered a dose of 250 mg, thrice daily for one week to five patients. This resulted in significant reductions in bleeding scores and pocket depths, as well as gains in attachment levels, and these improvements were sustained six months after therapy. In three of the patients, mechanical debridement was undertaken and this contributed to the improvement of the periodontal condition. It was also found that metronidazole significantly reduced the proportions of the anaerobe *Bacteroides asaccharolyticus* and spirochaetes for six months after treatment, although the overall effect of the drug on the total anaerobic flora was not established.

The clinical, histopathological, and bacteriological benefit of metronidazole therapy is more pronounced when concurrent scaling, root planing, and oral hygiene instruction are undertaken (Lindhe *et al.* 1983*b*) Metronidazole therapy alone can significantly reduce or eliminate obligate anaerobes, but if facultative anaerobes remain unaffected by the drug, then the effect on clinical measures of disease should be limited. Despite this, however, a one-week course of metronidazole in the absence of other treatment can lead to a resolution of bleeding, a reduction in pocket depths, and less crevicular fluid flow (Lekovic *et al.* 1983). This is particularly evident in deeper pockets, which become shallower, although metronidazole can also prevent shallow sites (1–3 mm depths) from losing attachment (Watts *et al.* 1986). A single-dose (2 g) regime of metronidazole, however, is ineffective, both clinically and microbiologically, in the treatment of adult periodontitis (Walsh *et al.* 1986).

The severity of the periodontal destruction may therefore be an important consideration in the use of metronidazole. Advanced and refractory periodontitis responds well to the drug when it is used as an adjunct to traditional therapeutic measures (Lindhe *et al.* 1983*b*; Loesche *et al.* 1984; Lundstrom *et al.* 1984). However, in a study of mentally retarded adolescents, Clark *et al.* (l983) found that a week's course of metronidazole in the absence of root planing had no effect upon clinical measures despite a significant reduction of spirochaetes. In this study, the severity of periodontitis at baseline was not made clear, but the age group of the subjects suggests that advanced periodontal destruction would have been unlikely. A greater proportion of facultative anaerobes may have been present and would have remained unaffected by the drug therapy. Additional evidence for this possiblity was presented in a later study in which metronidazole was used as an adjunct to oral hygiene instruction and mechanical debridement in patients suffering from varying severities of periodontal disease. The drug had no effect on gingival bleeding beyond that which was achieved by the routine treatments. However, significantly greater reductions in pocket depths were achieved by the use of metronidazole in patients with severe periodontitis (Joyston-Bechal *et al.* 1984), although the effect was no longer apparent after three years (Joyston-Bechal *et al.* 1986). Metronidazole also appears to be of no benefit either as an adjunct to subgingival soft-tissue curettage in shallow

pockets (Sterry *et al.* 1985), or as part of a maintenance regime for periodontally stable sites (Giedrys-Leeper *et al.* 1985).

A problematical group of periodontal patients are those with advanced disease but who do not respond to oral hygiene instruction. In a study of 10 such patients, Jenkins *et al.* (1989) showed that a week's course of metronidazole resulted in significant improvements in pocket depths and attachment levels. They concluded, however, that these changes, which occurred in the absence of improvement in either plaque indices or inflamed gingival units, were not of sufficient clinical magnitude to warrant administration of a medically important drug.

Finally, metronidazole has also been found to be very effective, when combined with amoxycillin, in eliminating *A. actinomycetemcomitans* in patients suffering from LJP (van Winkelhoff *et al.* 1989). A seven-day regimen of metronidazole, 250mg, and amoxycillin, 750 mg, both thrice daily and combined with subgingival debridement, led to almost total elimination of the actinobacillus for up to 11 months after therapy. In view of the potential role of this organism in aggressive forms of periodontal disease, the achievement of undetectable levels over long periods of time must be considered a primary aim of treatment.

10.5.4 LOCAL DELIVERY OF METRONIDAZOLE

Investigations of topical applications of metronidazole have used pulsed-jet irrigators, acrylic resin strips, and dialysis tubing (Yeung *et al.* 1983; wan Yusof *et al.* 1984; Aziz-Gandour and Newman 1986) and these methods of delivery give beneficial effects in reducing clinical signs of periodontal inflammation. Furthermore, the release kinetics of metronidazole from ethyl cellulose strips are such that a dose of 2 mg can be provided locally within a pocket and released over three days. Such sustained-release devices would produce bactericidal levels of the drug in pockets without exposing patients to large systemic doses of metronidazole (Golomb *et al.* 1984).

10.5.5 METRONIDAZOLE AND ACUTE NECROTIZING ULCERATIVE GINGIVITIS (ANUG)

The observation that metronidazole is effective in the treatment of ANUG resulted from the fortuitous observation of a patient who was receiving the medication for trichomonal vaginitis (Shinn 1962). This finding was later confirmed by the results of clinical trials which established that a seven day course of systemic metronidazole (200 mg thrice daily) was enough to eliminate clinical signs and symptoms of infection (Shinn *et al.* 1965; Proctor and Baker 1971).

Gingival ulceration, bleeding, pain, and halitosis usually resolve rapidly within about 48–72 of starting metronidazole treatment. These clinical changes are accompanied by the rapid disappearance of the infecting spirochaetes and fusobacteria that are characteristic of this acute disease (Shinn *et al.* 1965; Stephen *et al.* 1966). However, once the acute phase of the disease has been controlled, then mechanical debridement should be carried out immediately. Failure to do so will result inevitably in recurrence of the infection and perhaps, therefore, unnecessary repeated administration of the antimicrobial.

10.6 THE MACROLIDES

The macrolide antibiotics, which represent the metabolic products of various subspecies of *Streptomyces* organisms, are so called because of a common macrocyclic lactone ring to which one or more deoxy sugars are attached. Macrolides are bacteriostatic drugs but can be bactericidal if high concentrations are achieved.

10.6.1 PHARMACODYNAMICS

Macrolides bind to the ribosomal subunits of susceptible micro-organisms and block the translocation process of protein synthesis. Gram-positive organisms are more sensitive to macrolides than are Gram-negative organisms because their cell walls are more readily permeable to the drugs. The overall spectrum of activity of macrolides is similar to that of benzyl penicillin and the drugs are often used in patients with a history of hypersensitivity to penicillins.

10.6.2 PHARMACOKINETICS

Erythromycin is the most frequently prescribed macrolide and is administered as enteric-coated capsules because of its susceptibility to gastric acid. Food in the stomach delays absorption of the stearate salts and peak plasma concentrations of about 0.5 µg/ml are reached approximately 4 after a 25 mg dose. Estolate salts are more completely absorbed and are less affected both by acid and the food content of the stomach. Erythromycin salts are widely distributed throughout body tissues. The greater part of the drug is broken down in the body and a small proportion is excreted in the urine and bile products.

Another macrolide that has been researched in periodontal trials is spiramycin. This antimicrobial is also irregularly absorbed from the gastro intestinal tract and is widely distributed in the body. High tissue concentrations are achieved and are maintained beyond the peak plasma levels. Animal experiments have shown that spiramycin can be detected in gingiva for at least seven days after the last dose (Leung *et al.* 1972). High concentrations have also been reported in saliva and salivary glands (Yankell *et al.* 1971; de Vries and Francis 1975). The excretion of spiramycin is similar to that of erythromycin.

10.6.3 MACROLIDES AND PERIODONTAL DISEASES

Harvey (1961) presented the details of seven cases of periodontal infection that had been controlled by a short course of spiramycin. He recommended using the drug when patients were allergic to penicillin or had penicillin-resistant organisms in the mouth.

In other controlled studies, spiramycin has been shown to significantly reduce signs of gingival inflammation including pocket depths, gingival indices, and crevicular fluid flow over short periods of up to four weeks (Winer *et al.* 1966; Mills *et al.* 1979; Sznajder *et al.* 1987). The drug also has an effect in reducing plaque formation when measured by plaque height (Mills *et al.* 1979) or wet weight (Rozanis *et al.* 1979). Furthermore, a two-week course of 2 g spiramycin daily can modify the microbial composition of plaque by reducing the proportions of motile rods and spirochaetes, with the latter exhibiting great susceptibility to the drugs. These findings, taken with the fact that spiramycin has not been widely prescribed by the medical profession led Sznajder *et al.* (1987) to suggest that it is a potentially attractive antibiotic for use in the management of periodontal disease.

The periodontal effects of spiramycin have been compared to those of erythromycin in patients suffering from severe or advanced periodontal disease (Mills *et al.* 1979). Generally, spiramycin was twice as effective as erythromycin. For example, pocket depths were reduced by 30 per cent in patients taking spiramycin whereas erythromycin produced a reduction of 15 per cent. Spiramycin reduced crevicular fluid flow by 40 per cent compared to 15 per cent for erythromycin. The reason for this finding is not clear, although the investigators suggested that the smaller molecular size of the active ingredient of spiramycin would facilitate its appearance in crevicular fluid and thereby enhance its periodontal effects.

10.7 LINCOMYCIN AND CLINDAMYCIN

Clindamycin is a derivative of lincomycin that is more active and has fewer side-effects than the parent drug. Both are active against Gram-positive bacteria, and clindamycin is effective against certain periodontal pathogens such as *Bact. melaninogenicus* and *Fusobacterium*.

10.7.1 PHARMACODYNAMICS

The mechanism of action of clindamycin and lincomycin is identical to that of the macrolides. The drugs bind to ribosomal subunits of susceptible organisms to prevent translocation and inhibit polypeptide synthesis.

10.7.2 PHARMACOKINETICS

Clindamycin is almost completely absorbed after oral administration to produce a peak blood concentration in about 45–60 min. The half-life of the drug is about 3 h and it is well distributed throughout the tissues including bone. Clindamycin also accumulates in polymorphonuclear leukocytes. The peak concentration of clindamycin in crevicular fluid after a 300 mg oral dose is about 2 µg/ml and comparable to that achieved in plasma. Most of the drug is metabolized and excreted in the urine and bile.

The level of clindamycin in crevicular fluid is sustained above 1 μg/ml for up to 6 h (plasma, 2 h) and this concentration is considered adequate to inhibit most of the bacteria associated with periodontal diseases (Walker *et al.* 1981*a*).

10.7.3 LINCOMYCIN/CLINDAMYCIN AND PERIODONTAL DISEASES

Due to the potential severity of the side-effects that can accompany the use of these drugs (see Table 10.2, p.181), their use in the treatment of periodontal disease has been limited. Short-term, clinical and microbiological studies have shown that clindamycin is beneficial in controlling advanced periodontal infections (Luthiger 1983; Ohta 1984). Furthermore, a long-term (12 months) evaluation of the clinical effects of a seven-day course of clindamycin also reported impressive results in patients with 'refractory' periodontitis. Suppuration, bleeding on probing, gingival redness, pocket depth, and loss of attachment were all significantly reduced in patients who had failed to respond to other modes of treatment including tetracycline therapy (Gordon *et al.* 1985).

However, although these findings suggest that clindamycin does have a role in periodontal therapy, we consider that the risk of inducing a severe colitis does not warrant using the drug to manage what is, essentially, a local infection. This principle is strengthened by the observations outlined in earlier sections that refractory and aggressive forms of periodontal disease can be successfully managed using other antibiotics.

10.8 OTHER ANTIBIOTICS

Despite its popularity in general medicine, penicillin has been infrequently researched as an adjunct to periodontal therapy. One of the earliest reports suggested that the topical application of aqueous penicillin might be valuable in treating acute ulcerative infections (Schuessler *et al.* 1945). However, the possibility of sensitization and the discovery of metronidazole have made obsolete this particular indication.

Systemic phenoxymethylpenicillin has apparently been used successfully as part of a surgical regimen in the treatment of juvenile periodontitis (Hoge and Kirkham 1980). However, later results from a controlled clinical trial indicated that the adjunctive use of phenoxymethylpenicillin does not enhance treatment of juvenile periodontitis by root planing and flap surgery (Kunihira *et al.* 1985).

Niridazole is an antiparasitic agent that has been compared *in vitro* to metronidazole and tetracycline for potential use in periodontal treatment. Anaerobic bacteria, including species of *Bacteroides*, *Wolinella* and *Fusobacterium*, were susceptible to low concentrations of niridazole. Furthermore, unlike metronidazole, niridazole was effective against a number of facultative anaerobes (Wade and Addy 1987). These findings suggest that the drug may have potential as a therapeutic agent in periodontal treatment.

10.9 CONTRAINDICATIONS AND UNWANTED EFFECTS

Antibiotics are amongst the most widely prescribed pharmaceutical agents in modern medicine. Although only a small number of these drugs have been used in the treatment of periodontal diseases, it is essential that the main contraindications for their use and their possible unwanted effects are known to the periodontist.

Generally, the contraindications for use are related to the impaired metabolism and excretion of the drugs. Consequently, disease or impaired function of the hepatic or renal tracts should warrant caution in prescribing systemic antibiotics. When penicillins are prescribed it is vitally important to determine whether or not there is a history of hypersensitivity to the drug. The unwanted effects of penicillin are often mild and characterized by rashes, urticaria, joint pains, and dermatitis, although severe anaphylactic reactions have been reported and can be fatal in about 10 per cent of cases.

The contraindications and unwanted effects of the groups of antibiotics that have been most frequently researched and recommended as adjunctive regimens in periodontal treatment are summarized in Table 10.2, p.181.

10.10 INDICATIONS FOR ANTIBIOTICS IN PERIODONTAL THERAPY

The results of the clinical trials discussed above suggest that there is an important role for antibiotic therapy as an adjunct to periodontal treatment. In accordance with the general principles of prescribing antibiotics, however, it is essential that the drugs are administered only after careful case selection, and antibiotic therapy should not be a substitute for the routine and time-honoured treatment regimens.

We consider that the following periodontal disease states would justify the adjunctive use of antibiotics:

1. In severe cases of ANUG, especially if there are signs of systemic involvement, metronidazole can quickly alleviate the symptoms, which then permits thorough mechanical debridement to be carried out. Broad-spectrum penicillins, which are frequently used in the treatment of more severe infections than those of the gingiva, should not be prescribed.

2. Occasionally, the local infection of a periodontal abscess can spread within tissue planes to cause marked facial swelling and systemic involvement. These cases are rare as periodontal infections frequently drain through the gingival crevice into the mouth. However, when these circumstances do arise, a broad-spectrum antibiotic should be prescribed to control the infection. Furthermore, careful clinical and radiographic examinations must be undertaken to establish whether the lesion is wholly periodontal in origin or whether there is pulpal involvement of the associated teeth.

3. Multiple abscess formation and gross periodontal infection would necessitate the administration of a broad-spectrum antibiotic such as tetracycline to control the condition. A number of medical conditions (e.g. diabetes mellitus, see Chapter 3) can

predispose to advanced periodontal destruction with abscess formation and whenever these signs present the clinician should investigate further for underlying medical problems.

4. Antibiotic therapy is warranted in moderate or advanced cases of periodontal disease, which, despite thorough non-surgical management and good plaque control, continue to show breakdown and loss of attachment. These so-called refractory cases can benefit from a short course of antibiotic therapy. Ideally, the drug of choice should be determined from sampling the cultivable pocket flora from which the predominant populating organisms can be identified. Subsequent microbiological monitoring of pockets will then prove to be invaluable and to assess whether or not the antibiotic regimen has been successful.

5. Antibiotic therapy is recommended in the management of cases of LJP either in combination with flap surgery or a non-surgical treatment programme. Such regimens are discussed in more detail in Chapter 5.

REFERENCE

Addy, M., Rawle, L., Handley, R., Newman, H. N. and Coventry, J. F. (1982). Development and *in vitro* evaluation of acrylic strips and dialysis tubing for local drug delivery. *Journal of Periodontology*, **53**, 693–9.

Altman, E. G. (1980). Rational use of metronidazole. *Australian Dental Journal*, **25**, 135–8.

Aziz-Gandour, I. A. and Newman, H. N. (1986). The effects of a simplified oral hygiene regime plus supragingival irrigation with chlorhexidine or metronidazole on chronic inflammatory periodontal disease. *Journal of Clinical Periodontology*, **13**, 228–36.

Bader, H. I. and Goldhaber, P. (1965). The passage of intravenously administered tetracycline into the gingival sulcus of dogs. *Journal of Oral Therapeutics and Pharmacology*, **2**, 324–9.

Baker, P. J., Evans, R. T., Coburn, R.A., and Genco, R. J. (1983). Tetracycline and its derivatives strongly bind to and are released from the tooth surface in active form. *Journal of Periodontology*, **54**, 580–5.

Baker, P. J., Evans, R. T., Slots, J., and Genco, R. J. (1985). Susceptibility of human oral anaerobic bacteria to antibiotics suitable for topical use. *Journal of Clinical Periodontology*, **12**, 201–8.

Britt, M. R. and Pohlod, D. J. (1986). Serum and crevicular fluid concentrations after a single oral dose of metronidazole. *Journal of Periodontology*, **57**, 104–7.

Christersson, L. A., Slots, J., Rosling, B. G., and Genco, R. J. (1985). Microbiological and clinical effects of surgical treatment of localised juvenile periodontitis. *Journal of Clinical Periodontology*, **12**, 465–76.

Ciancio, S. G. (1976). Tetracyclines in periodontal therapy. *Journal of Periodontology*, **47**, 155–9.

Ciancio, S., Singh, S., Genco, R., Krygier, G., and Mather, M. L. (1976). Analysis of tetracycline in human gingival fluid: methodology and results. *Journal of Dental Research*, **55**, B164 (abstr. 411).

Ciancio, S. G., Mather, M. L., and McMullen, J. A. (1980). An evaluation of minocycline in patients with periodontal disease. *Journal of Periodontology*, **51**, 530–4.

Ciancio, S. G., Slots, J., Reynolds, H. S., Zambon, J. J., and McKenna, J. D. (1982). The effect of short-term administration of minocycline HCl on gingival inflammation and subgingival microflora. *Journal of Periodontology*, **53**, 557–61.

Clark, D. C., Shenker, S., Stulginski, P., and Schwartz, S. (1983). Effectiveness of routine periodontal treatment with and without adjunctive metronidazole therapy in a sample of mentally retarded adolescents. *Journal of Periodontology*, **54**, 658–65.

De Vries, J. and Francis, L. E. (1975). Antibiotic therapy for the practising dentist. Spiramycin and general discussion. *Journal of the Canadian Dental Association*, **41**, 101–2.

Fasciano, R. W. and Fazio, R. C. (1981). Periodontal regeneration with long term tetracycline therapy. *Quintessence International*, **12**, 1081–8.

Genco, R. J. (1981). Antibiotics in the treatment of human periodontal disease. *Journal of Periodontology*, **52**, 545–58.

Genco, R. J., Cianciola, L. J., and Rosling, B. (1981). Treatment of localised juvenile periodontitis. *Journal of Dental Research*, **60**, 527 (abstr. 872).

Giedrys-Lepeper, E., Selipsky, H., and Williams, B. L. (1985). Effects of short-term administration of metronidazole on the subgingival microflora. *Journal of Clinical Periodontology*, **12**, 797–814.

Gillett, R. and Johnson, N. W. (1982). Bacterial invasion of the periodontium in a case of juvenile periodontitis. *Journal of Clinical Periodontology*, **9**, 93–100.

Golomb, G., Friedman, M., Soskolne, A., Stabholz, A., and Sela, M. N. (1984). Sustained release device containing metronidazole for periodontal use. *Journal of Dental Research*, **63**, 1149–53.

Golub, L. M. *et al.* (1983). Minocycline reduces gingival collagenolytic activity during diabetes: preliminary observations and a proposed new mechanism of action. *Journal of Periodontal Research*, **18**, 516–24.

Golub, L. M. *et al.* (1984). Tetracyclines inhibit tissue collagenase activity. A new mechanism in the treatment of periodontal disease. *Journal of Periodontal Research*, **19**, 651–5.

Golub, L. M., Goodson, J. M., Lee, H. M., Vidal, A. M., McNamara, T. F., and Ramamurthy, N. S. (1985a). Tetracyclines inhibit tissue collagenases. Effects of ingested low-dose and local delivery systems. *Journal of Periodontology*, **56**, (Suppl. 11), 93–7.

Golub, L. M. *et al.* (1985b). Further evidence that tetracyclines inhibit collagenase activity in human crevicular fluid and from other mammalian sources. *Journal of Periodontal Research*, **20**, 12–23.

Golub, L. M., McNamara, T. F., D'Angelo, G., Greenwald, R. A., and Ramamurthy, N. S. (1987). A non-antibacterial, chemically-modified tetracycline inhibits mammalian collagenase activity. *Journal of Dental Research*, **66**, 1310–14.

Goodson, J. M., Haffajee, A., and Socransky, S. S. (1979). Periodontal therapy by local delivery of tetracycline. *Journal of Clinical Periodontology*, **6**, 83–92.

Goodson, J. M., Holborow, D., Dunn, R. L., Hogan, P., and Dunham, S. (1983). Monolithic tetracycline-containing fibers for controlled delivery to periodontal pockets. *Journal of Periodontology*, **54**, 575–9.

Gordon, J. M., Walker, C. M., Murphy, J. C., Goodson, J. M., and Socransky, S. S. (1980). Concentration of tetracycline in human crevicular fluid after single and multiple doses. *Journal of Dental Research*, **57**, (spec. iss. A), abstr. 977.

Gordon, J. *et al.* (1985). Efficacy of clindamycin hydrochloride in refractory periodontitis. *Journal of Periodontology*, **56** (Suppl. 11), 75–80.

Harvey, R. F. (1961). Clinical impressions of a new antibiotic in periodontitis: spiramycin. *Journal of the Canadian Dental Association*, **27**, 576–85.

Hawley, R. J., Lee, L. N., and LeBlanc, D. J. (1980). Effects of tetracycline on the streptococcal flora of periodontal pockets. *Antimicrobial Agents and Chemotherapy*, **17**, 372–8.

Hellden, L. B., Listgarten, M. A., and Lindhe, J. (1979). The effect of tetracycline and/or scaling on human periodontal disease. *Journal of Clinical Periodontology*, **6**, 222–30.

Hoerman, K. C., Lang, R. L., Klapper, L., and Beery, J. (1985). Local tetracycline therapy of the periodontium during orthodontic treatment. *Quintessence International*, **16**, 161–6.

Hoge, H. W. and Kirkham, D. B. (1980). Periodontosis: treatment results in a 15-year-old girl. *Journal of the American Dental Association*, **101**, 795–7.

Jenkins, W. M. M., MacFarlane, T. W., Gilmour, W. H., Ramsay, I., and MacKenzie, D. (1989). Systemic metronidazole in the treatment of periodontitis. *Journal of Clinical Periodontology*, **16**, 443–50.

Joyston-Bechal, S., Smales, F. C., and Duckworth, R. (1984). Effect of metronidazole on chronic periodontal disease in subjects using a topically applied chlorhexidine gel. *Journal of Clinical Periodontology*, **11**, 53–62.

Joyston-Bechal, S., Smales, F. C., and Duckworth, R. (1986). A follow-up study three years after metronidazole therapy for chronic periodontal disease. *Journal of Clinical Periodontology*, **13**, 944–9.

Kornman, K. S. and Karl, E. H. (1982). The effect of long-term, low-dose tetracycline therapy on the subgingival microflora in refractory adult periodontitis. *Journal of Periodontology*, **53**, 604–10.

Kunihira, D. M., Caine, F. A., Palcanis, K. G., Best, A. M., and Ranney, R. R. (1985). A clinical trial of phenoxymethyl penicillin for adjunctive treatment of juvenile periodontitis. *Journal of Periodontology*, **56**, 352–8.

Lekovic, V., Kenney, E. B., Carranza, F. A., and Endres, B. (1983). The effect of metronidazole on human periodontal disease. A clinical and bacteriological study. *Journal of Periodontology*, **54**, 476–80.

Leung, F. C., Gardner, J. M., Paor, W. S., and Yankell, S. L. (1972). Spiramycin excretion in animals. II. Repeated oral doses in rats. *Journal of Dental Research*, **51**, 712–15.

Lindhe, J. and Liljenberg, B. (1984). Treatment of localised juvenile periodontitis. *Journal of Clinical Periodontology*, **11**, 399–410.

Lindhe, J., Heijl, L., Goodson, J. M., and Socransky, S. S. (1979). Local tetracycline delivery using hollow fibre devices in periodontal therapy. *Journal of Clinical Periodontology*, **6**, 141–9.

Lindhe, J., Liljenberg, B., and Adielsson, B. (1983a). Effect of long-term tetracycline therapy on human periodontal disease. *Journal of Clinical Periodontology*, **10**, 590–601.

Lindhe, J., Liljenberg, B., Adielson, B., and Borjesson, J. (1983b). Use of metronidazole as a probe in the study of human periodontal disease. *Journal of Clinical Periodontology*, **10**, 100–12.

Listgarten, M. A. (1976). Structure of the microbial flora associated with periodontal disease and health in man. A light and electron microscopic study. *Journal of Periodontology*, **47**, 1–18.

Listgarten, M. A., Lindhe, J., and Hellden, J. (1978). Effect of tetracycline and/or scaling on human periodontal disease. Clinical, microbiological and histological observations. *Journal of Clinical Periodontology*, **5**, 246–71.

Loesche, W. J., Syed, S. A., Morrison, E. C., Laughan, B., and Grossman, N. S. (1981). Treatment of periodontal infections due to anaerobic bacteria with short-term treatment with metronidazole. Journal of Clinical Periodontology, **8**, 29–44.

Loesche, W. J., Syed, S. A., Morrison, E. C., Kerry, G. A., Higgins, T., and Stoll, J. (1984). Metronidazole in periodontitis. I. Clinical and bacteriological results after 15 to 30 weeks. *Journal of Periodontology*, **55**, 325–35.

Lundstrom, A., Johansson, L. A., and Hamp, S. E. (1984). Effect of combined systemic antimicrobial therapy and mechanical plaque control in patients with recurrent periodontal disease. *Journal of Clinical Periodontology*, **11**, 321–30.

Luthiger, U. (1983). Clindamycin and penicillin V in the treatment of periodontal infections. A randomised study. *Swiss Dent (Zurich)*, **4**, 41–3.

Mandell, R. L. and Socransky, S. S. (1988). Microbiological and clinical effects of surgery plus doxycycline on juvenile periodontitis. *Journal of Periodontology*, **59**, 373–9.

Mandell, R. L., Tripodi, L. S., Savitt, E., Goodson, J. M., and Socransky, S. S. (1986). The effect of treatment on *Actinobacillus actinomycetemcomitans* in localised juvenile periodontitis. *Journal of Periodontology*, **57**, 94–9.

Mills, W. H., Thompson, G. W., and Beagrie, G. S. (1979). Clinical evaluation of Spiramycin and Erythromycin in control of periodontal disease. *Journal of Clinical Periodontology*, **6**, 308–16.

Mitchell, D. A. (1984). Metronidazole: its use in clinical dentistry. *Journal of Clinical Periodontology*, **11**, 145–58.

Moskow, B. S. (1986). Repair of an extensive periodontal defect after tetracycline administration. A case report. *Journal of Periodontology*, **57**, 29–34.

Notten, F., Oosten, A. K-V., and Mikx, F. (1982). Capillary agar diffusion assay for measuring metronidazole in human gingival crevice fluid. *Antimicrobial Agents and Chemotherapy*, **21**, 836–7.

Novak, M. J., Polson, A. M., and Adair, S. M. (1988). Tetracycline therapy in patients with early juvenile periodontitis. *Journal of Periodontology*, **59**, 366–72.

Ohta, Y. (1984). Microbiological study on the periodontal lesions in advanced periodontitis. Changes in the regional flora and clinical features caused by short-term treatment with clindamycin. *Skikwa Gakuho*, **8**, 1209–23.

Pascale, D., Gordon, J., Lamster, I., Mann, P., Sieger, M., and Arndt, W. (1986). Concentration of doxycycline in human crevicular fluid. *Journal of Clinical Periodontology*, **13**, 841–4.

Pitcher, G. R., Newman, H. N., and Strahan, J. D. (1980). Access to subgingival plaque by disclosing agents using mouthrinsing and direct irrigation. *Journal of Clinical Periodontology*, **7**, 300–8.

Ponitz, D. P., Gershkoff, A., and Wells, H. (1970). Passage of orally administered tetracycline into the gingival crevice around natural teeth and around protruding subperiosteal implant abutments in man. *Dental Clinics of North America*, **14**, 125–36.

Proctor, D. B. and Baker, C. G. (1971). Treatment of acute ulcerative gingivitis with metronidazole. *Journal of the Canadian Dental Association*, **37**, 376–80.

Rams, T. E. and Keyes, P. H. (1983). A rationale for the management of periodontal diseases: effects of tetracycline on subgingival bacteria. *Journal of the American Dental Association*, **107**, 37–41.

Reynolds, H. S., Ciancio, S. G., Meyers, M. D., Evans, R. T., and Slots, J. (1981). *In vitro* antimicrobial susceptibility of minocycline (Minocin) against oral bacteria. *Journal of Dental Research*, **60** (Spec. Iss. A), 527 (abstr. 870).

Rood, J. P. (1980). The value of metronidazole in dental and oral surgery. *Dental Update*, **7**, 293–300.

Rozanis, J., Johnson, R. W., Satiul Haq, M., and Schofield, I. D. F. (1979). Spiramycin as a selective dental plaque control agent. *Journal of Periodontal Research*, **14**, 55–64.

Saglie, R., Newman, M. G., Carranza, F. A., and Pattison, G. L. (1982). Bacterial invasion of gingiva in advanced periodontitis in humans. *Journal of Periodontology*, **53**, 217–22.

Schuessler, C. F., Fairchild, J. M., and Stransky, I. M. (1945). Penicillin in the treatment of Vincent's infection. *Journal of the American Dental Association*, **32**, 551–4.

Scopp, I. W., Froum, S. J., Sullivan, M., Kazandgjian, G., Wank, D., and Fine, A. (1980). Tetracycline: a clinical study to determine its effectiveness as long-term adjunct. *Journal of Periodontology*, **51**, 328–30.

Shinn, D. L. S. (1962). Metronidazole in acute ulcerative gingivitis. *Lancet*, **i**, 1191.

Shinn, D. L. S., Squires, S., and MacFadzean, J. A. (1965). The treatment of Vincent's disease with metronidazole. *Dental Practice*, **15**, 275–80.

Slots, J. and Rosling, B. G. (1983). Suppression of the periodontopathic microflora in localised juvenile periodontitis by systemic tetracycline. *Journal of Clinical Periodontology*, **10**, 465–86.

Slots, J., Mashimo, P., Levine, M. J., and Genco, R. J. (1979). Periodontal therapy in humans. I. Microbiological and clinical effects of a single course of periodontal scaling and root planing and of adjunctive tetracycline therapy. *Journal of Periodontology*, **50**, 495–509.

Slots, J., Evans, R. T., Lobbins, P. M., and Genco, R. J. (1980a). *In vitro* microbial susceptibility of *Actinobacillus actinomycetemcomitans*. *Antimicrobial Agents and Chemotherapy*, **18**, 9–12.

Slots, J., Reynolds, H. S., and Genco, R. J. (1980*b*). *Actinobacillus actinomycetemcomitans* in human periodontal disease: a cross-sectional microbiological investigation. *Infection and Immunity*, **29**, 1013–20.

Stephen, K. W., McLathie, M. F., Mason, D. K., Noble, H. W., and Stevenson, D. M. (1966). Treatment of acute ulcerative gingivitis (Vincent's type). *British Dental Journal*, **121**, 313–22.

Sterry, K. A., Langeroudi, M., and Dolby, A. E. (1985). Metronidazole as an adjunct to periodontal therapy with sub-gingival curettage. *British Dental Journal*, **158**, 176–8.

Sznajder, N., Piovano, S., Bernat, M. I., Fores, L., Macchi, R., and Carraro, J. J. (1987). Effect of spiramycin therapy on human periodontal disease. *Journal of Periodontal Research*, **22**, 255–8.

Theilade, E. (1986). The non-specific theory in microbial aetiology of inflammatory periodontal diseases. *Journal of Clinical Periodontology*, **13**, 905–11.

Van Palenstein Heldermann, W. H. (1986). Is antibiotic therapy justified in the treatment of human chronic inflammatory periodontal disease? *Journal of Clinical Periodontology*, **13**, 932–8.

Van Winkelhoff, A. J., Rodenburg, J. P., Goene, R. J., Abbas, F., Windel, E. G., and de Graff, J. (1989). Metronidazole plus amoxycillin in the treatment of *Actinobacillus actinomycetemcomitans* associated periodontitis. *Journal of Clinical Periodontology*, **16**, 128–31.

Wade, W. G. and Addy, M. (1987). Comparison of *in vitro* activity of niridazole, metronidazole and tetracycline against subgingival bacteria in chronic periodontitis. *Journal of Applied Bacteriology*, **63**, 455–7.

Walker, C. B., Gordon, J. M., Cornwall, H. A., Murphy, J. C., and Socransky, S. S. (1981*a*). Gingival crevicular fluid levels of clindamycin compared with its minimal inhibitory concentrations for periodontal bacteria. *Antimicrobial Agents and Chemotherapy*, **19**, 867–71.

Walker, C. B., Gordon, J. M., McQuilkin, S. J., Niebloom, T. A., and Socransky, S. S. (1981*b*). Tetracycline: levels achievable in gingival crevice fluid and *in vitro* effect on subgingival organisms. II. Susceptibilities of periodontal bacteria. *Journal of Periodontology*, **52**, 613–16.

Walker, C. B., Gordon, J. M., and Socransky, S. S. (1983). Antibiotic susceptibility testing of subgingival plaque samples. *Journal of Clinical Periodontology*, **10**, 422–32.

Walsh, M. M. *et al.* (1986). Clinical and microbiologic effects of single-dose metronidazole or scaling and root planing in treatment of adult periodontitis. *Journal of Clinical Periodontology*, **13**, 151–7.

Wan Yusof, W. Z. (1984). Subgingival metronidazole in dialysis tubing and subgingival chlorhexidine irrigation in the control of chronic inflammatory periodontal disease. *Journal of Clinical Periodontology*, **11**, 166–75.

Watts, T., Palmer, R., and Floyd, P. (1986). Metronidazole: a double-blind trial in untreated periodontal disease. *Journal of Clinical Periodontology*, **13**, 939–43.

Weeks, D. B. (1980). Tetracycline in the treatment of periodontal disease: review of current literature. *Journal of the American Dental Association*, **101**, 935–6.

Williams, B. L., Pantalone, R. M., and Sherris, J. C. (1976). Subgingival microflora and periodontitis. *Journal of Periodontal Research*, **11**, 1–18.

Williams, B. L., Osterberg, S. K-A., and Jorgensen, J. (1979). Subgingival microflora of periodontal patients in tetracycline therapy. *Journal of Clinical Periodontology*, **6**, 210–21.

Winer, R., Cohen, M. M., and Chauncey, M. H. (1966). Antibiotic therapy in periodontal disease. *Journal of Oral Therapeutics and Pharmacology*, **2**, 403–10.

Wolff, L. F., Liljemark, W. F., Bloomqvist, C. G., Philstrom, B. L., Schaffer, E. M., and Bandt, C. L. (1985). The distribution of *Actinobacillus actinomycetemcomitans* in human plaque. *Journal of Periodontal Research*, **20**, 237–50.

Yankell, S. L., Leung, F. C., Gardner, J. M., and Paor, W. S. (1971). Spiramycin excretion in animals. I. A single oral dose in rats. *Journal of Dental Research*, **50**, 1359.

Yeung, F. I., Newman, H. N., and Addy, M. (1983). Subgingival metronidazole in acrylic resin vs. chlorhexidine irrigation in the control of chronic periodontitis. *Journal of Periodontology*, **54**, 651–7.

Zambon, J. J., Christersson, L. A., and Slots, J. (1983). *Actinobacillus actinomycetemcomitans* in human periodontal disease. Prevalence in patient groups and distribution of biotypes and serotypes within families. *Journal of Periodontology*, **54**, 707–11.

11. Anti-inflammatory drugs and periodontal disease[†]

11.1 INTRODUCTION

The development of all periodontal diseases is a consequence of the inflammatory and immunological reactions of the host to bacterial plaque on the tooth surface. Any drug that has anti-inflammatory properties, therefore, should be capable of modifying the host's reactions to the bacterial insult and so have a clinical effect upon the progression of the disease. In this chapter, the anti-inflammatory drugs and their effects on periodontal diseases will be considered in two broad categories: corticosteroids and the non-steroidal anti-inflammatory drugs.

11.2 CORTICOSTEROIDS

The physiological functions and effects of the endogenous corticosteroids (glucocorticoids and mineralocorticoids) are numerous and widespread. These hormones influence carbohydrate, lipid, and protein metabolism; electrolyte and water balance; and have a direct influence on the functions of the cardiovascular system, skeletal muscle, the kidneys, and other organs and tissues. In states of adrenal insufficiency the physiological levels of corticosteroids need to be replenished by substitution therapy. Such regimens are well documented in standard medical texts and will not be considered further. However, it is the pharmacological actions of the synthetic glucocorticoids that may influence inflammatory changes in the periodontium and it is these actions that will be considered in detail.

11.2.1 PHARMACODYNAMICS OF THE GLUCOCORTICOIDS

Glucocorticoids and their synthetic analogous can inhibit both the early and late stages of the inflammatory process, such as capillary dilatation, leukocyte chemotaxis, fibroblast proliferation, and collagen deposition, irrespective of the inciting agent. Clinically, the anti-inflammatory effects are palliative, as the aetiological factors of the underlying disease process often remain unaffected. An important anti-inflammatory action of glucocorticoids is the ability to inhibit the migration of neutrophils, monocytes, and macrophages to the site of inflammation (Ward 1966; Parrillo and Fauci 1979).

[†] The text for this chapter is reproduced from Heasman, P. A. (1988). Journal of Dentistry, **16**, 247–57. By permission of the publisher, Butterworth & Company Limited.

Glucocorticoids block the effects of certain lymphokines (for example, macrophage inhibition factor) on their target cells, thereby preventing local accumulation of the cells at the inflammatory site (Balow and Rosenthal 1973; Weston et al. 1973). They also interfere with the cytotoxic potential of macrophages (Dimitriu 1976).

Evidence now suggests that glucocorticoids induce the synthesis of a protein (macrocortin) that can inhibit the enzyme phospholipase A_2 and so diminish the release of arachidonic acid from phospholipids (Blackwell et al. 1980). As a result of this action, the formation of the eicosanoids (prostaglandins, leukotrienes, hydroxy fatty acids, and related compounds), which play vital roles in chemotaxis and inflammation, will be reduced.

Glucocortocoids may also have significant effects upon the lymphoid system and immune response. However, many of these effects have been demonstrated in vitro and at unrealistically high concentrations of steroids. One response that is inhibited by low concentrations of glucocorticoids in vitro is T-cell proliferation as stimulated by mitogens or mixed leukocyte populations. This effect is due to the inhibition of interleukin-1 release by macrophages. A deficiency of interleukin-1 precludes the formation of inter-leukin-2, which acts as an intermediate stimulant of T-cell proliferation (Gillis et al. 1979; Smith 1980).

The pharmacological properties of the corticosteroids ensure their common use in the treatment and palliation of such diseases as rheumatoid arthritis, osteoarthritis, collagen disorders, allergic and hypersensitivity problems, ocular, skin and renal disease, and disorders of the gastrointestinal tract. For the treatment of such conditions, long-term administration of corticosteroids may be necessary and under these circumstances the anti-inflammatory and immune properties of this group of drugs may extend to inhibit or influence the progression of plaque-associated periodontal disease (Waterhouse 1969). It is also possible that by interfering with the synthesis of new protein and accelerating the catabolism of existing bone matrix (Jenkins 1978), prolonged therapy with corticosteroids may favour osteoporosis of bone, including that of the maxilla and mandible.

11.2.2 GLUCOCORTICOIDS AND THE PERIODONTAL TISSUES

Animal experiments

Histological evidence for the effects of corticosteroids upon the periodontal tissues has emerged almost exclusively from animal experiments. Applebaum and Seelig (1955) observed microscopic changes in the teeth and periodontal ligaments of rats after adrenalectomy or cortisone treatment. Supporting bone was lost from the molars and a detailed study at high magnification revealed abnormal changes in the alveolar bone of the rats given cortisol. Glickman *et al.* (1952, 1953) reported osteoporosis of alveolar bone in white mice after daily intramuscular injections of cortisone 0.5 mg for 43 days. Histological changes in the periodontium included a reduction in the number of osteoblasts, the intercellular matrix, the height of alveolar bone, the number of fibroblasts, and of collagen fibres. There was also an increase in oedema of the periodontal membrane when comparisons were made with control groups. The suggested mechanisms by which the cortisone injections induced such changes were by accentuated catabolism or reduced production of periodontal protein matrix. Similar observations were made when the dose of cortisone was reduced to 0.25 mg daily (Glickman and Shklar 1954) or increased to 3.0 mg daily in rats (Goldsmith and Stahl 1953).

The relative effects of cortisone injections and aggravating local factors on the periodontal structures of the albino rat were studied by Labelle and Schaffer (1967). Ligatures were placed around maxillary second molars on one side of the jaw in 24 rats, half of which were given daily intramuscular injections of 2.5 mg cortisone acetate. Histologic examination of the tissues was made after five weeks. The experimental design grouped the observations of periodontal structures into four categories: injected rats, with and without ligatures on molars; non-injected controls, with and without ligatures. The results showed that all periodontal tissues were affected to some degree by cortisone, with a marked reduction in the numbers and size of osteoblasts and fibroblasts. Periodontal tissues from ligated molars of injected rats showed few additional changes when compared to the non-ligated side. However, the periodontal tissues of ligated teeth of non-injected rats showed a marked inflammatory reaction. It was concluded that although cortisol does produce changes in the periodontium, these changes are not influential on the production of periodontal disease.

An ultrastructural study involving rats injected daily with hydrocortisone acetate, 12.5 mg, confirmed previous observations and added that there was a reduction in the area of extracellular matrix occupied by oxytalan fibres (Bond 1986). A reduced rate of eruption of the continuously growing incisor was also found in the cortisol-treated rats.

Observations on humans

Clinical observations on the gingival tissues of 100 bedridden and out-patients who were receiving long-term corticosteroid therapy were compared with those from 101 control patients (Krohn 1958). Regardless of steroid therapy, the inflammatory changes were more severe in those subjects with poorer oral hygiene and the gingival inflammation and periodontal destruction were more dependent upon plaque control than upon corticosteroid dosage.

Topical applications of corticosteroids to the inflamed marginal gingivae of patients with periodontal disease resulted in a reduction of inflammation and sulcus bleeding, with no effect on the progression of periodontitis (Stawinski 1960; Haim 1962). However, Iusem *et al.* (1956) injected cortisol preparations directly into the gingival tissues of five patients with periodontal disease and showed, histologically, reduced capillary permeability, fewer plasma cells in the granulation tissue, inhibition of collagen synthesis, and clinical improvement in haemorrhagic and hyperplastic gingivitis.

There are several studies on the prevalence of gingival and periodontal disease in groups of patients on prolonged immunosuppressive therapy after renal transplantation. Their findings are discussed in Chapter 3.

The effects of prednisone therapy upon gingival inflammation and periodontal bone loss have been studied in a group of patients suffering from multiple sclerosis who had been on steroid therapy for up to four years (Safkan and Knuuttila 1984). Comparisons were made between this group, a group of patients who suffered from neurological disorders but were not receiving steroids, and healthy controls. There were no differences in the frequency and severity of periodontal disease between the groups and it was concluded that corticosteroid therapy over 1–4 years had no influence on the measures of periodontal diseases in patients suffering from neurological disorders.

11.2.3 SUMMARY

It appears that despite the obvious histological and ultrastructural changes in the periodontal tissues of rats and mice after systemic cortisone therapy, the observations of periodontal health status after long-term corticosteroid therapy in humans remain equivocal. The reasons for these inconsistent findings may include insufficient dosage, inadequate observation periods, interspecies variation, and possible interactions among the combinations of drugs used in immunosuppressed patients.

11.3 NON-STEROIDAL ANTI-INFLAMMATORY DRUGS (NSAIDs)

The NSAIDs are a heterogeneous group of compounds whose analgesic, antipyretic, and anti-inflammatory properties result from pharmacological mechanisms that are different from those of the anti-inflammatory steroids and the opioid analgesics. The majority of NSAIDs are weak organic acids and are often referred to as aspirin-like drugs, a term derived from their prototype, acetylsalicylic acid.

The main therapeutic indications for the use of NSAIDs in medicine are as analgesics against low-to-moderate pain, as antipyretics to reduce body temperature in mild febrile states, and as anti-inflammatory agents, which is where this group of drugs have their main clinical application. NSAIDs are used, usually in combination with one another, in the treatment of musculoskeletal disorders such as rheumatoid arthritis, osteoarthritis, and ankylosing spondylitis. The commonly prescribed NSAIDs and their therapeutic indications are shown in Table 11.1

Table 11.1 Non-steroidal anti-inflammatory drugs and their main therapeutic indications

Drugs	Indications
Salicylates Aspirin Benoryate Diflusinal	Rheumatoid arthritis, osteoarthritis and other painful musculoskeletal disorders
Arylalcanoic acid derivatives Phenylacetic acid derivatives Aclofenac Diclofenac Fenclofenac	Rheumatoid arthritis, osteoarthritis, Still's disease and other general muskuloskeletal disorders
Phenylpropionic acid derivatives Fenoprofen Ibuprofen Ketoprofen Naproxen Flurbiprofen Oxicam (piroxicam)	Rheumatoid arthritis, osteoarthritis, soft tissue injuries and ankylosing spondylitis Rheumatoid arthritis, acute gout, osteoarthritis and, ankylosing spondylitis
Pyrazoles Azapropazone Feprazone Sulindac	Rheumatoid arthritis, acute gout, osteoarthritis and ankylosing spondylitis
Pyrazolone compounds Phenylbutazone* Indomethacin Tolmetin	Rheumatoid arthritis, osteoarthritis, ankylosing spondylitis, lumbago and acute periarticular disease
Anthranilic acid derivatives Mefenamic acid Flufenamic acid	Rheumatoid arthritis, Still's disease and osteoarthritis

*In the United Kingdom this drug can only be prescribed in hospital practice.

The main side-effect of the NSAID group of drugs is a high incidence of gastrointestinal irritation (Davenport 1964). Damage to the gastric mucosa is related to prostaglandin inhibition. Prostaglandins appear to protect the lining of the gastrointestinal tract from acid attack (Kollberg et al. 1981). Therefore, when prostaglandin synthesis is inhibited the lining mucosa is more vulnerable to ulceration.

11.3.1 PHARMACODYNAMICS

NSAIDs exert their pharmacological properties by inhibiting the synthesis and release of the prostaglandins and other eicosanoids (Ferreira et al. 1971; Smith and Willis 1971; Vane 1971). Prostaglandins are synthesized from arachidonic acid by all mammalian tissue cells except erythrocytes. Prostaglandins and other eicosanoids are derived from fatty acids and cell membrane phospholipids. Mechanical or chemical stimuli activate the enzyme phospholipase A$_2$; the enzyme acts on the fatty acids to form arachidonic acid (Fig. 11.1).

The free arachidonic acid serves as the substrate for the enzyme cyclo-oxygenase, which converts arachidonate, via unstable intermediates, to prostacyclin, thromboxane, and prostaglandins of the D, E, and F series. An alternative pathway for arachidonic acid metabolism has been described (Samuelsson 1981). The enzyme lipoxygenase acts upon the arachidonate to form a range of hydroperoxy-eicosatetraenocic acids (HPETES), which may be reduced to form the corresponding hydroxyeicosatetraenoic acids (HETES). Leukotrienes are derived by the action of 5-lipoxygenase on arachidonate to form 5-HPETE.

Before detailed consideration is given to the effects of NSAIDs on periodontal inflammation it is relevant to discuss the evidence that implicates eicosanoid molecules in inflammation, bone resorption, and, more specifically, periodontal disease.

11.3.2 THE ROLE OF EICOSANOIDS IN INFLAMMATION

Generally, eicosanoids appear to have two separate roles in inflammation. First, they promote its development and secondly they modulate and regulate inflammatory cell function (Gordon et al. 1976).

Inflamed tissues contain significantly higher levels of eicosanoids than do non-inflamed tissues (Eakins et al. 1972; Jorgensen and Sondergaard 1976) and the prostaglandins, in particular, have been associated with vascular changes, local oedema, redness, and pain found in the development of inflammation (Crunkhorn and Willis 1969, 1971; Vane 1976; Kuehl et al. 1977). Prostaglandins have a direct influence on the degree of vasodilatation but cannot alone cause oedema and pain. Prostaglandins can increase pain and oedema when they have been induced by other mediators such as histamine, bradykinin, and fragments of the complement system (Williams and Peck 1977; Williams 1983). This accounts for the ability of cyclo-oxygenase inhibitors to reduce swelling and redness associated with inflammation. This potentiation of the inflammatory response by prostaglandins (PG) has a ranking order of PGE$_1$ > PGE$_2$ > PGF$_1$ > PGF$_2$ (Williams and Morley 1973). Some lipoxygenase products, including the leukotrienes, may also affect vascular permeability (Samuelsson 1983).

Eicosanoids are capable of influencing the activities of inflammatory cells in a number of ways. The main effect of prostaglandins on polymorphonuclear leukocytes is to inhibit lysosomal enzyme release during phagocytosis, although they have also been associated with enhanced chemotaxis and chemokinesis (Estensen et al. 1973; Lewis 1983).

Prostaglandins can affect macrophage proliferation and function, and the effects can be stimulatory or inhibitory (Stenson and Parker 1980). Prostaglandins can inhibit clonal proliferation of macrophage stem cells, and also inhibit the spreading and migration of mature macrophages. Stimulatory effects include augmentation of phagocytosis and increased numbers of cell-surface antibody receptors.

Less is known of the effects of lipoxygenase products on macrophages, although there is some evidence to suggest

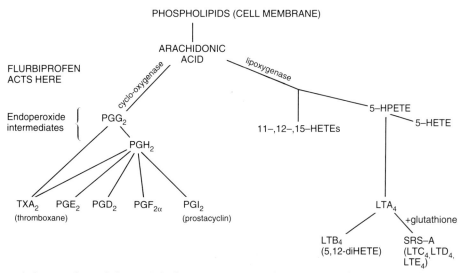

Fig. 11.1 Pathways of arachidonic acid metabolism: LT, leukotriene; PG, prostaglandin; SRS-A, slow reacting substance A.

that the leukotrienes may have a role in the activation of macrophages (Lewis 1983).

The effects of prostaglandins on lymphocytes are to suppress cell transformation (Mihas *et al.* 1975), lymphokine production (Gordon *et al.* 1976) and T-cell mitogenesis (Goodwin *et al.* 1977). Eicosanoids, therefore, have wide and varied effects upon inflammatory processes that are strongly associated with periodontal disease. The hallmark of periodontal destruction, however, is bone resorption and there is much evidence also to implicate the eicosanoids in this process.

11.3.3 THE ROLE OF EICOSANOIDS IN BONE RESORPTION

Reports in the early 1970s that the local production of prostaglandins in tissues may stimulate bone resorption in osteolytic disease processes were of particular interest to periodontal researchers. Such mediators of bone loss may be similar or identical to those responsible for the loss of alveolar bone in chronic periodontal disease.

The prostaglandins can influence bone in a number of ways and may induce bone resorption by facilitating the release of osteoclast activating factor from lymphocytes (Yoneda and Mundy 1979). However, many prostaglandins have been shown to stimulate bone resorption directly in organ culture, with PGE$_2$ being the most potent (Klein and Raisz 1970; Goodson *et al.* 1974; Raisz *et al.* 1974; Dietrich *et al.* 1975; Rifkin *et al.* 1980). Furthermore, Robinson *et al.* (1975) reported that synovial tissue from patients with rheumatoid arthritis produced a potent, bone resorption-stimulating factor in tissue culture and this was identified as PGE$_2$. Prostaglandin E$_2$ has also been shown to inhibit bone collagen formation, which may result in the inhibition of the repair of resorbed bone (Raisz and Koolemans-Beynen 1974).

There are some lesions that demonstrate an ability to resorb bone and these include dental cysts, granulomas, and ameloblastomas. Prostaglandins have been identified as the primary bone-resorbing factor in these, and the resorption can be blocked by certain cyclo-oxygenase inhibiting drugs (Harris and Goldhaber 1973; Harris *et al.* 1973; Oguntebi *et al.* 1988).

Thus, within a relatively short period of time, a clear relationship has been demonstrated between the production of certain prostaglandins and the resorption of bone in several osteolytic disorders. It may be supposed, therefore, that the control of such disease processes may be achieved by using NSAIDs to block the further production of the responsible eicosanoids. Before considering the use of NSAIDs in the treatment of gingival inflammation and alveolar bone loss, the specific role of the eicosanoids in periodontal disease will be reviewed.

11.3.4 THE ROLE OF EICOSANOIDS IN PERIODONTAL DISEASE

A considerable amount of research has established that significantly higher levels of prostaglandins are present in inflamed bovine (Goodson and Brunetti 1974) and human (Goodson 1973; Goodson *et al.* 1974; Albers *et al.* 1975; El Attar 1976; El Attar and Lin 1980; Ohm *et al.* 1984) periodontal tissues when compared to healthy gingiva.

El Attar (1976) measured the PGE$_2$ levels in 12 normal and 24 chronically inflamed samples of human gingival tissue and found an 18-fold increase of the prostaglandin in the inflamed tissues. The findings were later confirmed (Holmes and El Attar 1977) and the increased amounts of PGE$_2$ were localized specifically to the monocyte population (Albers *et al.* 1975). Another group of workers (Loning *et al.* 1980) suggested that the local reaction of progressive periodontal disease may be influenced by macrophage-derived factors such as lysosomal enzymes and prostaglandins. They reported that prostaglandin levels are markedly elevated in established gingival lesions and that prostaglandin E was located mainly in macrophages.

Many studies have now implicated prostaglandin E as a mediator of periodontal inflammation as well as introducing a role for prostaglandin F in the overall disease process. It has been suggested that prostaglandin E acts as a pro-inflammatory mediator to increase vascular permeability whereas prostaglandin F inhibits vascular permeability and moderates the severity of the disease (Crunkhorn and Willis 1971; Willoughby 1972).

Advanced periodontal lesions in humans have been studied to determine whether there were any differences in prostaglandin levels between superficial (gingival) and deep (periodontal) lesions. Detectable levels of PGE_2 were found in half of eight superficial samples studied and in two-thirds of the deep tissues, which suggests that the presence of PGE_2 may be a feature of both gingivitis and periodontitis (Dewhirst *et al.* 1983).

The presence of PGE_2 in gingival crevicular fluid of patients suffering from either adult or juvenile periodontitis has been demonstrated by Offenbacher *et al.* (1984), who showed a highly significant correlation between levels of PGE_2 in crevicular fluid and periodontal connective tissue. The concentrations of PGE_2 were almost three times greater in juvenile than in adult periodontitis, and further work now suggests that levels of PGE_2 are significantly elevated at sites of ongoing, connective-tissue attachment loss. These levels may be useful as markers for potentially 'active' periodontal lesions and there is now evidence from studies of disease progression in monkeys that high levels of PGE_2 (and thomboxane B_2) are associated with ongoing attachment loss and alveolar bone resorption (Offenbacher *et al.* 1989).

In addition to prostaglandin E, several other products of arachidonic acid metabolism via the cyclo-oxygenase pathway have been isolated in the diseased periodontium. These include the hydrolysis product of prostacyclin metabolism (6-keto-$PGF_1\alpha$ which may play an important part in bone resorption, as well as thromboxane B_2 and other endoperoxide metabolites of prostaglandin metabolism (Wong *et al.* 1980; Dewhirst *et al.* 1983; Ohm *et al.* 1984).

The conversion of arachidonic acid through the lipoxygenase pathway may also be important in the pathogenesis of periodontal disease, as a number of hydroxy fatty acid products have been identified in the diseased periodontium. Extracts of inflamed gingiva convert arachidonate to the non-prostaglandin metabolite 12-hydroxyeicosatetraenoic acid (12-HETE), which is the major product of arachidonic acid metabolism in diseased gingiva (Sidhagen *et al.* 1982; El Attar and Lin 1983). Indeed, both 12-HETE and 15-HETE are important mediators of inflammation in the tissues of patients with advanced periodontal disease (El Attar *et al.* 1986).

There is, therefore, a substantial amount of evidence that implicates the products of arachidonic acid metabolism in the pathogenesis of gingivitis and periodontitis, and most workers have suggested that the cyclo-oxygenase product, PGF_2, is potentially the most significant mediator of disease progression. It is now relevant to examine the possibility that blockage of this latter pathway, using NSAIDs as inhibitors of the enzyme cyclo-oxygenase, may have a controlling influence on the disease process. Although the use of NSAIDs in the treatment of periodontal disease is so far experimental, the research in this area is promising and the prospects for using NSAIDs in the prevention and treatment of the disease are very exciting.

11.3.5 NSAIDs AND PERIODONTAL DISEASES

The results of the work discussed so far show that the eicosanoids may have an important role in the pathogenesis of periodontal disease. If this hypothesis is accepted, then the introduction of NSAIDs to inhibit arachidonic acid metabolism by blocking the cyclo-oxygenase pathway would be a logical innovation. Indeed, the results of both ongoing and earlier research indicate quite clearly that a role does exist for NSAIDs in the management of periodontal inflammation.

In vitro models

The first evidence that NSAID block prostaglandin production in gingival tissues was produced by Gomes and co-workers who, in 1976, demonstrated that inflamed gingival fragments taken from monkeys consistently released prostaglandins in to the culture medium, and that the pyrazole compound indomethacin reduced the amount of prostaglandin released by at least 90 per cent. Furthermore, the NSAIDs indomethacin, ibuprofen, piroxicam, flurbiprofen, and zomepirac sodium have been shown, in gingival homogenates, to have a significant inhibitory effect on the production of prostaglandin and 12-HETE when compared to control systems (El Attar *et al.* 1983, 1984). It was concluded that, as the major mediators of gingival inflammation may include products of the lipoxygenase pathway, those NSAIDs that are equally efficacious in inhibiting both the cyclo-oxygenase and lipogenase pathways may have a definite advantage over cyclo-oxygenase inhibitors alone (El Attar *et al.* 1984). Later reports on animals indicate that specific cyclo-oxygenase inhibitors are very effective in controlling periodontal attachment loss and alveolar bone resorption.

Animal experiments

The efficacy of indomethacin in the suppression of gingival inflammation and alveolar bone resorption has been studied in a ligature-induced periodontitis in beagles by Nyman and his group (Nyman *et al.* 1979). The results of this now classical work were that twice-daily oral doses of indomethacin interfered with the periodontal response to ligation, and that indomethacin delayed the onset and suppressed the magnitude of the acute inflammatory reaction and also reduced the amount of alveolar bone resorption during the study period.

The same model of periodontitis was later used to study further the bone-resorbing potential of inflamed periodontal tissues and to compare the effects of systemic NSAID (indomethacin) and antimicrobial (metronidazole) therapy (Nuki *et al.* 1981). Bone resorption was suppressed by metronidazole but unaffected by indomethacin and it was suggested that the effects of the antimicrobial were due to a change in the flora of the gingival crevice. These results contrast with those of Nyman's group, who reported that indomethacin did have a beneficial effect in preventing bone resorption. The drug therapy in Nuki's study, however, was only given for a short time (7 days) during the experiment, and such dosing may well be insufficient to produce significant, clinical changes in the levels of alveolar bone.

The effects of indomethacin on alveolar bone loss in experimental periodontitis have also been studied in the squirrel monkey (Weaks-Dybvig *et al.* 1982). The loss of alveolar bone height and mass seen in control animals was abolished in monkeys dosed with indomethacin. Histopathological examination of periodontal tissues from the indomethacin group showed a suppression of the large increase in osteoclast density that was evident in the controls.

The effects of indomethacin on bone destruction in periodontal disease in hamsters have been compared to those of calcitonin, a hormonal inhibitor of osteoclast resorption. Indomethacin was found to reduce the alveolar bone loss by 28 per cent and the number of osteoclasts per mm^2 by 55 per cent in diseased animals, but the changes were not statistically significant. Calcitonin, however, significantly reduced bone loss and decreased the number of osteoclasts to control levels (Lasfargues and Saffar 1983). Therefore, although indomethacin does appear to have an effect on bone resorption, the hormone calcitonin is more effective.

In 1984, Williams and his group published some observations on the effects of the phenylpropionic acid derivative flurbiprofen on periodontal disease. They compared the effects of non-surgical and surgical management of naturally occurring periodontal disease in beagles when each mode of therapy was combined with either flurbiprofen or placebo therapy over a 12-month period. The results indicated that daily administration of flurbiprofen significantly decreased the rate of alveolar bone loss at 3, 6, 9 and 12 months in comparison to baseline rates in both surgically and non-surgically treated groups. In contrast, the rate of bone loss in the placebo-treated dogs did not decrease during the treatment period, except at 9 months in the surgically treated group; and this reduction was not maintained at 12 months. A further, important finding from this study was that flurbiprofen therapy did not appear to affect gingival inflammation (Williams *et al.* 1984).

The doses of flurbiprofen used were approximately 1/200 of the doses used clinically in the treatment of human arthritis and ankylosing spondylitis. It was therefore concluded that doses of the cyclo-oxygenase inhibitor that are unable to control the (gingival) inflammatory response can have dramatic effects upon the rate of bone loss, even in cases where local, supplemental treatment was withheld.

The study was continued over a six-month, post-treatment period after the withdrawal of the flurbiprofen (Jeffcoat *et al.* 1986). The decreased rate of bone loss that had been found in the flurbiprofen group was sustained through three months of the post-treatment period but was lost six months after the termination of flurbiprofen therapy.

In a similar experiment the effect of another propionic acid derivative, ibuprofen, upon periodontal disease was studied in beagles over a 13-month period (Williams *et al.* 1987a, 1988a). The dogs were given either a sustained-release ibuprofen preparation or a standard oral preparation, and a further group acted as untreated controls. In the untreated animals the rate of bone loss during the treatment period did not change significantly from baseline, although the rate was increased. In the dogs receiving standard or

sustained-release ibuprofen the rate of bone loss in the treatment period was significantly less than that during the pre-treatment period. Furthermore when the rate of bone loss in the control dogs was compared with the rate of bone loss in the ibuprofen-treated dogs, the latter had significantly less bone loss. The sustained-release ibuprofen preparation, which gave consistently greater blood levels over 24 h, was overall more effective in preventing bone loss. Indeed, the encouraging results of the flurbiprofen studies that were reported earlier by this group may be related to the long half-life (36 h) of flurbiprofen in dogs. It may be suggested that, for the most effective inhibition of bone resorption, a sustained-release preparation of a drug with a relatively long half-life should be used.

Recently published work from the Harvard Centre (Williams *et al.* 1987b) has compared the effects of both flurbiprofen and the pyrazolone indomethacin on the progression of bone loss in beagles over a 12-month period. The design of the experiment was similar to that used earlier but with dogs dosed daily with either indomethacin or flurbiprofen in addition to the controls. However, in this investigation, radioimmunoassay was used to measure levels of PGE$_2$, PGE$_2\alpha$ thromboxane B$_2$, and 6-keto-PGE$_1\alpha$, in crevicular fluid, both before and after NSAID therapy (Williams *et al.* 1988b). The levels of PGE$_2$, PGF$_2$ and thromboxane B$_2$ in crevicular fluid were similarly and significantly decreased by indomethacin and flurbiprofen, and the levels of 6-keto-PGF$_1$ were not altered. In addition, flurbiprofen significantly decreased bone resorption from baseline whereas indomethacin did not. However, the indomethacin-treated animals did not show the striking increase in bone resorption during the treatment phase that was found in the control group. The conclusion was that both drugs inhibit eicosanoids in crevicular fluid in a similar manner, but not the rate of bone loss.

Several interesting issues have arisen from this work. It is clear from the reduced levels of eicosanoids that both drugs inhibit the cyclo-oxygenase pathway but it is difficult to appreciate why the levels of the prostacyclin metabolite, 6-keto-PGF$_1$, remain unchanged. It is possible that the presence of prostacyclin in the periodontal tissues may reflect their vascularization and not be related to inflammation *per se*.

Although both drugs had similar effects on the eicosanoids that were assayed, it is quite conceivable that other, unmeasured metabolites are responsible for the bone resorption. Such metabolites may be inhibited by flurbiprofen but not by indomethacin and, therefore, explain the differential effects of these drugs on bone loss. Further work is required to confirm or refute this hypothesis. Finally, perhaps the most stimulating consideration is that the actions and mechanisms by which flurbiprofen inhibits alveolar bone resorption in beagles are unrelated to its potential to inhibit cyclo-oxygenase and may involve some other, as yet unknown, biological effect (Doppelt *et al.* 1987). Similar investigations into the effect of flurbiprofen on spontaneous and ligature-induced periodontitis in the rhesus monkey have been undertaken by Offenbacher and co-workers. Two groups of monkeys were treated with different doses of flurbiprofen (0.3 mg/kg/day and 8.0 mg/kg/day) and a third group acted as controls. At the six-month assessment there was a similar and statistically significant inhibition of attachment loss, gingival redness, and bleeding on probing in both flurbiprofen-treated groups and this finding was not dependent upon the marked differences in plasma levels of the drug in these two groups (0.22 µg/ml and 3.2 µg/ml). All the control animals continued to lose attachment throughout the study (Offenbacher *et al.* 1987).

One of the most notable differences between Offenbacher's findings and those of Williams' group is the reduction in gingival index scores and bleeding on probing that followed flurbiprofen therapy, as reported by Offenbacher *et al.* (1987). Williams *et al.* (1984) found that flurbiprofen had no effect on gingival inflammation. Perhaps the most obvious explanation for this inconsistency (other than differences in response between species) is the differences in the doses of flurbiprofen: those used in Offenbacher's work were between 15 and 400 times those used in the Williams' experiment and the higher plasma levels of flurbiprofen that would have been achieved by Offenbacher may have led to distinct anti-inflammatory effects within the inflamed gingival environment. The smaller doses used by the Williams' group may have been insufficient to inhibit significantly the inflammatory response by blocking the cyclo-oxygenase enzyme. They may, however, have been capable, through unknown mechanisms, of inhibiting alveolar bone loss.

Later work by Offenbacher's group, again using monkeys, showed that there is a significant, dose-related inhibition of clinical attachment and radiographic bone loss in flurbiprofen-treated animals. Furthermore, it appeared that these effects were related to a selective inhibition of the synthesis of PGE_2 and thromboxane B_2 (Offenbacher *et al.* 1988).

Topical applications of NSAIDs have also been investigated in animals. The effects of a substituted oxalopyridine derivative on ligature-induced periodontal disease have been studied in the squirrel monkey (Vogel *et al.* 1986). The NSAID, which was applied topically for 14 days, was found to inhibit gingival inflammation and loss of attachment when compared to both placebo and systemically administered indomethacin. However, both the topical NSAID and systemic indomethacin were found to inhibit bone loss and these findings suggest that routes of administration of NSAIDs, other than systemic dosing, may also be consistent with inhibition of bone resorption. Indeed, there is evidence to suggest that flurbiprofen can be absorbed through the oral tissues (Stalker *et al.* 1987). It has yet to be established, however, whether the specific actions of the drug result from a 'true' topical effect or from it being absorbed into the circulation and thereby exerting its effect systemically.

The other finding from Vogel's work was that systemic indomethacin was able significantly to inhibit bone loss in monkeys. This contrasts with the findings of Williams *et al.* (1987*b*), although there are too many variables between the studies (dose of indomethacin, animal species, length of dosing) for any meaningful conclusions to be drawn. The daily application of a topical gel that contained 0.3 mg flurbiprofen has also been shown to inhibit the rate of alveolar bone resorption in beagle dogs (Williams *et al.* 1988*c*). Additional observations, however, were that the

plasma levels of flurbiprofen in the beagles to which the gel was applied were similar to those that could be achieved after an oral dose and swallowing of the drug, and that absorption through the mucous membranes could not be ruled out.

Nevertheless, when these observations are considered with those of previous studies it becomes clear that relatively small doses of NSAIDs, and in particular flurbiprofen, have profound effects upon the rate of alveolar bone resorption in ligature-induced periodontitis in animals. The application of such therapeutic methods to the management of human periodontal disease demands investigation.

Human studies

The first observations of the effects of NSAIDs upon human periodontal tissues were made in an epidemiological, cross-sectional study in which the periodontal status of subjects who had been taking a variety of NSAIDs for at least one year was compared to that of a control group (Waite *et al.* 1981). There were significantly lower gingival indices and probing depths in the test subjects, and there was also a trend towards a reduced loss of connective tissue attachment in this group. It appeared that NSAIDs may influence the response of the periodontal tissues to plaque by reducing the concentrations of prostaglandins in the tissues, although there were no laboratory investigations to confirm this supposition.

In a similar study, Feldman *et al.* (1983) investigated, radiographically, the height of alveolar bone in 75 patients with rheumatoid arthritis who each had at least a five-year history of regularly taking aspirin and/or indomethacin, and compared these observations with those on an age-matched control group of volunteers. A significantly greater number of sites with more than 10 per cent bone loss were found in the controls, and it was suggested that the NSAIDs were responsible for the inhibition of the bone resorption.

Although the results of these two studies are most interesting, neither conclusively demonstrates that it is the NSAIDs which are responsible for the inhibition of attachment and bone loss. In fact, if these results are considered independently of the work on animals, it may be suggested that less bone loss is seen in patients who suffer from rheumatoid arthritis, possibly as a result of altered immune mechanisms.

A number of studies, however, have been directed towards establishing whether or not NSAIDs have anti-inflammatory actions upon the severity of gingival inflammation. Vogel *et al.* (1984) compared the effects of a systemic NSAID (sulindac) with a topical steroid gel (fluocinonide) upon experimental gingivitis in human volunteers. Sulcular fluid flow and bleeding were used as indicators of disease activity and the results showed that the topical steroid significantly inhibited gingival inflammation whereas the systemic NSAID had no apparent effect.

The issue is complicated further when the findings of later studies are considered. Reiff *et al.* (1987) investigated the effects of solutions of aspirin, buffered aspirin, and buffer alone upon established gingival inflammation in human volunteers. After twice-daily rinses over 21 days the sulcular bleeding index was reduced significantly in each of the above groups, although little improvement was found after rinsing with water alone.

In a double-blind, cross-over study, Heasman *et al.* (1987) investigated the effects of topical flurbiprofen and a placebo on the development of an experimental gingivitis in volunteers who had abstained from toothbrushing for 17 days. The volunteers acted as their own controls as the active and placebo solutions were applied subgingivally to separate quadrants of the maxilla. There were no significant differences between the treatments for gingival index, probing pocket depths, or papillary bleeding index. However, no allowances had been made for the possibility of absorption of flurbiprofen through the oral mucous membrane. Further irrigations were undertaken and plasma assays showed that flurbiprofen was present within the range 0.24–0.66 µg/ml and it was suggested that systemic absorption of flurbiprofen may have influenced the gingival response on both sides of the jaw.

More conclusive evidence for the effect of flurbiprofen on established gingivitis was demonstrated in a later study (Heasman and Seymour 1989) when volunteers abstained from tooth-cleaning for 21 days and were then allocated to one of three treatment groups. One group received oral flurbiprofen (100 mg/day) as an adjunct to toothbrushing, a second group received placebo as an adjunct to toothbrushing, and the third group received oral flurbiprofen only. The treatment in all groups continued for six days. There were significant reductions in gingival indices and sulcular fluid flow in all three groups after treatment, although no changes were found in pocket probing depths. There were no significant differences between any of the treatments. It was concluded that systemic flurbiprofen can significantly reduce the signs of an experimental gingivitis over six days and this effect may be seen when the drug is used alone or as an adjunct to toothbrushing.

The effects of short-term administration of flurbiprofen on patients with refractory periodontitis have been described by the Harvard workers (Jeffcoat *et al.* 1988). Sensitive radiographic techniques were used to analyse changes in alveolar bone levels in patients who had been prescribed flurbiprofen (50 mg, twice daily) for two months. The study patients (and a control group who were given a placebo) also received supragingival scaling and plaque-control therapy. After two months there were significantly fewer sites that had lost alveolar bone in the flurbiprofen-treated group, and, in this group, there were some sites that had actually gained bone.

The same workers have reported on a three year study of the longer-term effects of system flurbiprofen therapy on a human periodontitis (Williams *et al.* 1987c). A group of patients was given flurbiprofen 50 mg twice daily for 24 months, while a second group received placebo. The available results show that the rate of bone loss in the flurbiprofen-treated group was significantly less than that in the placebo-treated group after 12 and 18 months of treatment. At 24 months, there was no difference in the rate of bone loss between the groups, and this could be explained by a lack of compliance by the patients taking the NSAID.

Conversely, there might have been a true loss of the effect of flurbiprofen, such that other pathways of bone resorption became active.

Comment

When the results of the volunteer and the animal studies are considered together it becomes apparent that the effects of flurbiprofen (and other NSAIDs) upon periodontal and gingival disease may result from two totally independent actions.

First, it is clear from the work of Williams and co-workers that flurbiprofen, when used in relatively small doses, can significantly inhibit alveolar bone loss in beagles without affecting the degree of gingival inflammation. This action was initially believed to be due to the drugs capacity to inhibit the cyclo-oxygenase enzyme. However, if this was the mechanism of action, similar effects would be expected to result from the use of other cyclo-oxygenase inhibitors, such as indomethacin, and Williams' group has demonstrated that this is not the case (Williams *et al.* 1987b, 1988b). It is conceivable, therefore, that the flurbiprofen acts through an as yet unknown pathway to inhibit bone loss. This may be a direct action upon osteoclasts, an effect on bone matrix production, or an effect on the calcification process itself.

Secondly, it appears that when doses of NSAIDs are similar to those used in the management of musculoskeletal disorders, then significant changes in the severity of gingival inflammation do become apparent (Waite *et al.* 1981; Feldman *et al.* 1983; Heasman and Seymour 1987). It can be supposed that these changes, which result from reductions in vascularity, capillary permeability, cellular chemotaxis, and enzyme release, are affected by the cyclo-oxygenase inhibiting power of the NSAID.

The length of time over which a NSAID should be given to obtain maximum effect has yet to be established. The findings of Williams' group indicate that the bone loss-inhibiting effects of flurbiprofen are lost shortly after cessation of the drug therapy. This would suggest that long-term and small-dose regimens may be necessary to prevent bone resorption over a period of time. The duration of the anti-inflammatory effects of cyclo-oxygenase blockers may also be limited. When the cyclo-oxygenase pathway of arachidonic acid metabolism is blocked, cellular stores of arachidonic acid substrate will increase. These stores may, eventually, be 're-metabolized' via the lipoxygenase pathway to produce leukotrienes and hydroxyeicosatetraenoic acids, which, like the prostaglandins, are potent mediators of inflammation.

11.3.6 SUMMARY

The results of the studies on animals demand that longitudinal investigations should be undertaken to establish the long-term effects of NSAIDs on human periodontal disease and particularly alveolar bone resorption.

The precise mechanism of action of NSAIDs in preventing bone loss needs to be established and then the dose, the frequency of dosing, and the most suitable method of administration of the drug can be determined. It would be unrealistic to expect patients with periodontal disease to undertake both regular and/or prolonged, systemic NSAID therapy, particularly as the disease is not outwardly disabling. However, if relatively small but active amounts of a NSAID, such as flurbiprofen, could be incorporated into a gel or a toothpaste for topical application, then the compliance of the patient would be more favourable.

We hope that the findings which will emanate from studies of NSAIDs and periodontitis over the next few years will provide new methods to prevent and control the onset and progression of a disease that currently is a major cause of tooth loss in later life.

REFERENCES

Albers, von, H. K., Loning, T., and Lisboa, B. P. (1975). Biochemische und morphologische untersuchungen uber die prostaglandine E und F der normalen und entzundlicy veranderten gingiva. *Deutsche Zahnaerztliche Zeitschrift*, **34**, 440–3.

Applebaum, E. and Seelig, A. (1955). Histologic changes in the jaws and teeth of rats following nephritis, adrenalectomy and cortisone treatment. *Oral Surgery, Oral Medicine, Oral Pathology*, **8**, 881–91.

Balow, J. E. and Rosenthal, A. S. (1973). Glucocorticoid suppression of macrophage migration inhibitory factor. *Journal of Experimental Medicine*, **137**, 1031–9.

Blackwell, H. J., Carnuccio, R., Dirosa, M., Flower, R. J., Parente, L., and Perisco, P. (1980). Macrocortin: a polypeptide causing the anti-phospholipase effect of glucocorticoids. *Nature*, **287**, 147–9.

Bond, H. R. (1986). A quantitative assessment of the effects of cortisol on the ultrastructure of the periodontal ligament. *Journal of Dental Research*, **65**, 492 (abstr. 37).

Crunkhorn, P. and Willis, A. L. (1969). Actions and interactions of prostaglandins administered intradermally in rat and in man. *British Journal of Pharmacology*, **36**, 216–17.

Crunkhorn, P. and Willis, A. L. (1971). Cutaneous reactions to intradermal prostaglandins. *British Journal of Pharmacology*, **41**, 49–56.

Davenport, H. W. (1964). Gastric mucosal injury by fatty acid acetyl-salicylic acids. *Gastroenterology*, **46**, 245–53.

Dewhirst, F. E., Moss, D. E., Offenbacher, S., and Goodson, J. M. (1983). Levels of PGE_2, thromboxane and prostacyclin in periodontal tissue. *Journal of Periodontal Research*, **18**, 156–63.

Dietrich, J. W., Goodson, J. M., and Raisz, L. G. (1975). Stimulation of bone resorption by various prostaglandins in organ culture. *Prostaglandins*, **10**, 231–8.

Dimitriu, A. (1976). Suppression of macrophage arming by corticosteroids. *Cellular Immunology*, **21**, 79–87.

Doppelt, S. H., Augustine, A., and Mankin, H. J. (1987). Effects of flurbiprofen on inhibiting bone resorption – an *in vivo* study. Orthopaedic Research Society Annual Meeting, Washington.

Eakins, K. E., Whitelock, R. A. F., Bennet, A., and Martinet, A. C. (1972). Prostaglandin-like activity in ocular inflammation. *British Medical Journal*, **3**, 452–3.

El Attar, T. M. A. (1976). PGE_2 in human gingiva in health and disease and its stimulation by female sex steroids. *Prostaglandins*, **11**, 331–42.

El Attar, T. M. A. and Lin, H. S. (1980). Cyclic AMP and prostaglandins in periodontal disease. In *Advances in prostaglandin and thromboxane research*, Vol. 8 (B. Samuelsson, P. W. Ramwell, and R. Paoletti), pp. 1739–40. Raven Press, New York.

El Attar, T. M. A. and Lin, H. S. (1983). Relative conversion of arachidonic acid through lipoxygenase and cyclo-oxygenase pathways by homogenates of diseased periodontal tissues. *Journal of Oral Pathology*, **12**, 7–10.

El Attar, T. M. A., Lin, H. S., and Tira, D. E. (1983). The effect of non-steroidal anti-inflammatory drugs on the metabolism of [14] C-arachidonic acid by human gingival tissue *in vitro*. *Journal of Dental Research*, **62**, 975–9.

El Attar, T. M. A., Lin, H. S., and Tira, D. E. (1984). Arachidonic acid metabolism in inflamed gingiva and its inhibition by anti-inflammatory drugs. *Journal of Periodontology*, **55**, 536–9.

El Attar, T. M. A., Lin, H. S., Killoy, W. J., Van Der Hoek, J. V., and Goodson, J. M. (1986). Hydroxy fatty acids and prostaglandin formation in diseased human periodontal pocket tissue. *Journal of Periodontal Research*, **21**, 169–76.

Estensen, R. D., Hill, R. R., Quie, P. G., Hogan, N., and Golberg, N. D. (1973). Cyclic GMP and cell movement. *Nature*, **245**, 458–60.

Feldman, R. S., Szeto, B., Cauncey, H. H., and Goldhaber, P. (1983). Non-steroidal anti-inflammatory drugs in the reduction of alveolar bone loss. *Journal of Clinical Periodontology*, **10**, 131–6.

Ferreira, S. H., Moncada, S., and Vane, J. R. (1971). Indomethacin and aspirin abolish prostaglandin release from the spleen. *Nature*, **231**, 237–9.

Gillis, S., Crabtree, G. R., and Smith, K. A. (1979). Glucocorticoid-induced inhibition of T-cell growth factor. *Journal of Immunology*, **123**, 1632–8.

Glickman, I. (1952). Interrelation of local and systemic factors in periodontal disease: bone factor concept. *Journal of the American Dental Association*, **45**, 422–9.

Glickman, I. and Shklar, G. (1954). Modification of the effect of cortisone upon alveolar bone by the systemic administration of oestrogen. *Journal of Periodontology*, **25**, 231–9.

Glickman, I., Stone, J. C. and Chawla, T. N. (1953). The effect of systemic administration of cortisone upon the periodontium of white mice. *Journal of Periodontology*, **24**, 161–6.

Goldsmith, E. D. and Stahl, S. S. (1953). Effects of long-term cortisone treatment on the supporting structures of the rat. *Journal of Dental Research*, **32**, 699 (abstr. 161).

Gomes, B. C., Hausmann, E., Weinfeld, M., and De Luca, C. (1976). Prostaglandins: bone resorption stimulating factors released from monkey gingiva. *Calcified Tissue Research*, **19**, 285–93.

Goodson, J. M. (1973). A potential role of prostaglandins in the aetiology of periodontal disease. In *Prostaglandins and cyclic AMP* (ed. R. H. Kahn, and W. E. M. Lands), pp. 215–16. Academic Press, New York.

Goodson, J. M. and Brunetti, A. (1974). Biosynthesis of PGE_2 by gingival homogenates. *Journal of Dental Research*, **53**, 181 (abstr. 506).

Goodson, J. M., Dewhirst, F. E., and Brunetti, A. (1974). Prostaglandin E_2 levels and human periodontal disease. *Prostaglandins*, **6**, 81–5.

Goodwin, J. S., Bankhurst, A. D., and Messner, R. P. (1977). Suppression of human T-cell mitogenesis by prostaglandins. *Journal of Experimental Medicine*, **146**, 1719–34.

Gordon, D., Bray, M. A., and Morley, J. (1976). Control of lymphokine secretion by prostaglandins. *Nature*, **262**, 401–2.

Haim, G. (1962). Therapeutic effect of hydrocortisone on diseases affecting the oral mucosa. *Dental Abstracts*, **7**, 112.

Harris, M. and Goldhaber, P. (1973). The production of a bone-resorbing factor by dental cysts *in vitro*. *British Journal of Oral Surgery*, **10**, 334–8.

Harris, M., Jenkins, M. V., Bennett, A., and Willis, M. R. (1973). Prostaglandin production and bone resorption by dental cysts. *Nature*, **245**, 213–15.

Heasman, P. A. and Seymour, R. A. (1989). The effect of a systemi-
cally-administered non-steroidal anti-inflammatory drug (flurbiprofen) on experimental gingivitis in humans. *Journal of Clinical Periodontology*, 16, 551–6.

Heasman, P. A. Seymour, R. A., and Boston, P. F. (1987). The effect of
a topical non-steroidal anti-inflammatory drug on the development
of experimental gigivitis in man. *Journal of Clinical Periodontology*, 16,
353–8.

Holmes, L. G. and El Attar, T. M. A. (1977). Gingival inflammation
assessed by histology, ³H-estrone metabolism and PGE₂ levels. *Journal
of Periodontal Research*, 12, 500–9.

Iusem, R., Ballestero, L. H., and Morris, B. (1956). Clinical experiences
with cortisone and ACTH in 5 cases of periodontal disease. *Journal of
Dental Research*, 32, 655–6.

Jeffcoat, M. K. *et al.* (1986). Flurbiprofen treatment of periodontal
disease in beagles. *Journal of Periodontal Research*, 21, 624–33.

Jeffcoat, M. K., Williams, R. C. Reddy, M. S., Rolla, A., English, R., and
Goldhaber, P. (1988). Short-term flurbiprofen administration for the
treatment of refractory periodontitis in humans. *Journal of Dental
Research*, 67, 371 (abstr. 2063).

Jenkins, G. N. (1978). The effects of hormones on the oral structures.
In *The physiology and biochemistry of the mouth*, (4th ed), pp. 215–37.
Blackwell Scientific, London.

Jorgensen, P. and Sondergaard, J. (1976). Biosynthesis of prostaglandins by human inflamed skin. *Acta Dermato-Venereologica*, 56,
11–13.

Klein, D. C. and Raisz, L. G. (1970). Prostaglandins; stimulation of
bone resorption in tissue culture. *Endocrinology*, 86, 1436–40.

Kollberg, B., Nordemar, R., and Johansson, C. (1981). Gastrointestinal
protection by low dose prostaglandin E in rheumatic disease. *Scandinavian Journal of Gastroenterology*, 16, 1005–8.

Krohn, S. (1958). Effect of the administration of steroid hormones on
the gingival tissues. *Journal of Periodontology*, 29, 300–6.

Kuehl, F. A., Humes, J. L., Egan, R. W., Ham, E. A., Beveridge, G. C.,
and Van Arman, C. G. (1977). Role of prostaglandin endoperoxide
PGG₂ in inflammatory processes. *Nature*, 265, 170–3.

Labelle, R. E. and Schaffer, E. M. (1967). The effects of cortisone and
induced local factors on the periodontium of the albino rat. *Journal of
Periodontology*, 37, 483–90.

Lasfargues, J. -J. and Saffar, J. L. (1983). Effect of indomethacin on bone
destruction during experimental periodontal disease in the hamster.
Journal of Periodontal Research, 18, 110–17.

Lewis, G. P. (1983). Immunoregulatory activity of metabolites of
arachidonic acid and their role in inflammation. *British Medical
Bulletin*, 39, 243–8.

Loning, T., Albers, Von H.-K., Lisboa, B. P., Burkhardt, A., and Caselitz, J.
(1980). PGE and the local immune response in chronic periodontal
disease. *Journal of Periodontal Research*, 15, 525–35.

Mihas, A. A., Gibson, R. G., and Hirschowitz, B. I. (1975). Suppression
of lymphocyte transformation by 16, [16] dimethyl prostaglandin E₂
and unsaturated fatty acids. *Proceedings of the Society of Experimental
Biology and Medicine*, 149, 1026–8.

Nuki, K., Soskolne, W. A., Raisz, L. G. Kornman, K. S., and Alander, C.
(1981). Bone resorbing activity of gingiva from beagle dogs following metronidazole and indomethacin therapy. *Journal of Periodontal
Research*, 16, 205–12.

Nyman, S., Schroeder, H. E., and Lindhe, J. (1979). Suppression of
inflammation and bone resorption by indomethacin during experimental periodontitis in dogs. *Journal of Periodontology*, 50, 450–61.

Offenbacher, S., Odle, B. M., Gray, R. C., and Van Dyke, T. E. (1984).
Crevicular fluid PGE levels as a measure of the periodontal disease
status of adult and juvenile periodontitis patients. *Journal of Periodontal Research*, 19, 1–13.

Offenbacher, S. *et al.* (1987). Effects of flurbiprofen on the progression
of periodontitis in *Macaca mulatta*. *Journal of Periodontal Research*, 22,
473–81.

Offenbacher, S. Odle, B., Braswell, L., Hall, C., and Johnson, H. (1988).
Effects of flurbiprofen on crevicular fluid cyclo-oxygenase metabolites in experimental periodontitis. *Journal of Dental Research*, 67, 370
(abstr. 2061).

Offenbacher, S., Odle, B., Braswell, L., Green, M., and Henninger, P.
(1989). Changes in cyclooxygenase metabolites in experimental
periodontitis in *Macaca mulatta*. *Journal of Periodontal Research*, 24,
63–74.

Oguntebi, B. R., Barker, B. F., Anderson, D. M., and Sakamura, J.
(1988). The effect of indomethacin on experimental chronic periapical lesions in rats. *Journal of Dental Research*, 67, 131 (abstr. 152).

Ohm, K., Albers, Von, H.-K., and Lisboa, B. P. (1984). Measurement of
8 prostaglandins in human gingival and periodontal disease using
high pressure liquid chromatography and radioimmunoassay. *Journal of Periodontal Research*, 19, 501–11.

Parrillo, J. E. and Fauci, A. S. (1979). Mechanisms of glucocorticoid
action on immune processes. *Annual Review of Pharmacology and
Toxicology*, 19, 179–201.

Raisz, L. G. and Koolemans-Beynen, E. R. (1974). Inhibition of bone
collagen synthesis by prostaglandin E₂ in organ culture. *Prostaglandins*, 8, 377–85.

Raisz, L. G., Sandberg, A. L., Goodson, J. M., Simmons, H. A., and
Mergenhagen, S. E. (1974). Complement dependent stimulation of
prostaglandin synthesis and bone resorbtion. *Science*, 185, 789–91.

Reiff, R. L., White, C. L., Overman, P. R., and El Attar, T. M. A. (1987).
Aspirin, buffered aspirin, buffer and water rinses in reducing gingival
inflammation. Abstracts of American Association of Dental Research
(Chicago meeting), p. 153 (abstr. 376).

Rifkin, B. R., Baker. R. L., and Colman, S. J. (1980). Effects of
prostaglandin E₂ on macrophages and osteoclasts in cultured foetal
long bones. *Cell and Tissue Research*, 207, 341–6.

Robinson, D. R., Tashjian, A. H., and Levine, L. (1975). Prostaglandin-
stimulated bone resorption by rheumatoid synovia. *Journal of Clinical
Investigation*, 56, 1181–8.

Safkan, B. and Knuuttila, M. (1984). Corticosteroid therapy and
periodontal disease. *Journal of Clinical Periodontology*, 11, 515–22.

Samuelsson, B. (1981). Prostaglandins, thromboxanes and leukotrienes: formation and biological roles. *Harvey Lectures*, 75, 1–40.

Samuelsson, B. (1983). Leukotrienes: mediators of immediate hypersensitivity reactions and inflammation. *Science*, 220, 568–75.

Sidhagen, B., Hamberg, M., and Fredholm, B. B. (1982). Formation of
12ʟ-hydroxyeicosatetraenoic acid (12-HETE) by gingival tissue.
Journal of Dental Research, 61, 761–3.

Smith, K. A. (1980). T-cell growth factor. *Immunological Review*, 51,
337–57.

Smith, J. B. and Willis, A. L. (1971). Aspirin selectively inhibits PG
production in human platelets. *Nature*, 231, 235–7.

Stalker, D. J., Pollock, S. R., and Albert, K. S. (1987). The *in-vivo*
assessment of buccal absorption of flurbiprofen. American Pharmaceutical Science Association Meeting, Chicago, Abstract 57.

Stawinski, K. (1960). Effects of corticol hormones in the treatment of
periodontal disease. *Dental Abstracts*, 5, 80.

Stenson, W. F. and Parker, C. W. (1980). Prostaglandins, macrophages and immunity. *Journal of Immunology*, 125, 1–5.

Vane, J. R. (1971). Inhibition of prostaglandin synthesis as a mechanism of action for the aspirin-like drugs. *Nature*, 231, 232–5.

Vane, J. R. (1976). Prostaglandins as mediators of inflammation. In
Advances in prostaglandin and thromboxane research, Vol. 2 (ed. B.
Samuelsson and R. Paoletti), pp. 791–801. Raven Press, New York.

Vogel, R. I., Cooper, S. A., Schneider, L. G., and Goteiner, D. (1984).
The effects of topical steroidal and systemic non-steroidal anti-
inflammatory drugs on experimental gingivitis in man. *Journal of
Periodontology*, 55, 247–51.

Vogel, R. I., Schneider, L., and Goteiner, D. (1986). The effects of a topically active non-steroidal anti-inflammatory drug on ligature-induced periodontal disease in the squirrel monkey. *Journal of Clinical Periodontology*, **13**, 139–44.

Waite, I. M., Saxton, C. A., Young, A., Wagg, B. J., and Corbett, M. (1981). The periodontal status of subjects receiving non-steroidal anti-inflammatory drugs. *Journal of Periodontal Research*, **16**, 100–8.

Ward, P. A. (1966). The chemosuppression of chemotaxis. *Journal of Experimental Medicine*, **124**, 209–29.

Waterhouse, J. P. (1969). Effects of endocrine secretions. In *Biology of the periodontium* (ed. A. H. Melcher and W. H. Bowen), pp. 476–80. Academic Press, London.

Weaks-Dybvig, M., Sanavi, F., Zander, H., and Rifkin, B. R. (1982). The effect of indomethacin on alveolar bone loss in experimental periodontitis. *Journal of Periodontal Research*, **17**, 90–100.

Weston, W. L., Mandel, M. J., Yeckley, J. A., Krueger, G. G., and Claman, H. N. (1973). Mechanism of cortisol inhibition of adoptive transfer of tuberculin sensitivity. *Journal of Laboratory and Clinical Medicine*, **82**, 366–71.

Williams, R. C., Jeffcoat, M. J., Kaplan, M. L., Goldhaber, P., Johnson, H. G., and Wechter, W. J. (1984). Flurbiprofen—a potent inhibitor of alveolar bone resorption in beagles. *Science*, **227**, 640–2.

Williams, R. *et al.* (1987a). Ibuprofen inhibits alveolar bone resorption in beagles. *Journal of Dental Research*, **66**, p. 356, Abstract 1997.

Williams, R. C. *et al.* (1987b). Indomethacin or flurbiprofen treatment of periodontitis in beagles: comparison of effect on bone loss. *Journal of Periodontal Research*, **22**, 403–7.

Williams, R. C. *et al.* (1987c). Three-year clinical trial of flurbiprofen treatment of human periodontitis: preliminary analysis. *Journal of Dental Research*, **67**, 370 (abstr. 2062).

Williams, R. C. *et al.* (1988a). Ibuprofen: an inhibitor of alveolar bone resorption in beagles. *Journal of Periodontal Research*, **23**, 225–9.

Williams, R. C. *et al.* (1988b). Indomethacin or flurbiprofen treatment of periodontitis in beagles: effect on crevicular fluid arachidonic acid metabolites compared with effect on alveolar bone loss. *Journal of Periodontal Research*, **23**, 134–8.

Williams, R. C. *et al.* (1988c). Topical flurbiprofen treatment of periodontitis in beagles. *Journal of Periodontal Research*, **23**, 166–9.

Williams, T. J. (1983). Interactions between prostaglandins, leukotrienes and other mediators of inflammation. *British Medical Bulletin*, **39**, 239–42.

Williams, T. J. and Morley, J. (1973). Prostaglandins as potentiators of increased vascular permeability in inflammation. *Nature*, **246**, 215–17.

Williams, T. J. and Peck, M. J. (1977). Role of prostaglandin-mediated vasodilation in inflammation. *Nature*, **270**, 530–2.

Willoughby, D. A. (1972). The inflammatory response. *Journal of Dental Research*, **51**, 226–7.

Wong, P. Y. K., Ross, J. R., and Sticht, F. D. (1980). Metabolism of arachidonic acid in inflamed human gingiva. I. Formation of 6-keto-PGF_1. *Journal of Dental Research*, **59**, 671–4.

Yoneda, T. and Mundy, G. R. (1979). Monocytes regulate osteoclast activating factor production by releasing prostaglandins. *Journal of Experimental Medicine*, **150**, 338–50.

Index